I0063756

Marine Glycosides

Marine Glycosides

Special Issue Editors

Thomas E Adrian
Francisco Sarabia
Ivan Cheng-Sanchez

MDPI • Basel • Beijing • Wuhan • Barcelona • Belgrade

MDPI

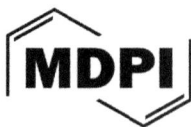

Special Issue Editors
Thomas E Adrian
Mohammed Bin Rashid University of Medicine and Health Sciences
Dubai, UAE

Francisco Sarabia
University of Malaga
Spain

Ivan Cheng-Sanchez
University of Malaga
Spain

Editorial Office
MDPI
St. Alban-Anlage 66
4052 Basel, Switzerland

This is a reprint of articles from the Special Issue published online in the open access journal *Marine Drugs* (ISSN 1660-3397) from 2017 to 2018 (available at: https://www.mdpi.com/journal/marinedrugs/special_issues/marine_glycosides)

For citation purposes, cite each article independently as indicated on the article page online and as indicated below:

LastName, A.A.; LastName, B.B.; LastName, C.C. Article Title. *Journal Name* **Year**, *Article Number*, Page Range.

ISBN 978-3-03897-902-9 (Pbk)
ISBN 978-3-03897-903-6 (PDF)

ⓒ 2019 by the authors. Articles in this book are Open Access and distributed under the Creative Commons Attribution (CC BY) license, which allows users to download, copy and build upon published articles, as long as the author and publisher are properly credited, which ensures maximum dissemination and a wider impact of our publications.

The book as a whole is distributed by MDPI under the terms and conditions of the Creative Commons license CC BY-NC-ND.

Contents

About the Special Issue Editors

Thomas E Adrian, Professor of Physiology, trained at the Royal Postgraduate Medical School (Imperial College School of Medicine) in London where he received his Ph.D. and M.R.C.Path. He moved to Yale University as director of the GI Surgical Research Laboratory, then to Creighton University in Omaha, Nebraska as Professor and head of the Physiology Division and Research Director in the Cancer Center, and then to Northwestern University School of Medicine in Chicago, where he was the Edward Elcock Professor and Director of Gastrointestinal Cancer Research. In 2006, he moved to Al Ain as Professor and Chairman of the Department of Physiology, College of Medicine at United Arab Emirates University. In 2018, he moved to the new College of Medicine at MBRU in Dubai. Professor Adrian has published more than 400 scholarly articles in peer-reviewed journals (Citations > 25,000; h-index = 80) and more than 80 reviews and book chapters.

Francisco Sarabia, Full Professor in Organic Chemistry, received his PhD degree from the University of Málaga (Spain) in 1994 under the supervision of Prof. López-Herrera. After postdoctoral research with Prof. K. C. Nicolaou at the Scripps Research Institute in La Jolla (1995–1997), he returned to the University of Málaga in 1998 as an Assistant Professor, where he was promoted to Full Professor in 2011. Prof. Sarabia was employed as a Visiting Professor at the Technological Institute of Zürich (ETH) in 1998 with Prof. A. Vasella, The Scripps Research Institute in 2001 with Prof. Nicolaou, and Scripps Florida in 2013 with Prof. W. R. Roush. His research interests include the total synthesis of natural products, the development of new synthetic methodologies, and the medicinal chemistry and discovery of new bioactive compounds of marine origin. He has been the Chairman of the Department of Organic Chemistry since 2014 and is responsible for the NMR facilities of the University of Málaga.

Ivan Cheng-Sanchez, Research Associate, was born in Málaga (Spain) in 1992. He received his B.Sc. in Chemistry in 2014 and his M.Sc. in Chemistry in 2015 from the University of Málaga after conducting research in the laboratories of Prof. F. Sarabia. In November 2015 he started his Ph.D. studies under the guidance of Prof. F. Sarabia at the same university. In 2017 he joined the laboratories of Prof. C. Nevado at the University of Zurich for three months, where he was involved in the synthesis of novel ATAD2 bromodomain inhibitors for cancer treatment. His research interests include the total synthesis of natural products, the design and synthesis of new bioactive agents inspired by natural products, and medicinal chemistry.

Preface to "Marine Glycosides"

This Special Issue of Marine Drugs highlights the chemistry, biology, and medicinal applications of recently discovered marine glycosides. Featuring a wide structural diversity and challenging molecular frameworks, these natural products exhibit a broad range of biological activities, which have propelled them as potential and promising leads in Medicinal Chemistry, prompting a great interest in scientific and medical circles. The papers included in this Special Issue have been written by authors who are leading experts in the field, and cover the isolation, structural elucidation, and/or biological evaluation of new glycosides of marine origin, including novel angucycline-, polyhydroxysteroidal-, steroidal saponin-, and sulfated triterpene-type glycosides, among others. The distribution of saponins and triterpene glycosides in sea cucumbers is also discussed. In addition, this Special Issue is supplemented by four reviews focused on the anticancer effects of Frondoside A, sea cucumber glycosides, marine carbohydrate-based compounds with medicinal properties, and the chemistry and biology of bioactive glycolipids of marine origin.

Thomas E Adrian, Francisco Sarabia, Ivan Cheng-Sanchez
Special Issue Editors

marine drugs

MDPI

Article

Poecillastrosides, Steroidal Saponins from the Mediterranean Deep-Sea Sponge *Poecillastra compressa* (Bowerbank, 1866)

Kevin Calabro [1,2], Elaheh Lotfi Kalahroodi [3], Daniel Rodrigues [3,4], Caridad Díaz [5],
Mercedes de la Cruz [5], Bastien Cautain [5], Rémi Laville [2], Fernando Reyes [5], Thierry Pérez [4],
Bassam Soussi [3,6,7] and Olivier P. Thomas [1,3,]*

[1] School of Chemistry, National University of Ireland Galway, University Road, H91 TK33 Galway, Ireland;
    KEVIN.CALABRO@nuigalway.ie
[2] Cosmo International Ingredients, 855 avenue du Docteur Maurice Donat, 06250 Mougins, France;
    remi.laville@airlquide.com
[3] Géoazur, Université Côte d'Azur, CNRS, OCA, IRD, 250 rue Albert Einstein, 06560 Valbonne, France;
    elaheh.lotfi-kalahroodi@univ-rennes1.fr (E.L.K.); daniel4rodrigues@gmail.com (D.R.);
    bassam.soussi@gu.se (B.S.)
[4] Institut Méditerranéen de Biodiversité et d'Ecologie marine et continentale,
    CNRS—Aix-Marseille University, IRD—University Avignon, Station Marine d'Endoume,
    rue de la batterie des lions, 13007 Marseille, France; thierry.perez@imbe.fr
[5] Fundación MEDINA, Centro de Excelencia en Investigación de Medicamentos Innovadores en Andalucía,
    Avda. del Conocimiento 34, Parque Tecnológico de Ciencias de la Salud, E-18016 Armilla, Granada, Spain;
    caridad.diaz@medinaandalucia.es (C.D.); mercedes.delacruz@medinaandalucia.es (M.d.l.C.);
    bastien.cautain@medinaandalucia.es (B.C.); fernando.reyes@medinaandalucia.es (F.R.)
[6] Department of Marine Sciences, University of Gothenburg, P.O. Box 460, SE40530 Gothenburg, Sweden
[7] Oman Centre for Marine Biotechnology, P.O. Box 236, PC 103 Muscat, Oman
*   Correspondence: olivier.thomas@nuigalway.ie; Tel.: +353-(0)91-493-563

Received: 17 May 2017; Accepted: 21 June 2017; Published: 26 June 2017

Abstract: The first chemical investigation of the Mediterranean deep-sea sponge *Poecillastra compressa* (Bowerbank, 1866) led to the identification of seven new steroidal saponins named poecillastrosides A–G (**1–7**). All saponins feature an oxidized methyl at C-18 into a primary alcohol or a carboxylic acid. While poecillastrosides A–D (**1–4**) all contain an *exo* double bond at C-24 of the side-chain and two osidic residues connected at O-2′, poecillastrosides E–G (**5–7**) are characterized by a cyclopropane on the side-chain and a connection at O-3′ between both sugar units. The chemical structures were elucidated through extensive spectroscopic analysis (High-Resolution Mass Spectrometry (HRESIMS), 1D and 2D NMR) and the absolute configurations of the sugar residues were assigned after acidic hydrolysis and cysteine derivatization followed by LC-HRMS analyses. Poecillastrosides D and E, bearing a carboxylic acid at C-18, were shown to exhibit antifungal activity against *Aspergillus fumigatus*.

Keywords: sponge; saponins; deep-sea; *Poecillastra compressa*

---

1. Introduction

In the marine environment, steroid and triterpenoid glycosides are widespread metabolites mainly produced by echinoderms [1–3], although saponins have also been isolated from other marine invertebrates such as octocorals or sponges [4,5]. To date, about 70 saponins have been reported from sponges [6] including sarasinosides from *Asteropus* spp. [7,8], *Melophlus* spp. [9,10], and *Lipastrotethya* sp. [11], ulososides from *Ulosa* sp. [12,13] and *Ectoplyasia ferox* [14], pandarosides and acanthifoliosides from *Pandaros acanthifolium* [15–18], wondosterols from the association of two sponges [19], eryilosides, sokodosides, nobiloside, and formosides from *Erylus* spp. [20–29], ptilosaponosides from *Ptilocaulis spiculifer* [30], mycalosides from *Mycale laxissima* [31,32], feroxosides from *Ectyoplasia ferox* [33], and silenosides from *Silene vulgaris* [34]. While some sponge saponins can be oxidized on the D ring or can contain unusual side chains, the aglycone of most of them belongs to the 30-norlanostane triterpenoid family, with steroidal saponins being rather rare for sponges. Some sponge saponins were subjected to different bioassays and they usually demonstrated interesting biological activities, mostly cytotoxicity against tumor cell lines [35–37].

In our continuous efforts to describe the chemical diversity of marine sponges from the Mediterranean, we undertook the first chemical study of the deep-sea Tetractinellid sponge *Poecillastra compressa* (Bowerbank, 1866). The genus *Poecillastra* is known to produce a broad range of secondary metabolites such as macrolactams [38,39], nitrosohydroxyalkylamines [40], sesquiterpenes, and steroids [41,42]. We report herein the isolation and structure elucidation of seven new steroidal glycosides named poecillastrosides A–G (**1**–**7**) from the deep-sea sponge *P. compressa* (Figure 1). Their structures were deduced from spectroscopic data including 1D- and 2D-NMR experiments as well as high-resolution mass spectra (HRESIMS) analyses. Three different aglycone moieties were identified, and oxidation at the C-18 position is a common feature among all isolated saponins. Poecillastroside A (**1**) contains an ergostane aglycone, whereas poecillastrosides B–D (**2**–**4**) contain a poriferastane, and poecillastrosides E–G (**5**–**7**) a cholestane with a cyclopropyl ring on the side-chain.

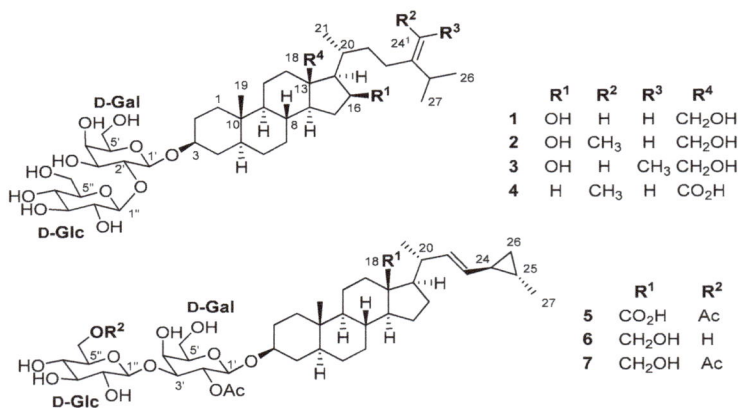

Figure 1. Structure of poecillastrosides A–G (**1**–**7**).

2. Results and Discussion

The freeze-dried sponge sample (43.1 g) was macerated and repeatedly extracted with a mixture of CH_2Cl_2/CH_3OH (1:1) under sonication. The extract (7.9 g) was fractionated by Reversed Phase C18 Vacuum Liquid Chromatography with solvent mixtures of decreasing polarity. The methanolic fraction was then purified by successive RP-Phenylhexyl and C18 HPLC yielding pure compounds **1**–**7**.

Compound **1** was isolated as a yellowish amorphous solid. Its molecular formula $C_{40}H_{68}O_{13}$ was determined by HRESIMS. The ^{1}H NMR spectrum of **1** suggested a steroidal saponin (Table 1). First, the characteristic anomeric signals at δ_H 4.49 (d, J = 7.6 Hz, 1H, H-1'), 4.56 (d, J = 7.9 Hz, 1H, H-1''), and δ_C 101.8 (C-1'), 105.2 (C-1'') evidenced the presence of two sugar residues. The ^{1}H NMR data of the steroid revealed one methyl singlet at δ_H 0.88 (s, 3H, H$_3$-19), three methyl doublets at δ_H 1.02 (d, J = 6.8 Hz, 3H, H$_3$-21) and 1.03 (d, J = 6.8 Hz, 6H, H$_3$-26 and -27), ten methylene groups, an oxygenated methylene with the AB system at δ_H 3.95 and 3.59, a 1,1-disubstituted olefin at δ_H 4.70 and 4.71 (H$_2$-24^1), seven methine groups, two oxygenated methines at δ_H 3.72 (m, 1H, H-3), 4.26 (td, J = 7.7, 3.7 Hz, 1H, H-16), and three quaternary carbons at C-10, C-13 and C-24. When compared to usual steroids, this aglycone lacks one characteristic methyl signal for C-18. A hydroxylation was proposed at this position based on the presence of an AB system at δ_H 3.59 (d, J = 11.5 Hz, 1H, H-18b) and 3.95 (d, J = 11.5 Hz, 1H, H-18a) and further key H-12b, H-14, H-17/C-18, and H_2-18/C-13, C-14, C-17 HMBC correlations. Another unusual feature for the steroid moiety was evidenced in the HSQC spectrum with signals of an oxygenated methine at δ_H 4.26 (td, J = 7.7, 3.7 Hz, 1H, H-16) and δ_C 72.8 (CH, C-16). The location of this hydroxyl group at C-16 was confirmed after interpretation of key H-16/H-17 and H-16/H-15a COSY and TOCSY correlations. While most of the relative configurations were in accordance with a common steroid core, the relative configuration at C-16 was established after examination of the NOESY spectrum. Absence of clear nuclear Overhauser effect (nOe) between H-16 and H-14 but also H-18 together with some overlap between H-17 and H-22 did not allow a straightforward determination of the relative configuration at this position. However, H-16/H-15a and H-8/H-15b nOes suggested a β orientation for the hydroxyl group at C-16. As a confirmation of this orientation, the coupling constant values of H-16 were in perfect accordance with those observed for the same signal of a closely related analogue weinbergsterol B, isolated from the sponge *Petrosia weinbergi* [43]. NMR signals of the sugar residues were assigned by extensive COSY, TOCSY, and HSQC interpretation. HMBC experiment evidenced H-5′/C-1′, H-1″/C-2′, H-5″/C-1″ long-range correlations, thus revealing the pyranose nature of these two sugars and their connection at C-2′. Finally, the connectivity of the sugar with the aglycone at C-3 was confirmed through the key HMBC H-1′/C-3 correlation. Moving to the relative configuration of the residues, the large coupling constants between H-1′/H-2′ and H-1″/H-2″ (7.9 and 7.6 Hz, respectively) were consistent with a β configuration for both anomeric centers. This interpretation was confirmed with the one-bond coupling constant $^1J_{CH} \approx 160$ Hz for the two anomeric positions [44]. In addition, the coupling constant values of $^3J_{H3'–H4'}$ 3.2 Hz and $^3J_{H5'–H4'}$ close to zero suggested an axial position for the hydroxyl at C-4 and, therefore, a β-galactopyranosyl residue attached at C-3 of the aglycone [45]. For the second sugar residue, all coupling constants were measured with values between 7 and 9 Hz which implies equatorial positions for all oxygen atoms and, therefore, a β-glucopyranosyl residue connected at C-2′ of the first residue.

Assuming a usual absolute configuration for the aglycone, we turned towards the pyranose moieties. After hydrolysis of the acetal bonds, the resulting monosaccharides were derivatized with L-cysteine methyl ester and phenylisothiocyanate in pyridine [46]. By comparison with standards, a D absolute configuration was assigned for both glucose and galactose monosaccharides.

Compound **2** was isolated as a yellowish amorphous solid. The molecular formula of **2** was determined by HRESIMS as $C_{41}H_{70}O_{13}$. The spectroscopic data were very similar to those of **1**, thereby suggesting that both compounds were close analogues. Examination of the ^1H NMR spectrum revealed the presence of an additional methyl group at δ_H 1.59 (d, J = 6.3 Hz, 3H, H_3-24^2) placed on the double bond at C-24^1, therefore, leading to a poriferastane skeleton. The relative configuration of **2** was found to be the same as that of poecillastroside A based on nOe correlations. A key H_3-24^2/H_2-23 nOe led us to assign the configuration of the double bond as *E*.

Compound **3** was isolated as a pale yellowish amorphous solid with the same molecular formula $C_{41}H_{70}O_{13}$. Both compounds **2** and **3** are, therefore, isomers. The ^1H NMR spectra were almost identical except for a deshielding of the signal corresponding to H-25, from δ_H 2.24 in **2** to δ_H 2.85 for **3**. We first supposed that a change in the configuration of the double had occurred. Due to the low amount of compound available, the corresponding carbons were not visible neither in the ^{13}C NMR spectrum nor in the HSQC, HMBC spectra. We, therefore, decided to enhance the sensitivity of the HSQC spectrum using the recently developed Pure Shift HSQC experiment [47]. Gratifyingly, we were then able to observe both HSQC spots corresponding to C-24^1 and C-25 (Figure S24). The shielding of the C-25 signal from δ_C 36.0 for **2** to δ_C 29.8 for **3** clearly confirmed a *Z* configuration for the double bond of **3**.

Table 1. NMR spectroscopic data for poecillastrosides A–D (**1–4**) in CD$_3$OD (500 MHz for ^{1}H NMR data and 125 MHz for ^{13}C NMR data).

No.	1 δH, mult. (J in Hz)	1 δC	2 δH, mult. (J in Hz)	2 δC	3 δH, mult. (J in Hz)	3 δC	4 δH, mult. (J in Hz)	4 δC
1	1.70, m / 0.98, m	38.1	1.69, m / 0.98, m	38.1	1.69, m / 0.98, m	38.1	1.69, m / 0.98, m	38.2
2	1.90, m / 1.50, m	30.5	1.90, m / 1.50, m	30.5	1.90, m / 1.50, m	30.5	1.92, m / 1.48, m	30.5
3	3.72, m	80.2	3.72, m	80.2	3.72, m	80.2	3.72, m	80.3
4	1.71, m / 1.34, m	35.5	1.71, m / 1.34, m	35.6	1.71, m / 1.34, m	35.5	1.70, m / 1.32, m	35.6
5	1.12, m	46.2	1.12, m	46.2	1.12, m	46.2	1.12, m	46.1
6	1.34, m / 1.32, m	29.9	1.34, m / 1.31, m	29.9	1.34, m / 1.31, m	29.8	1.32, m / 1.29, m	29.9
7	1.73, m / 0.94, m	33.3	1.74, m / 0.94, m	33.3	1.75, m / 0.95, m	33.3	1.74, m / 0.92, m	33.1
8	1.67, m	36.1	1.67, m	36.1	1.67, m	36.1	1.38, m	38.5
9	0.75, m	56.2	0.74, m	56.2	0.74, m	56.2	0.72, m	55.9
10		36.8		36.9		36.8		36.8
11	1.51, m / 1.31, m	22.8	1.52, m / 1.32, m	22.8	1.52, m / 1.32, m	22.8	1.63, m / 1.34, m	24.4
12	2.01, m / 1.11, m	38.9	2.01, m / 1.10, m	38.8	2.01, m / 1.10, m	38.8	2.64, m / 1.09, m	38.2
13		48.1		48.1		48.1		55.8
14	1.10, m	55.1	1.10, m	55.1	1.10, m	55.1	1.39, m	58.4
15	2.17, m / 1.34, m	38.5	2.16, m / 1.33, m	38.6	2.16, m / 1.33, m	38.6	1.81, m / 1.19, m	26.5
16	4.26, td (7.7, 3.7)	72.8	4.26, td (7.9, 3.7)	72.8	4.26, td (7.9, 3.7)	72.8	1.80, m / 0.89, m	24.4
17	1.19, m	62.3	1.19, m	62.3	1.19, m	62.3	1.48, m	57.4
18	3.95, d (11.6) / 3.59, d (11.6)	62.6	3.95, d (11.6) / 3.60, d (11.6)	62.6	3.95, d (11.6) / 3.60, d (11.6)	62.4		180.1
19	0.88, s	12.8	0.88, s	12.8	0.88, s	12.9	0.76, s	12.8
20	1.94, m	31.6	1.93, m	32.2	1.93, m	32.0	1.49, m	38.8
21	1.02, d (6.8)	19.0	1.07, d (6.7)	19.1	1.02, d (6.7)	19.1	1.09, d (6.3)	19.1
22	1.87, m / 1.21, m	35.5	1.73, m / 1.18, m	35.5	1.83, m / 1.18, m	36.8	1.45, m / 1.14, m	36.0
23	2.15, m / 1.98, m	32.4	2.13, m / 1.94, m	26.8	2.04, m / 1.83, m	29.1	2.07, m / 1.90, m	29.9
24		158.0		148.2		146.9		147.9
24^1	4.71, br s 4.70, br s	106.7	5.19, q (6.7)	116.6	5.17, q (6.7)	117.7	5.18, q (6.7)	116.8
24^2			1.59, d (6.3)	13.4	1.58, d (6.3)	12.8	1.56, d (6.7)	13.4
25	2.29, h (6.5)	34.8	2.24, m	36.0	2.85, m	29.8	2.19, m	35.6
26	1.03, d (6.8)	22.5	0.99, d (6.8)	22.7	0.99, d (6.8)	21.4	0.98, d (6.8)	22.7
27	1.03, d (6.8)	22.3	0.99, d (6.8)	22.6	0.99, d (6.8)	21.4	0.98, d (6.8)	22.6
1'	4.49, d (7.6)	101.8	4.49, d (7.6)	101.8	4.49, d (7.6)	101.8	4.48, d (7.5)	101.8
2'	3.70, m	80.8	3.69, t (10.2)	80.8	3.69, t (10.2)	80.8	3.70, t (10.2)	80.8
3'	3.65, dd (9.6, 3.3)	74.8	3.65, dd (9.6, 3.3)	74.8	3.65, dd (9.6, 3.3)	74.8	3.64, dd (9.5, 3.3)	74.8
4'	3.84, d (3.2)	70.0	3.84, d (3.2)	70.0	3.84, d (3.2)	70.0	3.84, d (3.1)	70.0
5'	3.50, t (6.1)	76.4	3.50, t (6.1)	76.4	3.50, t (6.1)	76.4	3.49, t (6.2)	76.4
6'	3.73, m / 3.71, m	62.7	3.73, m / 3.71, m	62.7	3.73, m / 3.71, m	62.7	3.73, m / 3.71, m	62.7
1"	4.56, d (7.9)	105.2	4.56, d (7.9)	105.2	4.56, d (7.9)	105.2	4.56, d (7.9)	105.2
2"	3.25, dd (9.1, 7.9)	75.8	3.25, dd (9.1, 7.9)	75.8	3.25, dd (9.1, 7.9)	75.8	3.25, dd (9.0, 7.8)	75.8
3"	3.37, t (8.8)	77.7	3.37, t (8.8)	77.7	3.37, t (8.8)	77.7	3.37, t (8.9)	77.7
4"	3.33, t (9.3)	71.4	3.33, t (9.3)	71.4	3.33, t (9.3)	71.4	3.33, t (9.4)	71.4
5"	3.29, m	78.4	3.29, m	78.4	3.29, m	78.4	3.28, m	78.4
6"	3.84, dd (11.2, 2.3) / 3.71, m	62.4	3.84, dd (11.1, 2.3) / 3.71, m	62.4	3.84, dd (11.1, 2.3) / 3.71, m	62.4	3.84, dd (13.5, 2.8) / 3.71, m	62.4

Compound **4** was isolated as a pale yellowish amorphous solid with a molecular formula C$_{41}$H$_{68}$O$_{13}$. The ^{1}H NMR spectrum of **4** was very similar to the one of **2** except for the absence of the signals corresponding to the AB system of H$_2$-18 and a shielding observed for δ_H 2.64 (m, 1H, H-12a). The only explanation consistent with all these observations, including the molecular formula, was the replacement of the hydroxyl group at C-18 by a carboxylic acid. This interpretation was further supported by a key H-17/C-18 HMBC correlation. Based on the chemical shift of the signal H-25 the configuration of the double bond was found to be the same as in **2**.

Compound **5** was isolated as a white amorphous solid with a molecular formula of C$_{43}$H$_{66}$O$_{15}$. Despite strong differences when compared with **1–4**, the NMR data of **5** evidenced that the molecule was a steroidal saponin (Table 2). The aglycone exhibited an unusual skeleton with the presence of a terminal methylated cyclopropyl ring on the lateral chain. This assumption was based on the shielded signals of H-25 and H-26 but also by COSY, HSQC, and HMBC data analyses with the key

H-27/C-24, H-27/C-26 HMBC correlations. Further analysis of ^{1}H NMR data revealed the *E* geometry of the olefinic bond ($J_{H-22,-23}$ = 15.2 Hz). No clear nOe correlations were observed for assessing the relative configuration around the cyclopropane ring. Gratifyingly, comparison with literature data and synthetic analogues of sterols with an identical side-chain led us to propose a *trans* configuration for the substituents at C-24 and C-25 of this ring [48–51]. To confirm this configuration in our case, we decided to look further into the coupling constants of the signals corresponding to the cyclopropane protons. Only the signals of the methylene and their multiplicity were clearly identified in the ^{1}H NMR spectrum (Figure 2). In the case of a *trans* configuration of the two substituents around the cyclopropane, H_a and H_b would have the same splitting pattern as they would have in the presence of a pseudo C2 axial symmetry perpendicular to the cyclopropane plane. The [3]J coupling constants between protons in a *cis* configuration are known to be between 8 and 10 Hz while values below 7 Hz are always observed when placed in a *trans* configuration. The multiplicity for both signals is observed as a doublet or triplet with coupling constants around 8 and 4 Hz, respectively. This same splitting pattern for both signals is only consistent for a *trans* configuration. Indeed, for a *cis* configuration, one of the two *gem* protons H_b would exhibit two large [3]J coupling constants of 8 Hz. We, therefore, confirm a *trans* configuration for the two substituents and estimate the *gem* [2]J coupling constants between H_a and H_b to be around 4 Hz. The presence of a carboxyl group at C-18 was inferred first from the HRESIMS data and then from the deshielding of H-12a, exactly in the same manner as for compound **4**. Another difference with **4** arose from the absence of the signal corresponding to the oxygenated methine at C-16. This feature was confirmed by COSY, HSQC, and HMBC correlations. Looking at the glycosidic part of the saponin, the relative configuration was similar to those of **1–4**, therefore, confirming one galactose linked to the aglycone and one glucose linked to the galactose. HMBC showed long-range correlations between H-1″/C-3′, H-2′/C_{Ac} (δ_C 172.2), and H-6″/C_{Ac} (δ_C 172.8), thereby indicating the presence of two acetyl groups at C-2′ and C-6″. Unlike compounds **1–4**, the glycosidic link between both sugar residues was placed at C-3′ of the galactose. Deshielding of the signal of C-3′ at δ_C 82.4 in the ^{13}C NMR spectrum confirmed this new substitution pattern.

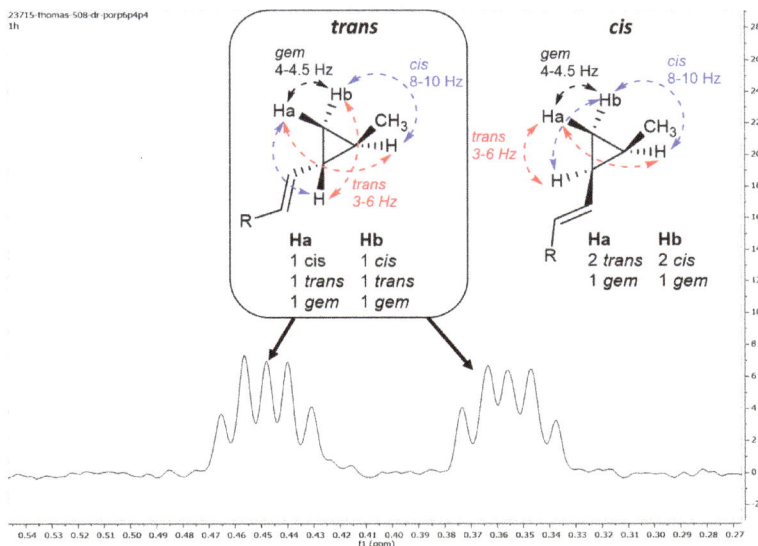

Figure 2. Assignment of the relative configuration of the disubstituted cyclopropane through ^{1}H NMR coupling constants [52].

Table 2. NMR spectroscopic data for poecillastrosides E–G (**5–7**) in CD$_3$OD (500 MHz for ^{1}H NMR data and 125 MHz for ^{13}C NMR data of **5**; 600 MHz for ^{1}H data and 150 MHz for ^{13}C data of **6** and **7**).

No.	5 δ_H, mult. (J in Hz)	5 δ_C	6 δ_H, mult. (J in Hz)	6 δ_C	7 δ_H, mult. (J in Hz)	7 δ_C
1	1.70, m / 0.97, m	38.0	1.72, m / 0.97, m	38.2	1.72, m / 0.98, m	38.2
2	1.85, m / 1.44, m	30.4	1.86, m / 1.46, m	30.7	1.87, m / 1.46, m	30.8
3	3.62, m	79.9	3.63, m	80.0	3.62, m	80.0
4	1.58, m / 1.17, m	35.8	1.58, m / 1.17, m	35.9	1.58, m / 1.19, m	36.0
5	1.12, m	46.0	1.09, m	46.1	1.10, m	46.1
6	1.32, m / 1.29, m	30.3	1.32, m / 1.29, m	29.9	1.31, m / 1.27, m	30.4
7	1.76, m / 0.94, m	33.1	1.68, m / 0.87, m	33.5	1.67, m / 0.87, m	33.5
8	1.53, m	38.8	1.43, m	37.1	1.43, m	37.0
9	0.73, m	55.9	0.68, m	56.0	0.68, m	56.0
10		36.7		36.8		36.8
11	1.63, m / 1.31, m	24.4	1.53, m / 1.36, m	22.3	1.53, m / 1.34, m	22.3
12	2.63, m / 1.10, m	38.4	2.44, d (12.8) / 0.94, m	35.9	2.44, dt (12.7, 3.4) / 0.94, m	35.9
13		55.6		47.9		47.9
14	1.38, m	58.4	1.11, m	57.6	1.12, m	57.6
15	1.75, m / 1.30, m	30.8	1.70, m / 1.30, m	29.9	1.71, m / 1.29, m	29.9
16	1.78, m / 1.53, m	25.8	1.54, m / 0.98, m	25.0	1.54, m / 0.98, m	24.9
17	1.46, m	57.3	1.15, m	58.2	1.16, m	58.1
18		180.1	3.65, d (11.5) / 3.45, d (11.6)	60.2	3.65, d (11.1) / 3.45, d (11.7)	60.4
19	0.73, s	12.7	0.83, s	12.7	0.83, s	12.7
20	1.92, m	42.4	2.26, m	41.7	2.26, m	41.7
21	1.07, d (6.3)	21.2	1.07, d (5.9)	22.1	1.07, d (6.4)	22.1
22	5.21, dd (15.1, 8.5)	134.6	5.22, dd (14.8, 9.0)	136.0	5.22, dd (15.2, 8.9)	136.0
23	4.90, m	132.4	4.94, dd (14.8, 8.1)	131.6	4.94, dd (15.2, 8.3)	131.6
24	0.96, m	23.4	0.93, m	23.4	0.93, m	23.4
25	0.62, m	15.5	0.62, m	15.5	0.62, m	15.5
26	0.44, td (9.0, 4.5) / 0.36, dt (9.0, 4.5)	15.2	0.45, m / 0.36, m	15.2	0.45, m / 0.35, m	15.2
27	1.03, d (5.9)	18.8	1.03, d (5.8)	18.9	1.03, d (5.9)	18.9
1′	4.56, d (8.0)	101.1	4.55, d (7.9)	101.2	4.56, d (8.0)	101.2
2′	5.11, dd (8.4, 8.1)	72.5	5.12, dd (9.0, 7.7)	72.6	5.11, dd (10.1, 8.0)	72.4
2′-Ac	2.06, s	21.2 / 172.2	2.06, s	21.2 / 171.2	2.06, s	21.2 / 172.2
3′	3.76, dd (10.2, 3.3)	82.4	3.80, dd (10.0, 2.8)	82.2	3.76, dd (10.1, 3.2)	82.4
4′	4.07, d (3.2)	70.2	4.11, d (3.1)	70.2	4.07, d (3.4)	70.2
5′	3.55, t (6.1)	76.4	3.56, t (6.2)	76.4	3.55, t (6.4)	76.4
6′	3.74, m / 3.73, m	62.3	3.74, m / 3.72, m	62.2	3.74, m / 3.72, m	62.1
1″	4.39, d (7.6)	106.0	4.38, d (7.9)	106.0	4.38, d (8.0)	106.0
2″	3.21, t (8.3)	74.6	3.19, t (8.3)	74.8	3.21, t (8.3)	74.7
3″	3.32, t (10.1)	77.7	3.35, m	77.9	3.33, m	77.9
4″	3.28, t (9.6)	71.6	3.28, m	71.3	3.29, m	71.5
5″	3.46, m	75.3	3.64, m	80.0	3.46, m	75.3
6″	4.38, d (11.9) / 4.20, dd (11.9, 6.1)	64.7	3.84, m / 3.67, m	62.5	4.38, dd (11.9, 2.7) / 4.20, dd (11.9, 6.2)	64.7
6″-Ac	2.06, s	20.8 / 172.8			2.06, s	20.8 / 172.8

Compound **6** was isolated as a white amorphous solid with a molecular formula of C$_{41}$H$_{66}$O$_{13}$. The spectroscopic data were very similar to those of **5**, thereby suggesting a close aglycone moiety. However, some changes were noticed by HSQC and HMBC analyses. Indeed, in the aglycone moiety, we observed the same AB system for H$_2$-18 as that present in compounds **1–3**. The long-range H-17/C-18 HMBC correlation confirmed the presence of an oxygenated methylene at C-13. In the D-β-glucose residue, the chemical shifts, and the COSY data were consistent with a terminal primary alcohol at C-6″, thereby implying the loss of the acetate at this position.

Compound **7** was isolated as a white amorphous solid with a molecular formula C$_{43}$H$_{68}$O$_{14}$. The ^{1}H NMR spectrum evidenced the fact that **7** is a close analogue of **6**. The long-range H-6″/C$_{Ac}$

(δ_C 172.8) HMBC correlation revealed the presence of an acetate group linked at O-6" as in compound **5**. The relative configuration of **7** was the same as those of **5** and **6**.

Poecillastrosides A–G were tested in a panel of antimicrobial and cytotoxicity assays, including antibacterial activity against Gram positive (methicillin resistant (MRSA) and methicillin sensitive (MSSA) *Staphylococcus aureus*), and Gram negative bacteria (*Escherichia coli*, *Klebsiella pneumoniae*, *Pseudomonas aeruginosa*, and *Acinetobacter baumannii*), antifungal activity against *Aspergillus fumigatus*, and cytotoxicity against the hepatic tumoral cell line hep_G2. Poecillastrosides D (**4**) (MIC$_{90}$ = 6 µg/mL) and E (**5**) (MIC$_{90}$ = 24 µg/mL) were the only two molecules active in the assay against *A. fumigatus*, revealing a key role of the carboxylic acid functionality at C-18 in the antifungal activity of this structural class. On the other hand, cytotoxicity assays also revealed weak activity of some members of the family against the hep_G2 human cell line, with IC$_{50}$ values of 38, 28, and 89 µg/mL for poecillastrosides B, C, and D (**2–4**), respectively. None of the compounds of this family displayed activity against the bacterial pathogens at the highest concentration tested (96 µg/mL for compound **1–5**, and 64 µg/mL for compounds **6** and **7**).

3. Material and Methods

3.1. General Experimental Procedures

Optical rotations were recorded with a PerkinElmer 343 polarimeter equipped with a 10 cm microcell and a sodium lamp. UV measurements were obtained by extraction of the Diode Array Detector (DAD) signal of the Ultra-High Pressure Liquid Chromatography (UHPLC) Dionex Ultimate 3000 (Thermo Scientific, Waltham, MA, USA). NMR experiments were performed on a 500 MHz (Advance, Bruker, Billerica, MA, USA) or a 600 MHz (Agilent, Santa Clara, CA, USA) spectrometer. Chemical shifts (δ in ppm) are referenced to the carbon (δ_C 49.0) and residual proton (δ_H 3.31) signals of CD$_3$OD. High-resolution mass spectra (HRESIMS) were obtained from a mass spectrometer Agilent 6540. HPLC separation and purification were carried out on a Jasco LC-2000 series equipped with a UV detector coupled with an Evaporative Light Scattering Detector, ELSD (Sedere, Alfortville, France).

3.2. Biological Material

Poecillastra compressa (Bowerbank, 1866) was collected in the Mediterranean Sea, off the French coasts, on 15 October 2014 at 200 m depth using a Remotely Operated Vehicle (Super Achille, COMEX S.A., Marseille, France). The voucher specimen "CS2ACHP09_ECH04" is kept at the Marine Station of Endoume (OSU Institut Pythéas, Marseille, France).

3.3. Extraction and Isolation

The dry sponge sample (43.1 g) was ground with a mortar and extracted with a mixture of CH$_3$OH/CH$_2$Cl$_2$ (1:1, *v/v*) at room temperature, yielding 7.9 g (18% yield from dry-weight) of extract after solvent evaporation. The crude extract was fractionated by RP-C18 vacuum liquid chromatography (elution with a decreasing polarity gradient of H$_2$O/CH$_3$OH from 1:0 to 0:1, then CH$_3$OH/CH$_2$Cl$_2$ from 1:0 to 0:1). The CH$_3$OH (422 mg) fraction was then subjected to RP-HPLC on a preparative phenylhexyl column, 250 mm × 19 mm, 5 µm (Xselect, Waters, Milford, CT, USA), using a mobile phase of water (A) and acetonitrile (B). The method was developed on 30 min acquisition time: isocratic 60% B for 15 min, then linear gradient to 98% B in 1 min, held at 98% B for 10 min, back to 60% B in 1 min, and held at that percentage of B for 3 min. Selected fractions from this chromatography were then purified by RP-HPLC on a semi-preparative HTec C18 column, 250 mm × 10 mm, 5 µm (Nucleodur, Macherey-Nagel, Düren, Germany), with the following methods for each subsequent purification: isocratic 47% B to afford pure **1** (4.3 mg, 9.98 × 10^{-3}% *w/w*), isocratic 49% B to afford **2** (6.2 mg, 1.44 × 10^{-2}% *w/w*) and **3** (1.4 mg, 3.49 × 10^{-3}% *w/w*), isocratic 50% B to afford **4** (1.6 mg,

$3.71 \times 10^{-3}\% \ w/w$), isocratic 51% B to afford **5** (0.9 mg, $2.09 \times 10^{-3}\% \ w/w$), and isocratic 53% B to afford **6** (0.7 mg, $1.62 \times 10^{-3}\% \ w/w$) and **7** (0.8 mg, $1.86 \times 10^{-3}\% \ w/w$).

Poecillastroside A (**1**): Yellow, amorphous solid; $[\alpha]_D^{20}$ +12.8 (*c* 0.1, CH_3OH); UV (DAD) λ_{max} 195 nm; ^1H NMR and ^{13}C NMR data, see Table 1; HRESIMS (−) *m/z* 755.4582 [M − H]$^-$ (calcd. for $C_{40}H_{67}O_{13}$, 755.4587, Δ − 0.7 ppm).

Poecillastroside B (**2**): Yellow, amorphous solid; $[\alpha]_D^{20}$ +13.2 (*c* 0.1, CH_3OH); UV (DAD) λ_{max} 210 nm; ^1H NMR and ^{13}C NMR data, see Table 1; HRESIMS (−) *m/z* 769.4743 [M − H]$^-$ (calcd. for $C_{41}H_{69}O_{13}$, 769.4744, Δ − 0.1 ppm).

Poecillastroside C (**3**): Yellow, amorphous solid; $[\alpha]_D^{20}$ +13.0 (*c* 0.1, CH_3OH); UV (DAD) λ_{max} 212 nm; ^1H NMR and ^{13}C NMR data, see Table 1; HRESIMS (−) *m/z* 769.4745 [M − H]$^-$ (calcd. for $C_{41}H_{69}O_{13}$, 769.4744, Δ + 0.1 ppm).

Poecillastroside D (**4**): Yellow, amorphous solid; $[\alpha]_D^{20}$ +8.9 (*c* 0.1, CH_3OH); UV (DAD) λ_{max} 222 nm; ^1H NMR and ^{13}C NMR data, see Table 1; HRESIMS (+) *m/z* 791.4567 [M + Na]$^+$ (calcd. for $C_{41}H_{68}NaO_{13}$, 791.4563, Δ + 0.5 ppm).

Poecillastroside E (**5**): White, amorphous solid; $[\alpha]_D^{20}$ −6.2 (*c* 0.1, CH_3OH); UV (DAD) λ_{max} 220 nm; ^1H NMR and ^{13}C NMR data, see Table 2; HRESIMS (+) *m/z* 845.4307 [M + Na]$^+$ (calcd. for $C_{43}H_{66}NaO_{15}$, 845.4299, Δ + 0.9 ppm).

Poecillastroside F (**6**): White, amorphous solid; $[\alpha]_D^{20}$ −27.3 (*c* 0.1, CH_3OH); UV (DAD) λ_{max} 222 nm; ^1H NMR and ^{13}C NMR data, see Table 2; HRESIMS (+) *m/z* 789.4405 [M + Na]$^+$ (calcd. for $C_{41}H_{66}NaO_{13}$, 789.4401, Δ + 0.5 ppm).

Poecillastroside G (**7**): White, amorphous solid; $[\alpha]_D^{20}$ −14.1 (*c* 0.1, CH_3OH); UV (DAD) λ_{max} 225 nm; ^1H NMR and ^{13}C NMR NMR data, see Table 2; HRESIMS (+) *m/z* 831.4518 [M + Na]$^+$ (calcd. for $C_{43}H_{68}NaO_{14}$, 831.4507, Δ + 1.3 ppm).

3.4. Determination of the Absolute Configuration of the Pyranoses

Hydrolysis of glycosides and derivatization of the subsequent monosaccharides were performed individually following previously described methodologies [46]. The monosaccharide derivatives separation was carried out by UHPLC-HRMS on Acquity BEH (Ethylene Bridged Hybrid) C18 1.7 μm, 2.1 mm × 100 mm (Waters). The column was heated at 40 °C. The eluent consisted of water with 0.1% formic acid (A) and acetonitrile/methanol/isopropanol (50:25:25, *v/v/v*) with 0.1% formic acid (B). The analysis was performed in isocratic mode at 13% B and at a flow rate of 360 μL/min. The injection volume was set at 3 μL. The identity of all monosaccharide derivatives was confirmed after extraction of the ion [M + H]$^+$ at *m/z* 433.1098 (Figure S55).

3.5. Evaluation of the Biological Activities

Compounds **1–7** were tested for their ability to inhibit the growth of Gram positive bacteria (*S. aureus* ATCC29213 (MSSA), and *S. aureus* MB5393 (MRSA)) and Gram negative bacteria (*E. coli* ATCC25922, *K. pneumoniae* ATCC700603, *P. aeruginosa* PAO1, and *A. baumannii* CL5973), and fungi (*A. fumigatus* ATCC46645), following previously described methodologies [53,54]. Cytotoxic activity against the hepatic human tumoral cell line hep_G2 was determined as previously reported [55].

4. Conclusions

Poecillastrosides A–G (**1–7**) share an unusual oxidized methyl at C-18, and they are the first saponins exhibiting this feature. The structures of poecillastrosides E–G (**5–7**) also incorporate a terminal methylated cyclopropyl ring already known in some sponge steroids and already investigated for biosynthetic studies [56]. This cyclopropanation process could lead to the cholestane skeleton, then ergostane, and finally poriferastane, all of them being present in the metabolome of this sponge. Many sterols containing a cyclopropyl ring have been isolated to date [57], but to our best knowledge, this is the first time that saponins containing a 3-membered ring on the side-chain have been reported. Poecillastrosides D (**4**) and E (**5**), bearing a carboxylic acid at C-18, were found to be the most bioactive compounds in the antimicrobial bioassays with an interesting antifungal activity against *Aspergillus fumigatus*.

Supplementary Materials: The following are available online at www.mdpi.com/1660-3397/15/7/199/s1: HRMS and ^{1}H, ^{13}C, COSY, TOCSY, HSQC, HMBC, and NOESY NMR data for compounds **1–7** as well as procedures for absolute configuration of compound **3**.

Acknowledgments: This work was partially funded by the Swiss company Ferring. The sampling was supported by the "Agence des Aires Marines Protégées (AAMP)", a French establishment dedicated to the protection of the marine environment. The authors are grateful to the COMEX crew who operated the MINIBEX vessel and its ROV SUPER ACHILLE. We are grateful to G. Genta-Jouve for fruitful discussions about the relative configuration of the cyclopropane. The company Cosmo International Ingredients supported the work of K. Calabro. R. Doohan (NUI Galway) is acknowledged for her help in the record of NMR spectra and H. Solanki for his help in the HRMS acquisition.

Author Contributions: O.P.T. conceived and designed the experiments; E.L.K., D.R. and K.C. performed the experiments; C.D., M.d.l.C., B.C. and F.R. performed the bioassays; K.C., O.P.T., R.L. and B.S. analyzed the data; T.P. collected and identified the biomaterial; K.C., F.R. and O.P.T. wrote the paper.

Conflicts of Interest: The authors declare no conflict of interest.

References

1. Stonik, V.A.; Kalinin, V.I.; Avilov, S.A. Toxins from sea cucumbers (holothuroids): Chemical structures, properties, taxonomic distribution, biosynthesis and evolution. *J. Nat. Toxins* **1999**, *8*, 235–248. [PubMed]
2. Makarieva, T.N.; Stonik, V.A.; Kapustina, I.I.; Boguslavsky, V.M.; Dmitrenoik, A.S.; Kalinin, V.I.; Cordeiro, M.L.; Djerassi, C. Biosynthetic studies of marine lipids. 42. Biosynthesis of steroid and triterpenoid metabolites in the sea cucumber *Eupentacta fraudatrix. Steroids* **1993**, *58*, 508–517. [CrossRef]
3. Burnell, D.J.; Apsimon, J.W. Chapter 6—Echinoderm Saponins. In *Marine Natural Products*; Scheuer, P.J., Ed.; Academic Press: Waltham, MA, USA, 1983; pp. 287–389.
4. Qi, S.; Zhang, S.; Huang, J.; Xiao, Z.; Wu, J.; Li, Q. Complete 1H and 13C NMR assignments of four new steroidal glycosides from a gorgonian coral *Junceella juncea. Magn. Reson. Chem.* **2005**, *43*, 266–268. [CrossRef] [PubMed]
5. Wang, S.-K.; Dai, C.-F.; Duh, C.-Y. Cytotoxic Pregnane Steroids from the Formosan Soft Coral *Stereonephthya crystalliana. J. Nat. Prod.* **2006**, *69*, 103–106. [CrossRef] [PubMed]
6. Ivanchina, N.V.; Kicha, A.A.; Stonik, V.A. Steroid glycosides from marine organisms. *Steroids* **2011**, *76*, 425–454. [CrossRef] [PubMed]
7. Kitagawa, I.; Kobayashi, M.; Okamoto, Y.; Yoshikawa, M.; Hamamoto, Y. Structures of Sarasinosides A1′, B1′, and C1′; New Norlanostane-Triterpenoid Oligoglycosides from the Palauan Marine Sponge *Asteropus sarasinosum. Chem. Pharm. Bull.* **1987**, *35*, 5036–5039. [CrossRef] [PubMed]
8. Espada, A.; Jiménez, C.; Rodríguez, J.; Crews, P.; Riguera, R. Sarasinosides D–G: Four new triterpenoid saponins from the sponge *Asteropus sarasinosum. Tetrahedron* **1992**, *48*, 8685–8696. [CrossRef]
9. Lee, H.-S.; Seo, Y.; Cho, K.W.; Rho, J.-R.; Shin, J.; Paul, V.J. New triterpenoid saponins from the sponge *Melophlus isis. J. Nat. Prod.* **2000**, *63*, 915–919. [CrossRef] [PubMed]
10. Dai, H.-F.; Edrada, R.A.; Ebel, R.; Nimtz, M.; Wray, V.; Proksch, P. Norlanostane triterpenoidal saponins from the marine sponge *Melophlus sarassinorum. J. Nat. Prod.* **2005**, *68*, 1231–1237. [CrossRef] [PubMed]
11. Lee, J.-H.; Jeon, J.-E.; Lee, Y.-J.; Lee, H.-S.; Sim, C.J.; Oh, K.-B.; Shin, J. Nortriterpene Glycosides of the Sarasinoside Class from the Sponge *Lipastrotethya* sp. *J. Nat. Prod.* **2012**, *75*, 1365–1372. [CrossRef] [PubMed]
12. Antonov, A.S.; Kalinovskii, A.I.; Stonik, V.A.; Evtushenko, E.V.; Elyakov, G.B. Structure of ulososide A, a new triterpenoid glycoside from the *Ulosa* sp. sponge. *Russ. Chem. Bull.* **1994**, *43*, 1265–1269. [CrossRef]

13. Antonov, A.S.; Kalinovsky, A.I.; Stonik, V.A. Ulososide B, a new unusual norlanostane-triterpene glycoside and its genuine aglycone from the Madagascar sponge *Ulosa* sp. *Tetrahedron Lett.* **1998**, *39*, 3807–3808. [CrossRef]

14. Colorado, J.; Muñoz, D.; Marquez, D.; Marquez, M.; Lopez, J.; Thomas, O.P.; Martinez, A. Ulososides and Urabosides—Triterpenoid Saponins from the Caribbean Marine Sponge *Ectyoplasia ferox*. *Molecules* **2013**, *18*, 2598–2610. [CrossRef] [PubMed]

15. Cachet, N.; Regalado, E.L.; Genta-Jouve, G.; Mehiri, M.; Amade, P.; Thomas, O.P. Steroidal glycosides from the marine sponge *Pandaros acanthifolium*. *Steroids* **2009**, *74*, 746–750. [CrossRef] [PubMed]

16. Regalado, E.L.; Tasdemir, D.; Kaiser, M.; Cachet, N.; Amade, P.; Thomas, O.P. Antiprotozoal Steroidal Saponins from the Marine Sponge *Pandaros acanthifolium*. *J. Nat. Prod.* **2010**, *73*, 1404–1410. [CrossRef] [PubMed]

17. Regalado, E.L.; Jimenez-Romero, C.; Genta-Jouve, G.; Tasdemir, D.; Amade, P.; Nogueiras, C.; Thomas, O.P. Acanthifoliosides, minor steroidal saponins from the Caribbean sponge *Pandaros acanthifolium*. *Tetrahedron* **2011**, *67*, 1011–1018. [CrossRef]

18. Regalado, E.L.; Turk, T.; Tasdemir, D.; Gorjanc, M.; Kaiser, M.; Thomas, O.P.; Fernandez, R.; Amade, P. Cytotoxic and haemolytic steroidal glycosides from the Caribbean sponge *Pandaros acanthifolium*. *Steroids* **2011**, *76*, 1389–1396. [CrossRef] [PubMed]

19. Ryu, G.; Choi, B.W.; Lee, B.H.; Hwang, K.-H.; Lee, U.C.; Jeong, D.S.; Lee, N.H. Wondosterols A–C, three steroidal glycosides from a Korean marine two-sponge association. *Tetrahedron* **1999**, *55*, 13171–13178. [CrossRef]

20. D'Auria, M.V.; Paloma, L.G.; Minale, L.; Riccio, R.; Debitus, C. Structure chacterization by two-dimensional NMR spectroscopy, of two marine triterpene oligoglycosides from a pacific sponge of the genus *Erylus*. *Tetrahedron* **1992**, *48*, 491–498. [CrossRef]

21. Gulavita, N.K.; Wright, A.E.; Kelly-Borges, M.; Longley, R.E.; Yarwood, D.; Sills, M.A. Eryloside E from an Atlantic sponge *Erylus goffrilleri*. *Tetrahedron Lett.* **1994**, *35*, 4299–4302. [CrossRef]

22. Stead, P.; Hiscox, S.; Robinson, P.S.; Pike, N.B.; Sidebottom, P.J.; Roberts, A.D.; Taylor, N.L.; Wright, A.E.; Pomponi, S.A.; Langley, D. Eryloside F, a novel penasterol disaccharide possessing potent thrombin receptor antagonist activity. *Bioorg. Med. Chem. Lett.* **2000**, *10*, 661–664. [CrossRef]

23. Shin, J.; Lee, H.-S.; Woo, L.; Rho, J.-R.; Seo, Y.; Cho, K.W.; Sim, C.J. New triterpenoid saponins from the sponge *Erylus nobilis*. *J. Nat. Prod.* **2001**, *64*, 767–771. [CrossRef] [PubMed]

24. Antonov, A.S.; Kalinovsky, A.I.; Stonik, V.A.; Afiyatullov, S.S.; Aminin, D.L.; Dmitrenok, P.S.; Mollo, E.; Cimino, G. Isolation and Structures of Erylosides from the Carribean Sponge *Erylus formosus*. *J. Nat. Prod.* **2007**, *70*, 169–178. [CrossRef] [PubMed]

25. Jaspars, M.; Crews, P. A triterpene tetrasaccharide, formoside, from the Caribbean Choristida sponge *Erylus formosus*. *Tetrahedron Lett.* **1994**, *35*, 7501–7504. [CrossRef]

26. Takada, K.; Nakao, Y.; Matsunaga, S.; van Soest, R.W.M.; Fusetani, N. Nobiloside, a New Neuraminidase Inhibitory Triterpenoidal Saponin from the Marine Sponge *Erylus nobilis*. *J. Nat. Prod.* **2002**, *65*, 411–413. [CrossRef] [PubMed]

27. Fouad, M.; Al-Trabeen, K.; Badran, M.; Wray, V.; Edrada, R.; Proksch, P.; Ebel, R. New steroidal saponins from the sponge *Erylus lendenfeldi*. *ARKIVOC* **2004**, *37*, 17–27.

28. Sandler, J.S.; Forsburg, S.L.; Faulkner, D.J. Bioactive steroidal glycosides from the marine sponge *Erylus lendenfeldi*. *Tetrahedron* **2005**, *61*, 1199–1206. [CrossRef]

29. Okada, Y.; Matsunaga, S.; van Soest, R.W.M.; Fusetani, N. Sokodosides, Steroid Glycosides with an Isopropyl Side Chain, from the Marine Sponge *Erylus placenta*. *J. Org. Chem.* **2006**, *71*, 4884–4888. [CrossRef] [PubMed]

30. Gabant, M.; Schmitz-Afonso, I.; Gallard, J.-F.; Menou, J.-L.; Laurent, D.; Debitus, C.; Al-Mourabit, A. Sulfated Steroids: Ptilosteroids A–C and Ptilosaponosides A and B from the Solomon Islands Marine Sponge *Ptilocaulis spiculifer*. *J. Nat. Prod.* **2009**, *72*, 760–763. [CrossRef] [PubMed]

31. Kalinovsky, A.I.; Antonov, A.S.; Afiyatullov, S.S.; Dmitrenok, P.S.; Evtuschenko, E.V.; Stonik, V.A. Mycaloside A, a new steroid oligoglycoside with an unprecedented structure from the Caribbean sponge *Mycale laxissima*. *Tetrahedron Lett.* **2002**, *43*, 523–525. [CrossRef]

32. Antonov, A.S.; Afiyatullov, S.S.; Kalinovsky, A.I.; Ponomarenko, L.P.; Dmitrenok, P.S.; Aminin, D.L.; Agafonova, I.G.; Stonik, V.A. Mycalosides B–I, Eight New Spermostatic Steroid Oligoglycosides from the Sponge *Mycale laxissima*. *J. Nat. Prod.* **2003**, *66*, 1082–1088. [CrossRef] [PubMed]

33. Campagnuolo, C.; Fattorusso, E.; Taglialatela-Scafati, O. Feroxosides A–B, two norlanostane tetraglycosides from the Caribbean sponge *Ectyoplasia ferox*. *Tetrahedron* **2001**, *57*, 4049–4055. [CrossRef]

34. Glensk, M.; Wray, V.; Nimtz, M.; Schöpke, T. Silenosides A–C, Triterpenoid Saponins from *Silene vulgaris*. *J. Nat. Prod.* **1999**, *62*, 717–721. [CrossRef] [PubMed]

35. Wang, W.; Hong, J.; Lee, C.-O.; Im, K.S.; Choi, J.S.; Jung, J.H. Cytotoxic Sterols and Saponins from the Starfish *Certonardoa semiregularis*. *J. Nat. Prod.* **2004**, *67*, 584–591. [CrossRef] [PubMed]

36. Wang, W.; Jang, H.; Hong, J.; Lee, C.-O.; Bae, S.-J.; Shin, S.; Jung, J.H. New cytotoxic sulfated saponins from the starfish *Certonardoa semiregularis*. *Arch. Pharm. Res.* **2005**, *28*, 285–289. [CrossRef] [PubMed]

37. Kicha, A.A.; Ivanchina, N.V.; Huong, T.T.T.; Kalinovsky, A.I.; Dmitrenok, P.S.; Fedorov, S.N.; Dyshlovoy, S.A.; Long, P.Q.; Stonik, V.A. Two new asterosaponins, archasterosides A and B, from the Vietnamese starfish *Archaster typicus* and their anticancer properties. *Bioorg. Med. Chem. Lett.* **2010**, *20*, 3826–3830. [CrossRef] [PubMed]

38. Rashid, M.A.; Gustafson, K.R.; Crouch, R.C.; Groweiss, A.; Pannell, L.K.; Van, Q.N.; Boyd, M.R. Application of High-Field NMR and Cryogenic Probe Technologies in the Structural Elucidation of Poecillastrin A, a New Antitumor Macrolide Lactam from the Sponge *Poecillastra* Species. *Org. Lett.* **2002**, *4*, 3293–3296. [CrossRef] [PubMed]

39. Takada, K.; Choi, B.W.; Rashid, M.A.; Gamble, W.R.; Cardellina, J.H.; Van, Q.N.; Lloyd, J.R.; McMahon, J.B.; Gustafson, K.R. Structural Assignment of Poecillastrins B and C, Macrolide Lactams from the Deep-Water Caribbean Sponge *Poecillastra* Species. *J. Nat. Prod.* **2007**, *70*, 428–431. [CrossRef] [PubMed]

40. Natori, T.; Kataoka, Y.; Kato, S.; Kawai, H.; Fusetani, N. Poecillanosine, a new free radical scavenger from the marine sponge *Poecillastra* spec. aff. *tenuilaminaris*. *Tetrahedron Lett.* **1997**, *38*, 8349–8350. [CrossRef]

41. Killday, K.B.; Longley, R.; McCarthy, P.J.; Pomponi, S.A.; Wright, A.E.; Neale, R.F.; Sills, M.A. Sesquiterpene-Derived Metabolites from the Deep Water Marine Sponge *Poecillastra sollasi*. *J. Nat. Prod.* **1993**, *56*, 500–507. [CrossRef] [PubMed]

42. Makarieva, T.N.; Stonik, V.A.; D'Yachuk, O.G.; Dmitrenok, A.S. Annasterol sulfate, a novel marine sulfated steroid, inhibitor of glucanase activity from the deep water sponge *Poecillastra laminaris*. *Tetrahedron Lett.* **1995**, *36*, 129–132. [CrossRef]

43. Sun, H.H.; Gross, S.S.; Gunasekera, M.; Koehn, F.E. Weinbersterol disulfates A and B, antiviral steroid sulfates from the sponge *Petrosia weinbergi*. *Tetrahedron* **1991**, *47*, 1185–1190. [CrossRef]

44. Tvaroska, I.; Taravel, F.R. Carbon-Proton Coupling Constants In The Conformational Analysis of Sugar Molecules. In *Advances in Carbohydrate Chemistry and Biochemistry*; Derek, H., Ed.; Academic Press: Waltham, MA, USA, 1995; Volume 51, pp. 15–61.

45. Stenutz, R. Coupling Constants of Pyranoses. Available online: http://www.stenutz.eu/sop/a704.html (accessed on 19 February 2017).

46. Wang, Y.-H.; Avula, B.; Fu, X.; Wang, M.; Khan, I.A. Simultaneous Determination of the Absolute Configuration of Twelve Monosaccharide Enantiomers from Natural Products in a Single Injection by a UPLC-UV/MS Method. *Planta Med.* **2012**, *78*, 834–837. [CrossRef] [PubMed]

47. Paudel, L.; Adams, R.W.; Király, P.; Aguilar, J.A.; Foroozandeh, M.; Cliff, M.J.; Nilsson, M.; Sándor, P.; Waltho, J.P.; Morris, G.A. Simultaneously Enhancing Spectral Resolution and Sensitivity in Heteronuclear Correlation NMR Spectroscopy. *Angew. Chem. Int. Ed.* **2013**, *52*, 11616–11619. [CrossRef] [PubMed]

48. Bonini, C.; Kinnel, R.B.; Li, M.; Scheuer, P.J.; Djerassi, C. Minor and trace sterols in marine invertebrates. 38. Isolation, structure elucidation, and partial synthesis of papakusterol, a new biosynthetically unusual marine sterol with a cyclopropyl-containing side chain. *Tetrahedron Lett.* **1983**, *24*, 277–280. [CrossRef]

49. Catalan, C.A.N.; Lakshmi, V.; Schmitz, F.J.; Djerassi, C. Minor and trace sterols in marine invertebrates. 39. 24ξ,25ξ-24,26-Cyclocholest-5-en-3β-ol, a novel cyclopropyl sterol. *Steroids* **1982**, *40*, 455–463. [CrossRef]

50. Fujimoto, Y.; Kimura, M.; Terasawa, T.; Khalifa, F.A.M.; Ikekawa, N. Stereocontrolled synthesis and determination of the C-24 and C-25 stereochemistry of glaucasterol. *Tetrahedron Lett.* **1984**, *25*, 1805–1808. [CrossRef]

51. Kobayashi, M.; Mitsuhashi, H. Marine sterols. XII. Glaucasterol, a novel C27 sterol with a unique side chain, from the soft coral *Sarcophyton glaucum*. *Steroids* **1982**, *40*, 665–672. [CrossRef]

52. Wiberg, K.B.; Nist, B.J. The Nuclear Magnetic Resonance Spectra of Cyclopropane Derivatives. *J. Am. Chem. Soc.* **1963**, *85*, 2788–2790. [CrossRef]

53. Audoin, C.; Bonhomme, D.; Ivanisevic, J.; Cruz, M.; Cautain, B.; Monteiro, M.; Reyes, F.; Rios, L.; Perez, T.; Thomas, O.P. Balibalosides, an Original Family of Glucosylated Sesterterpenes Produced by the Mediterranean Sponge Oscarella balibaloi. *Mar. Drugs* **2013**, *11*, 1477–1489. [CrossRef] [PubMed]

54. Braña, A.F.; Sarmiento-Vizcaíno, A.; Pérez-Victoria, I.; Otero, L.; Fernández, J.; Palacios, J.J.; Martín, J.; de la Cruz, M.; Díaz, C.; Vicente, F.; et al. Branimycins B and C, Antibiotics Produced by the Abyssal Actinobacterium Pseudonocardia carboxydivorans M-227. *J. Nat. Prod.* **2017**, *80*, 569–573. [CrossRef] [PubMed]

55. Cautain, B.; de Pedro, N.; Schulz, C.; Pascual, J.; Sousa, T.d.S.; Martin, J.; Pérez-Victoria, I.; Asensio, F.; González, I.; Bills, G.F.; et al. Identification of the Lipodepsipeptide MDN-0066, a Novel Inhibitor of VHL/HIF Pathway Produced by a New Pseudomonas Species. *PLoS ONE* **2015**, *10*, e0125221. [CrossRef] [PubMed]

56. Wessjohann, L.A.; Brandt, W.; Thiemann, T. Biosynthesis and Metabolism of Cyclopropane Rings in Natural Compounds. *Chem. Rev.* **2003**, *103*, 1625–1648. [CrossRef] [PubMed]

57. Gunasekera, S.P.; Cranick, S.; Pomponi, S.A. New Sterol Ester from a Deep Water Marine Sponge, *Xestospongia* sp. *J. Nat. Prod.* **1991**, *54*, 1119–1122. [CrossRef]

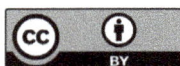

© 2017 by the authors. Licensee MDPI, Basel, Switzerland. This article is an open access article distributed under the terms and conditions of the Creative Commons Attribution (CC BY) license (http://creativecommons.org/licenses/by/4.0/).

marine drugs

MDPI

Article

Nine New Triterpene Glycosides, Magnumosides A₁–A₄, B₁, B₂, C₁, C₂ and C₄, from the Vietnamese Sea Cucumber *Neothyonidium* (=*Massinium*) *magnum*: Structures and Activities against Tumor Cells Independently and in Synergy with Radioactive Irradiation

Alexandra S. Silchenko [1], Anatoly I. Kalinovsky [1], Sergey A. Avilov [1], Vladimir I. Kalinin [1,*], Pelageya V. Andrijaschenko [1], Pavel S. Dmitrenok [1], Ekaterina A. Chingizova [1], Svetlana P. Ermakova [1], Olesya S. Malyarenko [1] and Tatyana N. Dautova [2]

[1]   G.B. Elyakov Pacific Institute of Bioorganic Chemistry, Far Eastern Branch of the Russian Academy of
      Sciences, Pr. 100-letya Vladivostoka 159, Vladivostok 690022, Russia; sialexandra@mail.ru (A.S.S.);
      kaaniv@piboc.dvo.ru (A.I.K.); avilov-1957@mail.ru (S.A.A.); pandriyashchenko@mail.ru (P.V.A.);
      paveldmt@piboc.dvo.ru (P.S.D.); martyyas@mail.ru (E.A.C.); svetlana_ermakova@hotmail.com (S.P.E.);
      vishchuk87@gmail.com (O.S.M.)
[2]   A.V. Zhirmunsky Institute of Marine Biology Far East Branch of Russian Academy of Sciences,
      Palchevsky St. 17, Vladivostok 690041, Russia; tndaut@mail.ru
*   Correspondence: kalininv@piboc.dvo.ru; Tel./Fax: +7-(423)2-31-40-50

Received: 25 July 2017; Accepted: 11 August 2017; Published: 16 August 2017

Abstract: Nine new sulfated triterpene glycosides, magnumosides A₁ (**1**), A₂ (**2**), A₃ (**3**), A₄ (**4**), B₁ (**5**), B₂ (**6**), C₁ (**7**), C₂ (**8**) and C₄ (**9**) as well as a known colochiroside B₂ (**10**) have been isolated from the tropical Indo-West Pacific sea cucumber *Neothynidium* (=*Massinium*) *magnum* (Phyllophoridae, Dendrochirotida) collected in the Vietnamese shallow waters. The structures of new glycosides were elucidated by 2D NMR spectroscopy and mass-spectrometry. All the isolated new glycosides were characterized by the non-holostane type lanostane aglycones having 18(16)-lactone and 7(8)-double bond and differed from each other by the side chains and carbohydrate moieties structures. Magnumoside A₁ (**1**) has unprecedented 20(24)-epoxy-group in the aglycone side chain. Magnumosides of the group A (**1–4**) contained disaccharide monosulfated carbohydrate moieties, of the group B (**5, 6**)—tetrasaccharide monosulfated carbohydrate moieties and, finally, of the group C (**7–9**)—tetrasaccharide disulfated carbohydrate moieties. The cytotoxic activities of the compounds **1–9** against mouse spleen lymphocytes, the ascites form of mouse Ehrlich carcinoma cells, human colorectal carcinoma DLD-1 cells as well as their hemolytic effects have been studied. Interestingly, the erythrocytes were more sensitive to the glycosides action than spleenocytes and cancer cells tested. The compounds **3** and **7** significantly inhibited the colony formation and decreased the size of colonies of DLD-1 cancer cells at non-cytotoxic concentrations. Moreover, the synergism of effects of radioactive irradiation and compounds **3** and **7–9** at subtoxic doses on proliferation of DLD-1 cells was demonstrated.

Keywords: *Neothyonidium magnum*; triterpene glycosides; magnumosides; sea cucumber; cytotoxic activity; radioactive irradiation

1. Introduction

The triterpene glycosides from sea cucumbers (class Holothurioidea) have a long history of investigation. These marine natural products are characterized by significant structural diversity [1–3] and taxonomic specificity which enables their use in resolving some systematic ambiguities [4–6]. Additionally, the triterpene glycosides exhibit a wide spectrum of biological activities [7,8], including anticancer effects against different cancer cell lines [9–14].

The glycosides from the sea cucumber *Neothyonidium* (=*Massinium*) *magnum* (Phyllophoridae, Dendrochirotida) have been previously investigated. The first studied sample of *N. magnum* was collected near the shores of New Caledonia [15]. The main component of glycosidic fraction, monosulfated tetraoside, "neothyonidioside", had the holostane-type aglycone with 9(11)- and 25(26)-double bonds and a 16-keto-group. Another sample of *N. magnum* was collected near Vietnam's shore [16]. The main component of its glycosidic fraction, neothyonidioside C, was different from "neothyonidioside" and characterized by the C-16-acetylated holostane-type aglycone having 7(8)- and 25(26)-double bonds. The carbohydrate chain of neothyonidioside C had the same set of monosaccharide residues as "neothyonidioside" but was disulfated.

Herein we report the results of investigation of *N. magnum* also collected in Vietnamese shallow waters but having the glycosides, magnumosides A_1–A_4 (**1–4**), B_1 (**5**), B_2 (**6**), C_1 (**7**), C_2 (**8**) and C_4 (**9**), which is significantly different from the compounds isolated previously. The structures of the glycosides were established based on ^{1}H and ^{13}C NMR spectra and 2D NMR (^{1}H,^{1}H-COSY, HMBC, HSQC, ROESY) and confirmed by HR-ESI mass spectrometry. The cytotoxic activities of **1–9** against mouse spleen lymphocytes, the ascites form of mouse Ehrlich carcinoma cells, mouse erythrocytes, and human colorectal adenocarcinoma DLD-1 cells were tested. The effects of compounds **1–9** on proliferation, colony formation of DLD-1 cells as well as the synergism of radioactive irradiation and compounds effects have been studied.

2. Results and Discussion

2.1. Structural Elucidation of the Glycosides

The sea cucumber *Neothyonidium* (=*Massinium*) *magnum* contains a very complicated mixture of glycosides, thus the isolation of individual compounds was rather labor-consuming and multistage. The concentrated ethanolic extract of *N. magnum* was chromatographed on a *Polychrom-1* column (powdered Teflon, Biolar, Olaine, Latvia). The glycosides were eluted with 50% EtOH and separated by chromatography on Si gel column using CHCl$_3$/EtOH/H$_2$O (100:100:17) and (100:125:25) as mobile phases. The obtained fractions were subsequently subjected to HPLC on a silica-based Supelcosil LC-Si (4.6 × 150 mm) column, on a reversed-phase semipreparative Supelco Ascentis RP-Amide (10 × 250 mm) column or analytical Diasfer *C-8* (4.6 × 250 mm) column to yield the magnumosides A_1 (**1**) (3.6 mg), A_2 (**2**) (5.0 mg), A_3 (**3**) (3.7 mg), A_4 (**4**) (8.0 mg), B_1 (**5**) (2.6 mg), B_2 (**6**) (1.8 mg), C_1 (**7**) (5.7 mg) and C_2 (**8**) (2.5 mg), C_4 (**9**) (15 mg) and colochiroside B_2 (**10**) (2.0 mg) (Figure 1). The known compound **10** was identified by comparison of its ^{1}H and ^{13}C NMR spectra with those reported for colochiroside B_2 (**10**, 3β-*O*-[3-*O*-methyl-β-D-glucopyranosyl-(1→3)-β-D-xylopyranosyl-(1→4)-β-D-quinovopyranosyl-(1→2)-4-*O*-sodium sulfate-β-D-xylopyranosyl]-16β-acetoxyholosta-25-hydroxy-7,23*E*-diene) from *Colochirus robustus* [17].

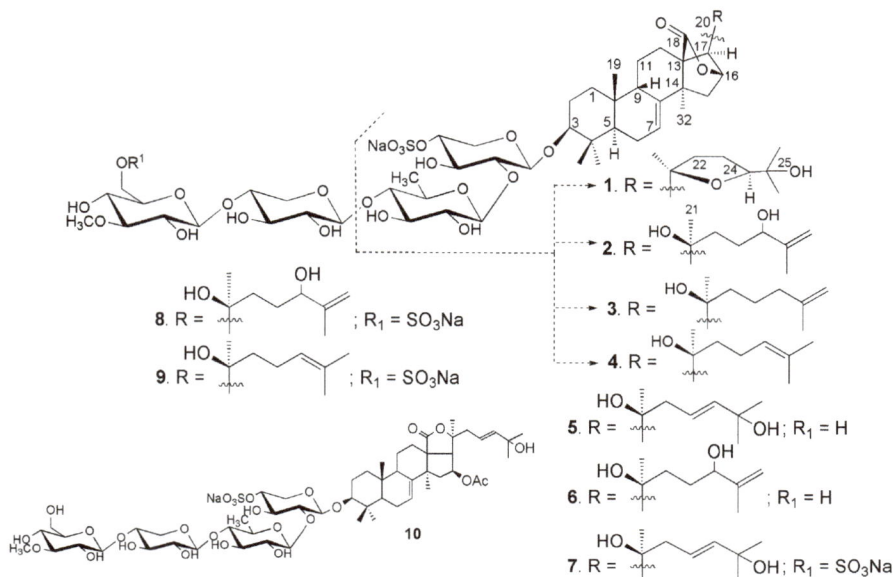

Figure 1. Chemical structure of the glycosides **1–10** isolated from *Neothyonidium magnum*.

The ^{1}H and ^{13}C NMR spectra of carbohydrate parts of magnumosides A$_1$–A$_4$ (**1–4**) were coincident to each other, indicating the identity of carbohydrate chains of these glycosides. The presence of two characteristic doublets at δ(H) 4.66 (J = 7.0 Hz) and 5.00 (J = 7.6 Hz) in the ^{1}H NMR spectra of the carbohydrate chains of **1–4** correlated by the HSQC spectra with the signals of anomeric carbons at δ(C) 104.8 and 105.2, correspondingly, were indicative of a disaccharide chain and β-configuration of glycosidic bonds. The ^{1}H,^{1}H-COSY and 1D TOCSY spectra of **1–4** showed the signals of two isolated spin systems assigned to the xylose and quinovose residues. The positions of interglycosidic linkages were confirmed by the ROESY and HMBC spectra of **1–4** (SM, Table 1) where the cross-peaks between H(1) of the xylose and H(3) (C(3)) of an aglycone and H(1) of the quinovose and H(2) (C(2)) of the xylose were observed. Thus, the carbohydrate chains of magnumosides of the group A (**1–4**) were identical to those of holothurins of the group B, that are characteristic glycosides for the representatives of the genus *Holothuria* and *Actinopyga* (Holothuriidae, Aspidochirotida) [1,18–20].

The molecular formula of magnumoside A$_1$ (**1**) was determined to be C$_{41}$H$_{63}$O$_{16}$SNa from the [M$_{Na}$ − Na]$^-$ ion peak at m/z 843.3838 (calc. 843.3842) in the (−)HR-ESI-MS. Analysis of the ^{1}H and ^{13}C NMR spectra (Tables 2 and 3) of the aglycone part of magnumoside A$_1$ (**1**) suggested the presence of an 18(16)-lactone that was deduced from the characteristic signals of carbons C(18) (δ(C) 180.9) and C(20) (δ(C) 81.9) and characteristic signals of oxygen-bearing methine CH-O(16) (δ(C) 79.6; δ(H) 4.84 (s)). The availability of an 18(16)-lactone and (S)-configuration of C(16) asymmetric center was confirmed by the absence of coupling constant $J_{17/16}$ for H(17) signal (δ(H) 2.48 (s)) in the ^{1}H NMR spectrum of **1** as well as by the presence of correlations H(16)/C(18) in the HMBC spectrum (Figure 2) and H(16)/H(21) in the ROESY spectrum (Figure 3). The signals of olefinic methine group H-C(7) (δ(C) 122.4; δ(H) 5.61 (dt, J = 2.3, 7.4 Hz)) and quaternary carbon C(8) (δ(C) 147.6) in the ^{13}C- and ^{1}H NMR spectra were indicative of 7(8)-double bond in the aglycone nucleus. The signal of oxygenated tertiary asymmetric carbon C(20) assigned by the characteristic for the aglycones of sea cucumber glycosides HMBC correlation H(21)/C(20) was observed at δ(C) 81.9. Its δ(C) value was similar to those values in onekotanogenin [21] and in colochiroside E [22] having the 18(16)-lactone and acetylated C(20) position. However, the presence of acetoxy-group in the aglycone of **1** was excluded by ESI mass spectrometry.

Table 1. ^{13}C and ^{1}H NMR chemical shifts of carbohydrate moieties of magnumosides of the group A (**1–4**), B (**5, 6**) and C (**7–9**) in C_5D_5N/D_2O (5:1), δ in ppm, *J* in Hz.

Position	1–4, δC [a]	1–4, δH [b]	5, 6, δC [a]	5, 6, δH [b]	7–9, δC [a]	7–9, δH [b]
Xyl (1→C-3)						
1	104.8 CH	4.66 (d, 7.0)	104.8 CH	4.65 (d, 7.3)	104.8 CH	4.65 (d, 7.0)
2	**82.3 CH**	4.00 (t, 8.7)	**82.2 CH**	4.00 (t, 8.7)	**82.3 CH**	3.98 (t, 8.8)
3	75.1 CH	4.24 (t, 8.7)	75.2 CH	4.25 (t, 8.7)	75.0 CH	4.24 (t, 8.8)
4	*76.1 CH*	5.01 m	*76.0 CH*	5.04 m	*76.1 CH*	4.99 m
5	63.9 CH$_2$	4.77 (dd, 5.2; 11.7) 3.72 (t, 11.7)	63.9 CH$_2$	4.77 (dd, 5.5; 11.9) 3.71 (dd, 9.6; 11.9)	63.9 CH$_2$	4.76 (dd, 5.4; 11.5) 3.71 (t, 11.8)
Qui (1→2Xyl)						
1	105.2 CH	5.00 (d, 7.6)	104.7 CH	5.00 (d, 7.8)	104.7 CH	4.98 (d, 7.7)
2	76.4 CH	3.90 (t, 9.3)	75.8 CH	3.88 (t, 9.1)	75.8 CH	3.87 (t, 8.6)
3	76.8 CH	4.04 (t, 9.3)	74.7 CH	3.97 (t, 9.1)	74.8 CH	3.95 (t, 9.0)
4	**76.1 CH**	3.61 (t, 8.7)	**85.6 CH**	3.51 (t, 9.1)	**85.6 CH**	3.50 (t, 9.0)
5	72.8 CH	3.66 (dd, 5.8; 8.7)	71.3 CH	3.65 (dd, 5.9; 9.6)	71.4 CH	3.63 (dd, 6.1; 9.3)
6	18.1 CH$_3$	1.53 (d, 5.9)	17.8 CH$_3$	1.61 (d, 5.9)	17.8 CH$_3$	1.60 (d, 6.1)
Xyl (1→4Qui)						
1			104.4 CH	4.77 (d, 7.7)	104.3 CH	4.76 (d, 7.7)
2			73.3 CH	3.89 (t, 8.6)	73.1 CH	3.85 (t, 8.6)
3			**86.4 CH**	4.12 (t, 8.6)	**87.0 CH**	4.04 (t, 8.8)
4			68.7 CH	3.94 m	68.7 CH	3.90 (t, 8.7)
5			65.8 CH	4.11 (dd, 5.6; 11.3) 3.59 (t, 10.8)	65.7 CH	4.11 (dd, 5.3; 11.8) 3.59 (t, 11.3)
MeGlc (1→3Xyl)						
1			104.4 CH	5.21 (d, 8.0)	104.6 CH	5.12 (d, 7.9)
2			74.5 CH	3.88 (t, 8.7)	74.3 CH	3.80 (t, 9.4)
3			87.0 CH	3.68 (t, 8.6)	86.4 CH	3.64 (t, 9.4)
4			70.4 CH	3.89 m	69.9 CH	3.96 (t, 9.4)
5			77.5 CH	3.90 m	75.5 CH	4.03 m
6			61.7 CH$_2$	4.38 (dd, 1.7; 11.5) 4.05 (dd, 5.9; 11.5)	67.1 CH$_2$	4.97 (d, 9.4) 4.72 (dd, 5.5; 11.0)
OMe			60.5 CH$_3$	3.80 s	60.5 CH$_3$	3.76 s

[a] Multiplicity by DEPT; [b] Multiplicity by 1D TOCSY; Bold—interglycosidic bond; Italic—sulfation.

Additionally, there was another downshifted resonance in the ^{13}C NMR spectrum of **1** at δ(C) 86.7 corresponding to the oxygen bearing methine carbon located at α-position to hydroxylated C-25. Its position as C(24) was deduced from the ^{1}H,^{1}H-COSY spectrum where the signals of isolated spin system from H(22) to H(24) were observed (Figure 2). Based on the NMR and ESI-MS data the presence of 20(24)-epoxy-group was suggested. The correlations from H-C(24) (δ(H) 3.97 (dd, *J* = 5.6; 9.3) to C(22), C(23), Me(26), Me(27); from H-C(22) to C(20), Me(21) and from Me(26)(27) to C(24) in the HMBC spectrum were in good agreement with this suggestion. Another downshifted signal (δ(C) 70.1) was assigned to the oxygen-bearing tertiary carbon positioned as C(25) that was deduced from the HMBC correlations Me(26)/C(25) and Me(27)/C(25). The multiplicity of the proton H(24), neighboring it, which was observed as doublet of doublets, confirmed this. The presence in the ^{1}H–^{1}H-COSY spectrum of the signals of four isolated spin systems confirmed the sequences of protons from H(1) to H(3); from H(5) to H(12); from H(15) to H(17) and finally from H(22) to H(24). The HMBC correlations Me(30)/C(4), Me(31)/C(4), Me(19)/C(10), Me(32)/C(13), C(14) and H(17)/C(20) allowed to elucidate the positions of quaternary carbons in the aglycone polycyclic nucleus.

Table 2. ^{1}H NMR data for the aglycones of compounds **1–9** in C_5D_5N/D_2O, δ in ppm, *J* in Hz.

Position	1 [a]	2, 6, 8 [b]	3 [b]	4, 9 [a]	5, 7 [b]
1	1.46 m	1.35 m	1.34 m	1.46 m	1.33 m
2	2.10 m, H_α	1.94 m, H_α	1.94 m, H_α	2.09 m, H_α	1.93 m, H_α
	1.89 m, H_β	1.74 m, H_β	1.73 m, H_β	1.87 m, H_β	1.73 m, H_β
3	3.26 (dd, 3.9, 11.6)	3.16 (dd, 3.8, 11.5)	3.16 (dd, 4.3, 11.7)	3.26 (dd, 4.1, 11.8)	3.16 (dd, 4.5, 11.4)
5	0.98 (dd, 3.3; 11.6)	0.86 (brd, 11.0)	0.86 (dd, 3.9; 11.7)	0.99 (dd, 3.6; 11.8)	0.86 (dd, 3.3; 11.9)
6	2.06 m, H_α	1.92 m, H_α	1.91 m, H_α	2.05 m, H_α	1.91 m, H_α
	1.96 m, H_β	1.82 m, H_β	1.81 m, H_β	1.97 m, H_β	1.81 m, H_β
7	5.61 (dt, 2.3; 7.4)	5.57 m	5.59 (brd, 7.4)	5.63 (dt, 2.4; 7.3)	5.56 (brd, 7.5)
9	3.18 (brd, 13.7)	3.03 (brd, 15.2)	3.02 (brd, 14.9)	3.23 (brd, 13.5)	3.02 (brd, 14.7)
11	2.03 m, H_β	1.93 m	1.94 m	2.03 m, H_β	1.95 m
	1.51 m, H_α	1.40 m	1.41 m	1.54 m, H_α	1.42 m
12	2.47 m, H_β	2.50 m, H_β	2.50 m	2.62 m, H_β	2.47 m, H_β
	2.03 m, H_α	2.14 m, H_α	2.09 m	2.14 m, H_α	2.10 m, H_α
15	2.12 (d, 13.2, H_β)	2.08 (d, 13.5, H_β)	2.10 (d, 13.5, H_β)	2.15 (d, 13.3, H_β)	2.08 (d, 13.8, H_β)
	1.89 (dd, 2.6; 13.5, H_α)	2.01 (dd, 2.0; 13.3, H_α)	2.05 (brd, 11.5, H_α)	1.94 (dd, 2.6; 13.4, H_α)	2.00 (dd, 2.6; 13.4, H_α)
16	4.84 br s	5.12 br s	5.08 br s	5.05 (d, 1.6)	5.14 br s
17	2.48 s	2.72 s	2.69 s	2.63 s	2.77 s
19	1.04 s	0.91 s	0.91 s	1.05 s	0.91 s
21	1.32 s	1.46 s	1.44 s	1.50 s	1.47 s
22	2.02 m	2.05 m	1.70 m	1.83 m	2.50 (br d, 6.9)
	1.73 m	1.83 m	—	1.80 m	—
23	2.08 m	2.06 m	1.72 m	2.40 m	5.92 (d, 15.8)
	1.87 m	1.97 m	1.62 m	2.31 m	—
24	3.97 (dd, 5.6; 9.3)	4.33 (t, 6.0)	2.00 (t, 7.4)	5.27 (t, 7.1)	6.13 (dt, 6.9; 8.0; 15.8)
26	1.31 s	5.16 br s	4.74 br s	1.70 s	1.48 s
	—	4.87 br s	4.73 br s	—	—
27	1.42 s	1.82 s	1.65 s	1.63 s	1.48 s
30	1.15 s	0.97 s	0.97 s	1.15 s	0.97 s
31	1.31 s	1.16 s	1.16 s	1.31 s	1.16 s
32	1.36 s	1.37 s	1.40 s	1.41 s	1.39 s

[a] ratio C_5D_5N/D_2O (4:1); [b] ratio C_5D_5N/D_2O (5:1).

The ROESY correlations (Figure 3) of **1** H(5)/H(3), H(5)/Me(31); H(9)/Me(19); H(17)/Me(21); (17)/Me(32) and Me(21)/H(12) confirmed the common elucidated earlier for the other sea cucumber glycosides (3*S*,5*R*,9*S*,10*R*,13*S*,14*S*,16*S*,17*R*,20*S*)-configurations [22–24] in magnumoside A$_1$ (**1**). The ROE correlations H(16)/H(24); H(17)/H(24) and Me(21)/Me(27) observed in the ROESY spectrum of **1** could be realized in the case of (24*S*)-configuration only. Moreover, the coupling constants of H(24) (dd, *J* = 5.6; 9.3 Hz) in the ^{1}H NMR spectrum were very close to the calculated ones, based on the dihedral angles values in MM2 optimized model of (20*S*),(24*S*)-isomer of **1**.

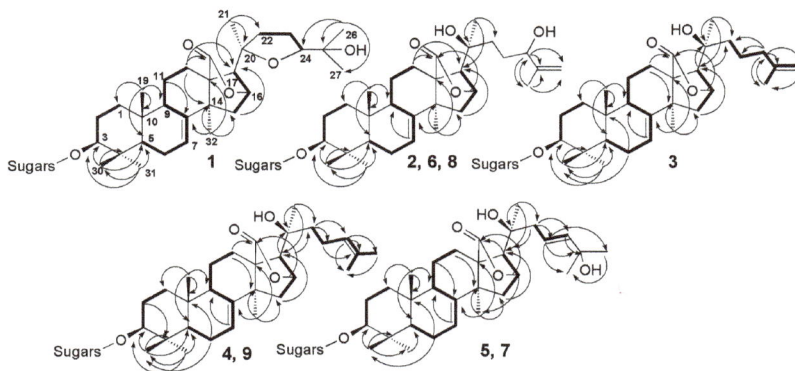

Figure 2. ^{1}H,^{1}H-COSY (—) and key HMBC (H→C) correlations for the aglycones of compounds **1–9**.

Table 3. ^{13}C NMR data for aglycones of compounds **1–8** in C_5D_5N/D_2O, δ in ppm, mult.

Position	1 [a]	2, 6, 8 [b]	3 [b]	4, 9 [a]	5, 7 [b]
1	35.8 CH$_2$	35.6 CH$_2$	35.6 CH$_2$	35.8 CH$_2$	35.6 CH$_2$
2	26.9 CH$_2$	26.7 CH$_2$	26.7 CH$_2$	26.9 CH$_2$	26.7 CH$_2$
3	88.8 CH	88.9 CH	89.0 CH	88.8 CH	89.0 CH
4	39.4 C	39.1 C	39.2 C	39.4 C	39.2 C
5	47.7 CH	47.5 CH	47.6 CH	47.6 CH	47.5 CH
6	23.2 CH$_2$	23.1 CH$_2$	23.1 CH$_2$	23.2 CH$_2$	23.1 CH$_2$
7	122.4 CH	122.3 CH	122.4 CH	122.4 CH	122.4 CH
8	147.6 C	147.6 C	147.6 C	147.8 C	147.6 C
9	46.1 CH	45.9 CH	46.0 CH	46.0 CH	45.9 CH
10	35.5 C	35.3 C	35.4 C	35.5 C	35.4 C
11	21.8 CH$_2$	21.7 CH$_2$	21.7 CH$_2$	21.9 CH$_2$	21.7 CH$_2$
12	20.1 CH$_2$	20.1 CH$_2$	20.2 CH$_2$	20.4 CH$_2$	20.1 CH$_2$
13	54.9 C	54.6 C	54.7 C	54.6 C	54.7 C
14	45.6 C	45.9 C	46.0 C	45.8 C	46.0 C
15	44.4 CH$_2$	44.2 CH$_2$	44.3 CH$_2$	44.5 CH$_2$	44.2 CH$_2$
16	79.6 CH	80.1 CH	80.1 CH	79.5 CH	80.1 CH
17	61.6 CH	62.2 CH	62.3 CH	62.2 CH	61.4 CH
18	180.9 C	182.6 C	182.6 C	181.6 C	182.8 C
19	23.9 CH$_3$	23.7 CH$_3$	23.8 CH$_3$	23.9 CH$_3$	23.8 CH$_3$
20	81.9 C	71.3 C	71.5 C	71.1 C	71.7 C
21	28.0 CH$_3$	26.0 CH$_3$	26.0 CH$_3$	26.5 CH$_3$	26.4 CH$_3$
22	37.7 CH$_2$	38.6 CH$_2$	42.0 CH$_2$	42.9 CH$_2$	45.8 CH$_2$
23	26.8 CH$_2$	29.4 CH$_2$	21.7 CH$_2$	22.7 CH$_2$	142.8 CH
24	86.7 CH	75.4 CH	38.1 CH$_2$	125.1 CH	121.9 CH
25	70.1 C	148.4 C	145.9 C	131.0 C	69.9 C
26	26.3 CH$_3$	110.6 CH$_2$	110.3 CH$_2$	25.5 CH$_3$	29.9 CH$_3$
27	26.7 CH$_3$	17.7 CH$_3$	22.2 CH$_3$	17.4 CH$_3$	29.9 CH$_3$
30	17.1 CH$_3$	17.0 CH$_3$	17.1 CH$_3$	17.1 CH$_3$	17.0 CH$_3$
31	28.5 CH$_3$	28.4 CH$_3$	28.5 CH$_3$	28.5 CH$_3$	28.5 CH$_3$
32	34.3 CH$_3$	34.3 CH$_3$	34.3 CH$_3$	34.3 CH$_3$	34.5 CH$_3$

[a] ratio C_5D_5N/D_2O (4:1); [b] ratio C_5D_5N/D_2O (5:1).

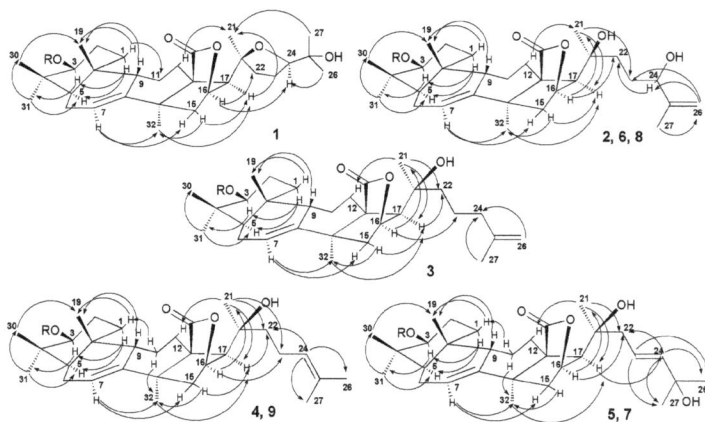

Figure 3. Key ROESY correlations for the aglycones of compounds **1–9**.

The carbohydrate chain structure of **1** was confirmed by the (−)ESI-MS/MS of the $[M_{Na} - Na]^-$ ion at m/z 843.4, where the peaks of fragment ions were observed at m/z 741.3 $[M_{Na} - Na - SO_3Na + H]^-$ and 697.3 $[M_{Na} - Na - Qui + H]^-$. The (+)ESI-MS/MS of the $[M_{Na} + Na]^+$ ion at m/z 889.4 demonstrated the peaks of ions at m/z: 769.4 $[M_{Na} + Na - NaHSO_4]^+$, 623.4 $[M_{Na} + Na - NaSO_4 - Qui]^+$, 491.3 $[M_{Na} + Na - NaSO_4 - Qui - Xyl]^+$.

Additionally, an unusual fragmentation pattern, characteristic for **1–9**, caused by the presence of 18(16)-lactone ring in their aglycones, was observed. In the (−)ESI-MS/MS of all biosides (magnumosides belonging to the group A) the ion peaks at *m/z* 497.2 appeared as a result of cleavage of B-ring of the aglycone, and 641.3 appeared as a result of D-ring cleavage, were observed (Figure 4).

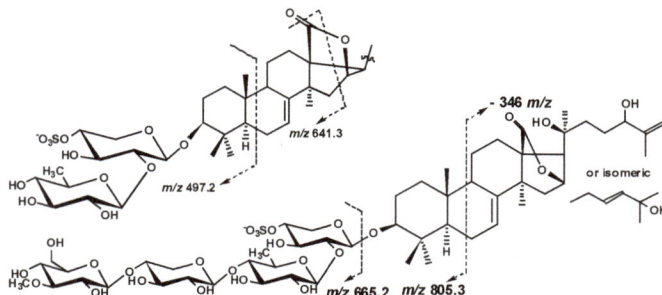

Figure 4. The aglycones fragmentation observed in the (−)ESI-MS/MS of compounds **1–9**.

Based on these results, the structure of magnumoside A$_1$ (**1**) was determined as 3β-*O*-[β-D-quinovopyranosyl-(1→2)-4-*O*-sodium sulfate-β-D-xylopyranosyl]-9β*H*,20(*S*),24(*S*)-epoxy-25-hydroxylanosta-7-ene-18(16)-lactone.

The molecular formula of magnumoside A$_2$ (**2**) was determined to be C$_{41}$H$_{63}$O$_{16}$SNa from the [M$_{Na}$ − Na]$^-$ molecular ion peak at *m/z* 843.3838 (calc. 843.3842) in the (−)HR-ESI-MS. Extensive analysis of the ^{1}H-, ^{13}C- (Tables 2 and 3) and 2D NMR spectra of the aglycone part of magnumoside A$_2$ (**2**) showed similarity of its polycyclic system to that of **1**. Indeed, the signals at δ(C) 182.6 (C(18)), 80.1 (C(16)), 62.2 (C(17)) as well as at δ(H) 5.12 (brs, H(16)) and 2.72 (s, H(17)) confirmed the presence of an 18(16)-lactone moiety, the signals at δ(C) 122.3 (C(7)) and 147.6 (C(8)) with corresponding proton signal at δ(H) 5.55–5.57 (m, H(7)) demonstrated the presence of 7(8)-double bond. However the signal of C(20) was high-shifted to δ(C) 71.3 when compared with that of **1** and was close to those of progenins obtained from cladoloside C by its alkaline treatment and having the identical to each other aglycone nuclei with hydroxylated C(20) position and non-shortened side chains [25]. The signals corresponding to the side chain of **2** formed the isolated spin system in the ^{1}H,^{1}H-COSY spectrum (Figure 2) from H(22) to H(24), indicating the latter signal was down-shifted to δ(H) 4.33 (brt, *J* = 6.0 Hz, H(24)) due to hydroxylation of this position and the multiplicity of the signal showed its vicinity to quaternary carbon C(25). The characteristic signals at δ(C) 148.4 (C(25)) and 110.6 (C(26)) with corresponding signals of olefinic protons at δ(H) 5.16 and 4.87 (each brs, H$_2$(26)) indicated the presence of terminal 25(26)-double bond. The HMBC correlations from Me(27) to C(24), C(25) and Me(26) corroborated the structure of the side chain (Figure 2). The ROESY correlations (Figure 3) H-C(5)/H-C(3), Me(31); H-C(9)/Me(19); H-C(16)/Me(21) and H-C(17)/Me(21); H-C(17)/Me(32) confirmed the common (3*S*,5*R*,9*S*,10*R*,13*S*,14*S*,16*S*,17*R*,20*S*)-configurations in lanostane-type aglycone of magnumoside A$_2$ (**2**) [22–24].

The absolute configuration of C(24) in **2** was determined by modified Mosher's method. Treatment of compound **2** with (−)-(*R*)- and (+)-(*S*)-MTPA chlorides gave (*S*)- and (*R*)-MTPA esters, correspondingly, and their ^{1}H,^{1}H-COSY spectra were analyzed. The Δ^{SR} signs were calculated and their values were negative for H(22) and H(23) and positive for H(26) and H(27), which allowed us to assign the (24*S*) configuration.

The (+)ESI-MS/MS of the [M$_{Na}$ + Na]$^+$ ion at *m/z* 889.4 demonstrated the peaks of fragment ions at *m/z*: 769.4 [M$_{Na}$ + Na − NaHSO$_4$]$^+$, 623.4 [M$_{Na}$ + Na − NaSO$_4$ − Qui]$^+$, 491.3 [M$_{Na}$ + Na − NaSO$_4$ − Qui − Xyl]$^+$, analogous to those for **1**, indicating the identity of their carbohydrate chains. The (−)ESI-MS/MS of **2** demonstrated the peak of fragment ion at *m/z* 697.3 [M$_{Na}$ − Na − Qui + H]$^-$

as well as the peaks at m/z 497.2 and 641.3 observed due to the aglycone cleavages mentioned above (Figure 4). Additionally, the peak $[M_{Na} - Na - C_6H_{12}O]^-$ was observed at m/z 743.3 in the (−)ESI-MS/MS of **2** due to the cleavage of the aglycone side chain by C-20–C-22 single bond.

All these data indicate that magnumoside A_2 (**2**) is 3β-O-[β-D-quinovopyranosyl-(1→2)-4-O-sodium sulfate-β-D-xylopyranosyl]-9βH,20(S),24(S)-dihydroxylanosta-7,25-diene-18(16)-lactone, having the new aglycone moiety.

Thus, applying Mosher's method for the aglycone of **2** corroborated the same (24S)-configuration in **1** proposed by the ROESY spectrum.

The molecular formula of magnumoside A_3 (**3**) was determined to be $C_{41}H_{63}O_{15}SNa$ from the $[M_{Na} - Na]^-$ molecular ion peak at m/z 827.3892 (calc. 827.3893) in the (−)HR-ESI-MS. The comparison of ^1H, ^{13}C NMR spectra (Tables 2 and 3) of its aglycone part with those of magnumoside A_2 (**2**) showed the closeness of the signals of the polycyclic systems indicating their identity. The signal of C(20) was observed at δ(C) 71.5 indicating the hydroxylation of this position. The protons of the aglycone side chain formed an isolated spin system H(22)/H(23)/H(24)/H(26)/H(27) in the ^1H,^1H-COSY spectrum of **3** (Figure 2) that allowed us to elucidate its structure as having a terminal double bond, for which signals were observed at δ(C) 145.9 (C(25)) and 110.3 (C(26)) in the ^{13}C NMR spectrum and at δ(H) 4.74 and 4.73 (each brs, H$_2$(26)) in the ^1H NMR spectrum. The ROESY correlations (Figure 3) confirmed the stereo structures of the aglycone polycyclic system and C(20)-chiral center of magnumoside A_3 (**3**) to be the same as in **2**.

The (+)ESI-MS/MS of **3** demonstrated the fragmentation of $[M_{Na} + Na]^+$ ion at m/z 873.4 resulting in the appearance of ion-peaks at m/z: 771.5 $[M_{Na} + Na - NaSO_3 + H]^+$, 753.5 $[M_{Na} + Na - NaHSO_4]^+$, 727.3 $[M_{Na} + Na - Qui + H]^+$, 607.4 $[M_{Na} + Na - NaSO_4 - Qui]^+$, 475.3 $[M_{Na} + Na - NaSO_4 - Qui - Xyl]^+$, analogous to those for **1** and **2**, indicating the identity of their carbohydrate chains. The characteristic peaks of fragment ions at m/z 497.2 and 641.3 were also observed in the (−)ESI-MS/MS of **3** (Figure 4).

All these data indicate that magnumoside A_3 (**3**) is 3β-O-[β-D-quinovopyranosyl-(1→2)-4-O-sodium sulfate-β-D-xylopyranosyl]-9βH,20(S)-hydroxylanosta-7,25-diene-18(16)-lactone.

The molecular formula of magnumoside A_4 (**4**) was determined to be the same as for **3** ($C_{41}H_{63}O_{15}SNa$) from the $[M_{Na} - Na]^-$ molecular ion peak at m/z 827.3892 (calc. 827.3893) in the (−)HR-ESI-MS. The comparison of ^1H, ^{13}C NMR spectra (Tables 2 and 3) of the glycosides **3** and **4** revealed the coincidence of the major part of the signals, except the signals assigned to C(23)–C(27). Actually, in the spectra of **4** the signals at δ(C) 125.1 (C(24)), 131.0 (C(25)) with corresponding olefinic proton signal at δ(H) 5.27 (t, J = 7.1 Hz, H(24)) were observed indicating the presence of 24(25)-double bond, which was confirmed by the HMBC and ROESY correlations (Figures 2 and 3). Thus, magnumosides A_3 (**3**) and A_4 (**4**) are the isomers by the double bond position that was corroborated by their ESI-MS spectra, demonstrating the presence of the ions with the same m/z values.

The fragmentation patterns in the (+) and (−)ESI-MS/MS of **4** were the same as for **3**, corroborating the identity of their carbohydrate chains and the isomerism of the aglycones.

Thus, magnumoside A_4 (**4**) is 3β-O-[β-D-quinovopyranosyl-(1→2)-4-O-sodium sulfate-β-D-xylopyranosyl]-9βH,20(S)-hydroxylanosta-7,24-diene-18(16)-lactone.

The ^1H and ^{13}C NMR spectra of carbohydrate parts of magnumosides B_1 (**5**) and B_2 (**6**) were coincident to each other showing the identity of carbohydrate chains of these glycosides. The presence of four characteristic doublets at δ(H) 4.65–5.21 (J = 7.3–8.0 Hz) in the ^1H NMR spectra of the carbohydrate chains of **5**, and **6** correlated by the HSQC spectra with the signals of anomeric carbons at δ(C) 104.4–104.8 were indicative of a tetrasaccharide chain and β-configuration of glycosidic bonds. The ^1H,^1H-COSY and 1D TOCSY spectra of **5** and **6** showed the signals of four isolated spin systems assigned to two xylose, one quinovose and 3-O-methylglucose residues. The positions of interglycosidic linkages were elucidated by the ROESY and HMBC spectra of **5** and **6** (Table 1) where the cross-peaks between H(1) of the first (xylose) residue and H(3) (C(3)) of an aglycone, H(1) of the second (quinovose) residue and H(2) (C(2)) of the first (xylose) residue, H(1) of the third (xylose) residue and H(4) (C(4)) of the second (quinovose) residue and H(1) of the terminal (3-*O*-methylglucose) residue and H(3) (C(3)) of the third (xylose) residue were observed. The signals of C(4) and C(5) of the first (xylose) residue were observed at δ(C) 76.0 and 63.9, correspondingly, indicating the presence of a sulfate group at C(4) of the sugar unit, analogically to the carbohydrate chains of magnumosides of the group A (**1–4**). The linear tetrasaccharide monosulfated carbohydrate chain of magnumosides of the group B (**5, 6**), having the xylose as third monosaccharide unit, were found earlier in "neothyonidioside" [15] isolated from another collection of *N. magnum*, also coincided with the sugar moiety of colochiroside B$_2$ (**9**) [17] found in the investigated sample of *N. magnum* and are widely distributed in the triterpene glycosides of sea cucumbers of the orders Aspidochirotida [2] and Dendrochirotida [2,8,26–28].

The molecular formula of magnumoside B$_1$ (**5**) was determined to be $C_{53}H_{83}O_{25}SNa$ from the $[M_{Na} - Na]^-$ molecular ion peak at *m/z* 1151.4954 (calc. 1151.4950) in the (−)HR-ESI-MS. The polycyclic system and hydroxylated C(20)-position of **5** were identical to those of **2–4** that was deduced from the comparison of their ^1H, ^{13}C NMR spectra (Tables 2 and 3). The olefinic carbons signals observed at δ(C) 142.8 (C(23)), 121.9 (C(24)) with corresponding protons signals at δ(H) 5.92 (d, *J* = 15.8 Hz, H(23)) and 6.13 (dt, *J* = 6.9; 8.0; 15.8 Hz, H(24)) and the signal of oxigenated tertiary carbon at δ(C) 69.9 (C(25)) in the ^{13}C and ^1H NMR spectra of **5**, correspondingly, were indicative for 23(24)*E*-en-25-ol fragment in the aglycone side chain. This structure was confirmed by the HMBC correlations from H-C(22) to C(23) and C(24), from H-C(23) to C(22), C(25), Me(26) and Me(27) and from Me(26) and Me(27) to C(23), C(24), C(25) (Figure 2). The ROESY correlations also corroborated the aglycone structure (Figure 3).

The (−)ESI-MS/MS of **5** demonstrated the fragmentation of $[M_{Na} - Na]^-$ ion at *m/z* 1151.4. The peaks of fragment ions were observed at *m/z*: 975.4 $[M_{Na} - Na - MeGlc + H]^-$, 843.4 $[M_{Na} - Na - MeGlc - Xyl]^-$, 697.3 $[M_{Na} - Na - MeGlc - Xyl - Qui + H]^-$ corroborating the sequence of sugars in the carbohydrate chain of **5**. The cleavage of the ring B of the aglycone led to the appearance of fragment ion-peak at *m/z* 805.3 $[M_{Na} - Na - C_{21}H_{30}O_4]^-$. Its further fragmentation led to the consequent loss of monosaccharide units and the ion-peaks were observed at *m/z* 629.2 $[M_{Na} - Na - C_{21}H_{30}O_4 - MeGlc + H]^-$, 497.2 $[M_{Na} - Na - C_{21}H_{30}O_4 - MeGlc - Xyl]^-$, 351.1 $[M_{Na} - Na - C_{21}H_{30}O_4 - MeGlc - Xyl - Qui + H]^-$.

All these data indicate that magnumoside B$_1$ (**5**) is 3β-*O*-[3-*O*-methyl-β-D-glucopyranosyl-(1→3)-β-D-xylopyranosyl-(1→4)-β-D-quinovopyranosyl-(1→2)-4-*O*-sodium sulfate-β-D-xylopyranosyl]-9βH,20(S),25-dihydroxylanosta-7,23E-diene-18(16)-lactone.

The molecular formula of magnumoside B$_2$ (**6**) was determined to be $C_{53}H_{83}O_{25}SNa$ from the $[M_{Na} - Na]^-$ molecular ion peak at *m/z* 1151.4945 (calc. 1151.4950) in the (−)HR-ESI-MS that was coincident with the formula of magnumoside B$_1$ (**5**). The analysis of the ^1H, ^{13}C NMR spectra of the aglycone part of **6** showed its identity to the aglycone part of magnumoside A$_2$ (**2**) (Tables 2 and 3). So, the glycosides **5** and **6** are the isomers by the positions of the double bond and hydroxyl group in the side chain.

The peaks of fragment ions in the (−)ESI-MS/MS of **6** were observed at the same *m/z* values as in the spectrum of **5**, corroborating the identity of carbohydrate chain structures of these compounds. The consequent fragmentation of the ion $[M_{Na} - Na - C_{21}H_{30}O_4]^-$ at *m/z* 805.3 in the spectrum of **6** that led to the loss of the aglycone and the ion-peak $[M_{Na} - Na - C_{30}H_{45}O_5]^-$ was observed at *m/z* 665.2.

Thus, magnumoside B$_2$ (**6**) is 3β-*O*-[3-*O*-methyl-β-D-glucopyranosyl-(1→3)-β-D-xylopyranosyl-(1→4)-β-D-quinovopyranosyl-(1→2)-4-*O*-sodium sulfate-β-D-xylopyranosyl]-9βH,20(S),24(S)-dihydroxylanosta-7,25-diene-18(16)-lactone.

The ^1H and ^{13}C NMR spectra of carbohydrate parts of magnumosides C$_1$ (**7**), C$_2$ (**8**) and C$_4$ (**9**) were coincident to each other and to those of neothyonidioside C, isolated earlier from this species [16], that indicated the identity of carbohydrate chains of these glycosides. The presence of four characteristic doublets at δ(H) 4.65–5.12 (*J* = 7.0–7.9 Hz) in the ^1H NMR spectra of the carbohydrate chains of **7–9** correlated by the HSQC spectra with the signals of anomeric carbons at δ(C) 104.3–104.8 were indicative of a tetrasaccharide chain and β-configuration of glycosidic bonds. The positions of interglycosidic linkages were elucidated based on the ROESY and HMBC spectra (SM, Table 1), where the cross-peaks analogical to **5**, and **6** were observed. The differences between the ^{13}C NMR spectra of magnumosides of the groups C (**7–9**) and B (**5**, **6**) were in the signals of C(5) and C(6) of terminal monosaccharide residue that were observed in the ^{13}C NMR spectra of **7–9** at δ(C) 75.5 and 67.1, correspondingly, due to the shifting effects of a sulfate group attached to C(6) of 3-O-methylglucose unit. Actually, magnumosides of the group C (**7–8**) are characterized by the linear tetrasaccharide disulfated carbohydrate chain, which have been found earlier in the glycosides of *Mensamaria intercedens* [29], *Pseudocolochirus violaceus* [30] and *Colochirus robustus* [17], representatives of the family Cucumariidae, order Dendrochirotida.

The molecular formula of magnumoside C_1 (**7**) was determined to be $C_{53}H_{82}O_{28}S_2Na_2$ from the $[M_{2Na} - Na]^-$ molecular ion peak at m/z 1253.4328 (calc. 1253.4337) in the (−)HR-ESI-MS. The aglycones of magnumoside C_1 (**7**) and B_1 (**5**) were identical to each other due to the coincidence of their ^{13}C NMR spectra (Tables 2 and 3) and their carbohydrate chains differed only by the quantity of sulfate groups. The (−)ESI-MS/MS of **7** where the peaks of fragment ions were observed at m/z 1133.4 $[M_{2Na} - Na - NaHSO_4]^-$, 957.4 $[M_{2Na} - Na - NaHSO_4 - MeGlc]^-$, 825.4 $[M_{2Na} - Na - NaHSO_4 - MeGlc - Xyl]^-$, 679.3 $[M_{2Na} - Na - NaHSO_4 - MeGlc - Xyl - Qui]^-$ corroborated the structure of carbohydrate chain. The cleavage of the ring B of the aglycone as well as the loss of one of the sulfate groups led to the appearance of fragment ion-peak at m/z 805.3 $[M_{2Na} - Na - NaSO_3 - C_{21}H_{30}O_4 + H]^-$. Its further fragmentation resulted in the loss of the aglycone, the ion-peak at m/z 665.2 $[M_{2Na} - Na - NaSO_3 - C_{30}H_{45}O_5]^-$, followed by the loss of sugar units, m/z: 533.1 $[M_{2Na} - Na - NaSO_3 - C_{30}H_{45}O_5 - Xyl]^-$, 387.1 $[M_{2Na} - Na - NaSO_3 - C_{30}H_{45}O_5 - Xyl - Qui]^-$, 255 $[M_{2Na} - Na - NaSO_3 - C_{30}H_{45}O_5 - Xyl - Qui - Xyl]^-$. The ion-peak at m/z 255 $[C_7H_{12}O_8SNa - Na - H]^-$ is also corresponded to the sulfated 3-O-methyl glucose residue.

Therefore, magnumoside C_1 (**7**) is 3β-O-[6-O-sodium sulfate-3-O-methyl-β-D-glucopyranosyl-(1→3) -β-D-xylopyranosyl-(1→4)-β-D-quinovopyranosyl-(1→2)-4-O-sodium sulfate-β-D-xylopyranosyl]-9βH,20(S),25-dihydroxylanosta-7,23E-diene-18(16)-lactone.

The molecular formula of magnumoside C_2 (**8**) coincided with that of **7** ($C_{53}H_{82}O_{28}S_2Na_2$) that was deduced from the $[M_{2Na} - Na]^-$ molecular ion peak at m/z 1253.4341 (calc. 1253.4337) in the (−)HR-ESI-MS. The aglycone of magnumoside C_2 (**8**) was identical to those of the magnumosides A_2 (**2**) and B_2 (**6**) that was suggested based on the coincidence of their ^{13}C NMR spectra (Tables 2 and 3). So, magnumoside C_2 (**8**) is additionally sulfated, by C(6) of 3-O-methylglucose residue, analog of magnumoside B_2 (**6**). The (−)ESI-MS/MS of **8** corroborated its isomerism to the magnumoside C_1 (**7**) since their fragmentation patterns were the same and the ion-peaks were characterized by the identical m/z values.

Thus, magnumoside C_2 (**8**) is 3β-O-[6-O-sodium sulfate-3-O-methyl-β-D-glucopyranosyl-(1→3)-β-D-xylopyranosyl-(1→4)-β-D-quinovopyranosyl-(1→2)-4-O-sodium sulfate-β-D-xylopyranosyl]-9βH,20(S),24(S)-dihydroxylanosta-7,25-diene-18(16)-lactone.

The NMR spectra of the aglycone moiety of magnumoside C_4 (**9**) were coincident to those of magnumoside A_4 (**4**) (Tables 2 and 3).

The molecular formula of magnumoside C_4 (**9**) was determined to be $C_{53}H_{82}O_{27}S_2Na_2$ from the $[M_{2Na} - Na]^-$ molecular ion peak at m/z 1237.4390 (calc. 1237.4388) in the (−)HR ESIMS. The peaks of fragment ions in the (−) ESI MS/MS of **9** were observed at m/z 1135.4 $[M_{2Na} - Na - NaSO_3 + H]^-$, 1117.4 $[M_{2Na} - Na - NaHSO_4]^-$, 959.4 $[M_{2Na} - Na - NaSO_4 - MeGlc]^-$, 827.4 $[M_{2Na} - Na - NaSO_4 - MeGlc - Xyl]^-$, 681.3 $[M_{2Na} - Na - NaSO_4 - MeGlc - Xyl - Qui]^-$ corroborated the structure of carbohydrate chain. The loss of the aglycone from the ion at m/z 1135.4 $[M_{2Na} - Na - NaSO_3 + H]^-$ led to the appearance of the ion-peak at m/z 665.2 $[M_{2Na} - Na - NaSO_3 - C_{30}H_{45}O_4]^-$, its further fragmentation resulted in the consequent loss of sugar units, m/z: 533.1 $[M_{2Na} - Na - NaSO_3 - C_{30}H_{45}O_4 - Xyl]^-$, 387.1 $[M_{2Na} - Na - NaSO_3 - C_{30}H_{45}O_4 - Xyl - Qui]^-$, 255 $[M_{2Na} - Na - NaSO_3 - C_{30}H_{45}O_4 - Xyl - Qui - Xyl]^-$. The ion-peak at m/z 255 $[C_7H_{12}O_8SNa - Na - H]^-$ is also corresponded to the sulfated 3-O-methyl glucose residue.

All these data indicate that magnumoside C_4 (**9**) is 3β-*O*-[6-*O*-sodium sulfate-3-*O*-methyl-β-D-glucopyranosyl-(1→3)-β-D-xylopyranosyl-(1→4)-β-D-quinovopyranosyl-(1→2)-4-*O*-sodium sulfate-β-D-xylopyranosyl]-9β*H*,20(*S*)-hydroxylanosta-7,24-diene-18(16)-lactone.

All the new glycosides, magnumosides A_1 (**1**), A_2 (**2**), A_3 (**3**), A_4 (**4**), B_1 (**5**), B_2 (**6**), C_1 (**7**), C_2 (**8**) and C_4 (**9**), isolated from *N. magnum*, are characterized by the presence of non-holostane-type aglycones with 18(16)-lactone moieties and non-shortened side chains. The aglycone of **1** having 20(24)-epoxy group in the side chain was found first in the triterpene glycosides of sea cucumbers. The aglycones, having 18(16)-lactone, are of rare occurrence in the sea cucumber glycosides. Such type aglycones were found in two variants: with shortened side chains, like in some glycosides from *Eupentacta fraudatrix* [31–33] and *Pentamera calcigera* [34]; and, that is more rare, with non-shortened side chains, like in psolusoside B from *Psolus fabricii* [21], colochiroside E from *Colochirus robustus* [22] and in magnumosides A_1 (**1**), A_2 (**2**), A_3 (**3**), A_4 (**4**), B_1 (**5**), B_2 (**6**), C_1 (**7**), C_2 (**8**) and C_4 (**9**).

These aglycones are strongly differing from the holostane-type aglycones found in isolated earlier glycosides, "neothyonidioside" and neothyonidioside C [15,16], from New-Caledonian and Vietnamese collections of *N. magnum*, correspondingly. In contrast, the aglycone of colochiroside B_2 (**10**) found in the investigated sample of *N. magnum* is biogenetically very close to that of neothyonidioside C which also has the holostane-type aglycone with 16-acetoxygroup and differs in the side chain structure. Furthermore, the monosulfated tetrasaccharide carbohydrate chain of **10** was identical to those of "neothyonidioside" and magnumosides of the group B (**5, 6**). The disulfated tetrasaccharide chain of magnumosides of the group C (**7–9**) was identical to that of neothyonidioside C. The finding of compound **10** in recent Vietnamese collection of *N. magnum* structurally close to found earlier glycosides from this species confirms the correctness of biological identification of the all studied samples. The predominance of non-holostane-type glycosides and the fact that neither "neothyonidioside" nor neothyonidioside C have been found in the studying sample of the animal could be explained by the changes in the quantitative and qualitative composition of different components of glycosidic fraction in the samples of one species collected in different places and seasons. The representative example of such changes demonstrated the components of glycosidic fraction of *Psolus fabricii*. Psolusoside A, a holostane glycoside was predominant in *P. fabricii* collected near the shore of the Onekotan Island of Kuril Ridge and non-holostane psolusoside B having a 18(16)-lactone was the minor one [35]. The opposite situation was observed in samples of *P. fabricii* collected in the Kraternaya Bay of Ushishir Islands of the Kuril Archipelago, where psolusoside A was found only in trace amount and psolusoside B was the predominant component [36].

The sets of magnumosides $A_2→B_2→C_2$ and $B_1→C_1$, in which the glycosides were characterized by the same aglycones and different carbohydrate chains within the set, demonstrated the biosynthetic transformations of the carbohydrate chains resulting in their elongation and additional sulfation. The biosynthetic modifications of the aglycones are mainly concerned with side chains transformations, when the double bonds and hydroxyls are introduced in different positions. The aglycone of magnumosides B_1 (**5**) and C_1 (**7**) with 23(24)-double bond and 20,25-hydroxyls is obviously could be the precursor of the unusual aglycone of magnumoside A_1 (**1**) with 20(24)-epoxy-25-hydroxy-fragment. The similar conversion of the aglycone having a linear side chain with a double bond and hydroxyl group to the aglycone having epoxy-group was observed in the process of obtaining the genins with 18(16)-lactone moieties by chemical transformations of the holostane aglycone of cladoloside C [25]. It was considered as a biomimetic reaction, modeling the biosynthetic process in the glycoside aglycones. The aglycone structure of colochiroside B_2 (**10**) is biogenetically related with the aglycones of **1**, **5** and **7**. It is known that the formation of 18(16)-lactone biosynthetically occurs in C(18)-carboxylated derivatives having both hydroxylated C(16) and C(20) positions. However, when the further oxidation (acetylation or carboxylation) of C(16) precedes the carboxylation of C(18) the holostane-type aglycones with functionality at C(16) are biosynthesized [37] (Figure 5). In the case of **10**, this process took place. Interestingly, the oxidative transformations of the side chain in biosynthesis of **10** may precede the lactonization.

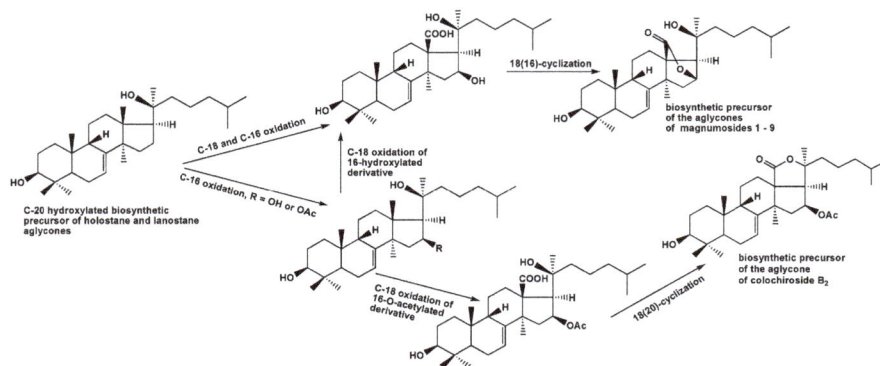

Figure 5. The hypothetic scheme of the aglycones biosynthesis of glycosides of *N. magnum*.

2.2. Biological Activities of Glycosides

2.2.1. Hemolytic and Cytotoxic Activities of the Glycosides 1–9 against Mouse Spleenocites and the Ascites Form of Mouse Ehrlich Carcinoma Cells

The cytotoxic action of the compounds **1–9** against mouse spleenocytes and the ascites form of mouse Ehrlich carcinoma cells as well as hemolytic action against mouse erythrocytes have been studied (Table 4). Magnumoside A$_1$ (**1**) was the only glycoside inactive in all tests that was caused by unusual aglycone structure having 18(16)-lactone in combination with 20(24)-epoxy-25-hydroxy-fragment. Magnumosides A$_2$ (**2**), B$_1$ (**5**) and B$_2$ (**6**) demonstrated moderate hemolytic activity and were non-cytotoxic up to the ultimate investigated concentration of 100 µM, that was explained by the presence of hydroxyls in their side chains [17,32,33]. However, magnumosides C$_1$ (**7**) and C$_2$ (**8**) that had aglycones identical to those of magnumosides B$_1$ (**5**) and B$_2$ (**6**) and differed from the latter compounds by the presence of the additional sulfate group were the exclusions from this relation and demonstrated significant effects in all tests. Moreover, magnumosides C$_1$ (**7**) and C$_4$ (**9**) turned out to be the most active compounds in this series. So, the activity-decreasing influence of hydroxyl-group in the side chain of **7** and **8** was counterbalanced by the additional sulfate group attached to C-6 of terminal monosaccharide residue of these compounds. On the whole, the erythrocytes were more sensitive to the glycosides action than the spleenocytes and cancer cells studied.

Table 4. Hemolytic activity of the glycosides **1–9** against mouse erythrocytes and cytotoxic activity against mouse spleenocytes and the ascites form of mouse Ehrlich carcinoma cells.

Compound	Hemolytic Activity, ED$_{50}$, µM/mL *	Cytotoxic Activity, IC$_{50}$, µM/mL **	
		spleenocytes	Ehrlich carcinoma cells
1	90.18 ± 1.57	>100.00	>100.00
2	33.33 ± 0.48	94.18 ± 1.18	>100.00
3	12.53 ± 0.29	19.20 ± 0.03	18.95 ± 0.03
4	20.12 ± 0.14	37.64 ± 0.00	28.37 ± 0.42
5	49.57 ± 0.63	>100.00	>100.00
6	58.11 ± 0.69	>100.00	>100.00
7	6.97 ± 0.14	8.97 ± 0.04	18.65 ± 0.00
8	16.20 ± 0.49	17.31 ± 0.43	37.52 ± 0.00
9	6.52 ± 0.16	12.23 ± 0.33	35.06 ± 0.18
Typicosid A$_1$	3.15 ± 0.12	9.92 ± 0.12	35.66 ± 0.11
Cucumarioside A$_2$-2	0.82 ± 0.02	1.21 ± 0.02	1.39 ± 0.015

* ED$_{50}$ is the effective dose of compound causing 50% of hemolysis of cells; ** IC$_{50}$ is a concentration of substance caused 50% reduction in cell viability.

2.2.2. The Effect of the Glycosides on Cell Viability of Human Colorectal Adenocarcinoma DLD-1 Cells

To determine cytotoxic effect of the compounds against human colorectal adenocarcinoma, DLD-1 cells were treated with various concentrations of **1–9** (0–100 μM) for 24 h and then cell viability was assessed by the MTS assay. It was showed that **1, 2, 4–6** did not possessed cytotoxic effect against DLD-1 cells that is in good correlation with the data on Echrlich carcinoma cells. The magnumoside A_3 (**3**), magnumoside C_1 (**7**), magnumoside C_2 (**8**) and magnumoside C_4 (**9**) decreased cell viability with IC_{50} value of 30.3, 34.3, 32.9, 37.1, and 33.9 μM, respectively (Table 5). Thus, for further experiments we chose the concentrations of investigated compounds lower than IC_{50}, at which no significant cytotoxic effect on DLD-1 cells was observed.

Table 5. The cytotoxic activity of the glycosides **1–9** against DLD-1 cells.

Glycoside	IC_{50}, μM *	Glycoside	IC_{50}, μM *
magnumoside A_1 (**1**)	>100	magnumoside B_2 (**6**)	>100
magnumoside A_2 (**2**)	>100	magnumoside C_1 (**7**)	32.9
magnumoside A_3 (**3**)	30.3	magnumoside C_2 (**8**)	37.1
magnumoside A_4 (**4**)	>100	magnumoside C_4 (**9**)	33.9
magnumoside B_1 (**5**)	>100	–	–

* IC_{50} is a concentration of substance caused 50% reduction in cell viability.

2.2.3. The Effect of the Glycosides on Formation and Growth of Colonies of Human Colorectal Adenocarcinoma DLD-1 Cells

The effect of **3, 7–9** on the colony formation of DLD-1 cells using soft agar assay has been studied. The magnumoside A_3 (**3**) and magnumoside C_1 (**7**) inhibited spontaneous colony formation by 22% and 26%, respectively, (Figure 6A) and, at the same time, they reduced colonies size of DLD-1 cancer cells by 49% and 43%, respectively, (Figure 6B). On the other hand, magnumosides C_2 (**8**) and C_4 (**9**) possessed slight inhibitory activity in this experiment (the percentages of inhibition were less than 20%) (Figure 6A,B).

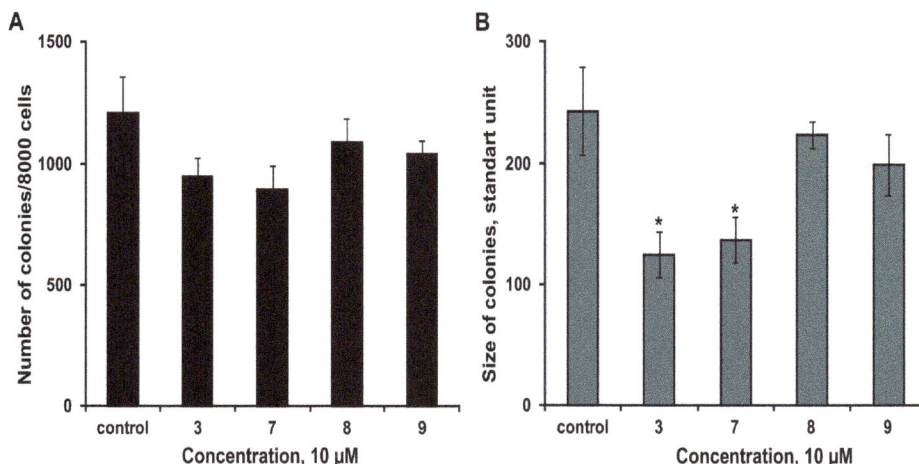

Figure 6. The effect of the glycosides **3, 7–9** on colony formation of DLD-1 cells. (**A**) The compounds decreased the number of colonies of cancer cells. (**B**) The compounds decreased the size of colonies of cancer cells. Data are shown as means ± standard deviation and the asterisks (* $p < 0.05$) indicates a significant decrease in colony formation of cells treated with the compounds compared with the control.

2.2.4. The Synergism of Radioactive Irradiation and the Compounds Effects on Proliferation and Colony Formation of Human Colorectal Adenocarcinoma Cells

At first, the individual effect of radiation or the compounds at concentration 2 μM on colony formation of DLD-1 cells was checked. The tested compounds did not influence the process of colonies formation at the dose of 2 μM. The number and size of colonies of DLD-1 cells were found to be decreased by 7% and 67%, respectively, after radiation exposure at dose of 4 Gy. Moreover, the synergism of effects of radioactive irradiation (4 Gy) and the compounds **3**, **7–9** (2 μM) was not observed (data not shown).

Nevertheless, the investigated compounds (2 μM) enhanced the antiproliferative effect from radioactive irradiation (4 Gy). Magnumoside C_4 (**9**) possessed the highest activity in this experiment; it increased the inhibitory effect from radiation on proliferation of DLD-1 cancer cells by 45%. Magnumoside A_3 (**3**), magnumoside C_1 (**7**) and magnumoside C_2 (**8**) enhanced the effect from radiation by more than 30% (Figure 7). Recently, it was reported that ginsenoside Rg3 isolated from the roots of *Panax ginseng* sensitized human lung carcinoma A549 and H1299 cells to γ-radiation and significantly enhanced the efficacy of radiation therapy in C57BL/6 mice bearing a Lewis lung carcinoma cell xenograft tumor [38]. Nevertheless, our finding of a synergism of the antiproliferative effect of the radioactive irradiation and a series of glycosides from *Neothyonidium magnum* on human tumor cells is the first study on sea cucumber triterpene glycosides.

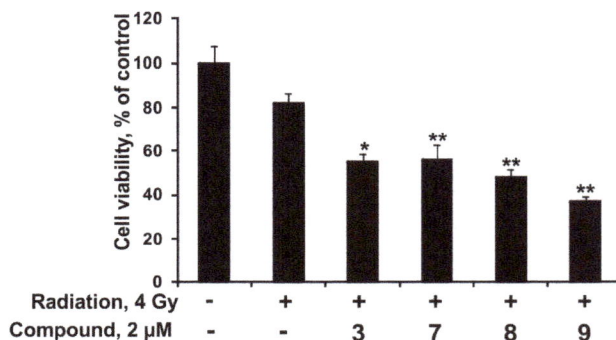

Figure 7. The effect of radioactive irradiation and a combination of radioactive irradiation and the compounds **3**, **7–9** on DLD-1 cancer cell proliferation. DLD-1 cells (8.0×10^3) were treated with radiation 4 Gy and the compounds **3**, **7–9** (2 μM) for 96 h. Cell viability was estimated using the MTS assay. Data are represented as the mean $\pm$ SD as determined from triplicate experiments. A Student's *t*-test was used to evaluate the data with the following significance levels: * $p < 0.05$, ** $p < 0.01$.

3. Experimental Section

3.1. General Experimental Procedures

Specific rotations were measured on Perkin-Elmer 343 polarimeter. NMR spectra were obtained on an AVANCE III-700 Bruker spectrometer (Bruker BioSpin, Fällanden, Switzerland) at 700.13 (^{1}H) and 176.04 (^{13}C) MHz, δ in ppm rel. to Me$_4$Si, *J* in Hz. ESI-MS/MS and HR-ESI-MS were run on an Agilent 6510 Q-TOF apparatus (Agilent Technologies, Santa Clara, CA, USA), sample concentration 0.01 mg/mL, in *m/z*. HPLC was carried out on an Agilent 1100 chromatograph equipped with a differential refractometer using Supelcosil LC-Si (4.6×150 mm, 5 μm) (Agilent Technologies, Santa Clara, CA, USA), Supelco Ascentis RP-Amide (10×250 mm, 5 μm) (Supelco Analytical, Bellefonte, PA, USA) and Diasfer *C-8* (4×250 mm, 5 μm) (Supelco Analytical, Bellefonte, PA, USA) columns.

Polychrom-1 (powdered Teflon, 0.25–0.50 mm; Biolar, Olaine, Latvia), silica gel KSK (50–160 μM, Sorbpolimer, Krasnodar, Russia) were used for column chromatography.

3.2. Animal Material

Specimens of the sea cucumber *Neothyonidium* (=*Massinium*) *magnum* (family Phyllophoridae; order Dendrochirotida) were collected during the expedition of Joint Russia-Vietnam laboratory of Marine Biology RAS-VAST in South China Sea in Nha Trang bay near Tam Island. Sampling was performed by SCUBA in July 2015 (collector T. Dautova) at a depth of 8 m. Sea cucumbers were identified by T. Dautova; voucher specimens are preserved in the collection of the Museum of A.V. Zhirmunsky Institute of Marine Biology, Vladivostok, Russia.

3.3. Extraction and Isolation

The sea cucumbers were minced and extracted twice with refluxing 60% EtOH. The dry weight of the residue was about 59.2 g. The combined extracts were concentrated to dryness in vacuum, dissolved in H_2O, and chromatographed on a *Polychrom-1* column (powdered Teflon, Biolar, Latvia). Eluting first of the inorganic salts and impurities with H_2O and then the glycosides with 50% EtOH gave 1800 mg of crude glycoside fraction. Then it was chromatographed on Si gel column using $CHCl_3$/EtOH/H_2O (100:100:17) followed by (100:125:25) as mobile phase to give fractions 1 (332 mg) and 2 (340 mg). The fraction 1 was additionally chromatographed on Si gel column with $CHCl_3$/EtOH/H_2O (100:75:10) as mobile phase to give three subfractions: 1.1 (95 mg), 1.2 (127 mg) and 1.3 (46 mg). Subfraction 1.1 was submitted to HPLC on silica-based column Supelcosil LC-Si (4.6 × 150 mm) with $CHCl_3$/MeOH/H_2O (65:20:2) as mobile phase to obtain fractions 1.1.1 (45 mg) and 1.1.2 (5 mg) that were sequentially submitted to HPLC on a reversed-phase semipreparative Supelco Ascentis RP-Amide column (10 × 250 mm) with different ratios of MeOH/H_2O/NH_4OAc (1 M water solution) as mobile phase. Fraction 1.1.1 chromatographed with the ratio (65/34/1) followed by the ratios (63/36/1) gave magnumosides A_3 (3) (3.7 mg) and A_4 (4) (8.0 mg); (58/41/1)—magnumoside A_1 (1) (3.6 mg). Fraction 1.1.2 chromatographed with the ratio (55/44/1) gave magnumoside A_2 (2) (5.0 mg).

Subfraction 1.3, obtained after chromatography on Si gel, was submitted to HPLC on Supelco Ascentis RP-Amide column (10 × 250 mm) with MeOH/H_2O/NH_4OAc (1 M water solution) (57/41/2) followed by (55/43/2) as mobile phase to give magnumosides B_1 (5) (2.6 mg), B_2 (6) (1.8 mg) and colochiroside B_2 (10) (2.0 mg).

The most polar fraction 2, obtained after the separation of crude glycoside fraction of Si gel column, was submitted to HPLC on Supelco Ascentis RP-Amide column (10 × 250 mm) with MeOH/H_2O/NH_4OAc (1 M water solution) (57/41/2) to give a set of subfractions. Subfraction 2.1 was submitted to HPLC on Diasfer C-8 (4.6 × 250 mm) column with AcN/H_2O/NH_4OAc (1 M water solution) (24/75/1) to obtain magnumoside C_1 (7) (5.7 mg). Subfraction 2.2 was submitted to HPLC in the same conditions to obtain magnumoside C_2 (8) (2.5 mg) and C_4 (9) (15 mg).

3.3.1. Magnumoside A_1 (1)

Colorless powder; $[\alpha]_D^{20}$ −48 (*c* 0.1, 50% MeOH); ^{1}H NMR data see Tables 1 and 2; ^{13}C NMR data see Tables 1 and 3; (−)HR-ESI-MS, *m/z*: 843.3838 [M_{Na} − Na]$^-$ (calcd for $C_{41}H_{63}O_{16}S^-$, 843.3842); (−)ESI-MS/MS, *m/z*: 843.4 [M_{Na} − Na]$^-$, 741.3 [M_{Na} − Na − SO_3Na + H]$^-$, 697.3 [M_{Na} − Na − Qui + H]$^-$, 641.3 [M_{Na} − Na − $C_{10}H_{18}O_4$]$^-$, 497.2 [M_{Na} − Na − $C_{21}H_{30}O_4$]$^-$. (+)ESI-MS/MS, *m/z*: 889.4 [M_{Na} + Na]$^+$, 769.4 [M_{Na} + Na − $NaHSO_4$]$^+$, 623.4 [M_{Na} + Na − $NaSO_4$ − Qui]$^+$, 491.3 [M_{Na} + Na − $NaSO_4$ − Qui − Xyl]$^+$.

3.3.2. Magnumoside A_2 (2)

Colorless powder; $[\alpha]_D^{20}$ −12 (*c* 0.1, 50% MeOH); ^{1}H NMR data see Tables 1 and 2; ^{13}C NMR data see Tables 1 and 3; (−)HR-ESI-MS, *m/z*: 843.3838 [M_{Na} − Na]$^-$, (calcd for $C_{41}H_{63}O_{16}S^-$, 843.3842),

(+)ESI-MS/MS, m/z: 889.4 $[M_{Na} + Na]^+$, 769.4 $[M_{Na} + Na - NaHSO_4]^+$, 623.4 $[M_{Na} + Na - NaSO_4 - Qui]^+$, 491.3 $[M_{Na} + Na - NaSO_4 - Qui - Xyl]^+$; (−)ESI-MS/MS, m/z: 843.4 $[M_{Na} - Na]^-$, 697.3 $[M_{Na} - Na - Qui + H]^-$, 743.3 $[M_{Na} - Na - C_6H_{12}O]^-$, 641.3 $[M_{Na} - Na - C_{10}H_{18}O_4]^-$, 497.2 $[M_{Na} - Na - C_{21}H_{30}O_4]^-$.

3.3.3. Magnumoside A_3 (3)

Colorless powder; $[\alpha]_D^{20}$ −63 (*c* 0.1, 50% MeOH); ^{1}H NMR data see Tables 1 and 2; ^{13}C NMR data see Tables 1 and 3. (−)HR-ESI-MS, m/z: 827.3892 $[M_{Na} - Na]^-$ (calcd for $C_{41}H_{63}O_{15}S^-$, 827.3893); (+)ESI-MS/MS, m/z: 873.4 $[M_{Na} + Na]^+$, 771.5 $[M_{Na} + Na - NaSO_3 + H]^+$, 753.5 $[M_{Na} + Na - NaHSO_4]^+$, 727.3 $[M_{Na} + Na - Qui + H]^+$, 607.4 $[M_{Na} + Na - NaSO_4 - Qui]^+$, 475.3 $[M_{Na} + Na - NaSO_4 - Qui - Xyl]^+$; (−)ESI-MS/MS, m/z 641.3 $[M_{Na} - Na - C_{10}H_{18}O_3]^-$, 497.2 $[M_{Na} - Na - C_{21}H_{30}O_3]^-$.

3.3.4. Magnumoside A_4 (4)

Colorless powder; $[\alpha]_D^{20}$ −98 (*c* 0.1, 50% MeOH); ^{1}H NMR: Tables 1 and 2; ^{13}C NMR data see Tables 1 and 3; (−)HR-ESI-MS, m/z: 827.3892 $[M_{Na} - Na]^-$ (calcd for $C_{41}H_{63}O_{15}S^-$, 827.3893); (+)ESI-MS/MS, m/z: 873.4 $[M_{Na} + Na]^+$, 771.5 $[M_{Na} + Na - NaSO_3 + H]^+$, 753.5 $[M_{Na} + Na - NaHSO_4]^+$, 727.3 $[M_{Na} + Na - Qui + H]^+$, 607.4 $[M_{Na} + Na - NaSO_4 - Qui]^+$, 475.3 $[M_{Na} + Na - NaSO_4 - Qui - Xyl]^+$; (−)ESI-MS/MS, m/z 641.3 $[M_{Na} - Na - C_{10}H_{18}O_3]^-$, 497.2 $[M_{Na} - Na - C_{21}H_{30}O_3]^-$.

3.3.5. Magnumoside B_1 (5)

Colorless powder; $[\alpha]_D^{20}$ −74 (*c* 0.1, 50% MeOH); ^{1}H NMR data see Tables 1 and 2; ^{13}C NMR data see Tables 1 and 3; (−)HR-ESI-MS, m/z: 1151.4954 $[M_{Na} - Na]^-$ (calcd for $C_{53}H_{83}O_{25}S^-$, 1151.4950); (−)ESI-MS/MS, m/z: 1151.4 $[M_{Na} - Na]^-$, 975.4 $[M_{Na} - Na - MeGlc + H]^-$, 843.4 $[M_{Na} - Na - MeGlc - Xyl]^-$, 697.3 $[M_{Na} - Na - MeGlc - Xyl - Qui + H]^-$, 805.3 $[M_{Na} - Na - C_{21}H_{30}O_4]^-$, 629.2 $[M_{Na} - Na - C_{21}H_{30}O_4 - MeGlc + H]^-$, 497.2 $[M_{Na} - Na - C_{21}H_{30}O_4 - MeGlc - Xyl]^-$, 351.1 $[M_{Na} - Na - C_{21}H_{30}O_4 - MeGlc - Xyl - Qui + H]^-$.

3.3.6. Magnumoside B_2 (6)

Colorless powder; $[\alpha]_D^{20}$ −57 (*c* 0.1, 50% MeOH); ^{1}H NMR: Tables 1 and 2; ^{13}C NMR data see Tables 1 and 3; (−)HR-ESI-MS, m/z: 1151.4954 $[M_{Na} - Na]^-$ (calcd for $C_{53}H_{83}O_{25}S^-$, 1151.4950); (−)ESI-MS/MS, m/z: 1151.4 $[M_{Na} - Na]^-$, 975.4 $[M_{Na} - Na - MeGlc + H]^-$, 843.4 $[M_{Na} - Na - MeGlc - Xyl]^-$, 697.3 $[M_{Na} - Na - MeGlc - Xyl - Qui + H]^-$, 805.3 $[M_{Na} - Na - C_{21}H_{30}O_4]^-$, 665.2 $[M_{Na} - Na - C_{30}H_{45}O_5]^-$.

3.3.7. Magnumoside C_1 (7)

Colorless powder; $[\alpha]_D^{20}$ −22 (*c* 0.1, 50% MeOH); ^{1}H NMR: Tables 1 and 2 (for carbohydrate chain); ^{13}C NMR data see Tables 1 and 3; (−)HR-ESI-MS, m/z: 1253.4328 $[M_{2Na} - Na]^-$ (calcd for $C_{53}H_{82}O_{28}S_2Na^-$, 1253.4337); (−)ESI-MS/MS, m/z: 1133.4 $[M_{2Na} - Na - NaHSO_4]^-$, 957.4 $[M_{2Na} - Na - NaHSO_4 - MeGlc]^-$, 825.4 $[M_{2Na} - Na - NaHSO_4 - MeGlc - Xyl]^-$, 679.3 $[M_{2Na} - Na - NaHSO_4 - MeGlc - Xyl - Qui]^-$, 805.3 $[M_{2Na} - Na - NaSO_3 - C_{21}H_{30}O_4 + H]^-$, 665.2 $[M_{2Na} - Na - NaSO_3 - C_{30}H_{45}O_5]^-$, 533.1 $[M_{2Na} - Na - NaSO_3 - C_{30}H_{45}O_5 - Xyl]^-$, 387.1 $[M_{2Na} - Na - NaSO_3 - C_{30}H_{45}O_5 - Xyl - Qui]^-$, 255 $[M_{2Na} - Na - NaSO_3 - C_{30}H_{45}O_5 - Xyl - Qui - Xyl]^-$.

3.3.8. Magnumoside C_2 (8)

Colorless powder; $[\alpha]_D^{20}$ −64 (*c* 0.1, 50% MeOH); ^{1}H NMR data see Tables 1 and 2; ^{13}C NMR data see Tables 1 and 3; (−)HR-ESI-MS, m/z: 1253.4328 $[M_{2Na} - Na]^-$ (calcd for $C_{53}H_{82}O_{28}S_2Na^-$, 1253.4337); (−)ESI-MS/MS, m/z: 1133.4 $[M_{2Na} - Na - NaHSO_4]^-$, 957.4 $[M_{2Na} - Na - NaHSO_4 - $

MeGlc]$^-$,825.4 [M$_{2Na}$ − Na − NaHSO$_4$ − MeGlc − Xyl]$^-$, 679.3 [M$_{2Na}$ − Na − NaHSO$_4$ −MeGlc − Xyl − Qui]$^-$, 805.3 [M$_{2Na}$ − Na − NaSO$_3$ − C$_{21}$H$_{30}$O$_4$ + H]$^-$, 665.2 [M$_{2Na}$ − Na − NaSO$_3$ − C$_{30}$H$_{45}$O$_5$]$^-$, 533.1 [M$_{2Na}$ − Na − NaSO$_3$ − C$_{30}$H$_{45}$O$_5$ − Xyl]$^-$, 387.1 [M$_{2Na}$ − Na − NaSO$_3$ − C$_{30}$H$_{45}$O$_5$ − Xyl − Qui]$^-$, 255 [M$_{2Na}$ − Na − NaSO$_3$ − C$_{30}$H$_{45}$O$_5$ − Xyl − Qui − Xyl]$^-$.

3.3.9. Magnumoside C$_4$ (9)

Colorless powder. $[\alpha]_D^{20}$ −52 (*c* 0.1, H$_2$O). NMR: See Tables 2 and 3. HR ESI MS (−) *m/z*: 1237.4390 (calc. 1237.4388) [M$_{2Na}$ − Na]$^-$; ESI MS/MS (−) *m/z*: 1135.4 [M$_{2Na}$ − Na − NaSO$_3$ + H]$^-$, 1117.4 [M$_{2Na}$ − Na − NaHSO$_4$]$^-$, 959.4 [M$_{2Na}$ − Na − NaSO$_4$ − MeGlc]$^-$, 827.4 [M$_{2Na}$ − Na − NaSO$_4$ − MeGlc − Xyl]$^-$, 681.3 [M$_{2Na}$ − Na − NaSO$_4$ −MeGlc − Xyl − Qui]$^-$, 665.2 [M$_{2Na}$ − Na − NaSO$_3$ − C$_{30}$H$_{45}$O$_4$]$^-$, 533.1 [M$_{2Na}$ − Na − NaSO$_3$ − C$_{30}$H$_{45}$O$_4$ − Xyl]$^-$, 387.1 [M$_{2Na}$ − Na − NaSO$_3$ − C$_{30}$H$_{45}$O$_4$ − Xyl − Qui]$^-$, 255 [M$_{2Na}$ − Na − NaSO$_3$ − C$_{30}$H$_{45}$O$_4$ − Xyl − Qui − Xyl]$^-$.

3.4. Preparation of the MTPA Esters of Compound 2

Two aliquots (0.6 mg) of compound **2** were treated with (−)-(*R*)- and (+)-(*S*)-α-methoxy-α-(trifluoromethyl)-phenylacetyl (MTPA) chloride (10 μL) in dry C$_5$D$_5$N (600 μL) for 2 h at r.t. in NMR tubes to give corresponding (*S*)- and (*R*)-MTPA esters. Data of 24-(*S*)-MTPA Ester of **2**. ^{1}H NMR (700 MHz): 1.66 (m, 1H of CH$_2$(22)), 1.79 (s, Me(27)), 1.85 (m, 1H of CH$_2$(22)), 2.07 (m, 1H of CH$_2$(23)), 2.23 (m, 1H of CH$_2$(23)), 5.04 (brs, 1H of CH$_2$(26)), 5.24 (brs, 1H of CH$_2$(26)), 5.75 (m, H-C(24)). Data of 24-(*R*)-MTPA Ester of **2**. ^{1}H NMR (700 MHz): 1.67 (s, Me(27)), 1.80 (m, 1H of CH$_2$(22)), 1.98 (m, 1H of CH$_2$(22)), 2.13 (m, 1H of CH$_2$(23)), 2.27 (m, 1H of CH$_2$(23)), 4.99 (brs, 1H of CH$_2$(26)), 5.14 (brs, 1H of CH$_2$(26)), 5.72 (m, H-C(24)).

3.5. Bioassay

3.5.1. Cell Culture

The spleenocytes from CD-1 line mice were used. The spleen was isolated from mice and homogenized. The spleenocytes were washed thrice and resuspended with RPMI-1640 medium contained gentamicine 8 μg/mL (Biolot, Saint Petersburg, Russia). The museum tetraploid strain of murine ascites Ehrlich carcinoma cells from the All-Russian cancer center RAMS (Moscow, Russia) was used. The cells of the ascites Ehrlich carcinoma were separated from ascites, which were collected on day 7 after inoculation in mouse CD-1 line. The cells were washed of ascites thrice and then resuspended in liquid media DMEM with L-Glutamine (Biolot, Saint Petersburg, Russia).

3.5.2. Cytotoxic Activity

The solutions of tested substances in different concentrations (20 μL) and cell suspension (200 μL) were added in wells of 96-well plate and incubated over night at 37 °C and 5% CO$_2$. After incubation the cells were sedimented by centrifugation, 200 μL of medium from each well were collected and 100 μL of pure medium were added. Then 10 μL of MTT solution 5 μg/mL (Sigma, St. Louis, MO, USA) were added in each well. Plate was incubated 4 h, after that 100 μL SDS-HCl were added to each well and plate was incubated at 37 °C 4–18 h. Optical density was measured at 570 nm and 630–690 nm. The activity of the substances was calculated as the ratio of the dead cells to general cells amount (ED$_{50}$). Typicoside A$_1$ [28] and cucumarioside A$_2$-2 [11] were used as positive controls.

3.5.3. Hemolytic Activity

Blood was taken from a CD-1 mouse. The erythrocytes were washed thrice with 0.9% NaCl, centrifuged (450 g) on a centrifuge LABOFUGE 400R (Heraeus, Hanau, Germany) for 5 min followed by re-suspending in phosphate-buffered saline (PBS), pH 7.2–7.4. Erythrocytes were used at a concentration provided an optical density of 1.5 at 700 nm for a non-hemolyzed sample. 20 μL of a water solution of test substance with a fixed concentration (0.12–100.00 μM) were added to a well of a 96-well plate containing 180 mL of the erythrocyte suspension and incubated for 1 h at 37 °C. The plates were centrifuged (900× *g*) on a LMC-3000 laboratory centrifuge (Biosan, Riga, Latvia) for 10 min. 10 µL of the supernatant were placed to special microplate with plate bottom for determination of the optical density on a spectrofotometer *Multiskan FC* at λ = 570 nm. ED$_{50}$ was calculated using SigmaPlot 3.02 software (Jandel Scientific, San Rafael, CA, USA). Triton X-100 (Biolot, Saint Petersburg, Russia) at concentration 1%, caused the hemolysis of 100% cells was used as positive control. The erythrocyte suspension in phosphate-buffered saline, pH 7.2–7.4 (PBS) with 20 µL of the solvent without a tested compound was used as negative control.

3.5.4. DLD-1 Human Colorectal Adenocarcinoma Cell Culture

Human colorectal adenocarcinoma cells DLD-1 were cultured in RPMI-1640 medium. Culture media was supplemented with 10% fetal bovine serum (FBS) and penicillin—streptomycin solution. Cells were maintained in a sterile environment and kept in an incubator at 5% CO$_2$ and 37 °C to promote growth. DLD-1 cells were sub-cultured every 3–4 days by their rinsing with phosphate buffered saline (PBS), adding trypsin to detach the cells from the tissue culture flask, and transferring 10–20% of the harvested cells to a new flask containing fresh growth media.

3.5.5. Cytotoxicity against DLD-1 Cells Assay

DLD-1 cells (1.0×10^4/well) were seeded in 96-well plates for 24 h at 37 °C in 5% CO$_2$ incubator. The cells were treated with the compounds **1–9** at concentrations range from 0 to 100 µM for additional 24 h. Subsequently, cells were incubated with 15 µL MTS reagent for 3 h, and the absorbance of each well was measured at 490/630 nm using microplate reader "Power Wave XS" (Bio Tek, Winooski, VT, USA). All the experiments were repeated three times, and the mean absorbance values were calculated. The results are expressed as the percentage of inhibition that produced a reduction in absorbance by compound's treatment compared to the non-treated cells (control).

3.5.6. Soft Agar Assay

DLD-1 cells (8.0×10^3) were seeded in 6-well plate and treated with the **3, 7–9** (10 µM) in 1 mL of 0.3% Basal Medium Eagle (BME) agar containing 10% FBS, 2 mM L-glutamine, and 25 µg/mL gentamicin. The cultures were maintained at 37 °C in a 5% CO$_2$ incubator for 14 days, and the cell's colonies were scored using a microscope "Motic AE 20" (Scientific Instrument Company, Campbell, CA, USA) and the Motic Image Plus computer program (Scientific Instrument Company, Campbell, CA, USA) [39].

3.5.7. DLD-1 Cell Proliferation Assay

DLD-1 cells (8×10^3) cells were seeded in 96-well plates in 200 mL of RPMI-1640/10%FBS medium at 37 °C in a 5% CO$_2$ incubator for 24 h. Then the cells were treated with 2 µM of **3, 7–9** for additional 24, 48, 72 or 96 h at 37 °C in a 5% CO$_2$ atmosphere. The reaction was terminated by adding MTS reagent to each well as described in the Section 3.5.5.

3.5.8. Radiation Exposure

Irradiation was delivered at room temperature using single doses of X-ray system XPERT 80 (KUB Technologies, Inc, Milford, CT, USA). The doses were from 4 to 8 Gy for colony formation assay. The absorber dose was measured using X-ray radiation clinical dosimeter DRK-1 (Akselbant, Moscow, Russia).

3.5.9. Cell Irradiation

DLD-1 cells (5.0×10^5) were plated at 60 mm dishes and incubated for 24 h. After the incubation, the cells were cultured in the presence or absence of 2 μM **3**, **7–9** for additional 24 h before irradiation at the dose of 4 Gy. Immediately after irradiation, cells were returned to the incubator for recovery. Three hour later, the cells were harvested and used for soft agar assay or proliferation assay to establish the synergism of radioactive irradiation and investigated compounds effects on colony formation or proliferation of tested cells.

3.5.10. Statistical Analysis

All assays were performed in triplicate. The results are expressed as the means ± standard deviation (SD). A Student's *t*-test was used to evaluate the data with the significance level of $p < 0.05$. The mean and standard deviation were calculated and plotted using SigmaPlot 3.02 Software (Jandel Scientific, San Rafael, CA, USA).

4. Conclusions

Summarizing the obtained data, three types of previously known carbohydrate chains, five new aglycones as well as one known aglycone have been found in the isolated glycosides 1–9. Magnumoside A_1 (1) has uncommon non-holostane aglycone with a unique for sea cucumber triterpene glycosides 20(24)-epoxy-25-hydroxy-fragment in the side chain. The biosythesis of the glycosides found in *N. magnum* has mosaic character, i.e., transformation in cyclic systems of aglycones and in their side chains as well as in carbohydrate chains (elongation and sulfation) proceed parallel and independently and they have the characteristics of a biosynthetic network. Disulfated glycosides 7 and 8 showed surprisingly high hemolytic and cytotoxic actions in spite of the presence of hydroxyl-groups in their side chains. The data concerning cytotoxic activities on DLD-1 human colorectal adenocarcinoma cells good correlated with the data on mouse ascites Echrlich carcinoma cells that confirmed the usefulness of the last model tumor for screening of substances that are cytotoxic against human tumor cells. The data concerning synergy of the activities of the glycosides 3 and 7–9 in subcytotoxic doses and subtoxic doses of radiation were obtained for the first time where magnumoside C_4 (9) revealed the highest increase of the inhibitory effect of radiation on cell proliferation of 45%. The substances having such effects allow a decrease in the effective doses of radiation that may be used for radiation therapy of human tumors. The search for substances with a similar mode of action among sea cucumber triterpene glycosides should be continued.

Acknowledgments: The chemical structure and part of bioassay were carried out at partial financial support of the Grant of the Russian Foundation of Basic Research No. 16-04-00010 for partial financial support. The studies of cytotoxic activities on a series of human cancer cell lines and it synergy with radioactive irradiation were supported by the Grant of the Russian Science Foundation No. 16-14-10131. The field work and identification processing of the animal samples were supported by APN (Asia Pacific Network for the Global Change Research) CAF2016-RR08-CMY-Dautova. The authors are very appreciative to Valentin A. Stonik (G.B. Elyakov Pacific Institute of Bioorganic Chemistry of the FEB RAS, Vladivostok, Russia) for reading, checking and discussion of the manuscript.

Author Contributions: Alexandra S. Silchenko and Vladimir I. Kalinin wrote the paper. Aleksandra S. Silchenko, Sergey A. Avilov conceived, designed and performed the experiments concerning isolation of the glycosides. Pelageya V. Andrijaschenko carried out some procedures of glycosides isolation. Anatoly I. Kalinovsky obtained and analyzed the NMR data. Alexandra S. Silchenko analyzed the NMR data. Pavel S. Dmitrenok performed the mass-spectrometry experiments and analyzed their results; Ekaterina A. Chingizova performed the bioassays; Olesya S. Malyarenko and Svetlana P. Ermakova performed the bioassays on DLD-1 cells; Tatiana N. Dautova collected and identified the animal material.

Conflicts of Interest: The authors declare no conflict of interest.

References

1. Stonik, V.A.; Kalinin, V.I.; Avilov, S.A. Toxins from the sea cucumbers (Holothuroids): Chemical structures, properties, taxonomic distribution, biosynthesis and evolution. *J. Nat. Toxins* **1999**, *8*, 235–248. [PubMed]
2. Kalinin, V.I.; Silchenko, A.S.; Avilov, S.A.; Stonik, V.A.; Smirnov, A.V. Sea cucumbers triterpene glycosides, the recent progress in structural elucidation and chemotaxonomy. *Phytochem. Rev.* **2005**, *4*, 221–236. [CrossRef]
3. Bahrami, Y.; Franko, C.M.M. Acetylated triterpene glycosides and their biological activity from Holothurioidea reported in the past six decades. *Mar. Drugs* **2016**, *14*, 147. [CrossRef] [PubMed]
4. Kalinin, V.I.; Avilov, S.A.; Silchenko, A.S.; Stonik, V.A. Triterpene glycosides of sea cucumbers (Holothuroidea, Echinodermata) as taxonomic markers. *Nat. Prod. Commun.* **2015**, *10*, 21–26. [PubMed]
5. Kalinin, V.I.; Silchenko, A.S.; Avilov, S.A. Taxonomic significance and ecological role of triterpene glycosides from Holothurians. *Biol. Bull.* **2016**, *43*, 532–540. [CrossRef]
6. Honey-Escandon, M.; Arreguin-Espinosa, R.; Solis-Martin, F.A.; Samyn, Y. Biological and taxonomic perspective of triterpenoid glycosides of sea cucumbers of the family Holothuriidae (Echinodermata, Holothuroidea). *Comp. Biochem. Physiol.* **2015**, *180B*, 16–39. [CrossRef] [PubMed]
7. Kalinin, V.I.; Aminin, D.L.; Avilov, S.A.; Silchenko, A.S.; Stonik, V.A. Triterpene glycosides from sea cucumbers (Holothurioidae, Echinodermata), biological activities and functions. In *Studies in Natural Product Chemistry (Bioactive Natural Products)*; Atta-ur-Rahman, Ed.; Elsevier Science Publisher: Amsterdam, The Netherlands, 2008; Volume 35, pp. 135–196.
8. Kim, S.K.; Himaya, S.W.A. Triterpene glycosides from sea cucucmbers and their biological activities. *Adv. Food Nutr. Res.* **2012**, *63*, 297–319.
9. Aminin, D.L.; Pislyagin, E.A.; Menchinskaya, E.S.; Silchenko, A.S.; Avilov, S.A.; Kalinin, V.I. Immunomodulatory and anticancer activity of sea cucumber triterpene glycosides. In *Studies in Natural Products Chemistry (Bioactive Natural Products)*; Atta-ur-Rahman, Ed.; Elsevier Science Publisher: Amsterdam, The Netherlands, 2014; Volume 41, pp. 75–94.
10. Careaga, V.P.; Maier, M.S. Cytotoxic triterpene glycosides from sea cucumbers. In *Handbook of Anticancer Drugs from Marine Origin*; Kim, S.-K., Ed.; Springer International Publishing: Cham, Switzerland, 2015; pp. 515–528.
11. Aminin, D.L.; Menchinskaya, E.S.; Pislyagin, E.A.; Silchenko, A.S.; Avilov, S.A.; Kalinin, V.I. Anticancer activity of sea cucumber triterpene glycosides. *Mar. Drugs* **2015**, *13*, 1202–1223. [CrossRef] [PubMed]
12. Janakiram, N.B.; Mohammed, A.; Rao, C. Sea cucumbers metabolites as potent anti-cancer agents. *Mar. Drugs* **2015**, *13*, 2909–2923. [CrossRef] [PubMed]
13. Fedorov, S.N.; Dyshlovoy, S.A.; Kuzmich, A.S.; Shubina, L.K.; Avilov, S.A.; Silchenko, A.S.; Bode, A.M.; Dong, Z.; Stonik, V.A. In vitro anticancer activities of some triterpene glycosides from holothurians of Cucumariidae, Stichopodidae, Psolidae, Holothuriidae and Synaptidae families. *Nat. Prod. Commun.* **2016**, *11*, 1239–1242.
14. Aminin, D.L.; Menchinskaya, E.S.; Pisliagin, E.A.; Silchenko, A.S.; Avilov, S.A.; Kalinin, V.I. Sea cucumber triterpene glycosides as anticancer agents. In *Studies in Natural Products Chemistry*; Atta-ur-Rahman, Ed.; Elsevier Science Publisher: Amsterdam, The Netherlands, 2016; Volume 49, pp. 55–105.
15. Zurita, M.B.; Ahond, A.; Poupat, C.; Potier, P. Invertebres marins du lagon Neo-Caledonien, VII. Etude structurale d'un nouveau saponoside sulfate extrait de l'holothurie *Neothyonidium magnum*. *J. Nat. Prod.* **1986**, *49*, 809–813. [CrossRef]
16. Avilov, S.A.; Kalinovskii, A.I.; Stonik, V.A. New triterpene glycoside from the holothurian *Neothyonidium magnum*. *Chem. Nat. Comp.* **1990**, *26*, 42–45. [CrossRef]
17. Silchenko, A.S.; Kalinovsky, A.I.; Avilov, S.A.; Andryjaschenko, P.V.; Dmitrenok, P.S.; Kalinin, V.I.; Yurchenko, E.A.; Dolmatov, I.Y. Colochirosides B_1, B_2, B_3 and C, novel sulfated triterpene glycosides from the sea cucumber *Colochirus robustus* (Cucumariidae, Dendrochirotida). *Nat. Prod. Commun.* **2015**, *10*, 1687–1694. [PubMed]
18. Silchenko, A.S.; Stonik, V.A.; Avilov, S.A.; Kalinin, V.I.; Kalinovsky, A.I.; Zaharenko, A.M.; Smirnov, A.V.; Mollo, E.; Cimino, G. Holothurins B_2, B_3 and B_4, New triterpene glycosides from Mediteranean sea cucumbers of the genus *Holothuria*. *J. Nat. Prod.* **2005**, *68*, 564–567. [CrossRef] [PubMed]
19. Zhang, S.L.; Li, L.; Sun, P.; Yi, Y.H. Lecanorosides A and B, two new triterpene glycosides from the sea cucumber *Actinopyga lecanora*. *J. Asian Nat. Prod. Res.* **2008**, *10*, 1097–1103. [CrossRef] [PubMed]

20. Han, H.; Zhang, W.; Liu, B.-S.; Pan, M.-X.; Wang, X.-H. A novel sulfated holostane glycoside from sea cucumber *Holothuria leucospilota*. *Chem. Biodivers.* **2010**, *7*, 1764–1769. [CrossRef] [PubMed]
21. Kalinin, V.I.; Kalinovskii, A.I.; Stonik, V.A. Onekotanogenin—A new triterpene genin from the holothurian *Psolus fabricii*. *Chem. Nat. Comp.* **1987**, *23*, 560–563. [CrossRef]
22. Silchenko, A.S.; Kalinovsky, A.I.; Avilov, S.A.; Andryjaschenko, P.V.; Dmitrenok, P.S.; Yurchenko, E.A.; Dolmatov, I.Y.; Dautov, S.S.; Stonik, V.A.; Kalinin, V.I. Colochiroside E, an usual non-holostane triterpene sulfated trioside from the sea cucumber *Colochirus robustus* and evidence of the impossibility of a 7(8)-double bond migration in lanostane derivatives having an 18(16)-lactone. *Nat. Prod. Commun.* **2016**, *11*, 741–746. [PubMed]
23. Ilyin, S.G.; Reshetnyak, M.V.; Afiyatullov, S.S.; Stonik, V.A.; Elyakov, G.B. The crystal and molecular structure of diacetate of holost-8(9)-en-3α,16β-diol. *Rep. USSR Acad. Sci.* **1985**, *284*, 356–359.
24. Ilyin, S.G.; Sharypov, V.F.; Stonik, V.A.; Antipin, M.Y.; Struchkov, Y.T.; Elyakov, G.B. The crystal and molecular structure of (23S)-acetoxy-9β-holost-7-en-3β-ol and stereochemical peculiarities of the double bond migration from 7(8) to 8(9) and 9(11)-positions in holostane-type triterpenoids. *Bioorg. Chem.* **1991**, *17*, 1123–1128.
25. Kalinovsky, A.I.; Silchenko, A.S.; Avilov, S.A.; Kalinin, V.I. The assignment of the absolute configuration of C-22 chiral center in the aglycones of triterpene glycosides from the sea cucumber *Cladolabes schmeltzii* and chemical transformations of cladoloside C. *Nat. Prod. Commun.* **2015**, *10*, 1167–1170. [PubMed]
26. Silchenko, A.S.; Kalinovsky, A.I.; Avilov, S.A.; Andryjaschenko, P.V.; Dmitrenok, P.S.; Kalinin, V.I.; Yurchenko, E.A.; Dolmatov, I.Y. Colochirosides A_1, A_2, A_3 and D, four novel sulfated triterpene glycosides from the sea cucumber *Colochirus robustus* (Cucumariidae, Dendrochirotida). *Nat. Prod. Commun.* **2016**, *11*, 381–387. [PubMed]
27. Silchenko, A.S.; Kalinovsky, A.I.; Avilov, S.A.; Andryjaschenko, P.V.; Dmitrenok, P.S.; Kalinin, V.I.; Yurchenko, E.A.; Dautov, S.S. Structures of violaceusosides C, D, E and G, sulfated triterpene glycosides from the sea cucumber *Pseudocolochirus violaceus* (Cucumariidae, Denrochirotida). *Nat. Prod. Commun.* **2014**, *9*, 391–399. [PubMed]
28. Silchenko, A.S.; Kalinovsky, A.I.; Avilov, S.A.; Andryjaschenko, P.V.; Dmitrenok, P.S.; Martyyas, E.A.; Kalinin, V.I.; Jayasandhya, P.; Rajan, G.C.; Padmakumar, K.P. Structures and biological activities of typicosides A_1, A_2, B_1, C_1 and C_2, triterpene glycosides from the sea cucumbers *Actinocucumis typica*. *Nat. Prod. Commun.* **2013**, *8*, 301–310. [PubMed]
29. Zou, Z.R.; Yi, Y.H.; Xu, Q.Z.; Wu, H.M.; Lin, H.W. A new disulfated triterpene glycoside from the sea cucumber *Mensamaria intercedens* Lampert. *Chin. Chem. Lett.* **2003**, *14*, 585–587.
30. Zhang, S.-Y.; Yi, Y.-H.; Tang, H.-F. Cytotoxic sulfated triterpene glycosides from the sea cucmber *Pseudocolochirus violaceus*. *Chem. Biodivers.* **2006**, *3*, 807–817. [CrossRef] [PubMed]
31. Avilov, S.A.; Kalinin, V.I.; Makarieva, T.N.; Stonik, V.A.; Kalinovskii, A.I. Structure of Cucumarioside G_2, a novel nonholostane glycoside from the sea cucumber *Eupentacta fraudatrix*. *J. Nat. Prod.* **1994**, *57*, 1166–1171. [CrossRef] [PubMed]
32. Silchenko, A.S.; Kalinovsky, A.I.; Avilov, S.A.; Andryjaschenko, P.V.; Dmitrenok, P.S.; Yurchenko, E.A.; Kalinin, V.I. Structures and cytotoxic properties of cucumariosides H_2, H_3 and H_4 from the sea cucumber *Eupentacta fraudatrix*. *Nat. Prod. Res.* **2012**, *26*, 1765–1774. [CrossRef] [PubMed]
33. Silchenko, A.S.; Kalinovsky, A.I.; Avilov, S.A.; Andryjaschenko, P.V.; Dmitrenok, P.S.; Martyyas, E.A.; Kalinin, V.I. Triterpene glycosides from the sea cucumber *Eupentacta fraudatrix*. Structure and cytotoxic action of cucumariosides A_2, A_7, A_9, A_{10}, A_{11}, A_{13} and A_{14}, seven new minor non-sulated tetraosides and an aglycone with an uncommon 18-hydroxy group. *Nat. Prod. Commun.* **2012**, *7*, 845–852. [PubMed]
34. Avilov, S.A.; Antonov, A.S.; Drozdova, O.A.; Kalinin, V.I.; Kalinovsky, A.I.; Stonik, V.A.; Riguera, R.; Lenis, L.A.; Jimenez, C. Triterpene glycosides from the Far-Eastern sea cucumber *Pentamera calcigera*. 1. Monosulfated glycosides and cytotoxicity of their unsulfated derivatives. *J. Nat. Prod.* **2000**, *63*, 65–71. [CrossRef] [PubMed]
35. Kalinin, V.I.; Kalinivskii, A.I.; Stonik, V.A. Psolusoside A—The main triterpene glycoside from the holothurian *Psolus fabricii*. *Chem. Nat. Compd.* **1985**, *21*, 197–202. [CrossRef]
36. Kalinin, V.I.; Kalinovskii, A.I.; Stonik, V.A.; Dmitrenok, P.S.; El'kin, Y.N. Structure of psolusoside B—A nonholostane triterpene glycoside of the holothurian genus *Psolus*. *Chem. Nat. Compd.* **1989**, *25*, 311–317. [CrossRef]

37. Silchenko, A.S.; Kalinovsky, A.I.; Avilov, S.A.; Andryjashenko, P.V.; Dmitrenok, P.S.; Kalinin, V.I.; Stonik, V.A. 3β-O-Glycosylated 16β-acetoxy-9β-H-lanosta-7,24-diene-3β,18,20β-triol, an intermediate metabolite from the sea cucumber *Eupentacta fraudatrix* and its biosynthetic significance. *Biochem. Syst. Ecol.* **2012**, *44*, 53–60. [CrossRef]

38. Wang, L.; Li, X.; Song, Y.M.; Wang, B.; Zhang, F.R.; Yang, R.; Wang, H.Q.; Zhang, G.J. Ginsenoside Rg3 sensitizes human non-small cell lung cancer cells to γ-radiation by targeting the nuclear factor-κB pathway. *Mol. Med. Rep.* **2015**, *12*, 609–614. [CrossRef] [PubMed]

39. Vishchuk, O.S.; Ermakova, S.P.; Zvyagintseva, T.N. The fucoidans from brown algae of Far-Eastern seas: Anti-tumor activity and structure-function relationship. *Food Chem.* **2013**, *141*, 1211–1217. [CrossRef] [PubMed]

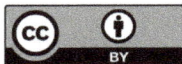

© 2017 by the authors. Licensee MDPI, Basel, Switzerland. This article is an open access article distributed under the terms and conditions of the Creative Commons Attribution (CC BY) license (http://creativecommons.org/licenses/by/4.0/).

marine drugs

MDPI

Article

Metabolite Profiling of Triterpene Glycosides of the Far Eastern Sea Cucumber *Eupentacta fraudatrix* and Their Distribution in Various Body Components Using LC-ESI QTOF-MS

Roman S. Popov [1], Natalia V. Ivanchina [1], Alexandra S. Silchenko [1], Sergey A. Avilov [1], Vladimir I. Kalinin [1], Igor Yu. Dolmatov [2,3], Valentin A. Stonik [1,3] and Pavel S. Dmitrenok [1,*]

[1] G.B. Elyakov Pacific Institute of Bioorganic Chemistry, Far Eastern Branch of Russian Academy of Sciences, 159 Prospect 100-letiya Vladivostoka, Vladivostok 690022, Russia; prs_90@mail.ru (R.S.P.); ivanchina@piboc.dvo.ru (N.V.I.); sialexandra@mail.ru (A.S.S.); avilov-1957@mail.ru (S.A.A.); kalininv@piboc.dvo.ru (V.I.K.); stonik@piboc.dvo.ru (V.A.S.)

[2] A.V. Zhirmunsky Institute of Marine Biology, National Scientific Center of Marine Biology, Far Eastern Branch of the Russian Academy of Sciences, 17 Palchevskogo St., Vladivostok 690041, Russia; idolmatov@mail.ru

[3] School of Natural Science, Far Eastern Federal University, 8 Sukhanova St., Vladivostok 690090, Russia

* Correspondence: paveldmt@piboc.dvo.ru; Tel.: +7-423-231-1132

Received: 18 August 2017; Accepted: 30 September 2017; Published: 2 October 2017

Abstract: The Far Eastern sea cucumber *Eupentacta fraudatrix* is an inhabitant of shallow waters of the south part of the Sea of Japan. This animal is an interesting and rich source of triterpene glycosides with unique chemical structures and various biological activities. The objective of this study was to investigate composition and distribution in various body components of triterpene glycosides of the sea cucumber *E. fraudatrix*. We applied LC-ESI MS (liquid chromatography–electrospray mass spectrometry) of whole body extract and extracts of various body components for metabolic profiling and structure elucidation of triterpene glycosides from the *E. fraudatrix*. Totally, 54 compounds, including 26 sulfated, 18 non-sulfated and 10 disulfated glycosides were detected and described. Triterpene glycosides from the body walls, gonads, aquapharyngeal bulbs, guts and respiratory trees were extracted separately and the distributions of the detected compounds in various body components were analyzed. Series of new glycosides with unusual structural features were described in *E. fraudatrix*, which allow clarifying the biosynthesis of these compounds. Comparison of the triterpene glycosides contents from the five different body components revealed that the profiles of triterpene glycosides were qualitatively similar, and only some quantitative variabilities for minor compounds were observed.

Keywords: sea cucumber; *Eupentacta fraudatrix*; triterpene glycoside; liquid chromatography–tandem mass spectrometry; metabolite profiling

---

1. Introduction

Sea cucumbers (Class Holothuroidea, Phylum Echinodermata) are widespread slow-moving marine animals. Metabolome of these animals is characterized by the high content of triterpene glycosides of a great structural diversity. Triterpene glycosides of sea cucumbers have unique chemical structures, significantly differing from those of terrestrial plants. These compounds possess a variety of biological and pharmacological effects including cytotoxic [1,2], antifungal [3,4], bactericidal, hemolytic, antiviral and antiparasitic properties [5]. Some glycosides are capable to induce apoptosis, inhibit the growth of tumor cells [6] and have immunomodulatory properties [7]. In addition, certain species of sea cucumbers are a valuable maricultural resource [8].

Majority of triterpene glycosides from sea cucumbers possess a lanostane-type aglycone with an 18(20)-lactone called as holostane derivatives. Individual triterpene aglycones differ from each other in the number and arrangement of oxygen substituents, double bonds and in the structure of the side chains demonstrating a significant natural diversity. Some triterpene glycosides have aglycones with 18(16)-lactone or without a lactone cycle. Usually, triterpene glycosides have a polycyclic nucleus with 7(8)- or 9(11)-double bond and oxygen-containing substituents, which may be bonded to C-12, C-17 or C-16. The side chains of aglycones may have one or more double bonds, hydroxyl or acetate groups and other substituents. Some glycosides have aglycones with shortened side chains.

The oligosaccharide chain of triterpene glycosides is attached to C-3 of the aglycone and may include up to six sugar units. Oligosaccharide chains with up to four monosaccharide units usually have a linear structure, while the penta- and hexaosides contain a branching at the first or second monosaccharide unit. Xylose (Xyl), glucose (Glc), quinovose (Qui), 3-O-methylglucose (MeGlc), and, rarely, 3-O-methylxylose (MeXyl) are the most common sugar residues in triterpene glycosides. The first unit in oligosaccharide chain is always xylose, quinovose (rarely glucose or xylose) is usually the second monosaccharide unit and glucose (or xylose) is the third [1,4]. The methylated monosaccharides always occupy the terminal position. Many glycosides have up to three sulfate groups at certain positions of the oligosaccharide chain.

It is supposed that triterpene glycosides have multiple defensive roles such as defense against predators, parasites and microorganisms. Indeed, a high percentage of these compounds in the Cuvierian tubules, that can be ejected toward a predator as well as their strong ichthyotoxic and membranolytic effects indicate their effective action against predators [9,10]. In addition, it is likely that glycosides play an important role in regulating the reproduction of sea cucumbers [11].

Triterpene glycosides display taxonomic specificity for different systematic groups of sea cucumbers. The level of this specificity may be different in various sea cucumbers taxa. The glycoside structures are specific for one genus or a group of genera for the sea cucumbers of the order Aspidochirotida. However, these compounds are usually species-specific for the representatives of the order Dendrochirotida [12].

Triterpene glycosides are usually present in extracts of sea cucumbers as complex mixtures. Minor compounds of these extracts remain largely unstudied, although knowledge about their chemical structures is also important for understanding of biosynthesis and biological roles of these compounds. Recent investigations have demonstrated the power of MS approaches for profiling and for studying of the body distribution of sea cucumber triterpene glycosides [13,14]. All sea cucumbers contain triterpene glycosides in their body walls and viscera; however, recent studies have demonstrated difference in content of these metabolites in the Cuvierian tubules and in the body wall. All the glycosides, detected in the body walls of *Holothuria forskali* were found to be also present in the Cuvierian tubules but the latter also contain specific congeners. Furthermore, profiles of triterpene glycosides in both analyzed body parts varied under stress condition [9,10,15].

The sea cucumber *Eupentacta fraudatrix* (Djakonov et Baranova) (=*Cucumaria fraudatrix* Djakonov et Baranova = *Cucumaria obunca* Lampert) (Family Sclerodactylidae, Order Dendrochirotida) is a common species in the shallow waters of the south part of the Sea of Japan and is a rich source of triterpene glycosides. *E. fraudatrix* is a well-studied species that is often used as a model organism in biological studies of various processes such as development [16,17], regeneration [18–20] and immunity [21–23]. The previous investigations of the sea cucumber *E. fraudatrix* have led to isolation of 37 triterpene glycosides comprising 15 non-sulfated tetraosides (cucumariosides A_1–A_{15} [24–26]), two non-sulfated triosides (cucumariosides B_1 and B_2 [27]), two non-sulfated pentaosides (cucumariosides C_1 and C_2 [28]), 4 sulfated tetraosides (cucumariosides G_1–G_4 [29–32]), eight sulfated pentaosides (cucumariosides H, H_2–H_8 [33–35]), two disulfated tetraosides (cucumariosides F_1 and F_2 [36]), and four disulfated pentaosides (cucumariosides I_1–I_4 [37,38]). The majority of the glycosides from

E. fraudatrix are characterized by the presence of 3-*O*-MeXyl residue as terminal unit in carbohydrate chain, which is considered a chemotaxonomic marker of the genus *Eupentacta*. Herein, we describe the application of LC-ESI MS for metabolic profiling, evaluation of the structural variability, structure elucidation and further refinement of known biosynthetic patterns of triterpene glycosides from the sea cucumber *E. fraudatrix*. In addition, triterpene glycosides from the body walls, gonads, aquapharyngeal bulbs, guts and respiratory trees were extracted separately and distribution of the detected compounds in various body components were analyzed.

2. Results and Discussion

2.1. Profiling and Structural Identification of the Triterpene Glycosides from E. fraudatrix

Profiling of triterpene glycosides from the whole body extract of the sea cucumber *E. fraudatrix* using LC-MS approach allowed numerous new as well as previously isolated triterpene glycosides to be characterized. The HPLC profile revealed at least 54 compounds, including 26 sulfated, 18 non-sulfated and 10 disulfated glycosides (Figures 1 and 2; Table 1; Figure S1; the numbers of the compounds correspond to the peak numbers on (−)LC-MS chromatogram).

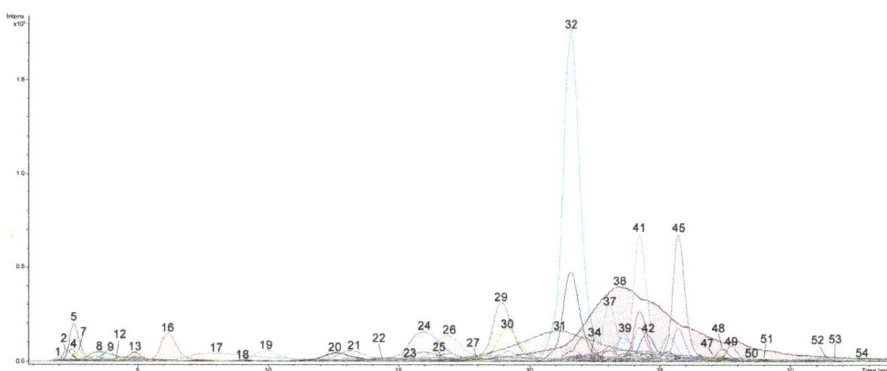

Figure 1. LC-ESI MS (liquid chromatography–electrospray mass spectrometry) total compounds chromatogram of detected triterpene glycosides in negative ion mode (sulfated, disulfated and non-sulfated glycosides were detected as $[M - Na]^-$, $[M - 2Na]^{2-}$ and $[M - H]^-$ ions) in ethanol extract of sea cucumber *Eupentacta fraudatrix*.

In positive ion mode, the majority of triterpene glycosides were detected within m/z range from 1000 to 1400 a.m.u. as $[M + Na]^+$ ions. However, stable peaks of $[M + Na]^+$ ions for disulfated glycosides were not observed in these conditions. In negative ion mode, sulfated and disulfated glycosides were detected as $[M - Na]^-$ and $[M - 2Na]^{2-}$ peaks, respectively, whereas non-sulfated compounds were detected as $[M - H]^-$ peaks.

The assignments of these compounds in all samples analyzed were based on the data of high resolution LC-MS and LC-MS/MS performed in both negative and positive ion modes. Elemental composition, determined on the base of high resolution data (mass accuracy tolerance < 2 ppm), fragmentation patterns of MS and MS/MS spectra, as well as chromatographic behavior of the corresponding compounds, allowed their structures to be proposed. It is known that triterpene glycosides are characterized by large structural variability. Generally, mass spectrometry does not permit to determine configuration of the unknown compounds. Besides, different epimeric monosaccharides as well as types of bonds between sugars cannot be strictly distinguished only by MS. However, the combination of the obtained data and biosynthetic considerations allows tentative structural assignments for the detected compounds.

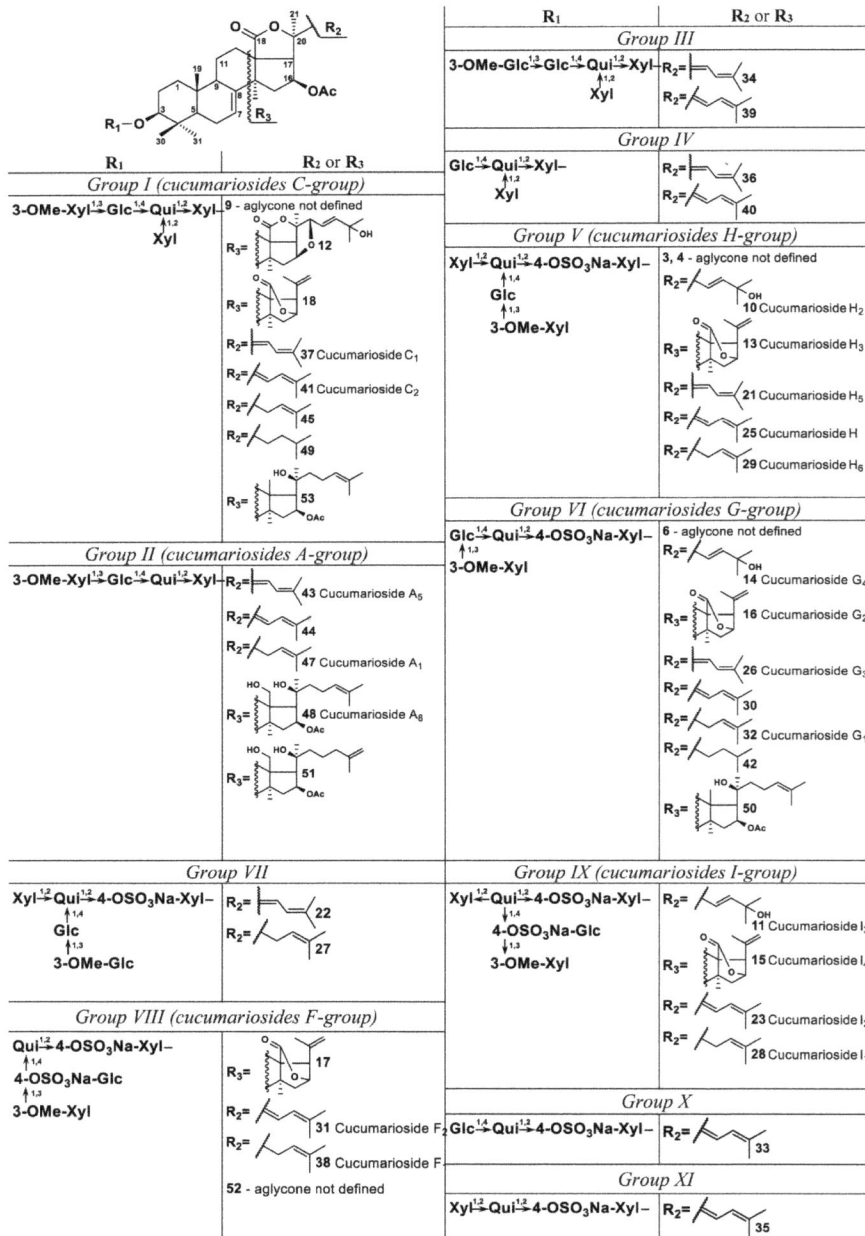

Figure 2. Structures of triterpene glycosides identified (**10**, **11**, **13**, **14**, **15**, **16**, **21**, **23**, **25**, **26**, **28**, **29**, **31**, **32**, **37**, **38**, **41**, **43**, **47**, and **48**) and proposed (**12**, **17**, **18**, **22**, **27**, **30**, **33**, **34**, **35**, **36**, **39**, **40**, **42**, **44**, **45**, **49**, **50**, **51**, and **53**) from the sea cucumber *E. fraudatrix* by LC–MS/MS method.

Table 1. Triterpene glycosides of the ethanol extract of the sea cucumber *E. fraudatrix* detected by LC-ESI MS and their concentrations in different organs.

No. [a]	R_t (min) [a]	Elemental Composition [b]	Measured m/z	Molecular Ion Type	Calculated m/z	Δ (ppm)	BW	GN	G	AB	RT	Identification (ChemSpider ID)
1	2.0	$C_{53}H_{85}O_{28}SNa$	1199.4788	$[M-Na]^-$	1199.4797	0.8	1.28	2.07	0.74	4.41	5.06	
2	2.3	$C_{58}H_{91}O_{31}SNa$	1315.5265	$[M-Na]^-$	1315.5271	0.4	2.06	3.89	2.02	10.76	12.19	
3	2.4	$C_{60}H_{93}O_{31}SNa$	1341.5430	$[M-Na]^-$	1341.5427	−0.2	0.58	3.02	0.51	2.15	1.98	
4	2.5	$C_{57}H_{85}O_{30}SNa$	1281.4854	$[M-Na]^-$	1281.4852	−0.2	3.12	7.12	2.21	11.88	16.15	
5	2.6	$C_{53}H_{85}O_{27}SNa$	1183.4848	$[M-Na]^-$	1183.4848	0.0	8.51	12.85	6.27	33.07	39.82	
6	2.7	$C_{55}H_{89}O_{27}SNa$	1209.4998	$[M-Na]^-$	1209.5004	0.5	0.89	4.65	0.61	2.50	2.50	
7	2.8	$C_{52}H_{77}O_{26}SNa$	1149.4426	$[M-Na]^-$	1149.4429	0.3	2.30	7.72	2.00	10.60	12.71	
8	3.5	$C_{53}H_{82}O_{30}S_2Na_2$	631.2170	$[M-2Na]^{2-}$	631.2172	0.3	7.23	13.08	5.68	26.16	27.96	
9	3.8	$C_{57}H_{86}O_{27}$	1201.5275	$[M-H]^-$	1201.5284	0.7	19.90	63.76	21.23	82.84	132.97	
10	4.0	$C_{60}H_{93}O_{30}SNa$	1325.5472	$[M-Na]^-$	1325.5478	0.4	2.05	3.45	2.13	3.96	3.21	Cucumarioside H2 * (ID29215132)
11	4.3	$C_{60}H_{92}O_{33}S_2Na_2$	702.2493	$[M-2Na]^{2-}$	702.2487	−0.9	5.40	5.53	5.24	4.21	3.49	Cucumarioside I3 * (ID30771157)
12	4.3	$C_{58}H_{90}O_{26}$	1201.5634	$[M-H]^-$	1201.5648	1.1	5.98	66.99	3.88	12.14	17.24	
13	5.0	$C_{53}H_{81}O_{27}SNa$	1181.4692	$[M-Na]^-$	1181.4691	0.0	67.31	65.70	56.11	38.44	22.47	Cucumarioside H3 * (ID29215133)
14	5.0	$C_{55}H_{85}O_{26}SNa$	1193.5051	$[M-Na]^-$	1193.5055	0.4	45.93	45.05	51.93	44.31	42.30	Cucumarioside G4 ** (ID29216498)
15	5.0	$C_{53}H_{90}O_{30}S_2Na_2$	630.2098	$[M-2Na]^{2-}$	630.2093	−0.7	31.18	68.95	44.00	19.20	11.98	Cucumarioside I4 * (ID30771158)
16	6.2	$C_{48}H_{73}O_{23}SNa$	1049.4268	$[M-Na]^-$	1049.4269	0.1	182.20	258.47	199.67	104.16	78.53	Cucumarioside G2 ** (ID16737749)
17	7.7	$C_{48}H_{72}O_{26}S_2Na_2$	564.1882	$[M-2Na]^{2-}$	564.1882	0.0	164.93	533.31	233.14	86.44	85.75	
18	9.1	$C_{53}H_{82}O_{24}$	1101.5126	$[M-H]^-$	1101.5123	−0.2	95.81	79.93	94.56	92.03	77.07	
19	9.9	$C_{60}H_{96}O_{31}SNa$	1367.5580	$[M-Na]^-$	1367.5584	0.3	131.88	158.75	151.50	88.37	59.04	
20	12.4	$C_{57}H_{87}O_{27}SNa$	1235.5156	$[M-Na]^-$	1235.5161	0.4	87.55	123.77	115.97	76.27	67.76	
21	13.0	$C_{60}H_{91}O_{29}SNa$	1307.5369	$[M-Na]^-$	1307.5372	0.2	102.46	101.10	101.29	75.06	56.43	Cucumarioside H5 * (ID29212282)
22	14.4	$C_{61}H_{90}O_{30}SNa$	1337.5472	$[M-Na]^-$	1337.5478	0.4	39.15	33.91	27.47	30.81	26.60	
23	14.5	$C_{60}H_{90}O_{32}S_2Na_2$	693.2437	$[M-2Na]^{2-}$	693.2434	−0.5	132.94	144.25	135.53	117.55	79.00	Cucumarioside I2 *
24	15.6	$C_{57}H_{86}O_{32}S_2Na_2$	657.2330	$[M-2Na]^{2-}$	657.2328	−0.3	164.12	260.64	225.03	129.11	119.00	
25	15.7	$C_{60}H_{91}O_{29}SNa$	1307.5370	$[M-Na]^-$	1307.5372	0.2	355.92	300.10	325.16	257.61	205.87	Cucumarioside H **
26	16.8	$C_{58}H_{83}O_{25}SNa$	1175.4946	$[M-Na]^-$	1175.4950	0.3	157.60	196.62	189.16	161.61	191.52	Cucumarioside G3 ** (ID29213085)
27	17.8	$C_{61}H_{95}O_{30}SNa$	1339.5629	$[M-Na]^-$	1339.5634	0.4	24.08	25.54	25.95	22.53	24.23	
28	18.1	$C_{60}H_{92}O_{32}S_2Na_2$	694.2512	$[M-2Na]^{2-}$	694.2512	0.3	188.33	207.58	222.25	202.43	149.95	Cucumarioside I1 * (ID30771156)
29	19.0	$C_{60}H_{90}O_{29}SNa$	1309.5524	$[M-Na]^-$	1309.5529	0.4	349.25	387.00	349.37	310.11	243.40	Cucumarioside H6 ** (ID29212283)
30	19.1	$C_{58}H_{83}O_{25}SNa$	1175.4946	$[M-Na]^-$	1175.4950	0.3	196.05	245.41	225.43	159.63	183.33	
31	20.8	$C_{55}H_{82}O_{28}S_2Na_2$	627.2223	$[M-2Na]^{2-}$	627.2223	−0.1	650.73	1465.87	1013.44	492.83	518.87	Cucumarioside F2 * (ID34981778)
32	21.5	$C_{55}H_{85}O_{25}SNa$	1177.5101	$[M-Na]^-$	1177.5106	0.4	1399.21	990.35	1149.58	1114.02	1446.29	Cucumarioside G1 ** (ID29212825)
33	21.8	$C_{49}H_{73}O_{21}SNa$	1029.4364	$[M-Na]^-$	1029.4371	0.6	3.49	4.46	4.22	3.38	2.41	
34	22.4	$C_{61}H_{94}O_{27}$	1257.5905	$[M-H]^-$	1257.5910	0.4	353.39	277.23	270.44	373.37	400.82	
35	22.4	$C_{48}H_{71}O_{20}SNa$	999.4257	$[M-Na]^-$	999.4265	0.8	4.00	4.03	4.08	3.80	3.78	
36	22.5	$C_{54}H_{82}O_{22}$	1081.5224	$[M-H]^-$	1081.5225	0.1	20.68	29.78	40.22	19.97	12.52	
37	23.1	$C_{60}H_{92}O_{26}$	1227.5799	$[M-H]^-$	1227.5804	0.4	2304.76	1883.92	1982.79	2465.98	2218.90	Cucumarioside C1 **
38	23.2	$C_{55}H_{84}O_{28}S_2Na_2$	628.2301	$[M-2Na]^{2-}$	628.2301	0.0	1397.27	1896.52	1889.40	1520.29	1581.81	Cucumarioside F1 * (ID34981780)
39	23.6	$C_{61}H_{94}O_{27}$	1257.5907	$[M-H]^-$	1257.5910	0.2	1232.75	844.94	836.78	1248.59	1121.92	
40	23.8	$C_{54}H_{82}O_{22}$	1081.5221	$[M-H]^-$	1081.5225	0.4	78.61	99.33	141.63	60.09	38.25	

Content of Detected Compounds in Different Organs (μg/g) [c]

Table 1. Cont.

No.[a]	Rt (min)	Elemental Composition [b]	Measured m/z	Calculated m/z	Molecular Ion Type	Δ (ppm)	Content of Detected Compounds in Different Organs (μg/g)[c]					Identification (ChemSpider ID)
							BW	GN	G	AB	RT	
41	24.2	$C_{60}H_{92}O_{26}$	1227.5796	1227.5804	[M − H]⁻	0.7	5042.17	3983.86	4978.07	4965.12	4323.97	Cucumarioside C_2 **
42	24.5	$C_{55}H_{87}O_{25}SNa$	1179.5253	1179.5263	[M − Na]⁻	0.8	107.49	63.87	80.66	86.34	113.97	
43	24.6	$C_{55}H_{86}O_{22}$	1095.5380	1095.5381	[M − H]⁻	0.1	30.86	30.40	35.66	40.90	55.20	Cucumarioside A_5 ** (ID29214535)
44	25.6	$C_{55}H_{84}O_{22}$	1095.5379	1095.5381	[M − H]⁻	0.2	12.26	15.38	19.73	17.26	25.04	
45	25.7	$C_{60}H_{94}O_{26}$	1229.5956	1229.5961	[M − H]⁻	0.4	3169.77	3565.18	3696.87	4227.02	3920.64	
46	26.6	$C_{47}H_{75}O_{18}SNa$	959.4674	959.4680	[M − Na]⁻	0.6	4.31	5.66	5.78	4.76	6.27	
47	27.1	$C_{55}H_{86}O_{22}$	1097.5534	1097.5538	[M − H]⁻	0.4	128.12	114.38	137.12	144.01	155.36	Cucumarioside A_1 * (ID29214532)
48	27.5	$C_{55}H_{90}O_{22}$	1101.5851	1101.5851	[M − H]⁻	0.0	38.22	39.78	38.21	45.55	54.26	Cucumarioside A_8 * (ID29215118)
49	27.7	$C_{60}H_{96}O_{26}$	1231.6110	1231.6117	[M − H]⁻	0.6	328.18	276.91	355.16	406.50	399.65	
50	28.5	$C_{55}H_{89}O_{24}SNa$	1165.5467	1165.5470	[M − Na]⁻	0.3	7.70	6.64	7.32	8.26	9.17	
51	28.9	$C_{55}H_{90}O_{22}$	1101.5843	1101.5851	[M − H]⁻	0.7	19.39	17.88	17.46	18.56	21.60	
52	31.3	$C_{55}H_{84}O_{27}S_2Na_2$	620.2328	620.2326	[M − 2Na]²⁻	−0.3	52.92	53.12	56.30	58.02	62.22	
53	31.4	$C_{60}H_{98}O_{25}$	1217.6314	1217.6324	[M − H]⁻	0.9	34.13	32.21	31.91	35.58	44.22	
54	32.6	$C_{56}H_{92}O_{23}$	1131.5951	1131.5957	[M − H]⁻	0.5	19.77	18.64	21.13	23.62	19.24	

[a] The compound's numbers correspond to the number of the peaks on (−)LC-MS chromatogram; [b] Formula calculated from the accurate mass; [c] Concentration is given as μg of compound on g of animal material; BW: body walls; GN: guts; G: gonads; G: guts; AB: aquapharyngeal bulbs; RT: respiratory trees; * Identification on basis of comparison of retention times, MS/MS data and elemental compositions with corresponding standards; ** Identification based on the elemental compositions and MS/MS data.

It is known that the majority of triterpene glycosides have a xylose at C-3 of the aglycone as the first monosaccharide unit, quinovose as the second monosaccharide unit, and glucose (or xylose) as the third monosaccharide unit in the main chain [1,4]. Methylated monosaccharides are always terminal units. Considering that the oligosaccharide chains of earlier isolated triterpene glycosides from this sea cucumber are closely related to each other and have general architecture 3-*O*-methyl-β-D-xylopyranosyl-(1→3)-β-D-glucopyranosyl-(1→4)-β-D-quinovopyranosyl-(1→2)-β-D-xylopyranosyl in the linear part of carbohydrate chains and may have β-D-xylopyranosyl-(1→2) in the branching at the second monosaccharide, some suggestions concerning structures of oligosaccharide chains of unknown glycosides may be proposed. In addition, most of the previously isolated glycosides of *E. fraudatrix* have a 16β-acetoxyholosta-7-ene aglycone. These common structural features give a possibility to propose structures for a series of newly identified glycosides.

The structures of detected glycosides were characterized by tandem MS. The (−)MS/MS provided many product ion series arising from the cleavages of both glycosidic bonds and bond of aglycone side chain. (+)MS/MS provided an intense B- and C-type product ion series (nomenclature according to Domon and Costello [39]) arising from the cleavages of glycosidic bonds with charge located on saccharide fragment (Table S1). These product ion series are characteristic and provided information about the sequence of monosaccharide units in carbohydrate chains. For example, the positive product ion spectrum of $[M + Na]^+$ precursor at m/z 1251.5776 (compound **41**) exhibits extensive fragmentation namely peaks at m/z 169.05 $[MeXyl + Na]^+$, 331.10 $[MeXyl + Glc + Na]^+$, 349.11 $[MeXyl + Glc + H_2O + Na]^+$, 389.14 $[MeXyl + Glc + C_3H_6O + Na]^+$, 417.14 $[MeXyl + Glc + C_4H_6O_2 + Na]^+$, 477.16 $[MeXyl + Glc + Qui + Na]^+$, 537.18 $[MeXyl + Glc + Qui + C_2H_4O_2 + Na]^+$, 609.20 $[MeXyl + Glc + Qui + Xyl + Na]^+$, 627.21 $[MeXyl + Glc + Qui + Xyl + H_2O + Na]^+$, 669.22 $[MeXyl + Glc + Qui + Xyl + C_2H_4O_2 + Na]^+$, 741.24 $[MeXyl + Glc + Qui + 2Xyl + Na]^+$, and 759.25 $[MeXyl + Glc + Qui + 2Xyl + H_2O + Na]^+$ (Figure 3). This fragmentation pattern corresponded to a branched non-sulfated oligosaccharide chain consisting of five monosaccharide units and compound **41** was identified as cucumarioside C_2.

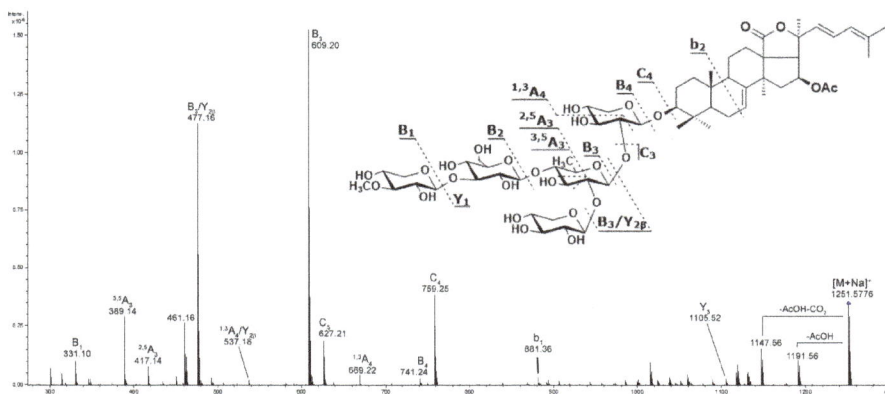

Figure 3. ESI MS/MS spectrum of $[M + Na]^+$ precursor ion at m/z 1251 identified as cucumarioside C_2 (**41**).

In some cases, several typical mass losses between the precursor and the fragment ions were detected in product ion spectra. These typical mass losses are related to the aglycone and provide information about the structure of nucleus and side chain. In MS/MS spectra of the majority of the glycosides, a mass loss of 60 Da between the precursor and the intense fragment ion was detected (for example, Figure S2). This corresponds to the loss of $C_2H_4O_2$ molecule (acetic acid) and is a characteristic of the glycosides containing an acetoxy group [40]. Next intense fragment ion with a mass loss 104 Da from the precursor corresponds to the loss of a $[C_2H_4O_2 + CO_2]$ fragment and is characteristic for the glycosides containing an acetoxy group and a 18(20)-lactone cycle. Analysis of the MS/MS spectra of a number of triterpene glycosides isolated earlier allowed to identify characteristic fragment peaks related with the cleavages of side chains. For example, (+)MS/MS spectra of the cucumarioside A_1 with 24-ene side chain have a mass loss of 228.1359 Da, corresponding to the loss of a $C_{12}H_{20}O_4$ fragment (Figure S2). The (+)MS/MS spectra of the glycosides with 22,24-diene system in the side chain display a characteristic mass loss of $C_{11}H_{17}O_4$ fragments (213.1121 Da). Otherwise, spectra of cucumarioside A_{15} with saturated side chain display a characteristic mass losses of fragments $C_{12}H_{22}O_4$ (230.1525 Da) and $C_{10}H_{10}O_4$ (204.1370 Da). These fragmentation patterns enable to propose structural features of aglycones for newly identified glycosides.

In accordance with the structures of oligosaccharide chains, all detected glycosides of *E. fraudatrix* can be divided into eleven groups (I–XI). Compounds of group I (**9**, **12**, **18**, **37**, **41**, **45**, **49**, and **53**) had branched non-sulfated oligosaccharide chain consisting of five monosaccharide units—methylated xylose, glucose, quinovose and xylose in the main chain and xylose as branching unit at the second monosaccharide. Such type of oligosaccharide chain corresponds to known cucumariosides of the C-group. Obtained data allowed to identify the glycosides **37** (m/z 1227.5799 [M − H]$^-$, calcd 1227.5804) as cucumarioside C_1 and **41** (m/z 1227.5796 [M − H]$^-$, calcd 1227.5804) as cucumarioside C_2 [28]. These compounds have similar holostane type aglycones having 16β-OAc and 7(8)-double bond in the nucleus and two double bonds in side chains which differ in the configuration of C-22 (22Z,24-diene system for cucumarioside C_1 and 22E,24-diene system for cucumarioside C_2). As a result, these compounds have similar MS/MS spectra, but their retention times differ (Rt of **37** is 23.1 min, and Rt of **41**—24.2 min). It was found that the glycosides with 22Z,24-diene system in the side chain have shorter retention time then analogous compounds with 22E,24-diene system. This made it possible to identify such pairs of similar compounds. In addition, (+)MS/MS spectra of **37** and **41** have characteristic mass losses of 204 Da and 213 Da, which confirm their structure. Compounds **45** (m/z 1229.5956 [M − H]$^-$, calcd 1229.5961) and **49** (m/z 1231.6110 [M − H]$^-$, calcd 1231.6117) differed in 2 and 4 Da, respectively, versus compounds **37** and **41**. Their MS/MS spectra were similar to the spectra of compounds **37** and **41**, but in (+)MS/MS spectrum of **45** a characteristic fragment peak [M + Na − $C_{12}H_{20}O_4$]$^+$ was detected at m/z 1025.4557, and in (+)MS/MS spectrum of **49** the fragment peaks [M + Na − $C_{12}H_{22}O_4$]$^+$ and [M + Na − $C_{10}H_{20}O_4$]$^+$ were detected at m/z 1025.4550 and 1051.4709, respectively. This indicates the presence of one double bond in **45** and no double bonds in the side chain of **49**. All these data revealed that **45** has a 16β-acetoxyholosta-7,24-diene aglycone and **49** has 16β-acetoxyholosta-7-ene aglycone. Structures of these two compounds are similar to known cucumariosides A_1 and A_{15}, respectively, with additional xylose as branching monosaccharide unit. Aglycone of glycoside **18** (m/z 1101.5126 [M − H]$^-$, calcd 1101.5123) has no fragmentation in tandem MS; HR MS and chromatographic behavior of this compound corresponds to that having a 23,24,25,26,27-pentanorlanostane aglycone with an 18(16)-lactone. Compound **12** (m/z 1201.5634 [M − H]$^-$, calcd 1201.5648) may has 16S,22R-epoxy-holosta-7,23E-diene-25-ol aglycone. Such aglycone was previously found in cucumarioside H_8, a sulfated derivative of **12** [33]. MS/MS data of **53** (m/z 1217.6314 [M − H]$^-$, calcd 1217.6324) showed that this compound has an aglycone with one oxygen less than some other aglycones of this group. The presence of a characteristic fragment peak [M + Na − $C_9H_{18}O$]$^+$ at m/z 1099.4918 may indicate that the aglycone of **53** has no γ-lactone moiety and probably has a structure of 16-acetoxy-20-hydroxy-lanosta-7,24-diene. The structure of the aglycone of glycoside **9** was not defined.

The compounds of group II (**43**, **44**, **47**, **48**, and **51**) have a linear non-sulfated oligosaccharide chain with four monosaccharides—methylated xylose, glucose, quinovose and xylose. Such type of oligosaccharide chain corresponds to known cucumariosides of the A-group. Glycoside **47** (m/z 1097.5534 [M − H]$^-$, calcd 1097.5538) was identified as cucumarioside A_1 based on comparison of its retention time, MS spectra and elemental composition with those of standard compound [24]. Glycoside **48** (m/z 1101.5851 [M − H]$^-$, calcd 1101.5851) was identified as cucumarioside A_8 by analogous way as for **47** [26]. The MS data obtained for compound **51** (m/z 1101.5843 [M − H]$^-$, calcd 1101.5851) were identical of those of cucumarioside A_8 indicating similarity of structures of **51** and **48**. Glycoside **51** may differ in configuration or position of the double bond in the side chain. We suggest that this glycoside contains a 20-hydroxy-25(26)-ene fragment in the aglycone. Glycoside **43** (m/z 1095.5380 [M − H]$^-$, calcd 1095.5381) was identified as cucumarioside A_5 based on MS spectra and elemental composition [24]. This metabolite has an aglycone with 22Z,24-diene system in the side chain. Compound **44** (m/z 1095.5379 [M − H]$^-$, calcd 1095.5381) is similar to **43**, but its retention time is higher. This may indicate that **44** has an aglycone with 22E,24-diene system in the side chain.

Fragmentation of oligosaccharide chain of glycosides of the group III (**34** and **39**) was similar to fragmentation of oligosaccharide chain of glycosides of the group I, but all fragment peaks in MS/MS spectra were shifted by 30 Da (Table S1). This may be due to the replacement of the terminal methylated xylose with a methylated glucose residue. Thus, group III includes compounds having non-sulfated main oligosaccharide chain with methylated glucose, glucose, quinovose and xylose monosaccharide units and xylose as branching unit. Data of glycosides **34** (m/z 1257.5905 [M − H]$^-$, calcd 1257.5910) and **39** (m/z 1257.5907 [M − H]$^-$, calcd 1257.5910) were similar to those of cucumariosides C_1 (**37**) and C_2 (**41**), respectively. This may indicate that glycosides **34** and **39** have the same 16β-acetoxyholosta-7-ene aglycone with 22Z,24-diene system for **34** and 22E,24-diene system for **39**. Actually, these compounds were isolated and their preliminary structures were confirmed by 1D NMR (Figures S6–S8).

Glycosides of group IV (**40** and **36**) have a non-sulfated oligosaccharide chain consisted of glucose, quinovose, and two xylose units. The presence of two Y-type fragment peaks at m/z 973.4761 [M + Na − Xyl]$^+$ and 943.4650 [M + Na − Glc]$^+$ in MS/MS of **40** indicates the oligosaccharide chain with two terminal non-methylated monosaccharides. Thus, the structure of the oligosaccharide chain of IV group glycosides was similar to those of I or III groups, without terminal methylated monosaccharide. Fragmentation pattern and HR MS data of compounds **36** (m/z 1081.5224 [M − H]$^-$, calcd 1081.5225) and **40** (m/z 1081.5221 [M − H]$^-$, calcd 1081.5225) corresponded to holostane type aglycones with 16β-OAc and 7(8)-double bond in the nucleus and side chain with two double bonds. Comparison of retention times of these glycosides indicates that **36** have 22Z,24-diene system and **40** have 22E,24-diene system in the side chains.

The group V (**3**, **4**, **10**, **13**, **21**, **25**, and **29**) include glycosides with branched pentasaccharide chain having one sulfate group at the first xylose unit and 3-O-methyl-xylose as a terminal monosaccharide unit and belong to the group of cucumariosides H. Structure of carbohydrate moieties were confirmed by tandem MS. Fragmentation of oligosaccharide chain of the glycosides of group V under collision induced dissociation (CID) conditions gave the intense characteristic product ion series of A-, B-and C-type ions (Table S1). Fragment ions C_4, B_4 and A_4 were mainly observed in desulfated form. In addition, CID spectra of sulfated glycosides provided characteristic product ion $^{1,5}A_4$, arising from the cleavage of the ring of sulfated xylose unit. Glycosides **10** (m/z 1325.5472 [M − Na]$^-$, calcd 1325.5478), **13** (m/z 1181.4692 [M − Na]$^-$, calcd 1181.4691), **21** (m/z 1307.5369 [M − Na]$^-$, calcd 1307.5372), **25** (m/z 1307.5370 [M − Na]$^-$, calcd 1307.5372), and **29** (m/z 1309.5524 [M − Na]$^-$, calcd 1309.5529) were identified as cucumariosides H_2, H_3, H_5, H, and H_6, respectively, based on the comparison of their retention times, MS spectra and elemental compositions with those of standard compounds [33–35]. Structures of glycosides **3** and **4** were not defined.

Glycosides of group VI (**6**, **14**, **16**, **26**, **30**, **32**, **42**, and **50**) belong to the group of cucumariosides G, having a linear tetrasaccharide chain with one sulfate group at the first xylose unit and 3-O-methyl-xylose as a terminal monosaccharide unit. MS/MS data obtained in both negative and positive ion modes and HR mass values allowed to identify glycosides **14** (m/z 1193.5051 [M − Na]$^-$, calcd 1193.5051) as cucumarioside G_4 [30], **16** (m/z 1049.4268 [M − Na]$^-$, calcd 1049.4269) as cucumarioside G_2 [32], **26** (m/z 1175.4946 [M − Na]$^-$, calcd 1175.4950) as cucumarioside G_3 [31], and **32** (m/z 1177.5101 [M − Na]$^-$, calcd 1177.5106) as cucumarioside G_1 [29]. Aglycone of **30** (m/z 1175.4946 [M − Na]$^-$, calcd 1175.4950) was identified as 16β-acetoxyholosta-7,22E,24-triene-3β-ol. Compound **42** (m/z 1179.5253 [M − Na]$^-$, calcd 1179.5263) probably has holostane type aglycone similar to aglycone of **49** with 16β-OAc and 7(8)-double bond in the nucleus and without double bonds in the side chain. Aglycone of **50** (m/z 1165.5467 [M − Na]⁻, calcd 1165.5470) is similar to the aglycone of **53** and has the structure 16-acetoxy-20-hydroxy-lanosta-7,24-diene. Structure of the aglycone of glycoside **6** was not defined.

Compounds of group VII (**22** and **27**) have branched oligosaccharide chain consisting of five monosaccharide units—3-O-methyl-glucose as a terminal monosaccharide, glucose, quinovose and sulfated xylose in main chain and xylose as branching unit at second monosaccharide. In MS/MS spectra of glycoside **22** (m/z 1337.5472 [M − Na]⁻, calcd 1337.5478) fragment peaks characteristic for a holostane aglycone with 16β-OAc and two double bonds in the side chain were detected. Obtained data indicated that **27** (m/z 1339.5629 [M − Na]⁻, calcd 1339.5634) probably has 16β-acetoxyholosta-7,24-diene aglycone.

The group VIII (**17**, **31**, **38**, and **52**) includes compounds with linear tetrasaccharide chain containing terminal 3-O-methyl-xylose, sulfated glucose, quinovose and sulfated xylose. These glycosides belong to the group of cucumariosides F. It should be noted that in the positive ion mode it was not possible to obtain stable ions [M + Na]⁺ for disulfated glycosides, so negative ion MS/MS spectra of [M − 2Na]²⁻ ions were used for analysis. Fragmentation of oligosaccharide chain of [M − 2Na]²⁻ ion in MS/MS spectra of disulfated glycosides under CID conditions gave the characteristic product ion series of A-, B- and Y-types ions, which were mainly observed in desulfated form (Table S1). All data allowed identifying glycosides **31** (m/z 627.2223 [M − 2Na]²⁻, calcd 627.2223) as cucumarioside F₂ and **38** (m/z 628.2301 [M − 2Na]²⁻, calcd 628.2301) as cucumarioside F₁ [36]. Glycoside **17** (m/z 564.1882 [M − 2Na]²⁻, calcd 564.1882) has 23,24,25,26,27-pentanorlanostane aglycone with an 18(16)-lactone. Structure of the aglycone of glycoside **52** was not defined.

Oligosaccharide chain of glycosides group IX (**11**, **15**, **23**, and **28**) belonging to the group of cucumariosides I, has a main chain with terminal 3-O-methyl-xylose, sulfated glucose, quinovose and sulfated xylose and xylose as branching monosaccharide unit. Glycosides **11** (m/z 702.2493 [M − 2Na]²⁻, calcd 702.2487), **15** (m/z 630.2098 [M − 2Na]²⁻, calcd 630.2093), **23** (m/z 693.2437 [M − 2Na]²⁻, calcd 693.2434), and **28** (m/z 694.2510 [M − 2Na]²⁻, calcd 694.2512) were identified as cucumariosides I₃, I₄, I₂, and I₁, respectively, based on the comparison of their retention times, MS spectra and elemental compositions with those of standard compounds [37,38].

Besides the described groups, two glycosides with trisaccharide chains were present in analyzed sample. In (−)MS/MS spectra of **33** (group X) (m/z 1029.4364 [M − Na]⁻, calcd 1029.4371) were detected fragment peaks at m/z 519.1029 [Glc + Qui + XylSO₃]⁻, 867.3829 [M − Na − Glc]⁻, and 721.3245 [M − Na − Glc − Qui]⁻. In (−)MS/MS spectra of **35** (group XI) (m/z 999.4257 [M − Na]⁻, calcd 999.4265) were detected fragment peaks at m/z 489.0899 [Xyl + Qui + XylSO₃]⁻ and 867.3832 [M − Na − Xyl]⁻. Both glycosides probably have the same holostane type aglycone with 16β-OAc and two double bonds in side chains (probably 22E,24-diene).

Thus, all glycosides of *E. fraudatrix* can be divided into eleven groups in accordance with structures of oligosaccharide chains. Five types of oligosaccharide chains were not found in *E. fraudatrix* previously. According to literature data, the majority of triterpene glycosides of *E. fraudatrix* have 3-O-MeXyl as terminal monosaccharide unit. We revealed new glycosides with terminal 3-O-MeGlc residue (**22**, **27**, **34**, and **39**); two of them (**34**, and **39**) were isolated, and their tentative structures are further supported by 1D NMR (Figures S6–S8).

The fact that not all previously isolated glycosides have been found by LC-MS approach in this study of *E. fraudatrix* could be explained by the changes in the quantitative and qualitative composition of different components of the glycosidic fraction in the samples of one species collected in different places and seasons. A representative example of such changes has been reported for the components of the glycosidic fraction of *Psolus fabricii*, where two different glycosides were predominant or minor in the samples collected near Onekotan Island or Ushishir Islands (Kuril Islands) [41,42]. Another example is given by the glycosides of *Massinium* (=*Neothynidium*) *magnum* where the structures of glycosides from various places or various times of collection were strongly different [43]. In addition, some earlier isolated cucumariosides of A-group may be artifacts formed during the isolation process [24].

Obtained data allowed us to propose a biosynthetic pathway for oligosaccharide chains in *E. fraudatrix* (Figure 4), in agreement with the biosynthetic pathway of oligosaccharide chains proposed earlier [27]. The elongation of the oligosaccharide chain occurs by the addition of monosaccharide residues to various positions of the forming oligosaccharide chain. This leads to the formation of glycosides with different oligosaccharide chains. Sulfatation of triterpene glycosides may occur at different stages of the forming of carbohydrate chains resulting in the appearance of sulfated oligosaccharide moieties comprised from two to six sugar units. From this viewpoint, cucumarioside B_2 [27] having the same but non-sulfated carbohydrate chain as **35** represents a biosynthetic precursor of the new glycoside **35**. Analogical relationships are observed in the series of isolated glycosides of *E. fraudatrix*: cucumariosides of C-group (I) → cucumariosides of H-group (V) → cucumariosides of I-group (IX); cucumariosides of A-group (II) → cucumariosides of G-group (VI) → cucumariosides of F-group (VIII); and also in the groups III → VII detected by ESI MS.

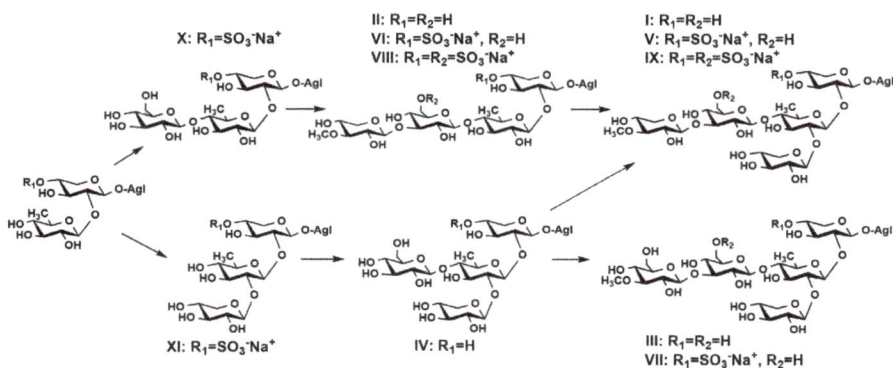

Figure 4. Hypothetic scheme of biosynthesis of oligosaccharide chains in *E. fraudatrix*.

2.2. Distribution of Detected Glycosides in the Different Body Components

Quantitative and qualitative analysis of detected triterpene glycosides in various body components of *E. fraudatrix* was also performed. We separately extracted triterpene glycoside mixtures from respiratory trees (RT), body walls (BW), gonad tubules (GN), guts (G) and aquapharyngeal bulbs (AB) and analyzed them by LC-ESI QTOF-MS. The profiling revealed that all the triterpene glycosides detected in the whole body extract were also present in all analyzed body parts.

The maximal content of overwhelming majority of the analyzed glycosides was observed in the body walls when compared with other body components of sea cucumber. This observation is a very good corroboration of a defensive role of triterpene glycosides. Since *E. fraudatrix* does not contain Cuvierian tubules, it accumulates the defensive molecules of triterpene glycosides in the body walls in order to indicate to predator its unpalatability. The main components of glycosidic fraction—cucumariosides C_1 (**37**) and C_2 (**41**), compounds **39** and **45**, as well as cucumariosides F_1 (**38**) and G_1 (**32**)—predominate in the body walls. These compounds contain pentasaccharide non-sulfated or tetrasaccharide mono- or disulfated carbohydrate chains making them highly hydrophilic substances and accelerating their diffusion to the surrounding water. Moreover, such compounds usually demonstrate significant membranolytic activities [1]. All these data also confirm the main external function of glycosides as chemical defense system.

The profiling of extracts from different body components revealed that relative amounts (normalized by sum and scaling) of most compounds were approximately the same (Figure 5; Figure S9).

However, several minor compounds were more typical for certain body components. Relative amounts of compounds **12**, **15**, **17** and some others (Figure 5; Figures S9 and S10) are significantly higher in gonads than in body walls or other organs. The analysis of their structures revealed that compounds **15** and **17** have non-holostane aglycones with shortened side chains thus having structural similarity with steroidal hormones of vertebrates. It is known that sex hormones of vertebrates are biosynthesized from cholesterol via the cleavage of its side chain through the oxidation of C-20 and C-22 positions [44]. Actually, compound **12** contains a oxygen-bearing substituent in C-22 position as well as a oxidized C-20 position that makes it a putative biosynthetic precursor of the aglycones with shortened side chains such as **15** and **17**. All these data are in good agreement with the earlier suggested internal biological function of the glycosides—the regulation of oocytes maturation in the sea cucumbers.

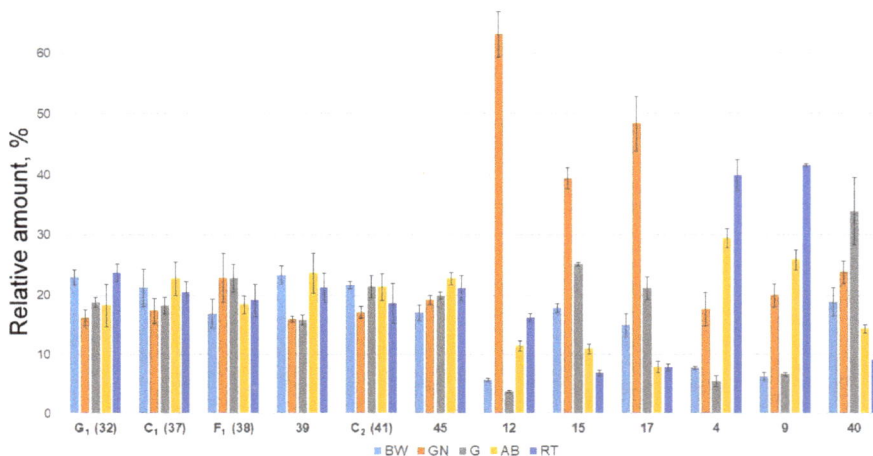

Figure 5. Relative quantities of triterpene glycosides cucumariosides G_1 (**32**), C_1 (**37**), F_1 (**38**) and C_2 (**41**), and compounds **39**, **45**, **12**, **15**, **17**, **4**, **9**, and **40** in respiratory trees (RT), gonads (GN), aquapharyngeal bulbs (AB), guts (G) and body walls (BW) (bar plots represent the concentration in μg/g animal material of metabolites (mean ± SD) scaled by 100%).

Interestingly, the glycosides of group IV (**36** and **40**) having peculiar "undeveloped" branched tetrasaccharide chains without methylated terminal sugar unit were characteristic for guts (Figure S11). There is a correlation between the contents of some glycosides in aquapharyngeal bulbs and respiratory trees (compounds **1**, **2**, **4**, **5**, **7**, **8**, and **9**; Figure S9) that may indicate additional biological functions of triterpene glycosides in the organism-producer, which have to be investigated.

3. Materials and Methods

3.1. Chemicals

Methanol (quality HPLC gradient grade) and water (quality UV-HPLC grade) were obtained from Panreac (Barcelona, Spain). All other chemicals and reagents were of analytical grade or equivalent. Cucumariosides A_1–A_4, A_6–A_{15} [24,25], H, H_2–H_8 [34,35,37], F_1–F_2 [36], I_1–I_4 [37,38] isolated early from the *E. fraudatrix* and typicoside A_2 isolated early from the sea cucumber *Actinocucumis typica* [45] were used as standards of triterpene glycosides. Structures of these compounds were established using different methods including high resolution NMR.

3.2. Animal Material

Specimens of the sea cucumber *Eupentacta fraudatrix* (Djakonov et Baranova) (family Sclerodactylidae, order Dendrochirotida) were collected at Amursky Bay (Peter the Great Gulf, the Sea of Japan) in April 2017 at a depth of 1.0–1.5 m. Species identification was carried out by Dr. I.Yu. Dolmatov (A.V. Zhirmunsky Institute of Marine Biology, National Scientific Center of Marine Biology, Far Eastern Branch of Russian Academy of Sciences, Vladivostok, Russia). Voucher specimen No. PIBOC-2017-04-EF is preserved in the collection the G.B. Elyakov Pacific Institute of Bioorganic Chemistry.

3.3. Sample Preparation and Solid-Phase Extraction (SPE)

Seven fresh animals (m = 3.9 ± 1.3 g) were chopped and extracted thrice with ethanol (totally 0.5 L, for 10 h). Other seven animals were dissected and separated into respiratory trees (RT, m = 1.7 g), body walls (BW, m = 10.2 g), gonad tubules (GN, m = 3.9 g), guts (G, m = 4.3 g) and aquapharyngeal bulbs (AB, m = 3.9 g). Metabolites from five different body components were extracted thrice with ethanol (totally 100 mL, for 10 h). Extracts were filtered, dried and reconstituted in 15 mL ethanol.

Two hundred microliters of the extract was centrifuged, and the supernatant was subjected solid-phase extraction (SPE). SPE cartridges (BondElut C18, 100 mg/1 mL, Agilent Technologies, Santa Clara, CA, USA) were fitted into stopcocks and connected to a vacuum manifold. The sorbent was conditioned with 3 mL of ethanol followed by 3 mL water. Care was taken that the sorbent did not become dry during conditioning. With the stopcocks opened and the vacuum turned on, the samples were loaded onto the cartridge. The 100 µL of extract were loaded into the SPE cartridge by drops. After sample addition, the SPE cartridge was washed with 1 mL of water. Glycosides were eluted with 1 mL of 100% ethanol. These extracts were dried and dissolved in 500 µL 80% MeOH in water (*v*/*v*) and subjected to LC-MS analyses.

3.4. LC-MS Analysis

Analysis was performed using an Agilent 1200 series chromatograph (Agilent Technologies, Santa Clara, CA, USA) connected to a Bruker Impact II Q-TOF mass spectrometer (Bruker Daltonics, Bremen, Germany). Zorbax Eclipse XDB-C18 column (1.0 × 150 mm, 3.5 µm, Agilent Technologies, Santa Clara, CA, USA) with Zorbax SB-C8 guard-column (2.1 × 12.5 mm, 5 µm, Agilent Technologies, Santa Clara, CA, USA) were used for chromatographic separation. The mobile phases were 0.1% formic acid in H_2O (eluent A) and 0.1% formic acid in MeOH (eluent B). The gradient program was as follows: isocratic at 60% of eluent B from start to 3 min, from 60% to 90% eluent B from 3 to 29 min, from 90% to 100% eluent B from 29 to 30 min, isocratic at 100% of eluent B to 35 min, from 100% to 60% eluent B from 35 to 38 min. After returning to the initial conditions, the equilibration was achieved after 15 min. Chromatographic separation was performed at a 0.1 mL/min flow rate at 40 °C. Injection volume was 1 µL.

The mass spectrometry detection has been performed using ESI ionization source. Optimized ionization parameters for ESI were as follows: a capillary voltage of ±4.0 kV, nebulization with nitrogen at 0.8 bar, dry gas flow of 7 L/min at a temperature of 200 °C. Metabolite profiles in positive ion mode were registered using post-column addition of 5×10^{-4} M sodium iodide at 60 µL/h flow rate for obtaining stabilized sodium adduct ions. Post-column infusion was performed with syringe pump via T-mixing tee. Based on the results of preliminary experiments, the mass spectra were recorded within *m*/*z* mass range of 100–1500 and 70–1500 for MS/MS spectra (scan time 1 s).

Collision induced dissociation (CID) product ion mass spectra were recorded in auto-MS/MS mode with a collision energy ranging from 75 to 125 eV (an exact collision energy setting depended on the molecular masses of precursor ions). The precursor ions were isolated with an isolation width of 4 Th.

The mass spectrometer was calibrated using the ESI-L Low Concentration Tuning Mix (Agilent Technologies, Santa Clara, CA, USA). Additionally a lock-mass calibration with hexakis (1H, 1H, 3H-tetrafluoropropoxy)phosphazine (922.0098 m/z in positive mode; 966.0007 m/z in negative mode; Agilent Technologies, Santa Clara, CA, USA) was performed using Calibrant Reservoir Kit (Bruker Daltonics, Bremen, Germany). The instrument was operated using the otofControl (ver. 4.0, Bruker Daltonics, Bremen, Germany) and data were analyzed using the DataAnalysis Software (ver. 4.3, Bruker Daltonics, Bremen, Germany).

All tests were performed at least in triplicate. The results are expressed as the mean ± standard deviation (SD).

3.5. Quantitative Analysis of Detected Triterpene Glycosides in Various Body Component

For quantitative analysis, we used cucumarioside A$_1$ from *E. fraudatrix* [24] as a reference standard for non-sulfated glycosides (R$_2$ = 0.988), typicoside A$_2$ from *Actinocucumis typica* [44] as a reference standard for monosulfated glycosides (R$_2$ = 0.999) and cucumarioside I$_2$ from *E. fraudatrix* [37] as a reference standard for disulfated glycosides (R$_2$ = 0.995). Standards at concentrations of 1.0, 2.5, 5.0, 10.0 and 50 µg/mL were used for building calibration curves (Figures S3–S5). All the experiments were carried out at least three times, LC-MS conditions are identical to those described above. As a result, the amounts of detected compounds were calculated through calibration curves. Results are shown in Table 1 as mean concentration in µg/g animal organs.

For comparative analysis of the content of triterpene glycosides in different organs of *E. fraudatrix* data pretreatment was performed. With the aim to make feature compounds more comparable to each other, the datasets were adjusted using scaling by 100% (for 100%—the total concentration of the compound in all organs). Results are shown in Figure 5 and Figures S9–S11 as the mean ± standard deviation (SD).

4. Conclusions

Profiling of *E. fraudatrix* was performed by LC-ESI MS. Analysis of chromatographic behavior, MS and MS/MS data allowed the structural identification of the triterpene glycosides to be performed. Totally, 54 triterpene glycosides were found and structures of 44 constituents were proposed based on LC-ESI MS, chromatographic behavior and biogenetic hypotheses. In accordance with the structures of oligosaccharide chains, all analyzed glycosides of *E. fraudatrix* can be divided into eleven groups, and five of them were found in *E. fraudatrix* for the first time. A theoretical scheme of biogenesis of oligosaccharide chains in the studied species was given. The comparison of the qualitative and quantitative contents from the five different body components revealed that the profiles of some triterpene glycosides differed in the body walls and gonads indicating different external and internal biological functions of these compounds. The predominance of the main highly hydrophilic and membranolytic glycosides of *E. fraudatrix* in the body walls confirms their defensive role. The presence of glycosides in all body components of *E. fraudatrix* indicates their multifunctionality.

Supplementary Materials: The following are available online at www.mdpi.com/1660-3397/15/10/302/s1, Table S1: Fragmentation of the different types of oligosaccharide chains determined in triterpene glycosides from the ethanol extract of the sea cucumber *E. fraudatrix*, Figure S1: LC-ESI MS base-peak chromatogram (a) and total compounds chromatogram (b) of ethanol extract of sea cucumber *Eupentacta fraudatrix* in negative ion mode, Figure S2: Fragment of ESI MS/MS spectrum of [M + Na]$^+$ precursor ion at m/z 1121 of cucumarioside A$_1$, Figure S3: Calibration curve for cucumarioside A$_1$ (ion [M − H]$^-$ at m/z 1097), Figure S4: Calibration curve for typicoside A$_2$ (ion [M − Na]$^-$ at m/z 1177), Figure S5: Calibration curve for cucumarioside I$_2$ (ion [M − 2Na]$^{2-}$ at m/z 693), Figure S6: ^{13}C NMR spectrum of glycoside **39**, Figure S7: ^{1}H NMR spectrum of glycoside **39**, Figure S8: ^{1}H NMR spectrum of glycoside **34**, Figure S9; Relative quantities of triterpene glycosides detected in *E. fraudatrix* in body walls (BW), gonads (GN), guts (G), aquapharyngeal bulbs (AB), and respiratory trees (RT) (bar plots represent the concentration in µg/g animal material of metabolites (mean ± SD) scaled by 100%), Figure S10: Relative quantities of triterpene glycosides grouped by aglycone structures detected in *E. fraudatrix* in respiratory trees (RT), gonads (GN), aquapharyngeal bulbs (AB), guts (G) and body walls (BW) (bar plots represent the concentration in µg/g animal material of metabolites (mean ± SD) scaled by 100%), Figure S11: Relative quantities of triterpene glycosides grouped by sugar moiety structures detected in *E. fraudatrix* in respiratory trees (RT), gonads (GN), aquapharyngeal bulbs (AB), guts (G) and body walls (BW) (bar plots represent the concentration in μg/g animal material of metabolites (mean ± SD) scaled by 100%).

Acknowledgments: The study was supported by Grant No. 16-13-10185 from the RSF (Russian Science Foundation).

Author Contributions: Roman S. Popov and Natalia V. Ivanchina conceived and designed the project, performed experiments, analyzed the data and wrote the manuscript; Alexandra S. Silchenko, Sergey A. Avilov and Vladimir I. Kalinin isolated standard compounds, discussed results and wrote the manuscript; Igor Yu. Dolmatov performed preparation of animal material; and Valentin A. Stonik and Pavel S. Dmitrenok supervised research and discussed results.

Conflicts of Interest: The authors declare no conflict of interest.

References

1. Kalinin, V.I.; Aminin, D.L.; Avilov, S.A.; Silchenko, A.S.; Stonik, V.A. Triterpene glycosides from sea cucumbers (Holothurioidea, Echinodermata), biological activities and functions. In *Studies in Natural Product Chemistry (Bioactive Natural Products)*; Atta-ur-Rahman, Ed.; Elsevier Science Publisher: Amsterdam, The Netherlands, 2008; Volume 35, pp. 135–196.

2. Careaga, V.P.; Maier, M.S. Cytotoxic triterpene glycosides from sea cucumbers. In *Handbook of Anticancer Drugs from Marine Origin*; Kim, S.-K., Ed.; Springer International Publishing: Cham, Switzerland, 2015; pp. 515–528.

3. Chludil, H.D.; Murray, A.P.; Seldes, A.M.; Maier, M.S. Biologically active triterpene glycosides from sea cucumbers (Holothuroidea, Echinodermata). In *Studies in Natural Products Chemistry*; Atta-ur-Rahman, Ed.; Elsevier Science Publisher: Amsterdam, The Netherlands, 2003; Volume 28, pp. 587–615.

4. Kim, S.K.; Himaya, S.W.A. Triterpene glycosides from sea cucumbers and their biological activities. *Adv. Food Nutr. Res.* **2012**, *63*, 297–319.

5. Maier, M.S.; Roccatagliata, A.J.; Kuriss, A.; Chludil, H.; Seldes, A.M.; Pujol, C.A.; Damonte, E.B. Two new cytotoxic and virucidal trisulfated triterpene glycosides from the antarctic sea cucumber *Staurocucumis liouvillei*. *J. Nat. Prod.* **2001**, *64*, 732–736. [CrossRef] [PubMed]

6. Aminin, D.L.; Menchinskaya, E.S.; Pisliagin, E.A.; Silchenko, A.S.; Avilov, S.A.; Kalinin, V.I. Anticancer activity of sea cucumber triterpene glycosides. *Mar. Drugs* **2015**, *13*, 1202–1223. [CrossRef] [PubMed]

7. Aminin, D.L.; Pislyagin, E.A.; Menchinskaya, E.S.; Silchenko, A.S.; Avilov, S.A.; Kalinin, V.I. Immunomodulatory and anticancer activity of sea cucumber triterpene glycosides. In *Studies in Natural Products Chemistry (Bioactive Natural Products)*; Atta-ur-Rahman, Ed.; Elsevier Science Publisher: Amsterdam, The Netherlands, 2014; Volume 41, pp. 75–94.

8. Bordbar, S.; Anwar, F.; Saari, N. High-value components and bioactives from sea cucumbers for functional foods—A review. *Mar. Drugs* **2011**, *9*, 1761–1805. [CrossRef] [PubMed]

9. Van Dyck, S.; Flammang, P.; Meriaux, C.; Bonnel, D.; Salzet, M.; Fournier, I.; Wisztorski, M. Localization of secondary metabolites in marine invertebrates: Contribution of MALDI MSI for the study of saponins in Cuvierian tubules of *H. forskali*. *PLoS ONE* **2010**, *5*, e13923. [CrossRef] [PubMed]

10. Van Dyck, S.; Caulier, G.; Todesco, M.; Gerbaux, P.; Fournier, I.; Wisztorski, M.; Flammang, P. The triterpene glycosides of *Holothuria forskali*: Usefulness and efficiency as a chemical defense mechanism against predatory fish. *J. Exp. Biol.* **2011**, *214*, 1347–1356. [CrossRef] [PubMed]

11. Aminin, D.L.; Anisimov, M.M. The influence of holotoxin A_1 to the Ca^{2+}-transport and meiotic maturation of oocytes from the sea cucumber *Stichopus japonicus*. *J. Evol. Biochem. Physiol.* **1990**, *26*, 9–13.

12. Kalinin, V.I.; Avilov, S.A.; Silchenko, A.S.; Stonik, V.A. Triterpene glycosides of sea cucumbers (Holothuroidea, Echinodermata) as taxonomic markers. *Nat. Prod. Commun.* **2015**, *10*, 21–26. [PubMed]

13. Van Dyck, S.; Gerbaux, P.; Flammang, P. Qualitative and quantitative saponin contents in five sea cucumbers from the Indian Ocean. *Mar. Drugs* **2010**, *8*, 173–189. [CrossRef] [PubMed]

14. Bondoc, K.G.V.; Lee, H.; Cruz, L.J.; Lebrilla, C.B.; Juinio-Mecez, M.A. Chemical fingerprinting and phylogenetic mapping of saponin congeners from three tropical holothurian sea cucumbers. *Comp. Biochem. Physiol. B* **2013**, *166*, 182–193. [CrossRef] [PubMed]

15. Van Dyck, S.; Gerbaux, P.; Flammang, P. Elucidation of molecular diversity and body distribution of saponins in the sea cucumber *Holothuria forskali* (Echinodermata) by mass spectrometry. *Comp. Biochem. Physiol. B* **2009**, *152*, 124–134. [CrossRef] [PubMed]

16. Dolmatov, I.Y.; Ivantey, V.A. Histogenesis of longitudinal muscle bands in holothurians. *Russ. J. Dev. Biol.* **1993**, *24*, 67–72.

17. Dolmatov, I.Y.; Yushin, V.V. Larval development of *Eupentacta fraudatrix* (Holothuroidea, Dendrochirota). *Asian Mar. Biol.* **1993**, *10*, 123–132.

18. Dolmatov, I.Y. Regeneration of the aquapharyngeal complex in the holothurian *Eupentacta fraudatrix* (Holothuroidea, Dendrochirota). In *Monographs in Developmental Biology*; Taban, C.H., Boilly, B., Eds.; Karger: Basel, Switzerland, 1992; Volume 23, pp. 40–50.

19. Mashanov, V.S.; Dolmatov, I.Y.; Heinzeller, T. Transdifferentiation in holothurian gut regeneration. *Biol. Bull.* **2005**, *209*, 184–193. [CrossRef] [PubMed]

20. Lamash, N.E.; Dolmatov, I.Y. Proteases from the regenerating gut of the holothurian *Eupentacta fraudatrix*. *PLoS ONE* **2013**, *8*, e58433. [CrossRef] [PubMed]

21. Zaika, O.A.; Dolmatova, L.S. Cooperative apoptosis of coelomocytes of the holothurian *Eupentacta fraudatrix* and its modulation by dexamethasone. *Adv. Biosci. Biotechnol.* **2013**, *4*, 908–917. [CrossRef]

22. Dolmatova, L.S.; Ulanova, O.A.; Dolmatov, I.Y. Comparative study of the effect of dexamethasone and new holothurians' extract on the level of the cytokine similar substances in certain immune cells types in the holothurian *Eupentacta fraudatrix*. *Pac. Med. J.* **2014**, 34–38.

23. Dolmatova, L.S.; Ulanova, O.A. Dexamethasone treatment in vitro resulted in different responses of two fractions of phagocytes of the holothurian *Eupentacta fraudatrix*. *Russ. J. Mar. Biol.* **2015**, *41*, 503–506. [CrossRef]

24. Silchenko, A.S.; Kalinovsky, A.I.; Avilov, S.A.; Andryjaschenko, P.V.; Dmitrenok, P.S.; Martyyas, E.A.; Kalinin, V.I. Triterpene glycosides from the sea cucumber *Eupentacta fraudatrix*. Structure and biological action of cucumariosides A_1, A_3, A_4, A_5, A_6, A_{12} and A_{15}, seven new minor non-sulfated tetraosides and unprecedented 25-keto, 27-norholostane aglycone. *Nat. Prod. Commun.* **2012**, *7*, 517–525. [PubMed]

25. Silchenko, A.S.; Kalinovsky, A.I.; Avilov, S.A.; Andryjaschenko, P.V.; Dmitrenok, P.S.; Martyyas, E.A.; Kalinin, V.I. Triterpene glycosides from the sea cucumber *Eupentacta fraudatrix*. Structure and cytotoxic action of cucumariosides A_2, A_7, A_9, A_{10}, A_{11}, A_{13} and A_{14}, seven new minor non-sulfated tetraosides and an aglycone with an uncommon 18-hydroxy group. *Nat. Prod. Commun.* **2012**, *7*, 845–852. [PubMed]

26. Silchenko, A.S.; Kalinovsky, A.I.; Avilov, S.A.; Andryjashenko, P.V.; Dmitrenok, P.S.; Kalinin, V.I.; Stonik, V.A. 3β-*O*-Glycosylated 16β-acetoxy-9β-H-lanosta-7,24-diene-3β,18,20β-triol, an intermediate metabolite from the sea cucumber *Eupentacta fraudatrix* and its biosynthetic significance. *Biochem. Syst. Ecol.* **2012**, *44*, 53–60. [CrossRef]

27. Silchenko, A.S.; Kalinovsky, A.I.; Avilov, S.A.; Andryjashenko, P.V.; Dmitrenok, P.S.; Martyyas, E.A.; Kalinin, V.I. Triterpene glycosides from the sea cucumber *Eupentacta fraudatrix*. Structure and biological activity of cucumariosides B_1 and B_2, two new minor non-sulfated unprecedented triosides. *Nat. Prod. Commun.* **2012**, *7*, 1157–1162. [PubMed]

28. Afiyatullov, S.S.; Kalinovskii, A.I.; Stonik, V.A. Structure of cucumariosides C_1 and C_2—2 New triterpene glycosides from the *Eupentacta fraudatrix* holothurian. *Khim. Prir. Soedin.* **1987**, *6*, 831–837. [CrossRef]

29. Afiyatullov, S.S.; Tishchenko, L.Ya.; Stonik, V.A.; Kalinovskii, A.I.; Elyakov, G.B. The structure of cucumarioside G_1—A new triterpene glycoside from the sea cucumber *Cucumaria fraudatrix*. *Khim. Prir. Soedin.* **1985**, *2*, 244–248.

30. Kalinin, V.I.; Avilov, S.A.; Kalinovskii, A.I.; Stonik, V.A.; Milgrom, Yu.M.; Rashkes, Ya.V. Cucumarioside G_4—A new triterpene glycoside from the holothurian *Eupentacta fraudatrix*. *Khim. Prir. Soedin.* **1992**, *6*, 600–603.

31. Kalinin, V.I.; Avilov, S.A.; Kalinovskii, A.I.; Stonik, V.A. Cucumarioside G_3—A minor triterpene glycoside from the holothurian *Eupentacta fraudatrix*. *Khim. Prir. Soedin.* **1992**, *6*, 635–636. [CrossRef]

32. Avilov, S.A.; Kalinin, V.I.; Makarieva, T.N.; Stonik, V.A.; Kalinovsky, A.I. Structure of cucumarioside G_2, a novel nonholostane glycoside from the sea cucumber *Eupentacta fraudatrix*. *J. Nat. Prod.* **1994**, *57*, 1166–1171. [CrossRef] [PubMed]

33. Kalinin, V.I.; Kalinovskii, A.I.; Afiyatullov, S.S. Triterpene glycosides of the holothurin *Eupentacta pseudoquinquisemita*. *Khim. Prir. Soedin.* **1988**, *2*, 221–225.

34. Silchenko, A.S.; Kalinovsky, A.I.; Avilov, S.A.; Andryjaschenko, P.V.; Dmitrenok, P.S.; Yurchenko, E.A.; Kalinin, V.I. Structure of cucumariosides H_5, H_6, H_7 and H_8, triterpene glycosides from the sea cucumber *Eupentacta fraudatrix* and unprecedented aglycone with 16,22-epoxy-group. *Nat. Prod. Commun.* **2011**, *6*, 1075–1082. [PubMed]

35. Silchenko, A.S.; Kalinovsky, A.I.; Avilov, S.A.; Andryjaschenko, P.V.; Dmitrenok, P.S.; Yurchenko, E.A.; Kalinin, V.I. Structures and cytotoxic properties of cucumariosides H_2, H_3 and H_4 from the sea cucumber *Eupentacta fraudatrix*. *Nat. Prod. Res.* **2012**, *26*, 1765–1774. [CrossRef] [PubMed]

36. Popov, R.S.; Avilov, S.A.; Silchenko, A.S.; Kalinovsky, A.I.; Dmitrenok, P.S.; Grebnev, B.B.; Ivanchina, N.V.; Kalinin, V.I. Cucumariosides F_1 and F_2, two new triterpene glycosides from the sea cucumber *Eupentacta fraudatrix* and their LC-ESI MS/MS identification in the starfish *Patiria pectinifera*, a predator of the sea cucumber. *Biochem. Syst. Ecol.* **2014**, *57*, 191–197. [CrossRef]

37. Silchenko, A.S.; Kalinovsky, A.I.; Avilov, S.A.; Andryjaschenko, P.V.; Dmitrenok, P.S.; Menchinskaya, E.S.; Aminin, D.L.; Kalinin, V.I. Structure of cucumarioside I_2 from the sea cucumber *Eupentacta fraudatrix* (Djakonov et Baranova) and cytotoxic and immunostimulatory activities of this saponin and relative compounds. *Nat. Prod. Res.* **2013**, *27*, 1776–1783. [CrossRef] [PubMed]

38. Silchenko, A.S.; Kalinovsky, A.I.; Avilov, S.A.; Andryjaschenko, P.V.; Dmitrenok, P.S.; Martyyas, E.A.; Kalinin, V.I. Triterpene glycosides from the sea cucumber *Eupentacta fraudatrix*. Structure and biological action of cucumariosides I_1, I_3, I_4, three new minor disulfated pentaosides. *Nat. Prod. Commun.* **2013**, *8*, 1053–1058. [PubMed]

39. Domon, B.; Costello, C.E. A systematic nomenclature for carbohydrate fragmentations in FAB-MS/MS spectra of glycoconjugates. *Glycoconj. J.* **1988**, *5*, 397–409. [CrossRef]

40. Antonov, A.S.; Kalinovsky, A.I.; Afiyatullov, S.S.; Leshchenko, E.V.; Dmitrenok, P.S.; Yurchenko, E.A.; Kalinin, V.I.; Stonik, V.A. Erylosides F_8, V_1–V_3, and W–W_2—New triterpene oligoglycosides from the Carribean sponge *Erylus goffrilleri*. *Carbohydr. Res.* **2017**, *449*, 153–159. [CrossRef] [PubMed]

41. Kalinin, V.I.; Kalinovskii, A.I.; Stonik, V.A. The structure of psolusoside A—The major triterpene glycoside of the sea cucumber *Psolus fabricii*. *Khim. Prir. Soedin.* **1985**, *2*, 212–217.

42. Kalinin, V.I.; Kalinovskii, A.I.; Stonik, V.A.; Dmitrenok, P.S.; Elkin, Y.N. Structure of psolusoside B—A nonholostane triterpene glycoside of the holothurian genus Psolus. *Khim. Prir. Soedin.* **1989**, *3*, 361–368. [CrossRef]

43. Silchenko, A.S.; Kalinovsky, A.I.; Avilov, S.A.; Kalinin, V.I.; Andrijaschenko, P.V.; Dmitrenok, P.S.; Chingizova, E.A.; Ermakova, S.P.; Malyarenko, O.S.; Dautova, T.N. Nine new triterpene glycosides, magnumosides A_1–A_4, B_1, B_2, C_1, C_2 and C_4, from the Vietnamese sea cucumber *Neothyonidium* (=*Massinium*) *magnum*: Structures and activities against tumor cells independently and in synergy with radioactive irradiation. *Mar. Drugs* **2017**, *15*, 256. [CrossRef] [PubMed]

44. Heftman, E.; Mosettig, E. *Biochemistry of Steroids*; Reinhold Publishing Corporation: New York, NY, USA, 1960; p. 231.

45. Silchenko, A.S.; Kalinovsky, A.I.; Avilov, S.A.; Andryjaschenko, P.V.; Dmitrenok, P.S.; Martyyas, E.A.; Kalinin, V.I.; Jayasandhya, P.; Rajan, G.C.; Padmakumar, K.P. Structures and biological activities of typicosides A_1, A_2, B_1, C_1 and C_2, triterpene glycosides from the sea cucumbers *Actinocucumis typica*. *Nat. Prod. Commun.* **2013**, *8*, 301–310. [PubMed]

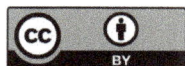

© 2017 by the authors. Licensee MDPI, Basel, Switzerland. This article is an open access article distributed under the terms and conditions of the Creative Commons Attribution (CC BY) license (http://creativecommons.org/licenses/by/4.0/).

marine drugs

MDPI

Review

Sea Cucumber Glycosides: Chemical Structures, Producing Species and Important Biological Properties

Muhammad Abdul Mojid Mondol [1], **Hee Jae Shin** [2,*], **M. Aminur Rahman** [3] and **Mohamad Tofazzal Islam** [4,*]

1   School of Science and Technology, Bangladesh Open University, Board Bazar, Gazipur 1705, Bangladesh; drmojidmondol@gmail.com
2   Marine Natural Products Laboratory, Korea Institute of Ocean Science and Technology, 787 Haeanro, Ansan 427-744, Korea
3   World Fisheries University Pilot Programme, Pukyong National University (PKNU), 45 Yongso-ro, Nam-gu, Busan 48513, Korea; aminur1963@gmail.com
4   Department of Biotechnology, Bangabandhu Sheikh Mujibur Rahman Agricultural University, Gazipur 1706, Bangladesh
*   Correspondence: shinhj@kiost.ac.kr (H.J.S.); tofazzalislam@yahoo.com (M.T.I.);
     Tel.: +82-31-400-6172 (H.J.S.); +880-2920-5310-14 (ext. 2252) (M.T.I.);
     Fax: +82-31-400-6170 (H.J.S.); +880-2920-5333 (M.T.I.)

Received: 27 June 2017; Accepted: 11 October 2017; Published: 17 October 2017

Abstract: Sea cucumbers belonging to echinoderm are traditionally used as tonic food in China and other Asian countries. They produce abundant biologically active triterpene glycosides. More than 300 triterpene glycosides have been isolated and characterized from various species of sea cucumbers, which are classified as holostane and nonholostane depending on the presence or absence of a specific structural unit $\gamma(18,20)$-lactone in the aglycone. Triterpene glycosides contain a carbohydrate chain up to six monosaccharide units mainly consisting of D-xylose, 3-O-methy-D-xylose, D-glucose, 3-O-methyl-D-glucose, and D-quinovose. Cytotoxicity is the common biological property of triterpene glycosides isolated from sea cucumbers. Besides cytotoxicity, triterpene glycosides also exhibit antifungal, antiviral and hemolytic activities. This review updates and summarizes our understanding on diverse chemical structures of triterpene glycosides from various species of sea cucumbers and their important biological activities. Mechanisms of action and structural–activity relationships (SARs) of sea cucumber glycosides are also discussed briefly.

Keywords: holostane; nonholostane; cucumarioside; cytotoxic; antifungal; glycosides

---

1. Introduction

Nature is the largest source of pharmaceutical lead drugs for the remedies of many diseases. Earlier scientists mainly focused on terrestrial samples (plants and microorganisms) for the discovery of lead bioactive compounds. With the passage of time, the search for new drugs or agrochemicals has been switching from land to ocean due to re-isolation of known natural products from terrestrial samples. Marine organisms produce diversified bioactive compounds because of large species biodiversities and living in extremely harsh environment.

Among so many sources, numerous bioactive metabolites have been isolated from marine invertebrates such as echinoderms with a broad spectrum of biological activities [1]. The echinoderms are divided into five classes, i.e., Holothuroidea (sea cucumbers), Asteroidea (starfishes), Echinoidea (sea urchins), Crinoidea (sea lilies), and Ophiuroidea (brittle stars and basket stars), which live exclusively in the marine habitat, distributed in almost all depths and latitudes, as well as reef environments or shallow shores [2,3]. The importance of these echinoderms as a potential source of bioactive compounds for the development of new therapeutic drugs/agrochemicals has been growing rapidly [1]. Compounds isolated from echinoderms showed numerous biological activities including antibacterial, anticoagulant, antifungal, antimalarial, antiprotozoal, anti-tuberculosis, anti-inflammatory, antitumor, and antiviral activities [1].

Sea cucumber traditionally has been used as tonic food in China and other Asian countries for thousands of years. Besides being used as food, sea cucumbers are also promising source of bioactive natural products which predominantly belong to triterpene glycosides exhibiting antifungal, cytotoxic, hemolytic, cytostatic, and immunomodulatory and antiviral activities [4]. Several monographs concerning the structures and biological properties of triterpene glycosides obtained from sea cucumbers have been published but not presented in a systematic way [5,6]. This report comprehensively reviews in depth structural features of sea cucumber glycosides with corresponding producing species. Important biological activities, mechanism of action, and structure–activity relationships (SARs) of the diverse glycosides produced by the different species of sea cucumber are also discussed briefly.

2. Taxonomy, Distribution and Nutritive Value of Sea Cucumbers

One of the predominant invertebrate lives in marine environment is sea cucumber, which belong to the class Holothuroidea under the phylum Echinodermata. Holothuroidea has been divided into three subclasses, Aspidochirotacea, Apodacea and Dendrochirotacea, and further into six orders, Apodida, Elasipodida, Aspidochirotida, Molpadida, Dendrochirotida and Dactylochirotida [7]. Majority of the harvestable species of sea cucumbers belong to three families, viz., Holothuriidae (genera *Holothuria* and *Bohadschia*), Stichopodidae (genera *Stichopus*, *Actinopyga*, *Thelenota*, *Parastichopus* and *Isostichopus*), and Cucumariidae (genus *Cucumaria*) [8].

Sea cucumbers are elongated tubular or flattened soft-bodied marine benthic invertebrates, typically with leathery skin, ranging in length from a few millimeters to a meter [9]. Holothuroids encompass 14,000 known species occur in most benthic marine habitats worldwide, in both temperate and tropical oceans, and from the intertidal zone to the deep sea, and are considered as the very important parts of oceanic ecosystem [10].

Economically, sea cucumbers are important in two reasons: first, some species produce triterpene glycosides that are interested to pharmaceutical companies finding their medical use and second, use as food item. About 70 species of sea cucumbers have been exploited worldwide; out of which 11 species have been found to be commercially important [11]. Sea cucumbers have been well recognized as a tonic and traditional remedy in Chinese and Malaysian literature for their effectiveness against hypertension, asthma, rheumatism, cuts and burns, impotency and constipation [12,13]. Nutritionally, sea cucumbers have an impressive profile of valuable nutrients such as vitamin A, vitamin B_1 (thiamine),vitamin B_2 (riboflavin), vitamin B_3 (niacin), and minerals, especially calcium, magnesium, iron and zinc [14,15].

3. Extraction, Purification and Characterization

To extract glycosides, first sea cucumbers will be freeze dried, then cut into pieces and extracted twice with refluxing EtOH. The combined extracts will be concentrated under reduced temperature and the residue will be dissolved in H_2O. Desalting will be carried out by passing this fraction through a Polychrom column (Teflon), eluting first the inorganic salts and crude polar impurities with H_2O and then the glycosides fraction with 50% EtOH. The fraction will be sub-fractionated by silica gel column chromatography using suitable gradient solvent system. The glycosides from each sub-fraction can be purified by reverse phase HPLC developing suitable solvent system (MeOH-H_2O).

Triterpene glycosides have two parts: carbohydrate and triterpene. The number of monosaccharide units present in the carbohydrate chain can be deduced by observing the number of anomeric carbons (~103 ppm) and protons (~5 ppm, d) resonances in ^{13}C and ^1H NMR spectra, respectively. The sequence of monosaccharide units in the carbohydrate chain can be established by the analysis of anomeric H/C correlations in the HMBC spectrum which can also be confirmed by NOE corrections between anomeric protons and MALDI-TOF mass spectroscopic data analysis. The position of attachment of glycone with aglycone can be confirmed by the HMBC experiment.

The presence of diverse types of monosaccharide units and their repetitions in the carbohydrate chain can be established by acid hydrolysis followed by GC-MS analysis of the corresponding aldononitrile peracetates [16]. The site of attachment of sulfate group at monosaccharide units can be determined by observing chemical shift of esterification carbon atoms. The chemical shifts of α (esterification) and β-carbons are shifted ~5 ppm downfield and ~2 ppm up field, respectively, compare to their corresponding nonsulfated derivatives.

The structure of the aglycone can be established based on its spectroscopic data (^{1}H NMR, ^{13}C NMR, COSY, HMBC, HSQC, and TOCSY) and by comparing with the literature data. Configuration can be determined by the analysis of NOE data, stable conformers, coupling constants and comparing chemical shifts of chiral centers with literature.

4. Structural Features of Triterpene Glycosides Isolated from Sea Cucumbers

Triterpene glycosides, also known as holothurins or saponins, are secondary metabolites typically produced by sea cucumbers (class Holothuroidea). These glycosides are amphiphilic in nature having two parts: aglycone (lipophilic, lipid-soluble) and glycone (hydrophilic, water-soluble). The majority of the glycosides contain so called holostane type aglycone comprise of lanostane-3β-ol with a γ(18,20)-lactone in the E-ring of the pentacyclic triterpene [(3β,20S-dihydroxy-5α-lanostano-γ(18,20)-lactone] (Figure 1). A few of the glycosides contain nonholostane type aglycone which do not have γ(18,20)-lactone in the tetracyclic triterpene.

The glycone parts may contain up to six monosaccharide units covalently connected to C-3 of the aglycone. The sugar moieties mainly consist of D-xylose (Xyl), D-quinovose (Qui), D-glucose (Glc), 3-O-methyl-D-glucose (MeGlc), 3-O-methyl-D-xylose (MeXyl) (Figure 2) and sometimes 3-O-methyl-D-quinovose (MeQui), 3-O-methyl-D-glucuronic acid (MeGlcA) and 6-O-acetyl-D-glucose (AcGlc). In the carbohydrate chain, the first sugar unit is always a xylose and a majority case second is quinovose, whereas 3-O-methyl-D-glucose and/or 3-O-methyl-D-xylose are always the terminal monosaccharide units. The presence of two quinovose residues in a carbohydrate chain is unique for sea cucumber and starfish glycosides.

In glycone part, the sugar units are generally arranged in a straight or branched chain (Figure 3). The majority of tetrasaccharides show a linear chain with the most common 3-O-Me-Glc-(1→3)-Glc-(1→4)-Qui-(1→2)-Xyl. Hexaglycosides are generally nonsulfated with a linear 3-O-Me-Glc (1→3)-Glc (1→4)-Xyl (2→1)-Qui (4→1)-Glc (3→1)-3-O-MeGlc unit. Pentasaccharides have a linear chain like tetrasaccharides but a branching at C-2 of quinovose (Figure 3).

Sixty percent of the triterpene glycosides isolated so far from sea cucumbers have sulfate groups linked to the monosaccharide units of the carbohydrate chain. Most of them are monosulfsated, but many di- and trisulfated glycosides have also been isolated. Most tetrasaccharides and pentasaccharides are sulfated at C-4 of xylose unit. In both the cases, additional sulfate groups at C-6 of the 3-O-methylglucose and glucose units have also been found. The term "Ds" stands for desulfated. Sea cucumber triterpene glycosides are chemotaxonomic markers specific for groups of genera within each family.

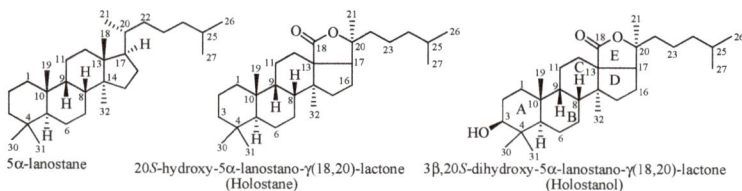

Figure 1. Structures of lanostane, holostane and holostanol.

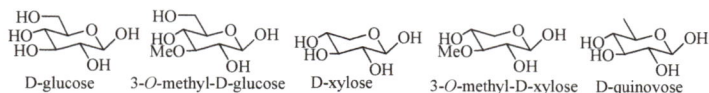

Figure 2. Common sugar units present in sea cucumber glycosides.

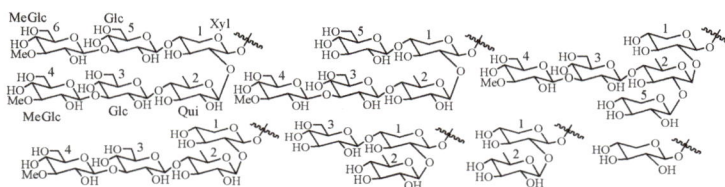

Figure 3. Some common carbohydrate architectures found in sea cucumber glycosides.

Triterpene glycosides can be classified as holostane type having 3β-hydroxy-5α-lanostano-γ(18,20)-lactone structural feature and nonholostane type do not have a γ(18,20)-lactone but have other structural features like holostane type glycosides.

4.1. Holostane Type Triterpene Glycosides

Depending on the position of double bond in the B and C ring of the aglycone (Figure 1), holostane type glycosides can be further subdivided into three groups: glycosides with 3β-hydroxyholost-7(8)-ene, 3β-hydroxyholost-9(11)-ene, and 3β-hydroxyholost-8(9)-ene aglycone skeletons. There are eight pentacyclic triterpene and 30 alkane side chain aglycone architectures commonly found in holostane type glycosides (Figure 4). In these architectures, certain functional groups are generally attached to the specific carbons: keto and β-acetoxy groups at C-16, and α-hydroxy group at C-12 and C-17.

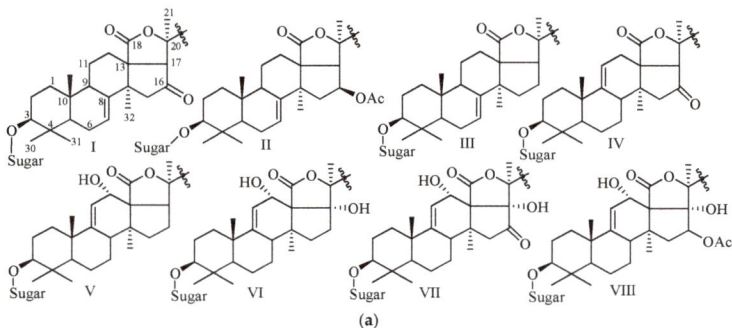

(a)

Figure 4. *Cont.*

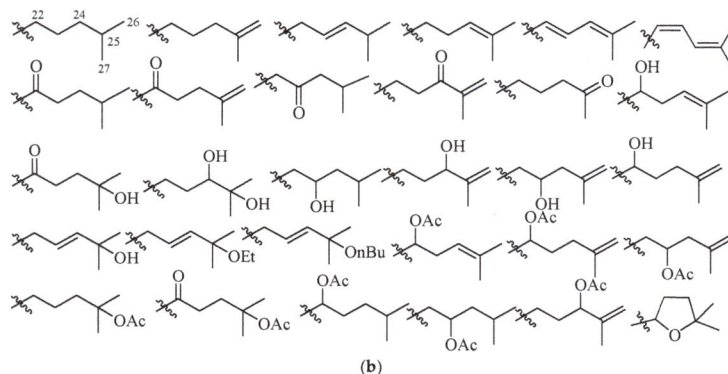

(b)

Figure 4. Pentacyclic triterpene and alkane side chain skeletons are commonly found in holostane type glycosides. (**a**) Pentacylic triterpene skeletons. Substitution by selective functional groups and unsaturation generally take place in the alkane side chain (2-methylpentane) attached to C-20 of the E-ring of aglycone; (**b**) Alkane side chain architectures.

4.1.1. 3β-Hydroxyholost-7(8)-ene Skeleton Containing Holostane Glycosides

Substantial number of triterpene glycosides in this category is produced by sea cucumbers. The species *Eupentacta fraudatrix*, *Holothuria lessoni*, *Bohadschia marmorata*, *Stichopus chloronotus* and *Staurocucumis liouvillei* produce most of the compounds in this group. For convenience, the large number of compounds in this category can be further subdivided into four groups depending on the number of sugar units.

Holostane Glycosides with 3β-Hydroxyholost-7(8)-ene Skeleton and Six Sugar Units

The name of the compounds in this group, their producing species, chemical structures and references are summarized in Table 1 and Figure 5. The most common features of glycosides in this category are the presence of α-acetoxy group at C-23, double bond at C-25(C-26) and terminal 3-*O*-methyl-D-glucose in carbohydrate chain. An interesting point to be noted in here is that the sulfate group is totally absent in this group of compounds.

Table 1. Name and producing species of glycosides with 3β-hydroxyholost-7(8)-ene and sixs ugar units.

Compound Name	Producing Species	Reference	Compound Name	Producing Species	Reference
Stichoposide C (**1**)	*Thelenota anax*	[17]	Stichoposide D (**2**)	*Thelenota anax*	[18]
Stichoposide E (**3**)	*Stichopus chloronotus*	[19]	Stichloroside A$_1$ (**4**)	*S. chloronotus*	[20]
Stichloroside A$_2$ (**5**)	*S. chloronotus*	[20]	Stichloroside B$_1$ (**6**)	*S. chloronotus*	[20]
Stichloroside B$_2$ (**7**)	*S. chloronotus*	[20]	Stichloroside C$_1$ (**8**)	*S. chloronotus*	[20]
Stichloroside C$_2$ (**9**)	*S. chloronotus*	[20]	Synallactoside A$_2$ (**10**)	*Synallactes nozawai*	[16]
Synallactoside B$_1$ (**11**)	*S. nozawai*	[16]	Variegatuside F (**12**)	*S. variegates*	[21]
Holotoxin E (**13**)	*S. japonicus*	[22]			

1 Stichoposide C $R^1 = CH_3$, $R^2 = H$, $R^3 = CH_2OH$
2 Stichoposide D $R^1 = R^3 = CH_2OH$, $R_2 = H$
3 Stichoposide E $R^1 = H$, $R^2 = R^3 = CH_2OH$

4 Stichloroside A_1 $R^1 = H$, $R^2 = CH_2OH$, $R^3 = CH_2OH$
5 Stichloroside A_2 $R^1 = H$, $R^2 = CH_2OH$, $R^3 = CH_2OH$, $\Delta^{25(26)}$
6 Stichloroside B_1 $R^1 = CH_2OH$, $R^2 = H$, $R^3 = CH_2OH$
7 Stichloroside B_2 $R^1 = CH_2OH$, $R^2 = H$, $R^3 = CH_2OH$, $\Delta^{25(26)}$
8 Stichloroside C_1 $R^1 = CH_3$, $R^2 = H$, $R^3 = CH_2OH$
9 Stichloroside C_2 $R^1 = CH_3$, $R^2 = H$, $R^3 = CH_2OH$, $\Delta^{25(26)}$
10 Synallactoside A_2 $R^1 = CH_3$, $R^2 = H$, $R^3 = H$, $\Delta^{25(26)}$
11 Synallactoside B_1 $R^1 = CH_3$, $R^2 = CH_3OH$, $R^3 = H$, $\Delta^{25(26)}$

12 Variegatuside F $R^1 = R^3 = CH_2OH$, $R^2 = H$, 23- ''''OH instead of ''''OAc
13 Holotoxin E $R^1 = CH_3$, $R^2 = H$, $R^3 = CH_2OH$, 16-=O, 23-H instead of ''''OAc, sugar unit 6=Glc, $\Delta^{25(26)}$

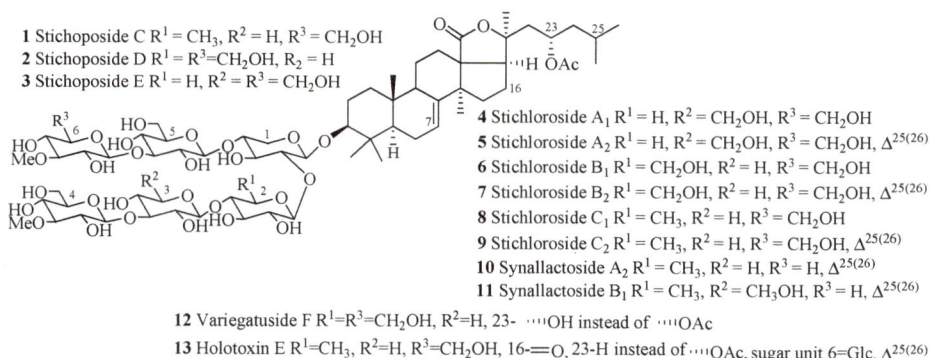

Figure 5. Chemical structures of holostane glycosides with 3β-hydroxyholost-7(8)-ene and six sugar units.

Holostane Glycosides with 3β-Hydroxyholost-7(8)-ene Skeleton and Five Sugar Units

The name of the compounds in this group, their producing species, chemical structures and references are summarized in Table 2 and Figure 6. The most common structural features in this group are the sulfate groups at C-4 of xylose and C-6 of glucose and methylglucose with either β-acetoxy or keto group at C-16 and C-25(26) double bond. A quite number of compounds contain a keto group at C-23. The rare structural features of triterpene glycoside are the presence of 16,22-epoxy group (**33**), ethoxy group (**29**) and methylglucuronic acid (**51**). Cucumarioside A_1-2 (**17**) is the only example of triterpene glycosides containing an acetate group at C-6 of the terminal sugar unit. Carbohydrate chain can be one branched (**14–48 and 52–54**) or straight (**49–51**). 3-O-methyl-D-xylose as a terminal monosaccharide unit that is a characteristic feature of all the glycosides isolated from *Eupentacta fraudatrix*.

Table 2. Name and producing species of glycosides with 3β-hydroxyholost-7(8)-ene and five sugar units.

Compound Name	Producing Species	Reference	Compound Name	Producing Species	Reference
Cucumarioside A_0-1 (**14**)	*Cucumaria japonica*	[23]	Cucumarioside A_0-2 (**15**)	*C. japonica*	[23]
Cucumarioside A_0-3 (**16**)	*C. japonica*	[23]	Cucumarioside A_1-2 (**17**)	*C. japonica*	[24]
Cucumarioside A_2-2 (**18**)	*C. japonica*	[25]	Cucumarioside A_2-3 (**19**)	*C. japonica*	[24]
Cucumarioside A_2-4 (**20**)	*C. japonica*	[24]	Cucumarioside A_2-5 (**21**)	*C. conicospermium*	[26]
Cucumarioside A_4-2 (**22**)	*C. japonica*	[24]	Cucumarioside A_6-2 (**23**)	*C. japonica*	[27]
Cucumarioside A_7-1 (**24**)	*C. japonica*	[28]	Cucumarioside A_7-2 (**25**)	*C. japonica*	[28]
Cucumarioside A_7-3 (**26**)	*C. japonica*	[28]	Cucumarioside H (**27**)	*E. fraudatrix*	[29]
Cucumarioside H_2 (**28**)	*E. fraudatrix*	[30]	Cucumarioside H_4 (**29**)	*E. fraudatrix*	[30]
Cucumarioside H_5 (**30**)	*E. fraudatrix*	[29]	Cucumarioside H_6 (**31**)	*E. fraudatrix*	[29]
Cucumarioside H_7 (**32**)	*E. fraudatrix*	[29]	Cucumarioside H_8 (**33**)	*E. fraudatrix*	[29]
Cucumarioside I_1 (**34**)	*E. fraudatrix*	[31]	Cucumarioside I_2 (**35**)	*E. fraudatrix*	[32]
Cucumarioside I_3 (**36**)	*E. fraudatrix*	[31]	Frondoside A (**37**)	*C. frondosa*	[33]
Frondoside B (**38**)	*C. frondosa*	[34]	Frondoside A_2-1 (**39**)	*C. frondosa*	[35]
Frondoside A_2-2 (**40**)	*C. frondosa*	[35]	Frondoside A_2-3 (**41**)	*C. frondosa*	[35]
Frondoside A_2-4 (**42**)	*C. frondosa*	[36]	Calcigeroside C_2 (**43**)	*P. calcigera*	[37]
Calcigeroside D_2 (**44**)	*P. calcigera*	[38]	Calcigeroside E (**45**)	*P. calcigera*	[38]
Colochiroside A (**46**)	*C. anceps*	[39]	Cucumarioside C_1 (**47**)	*E. fraudatrix*	[40]
Cucumarioside C_2 (**48**)	*E. fraudatrix*	[40]	Synallactoside B_2 (**49**)	*S. nozawai*	[16]
Synallactoside C (**50**)	*S. nozawai*	[16]	Synaptoside A (**51**)	*Synapta maculata*	[41]
Okhotoside A_2-1 (**52**)	*C. okhotensis*	[42]	Frondoside A_7-1 (**53**)	*C. frondosa*	[43]
Frondoside A_7-2 (**54**)	*C. frondosa*	[43]			

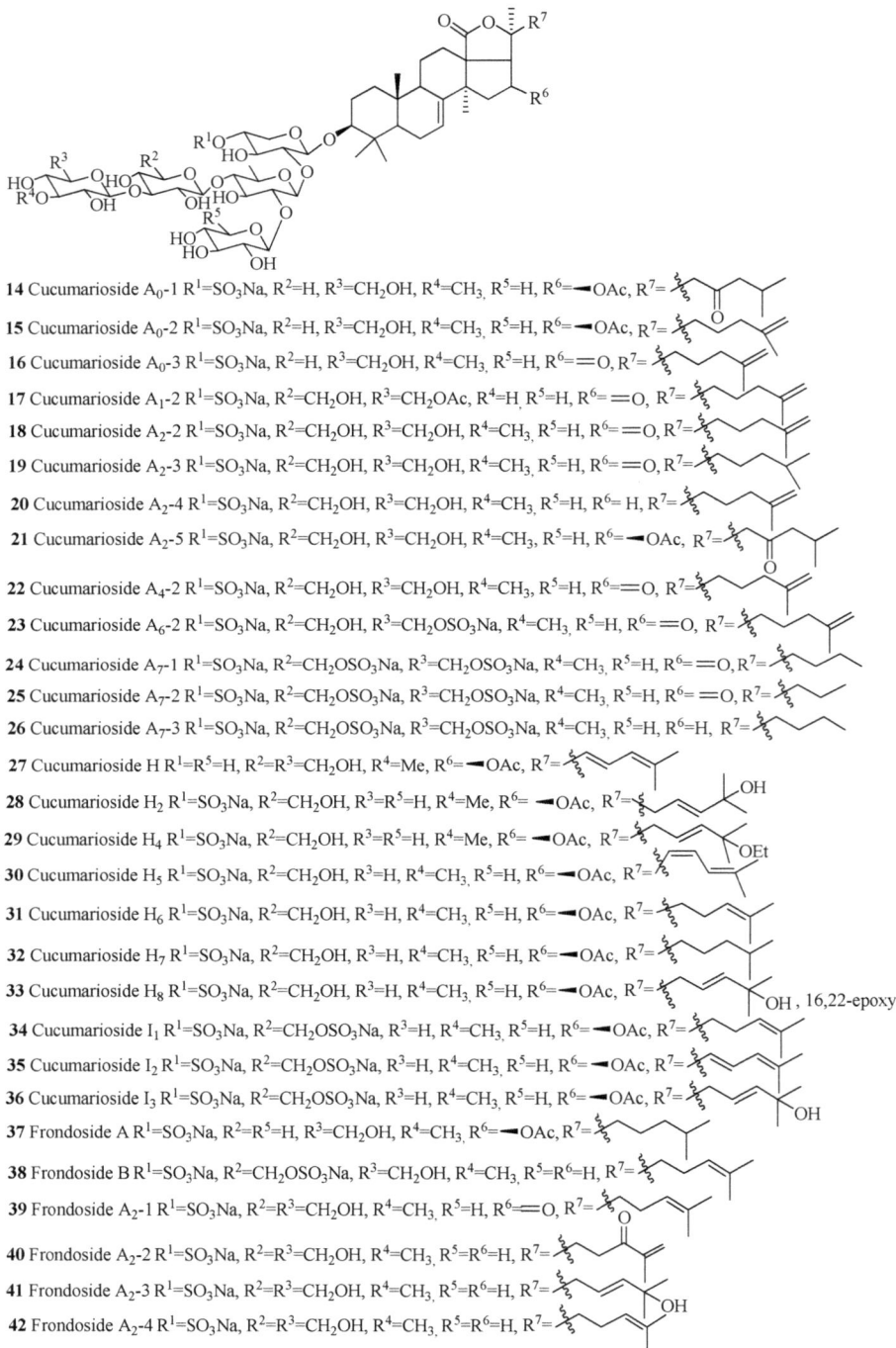

14 Cucumarioside A_0-1 R^1=SO_3Na, R^2=H, R^3=CH_2OH, R^4=CH_3, R^5=H, R^6=—OAc, R^7=

15 Cucumarioside A_0-2 R^1=SO_3Na, R^2=H, R^3=CH_2OH, R^4=CH_3, R^5=H, R^6=—OAc, R^7=

16 Cucumarioside A_0-3 R^1=SO_3Na, R^2=H, R^3=CH_2OH, R^4=CH_3, R^5=H, R^6==O, R^7=

17 Cucumarioside A_1-2 R^1=SO_3Na, R^2=CH_2OH, R^3=CH_2OAc, R^4=H, R^5=H, R^6==O, R^7=

18 Cucumarioside A_2-2 R^1=SO_3Na, R^2=CH_2OH, R^3=CH_2OH, R^4=CH_3, R^5=H, R^6==O, R^7=

19 Cucumarioside A_2-3 R^1=SO_3Na, R^2=CH_2OH, R^3=CH_2OH, R^4=CH_3, R^5=H, R^6==O, R^7=

20 Cucumarioside A_2-4 R^1=SO_3Na, R^2=CH_2OH, R^3=CH_2OH, R^4=CH_3, R^5=H, R^6=H, R^7=

21 Cucumarioside A_2-5 R^1=SO_3Na, R^2=CH_2OH, R^3=CH_2OH, R^4=CH_3, R^5=H, R^6=—OAc, R^7=

22 Cucumarioside A_4-2 R^1=SO_3Na, R^2=CH_2OH, R^3=CH_2OH, R^4=CH_3, R^5=H, R^6==O, R^7=

23 Cucumarioside A_6-2 R^1=SO_3Na, R^2=CH_2OH, R^3=CH_2OSO_3Na, R^4=CH_3, R^5=H, R^6==O, R^7=

24 Cucumarioside A_7-1 R^1=SO_3Na, R^2=CH_2OSO_3Na, R^3=CH_2OSO_3Na, R^4=CH_3, R^5=H, R^6==O, R^7=

25 Cucumarioside A_7-2 R^1=SO_3Na, R^2=CH_2OSO_3Na, R^3=CH_2OSO_3Na, R^4=CH_3, R^5=H, R^6==O, R^7=

26 Cucumarioside A_7-3 R^1=SO_3Na, R^2=CH_2OSO_3Na, R^3=CH_2OSO_3Na, R^4=CH_3, R^5=H, R^6=H, R^7=

27 Cucumarioside H R^1=R^5=H, R^2=R^3=CH_2OH, R^4=Me, R^6=—OAc, R^7=

28 Cucumarioside H_2 R^1=SO_3Na, R^2=CH_2OH, R^3=R^5=H, R^4=Me, R^6=—OAc, R^7=

29 Cucumarioside H_4 R^1=SO_3Na, R^2=CH_2OH, R^3=R^5=H, R^4=Me, R^6=—OAc, R^7=

30 Cucumarioside H_5 R^1=SO_3Na, R^2=CH_2OH, R^3=H, R^4=CH_3, R^5=H, R^6=—OAc, R^7=

31 Cucumarioside H_6 R^1=SO_3Na, R^2=CH_2OH, R^3=H, R^4=CH_3, R^5=H, R^6=—OAc, R^7=

32 Cucumarioside H_7 R^1=SO_3Na, R^2=CH_2OH, R^3=H, R^4=CH_3, R^5=H, R^6=—OAc, R^7=

33 Cucumarioside H_8 R^1=SO_3Na, R^2=CH_2OH, R^3=H, R^4=CH_3, R^5=H, R^6=—OAc, R^7= , 16,22-epoxy

34 Cucumarioside I_1 R^1=SO_3Na, R^2=CH_2OSO_3Na, R^3=H, R^4=CH_3, R^5=H, R^6=—OAc, R^7=

35 Cucumarioside I_2 R^1=SO_3Na, R^2=CH_2OSO_3Na, R^3=H, R^4=CH_3, R^5=H, R^6=—OAc, R^7=

36 Cucumarioside I_3 R^1=SO_3Na, R^2=CH_2OSO_3Na, R^3=H, R^4=CH_3, R^5=H, R^6=—OAc, R^7=

37 Frondoside A R^1=SO_3Na, R^2=R^5=H, R^3=CH_2OH, R^4=CH_3, R^6=—OAc, R^7=

38 Frondoside B R^1=SO_3Na, R^2=CH_2OSO_3Na, R^3=CH_2OH, R^4=CH_3, R^5=R^6=H, R^7=

39 Frondoside A_2-1 R^1=SO_3Na, R^2=R^3=CH_2OH, R^4=CH_3, R^5=H, R^6==O, R^7=

40 Frondoside A_2-2 R^1=SO_3Na, R^2=R^3=CH_2OH, R^4=CH_3, R^5=R^6=H, R^7=

41 Frondoside A_2-3 R^1=SO_3Na, R^2=R^3=CH_2OH, R^4=CH_3, R^5=R^6=H, R^7=

42 Frondoside A_2-4 R^1=SO_3Na, R^2=R^3=CH_2OH, R^4=CH_3, R^5=R^6=H, R^7=

Figure 6. *Cont.*

43 Calcigeroside C$_2$ R^1=SO$_3$Na, R^2=CH$_2$OH, R^3=H, R^4=CH$_3$ R^5=CH$_2$OH, R^6=H, R^7=

44 Calcigeroside D$_2$ R^1=SO$_3$Na, R^2=CH$_2$OSO$_3$Na, R^3=H, R^4=CH$_3$ R^5=CH$_2$OH, R^6=H, R^7=

45 Calcigeroside E R^1=SO$_3$Na, R^2=R^5=CH$_2$OH, R^3=CH$_2$OSO$_3$Na, R^4=CH$_3$ R^6=—OAc, R^7=

46 Colochiroside A R^1=SO$_3$Na, R^2=CH$_2$OSO$_3$Na, R^3=CH$_2$OH, R^4=CH$_3$, R^5=H, R^6===O, R^7=

47 Cucumarioside C$_1$ R^1=R^5=H, R^2=R^3=CH$_2$OH, R^4=CH$_3$, R^6= —OAc, R^7=

48 Cucumarioside C$_2$ R^1=R^5=H, R^2=R^3=CH$_2$OH, R^4=CH$_3$, R^6= —OAc, R^7=

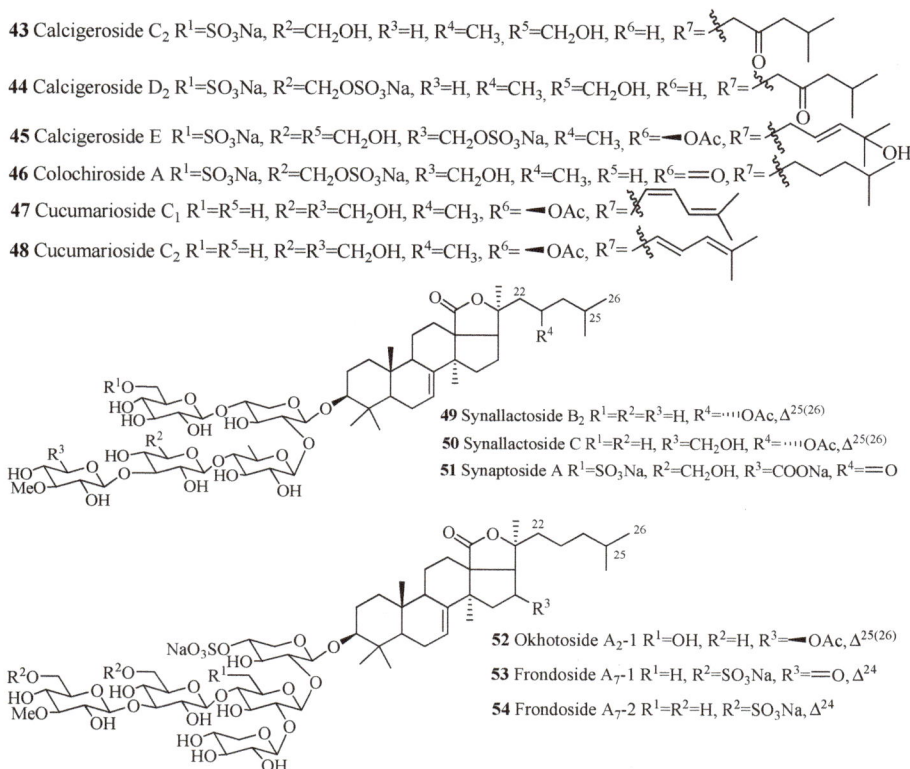

49 Synallactoside B$_2$ R^1=R^2=R^3=H, R^4=''''OAc, Δ$^{25(26)}$

50 Synallactoside C R^1=R^2=H, R^3=CH$_2$OH, R^4=''''OAc, Δ$^{25(26)}$

51 Synaptoside A R^1=SO$_3$Na, R^2=CH$_2$OH, R^3=COONa, R^4===O

52 Okhotoside A$_2$-1 R^1=OH, R^2=H, R^3=—OAc, Δ$^{25(26)}$

53 Frondoside A$_7$-1 R^1=H, R^2=SO$_3$Na, R^3===O, Δ^{24}

54 Frondoside A$_7$-2 R^1=R^2=H, R^2=SO$_3$Na, Δ^{24}

Figure 6. Chemical structures of holostane glycosides with 3β-hydroxyholost-7(8)-ene and five sugar units.

Holostane Glycosides with 3β-Hydroxyholost-7(8)-ene Skeleton and Four Sugar Units

Several compounds in this group were isolated from the species of *Staurocucumis liouvillei* and *Eupentacta fraudatrix* (Table 3). The most common characteristic of glycosides in the group is the presence of sulfate at C-4 of xylose and either keto or β-acetoxy group at C-16 (Figure 7). Some of the compounds in this series, especially liouvillosides, violaceusosides and cucumechinosides, may contain up to three sulfates in their carbohydrate chain. The presence of α-hydroxy at C-12 and C-17 (**78** and **79**), artifact *n*-butoxy (**113**) and ethoxy (**114**) groups at C-25, and three consecutive xylose sugar units in carbohydrate chain (**72**) are rare structural features in this category. Cucumariosides A$_1$ (**111**), A$_5$ (**115**) and A$_{11}$ (**118**) are the desulfated derivatives of cucumariosides G$_1$ (**123**), G$_3$ (**124**) and G$_4$ (**125**), respectively.

Table 3. Name and producing species of glycosides with 3β-hydroxyholost-7(8)-ene and four sugar units.

Compound Name	Producing Species	Reference	Compound Name	Producing Species	Reference
Liouvilloside A (**55**)	*Staurocucumis liouvillei*	[44]	Liouvilloside A$_1$ (**56**)	*S. liouviellei*	[45]
Liouvilloside A$_2$ (**57**)	*S. liouvillei*	[45]	Liouvilloside A$_3$ (**58**)	*S. liouvillei*	[45]
Liouvilloside A$_5$ (**59**)	*S. liouvillei*	[46]	Liouvilloside B (**60**)	*S. liouvillei*	[44]
Liouvilloside B$_1$ (**61**)	*S. liouvillei*	[45]	Liouvilloside B$_2$ (**62**)	*S. liouvillei*	[45]
Violaceuside A (**63**)	*P. violeceus*	[47]	Violaceuside B (**64**)	*P. violeceus*	[47]
Violaceuside I (**65**)	*P. violeceus*	[48]	Violaceuside II (**66**)	*P. violeceus*	[48]

Table 3. *Cont.*

Compound Name	Producing Species	Reference	Compound Name	Producing Species	Reference
Violaceuside III (67)	*P. violeceus*	[48]	Intercedenside A (68)	*M. intercedens*	[49]
Intercedenside B (67)	*Mensamria intercedens*	[49]	Intercedenside C (70)	*M. intercedens*	[49]
Intercedenside D (71)	*M. intercedens*	[50]	Intercedenside E (72)	*M. intercedens*	[50]
Intercedenside F (73)	*M. intercedens*	[50]	Intercedenside G (74)	*M. intercedens*	[50]
Intercedenside H (75)	*M. intercedens*	[50]	Intercedenside I (76)	*M. intercedens*	[50]
Patagonicoside A (77)	*Psolus patagonicus*	[51]	Patagonicoside B (78)	*P. patagonicus*	[52]
Patagonicoside C (79)	*P. patagonicus*	[52]	Philinopside A (80)	*P. quadrangularis*	[53]
Philinopside B (81)	*Pentacta quadrangularis*	[53]	Philinopside E (82)	*P. quadrangularis*	[54]
Philinopside F (83)	*P. quadrangularis*	[54]	Molliside A (84)	*A. mollis*	[55]
Molliside B$_2$ (85)	*Australostichopus mollis*	[55]	Eximisoside A (86)	*P. eximius*	[56]
Pseudostichoposide A (87)	*Pseudostichopus trachus*	[57]	Cucumarioside F$_1$ (88)	*E. fraudatrix*	[58]
Cucumarioside F$_2$ (89)	*E. fraudatrix*	[58]	Pseudocnoside A (90)	*P. leoninus*	[59]
Typicoside A$_1$ (91)	*Actinocucumis typica*	[60]	Typicoside A$_2$ (92)	*A. typica*	[60]
Typicoside B$_1$ (93)	*A. typica*	[60]	Typicoside C$_1$ (94)	*A. typica*	[60]
Typicoside C$_2$ (95)	*A. typica*	[60]	Frondoside A$_1$ (96)	*C. okhotensis*	[61]
Okhotoside A$_1$-1 (97)	*Cucumaria okhotensis*	[61]	Okhotoside B$_1$ (98)	*C. okhotensis*	[62]
Okhotoside B$_2$ (99)	*C. okhotensis*	[62]	Okhotoside B$_3$ (100)	*C. okhotensis*	[62]
Colochiroside A$_1$ (101)	*Colochirus robustus*	[63]	Colochiroside A$_2$ (102)	*C. robustus*	[63]
Colochiroside A$_3$ (103)	*C. robustus*	[63]	Colochiroside B$_1$ (104)	*C. robustus*	[64]
Colochiroside B$_2$ (105)	*C. robustus*	[64]	Colochiroside B$_3$ (106)	*C. robustus*	[64]
Violaceusosides C (107)	*P. violaceus*	[65]	Violaceusosides D (108)	*P. violaceus*	[65]
Violaceusosides E (109)	*P. violaceus*	[65]	Violaceusosides G (110)	*P. violaceus*	[65]
Cucumarioside A$_1$ (111)	*E. fraudatrix*	[66]	Cucumarioside A$_2$ (112)	*E. fraudatrix*	[67]
Cucumarioside A$_3$ (113)	*E. fraudatrix*	[66]	Cucumarioside A$_4$ (114)	*E. fraudatrix*	[66]
Cucumarioside A$_5$ (115)	*E. fraudatrix*	[66]	Cucumarioside A$_6$ (116)	*E. fraudatrix*	[66]
Cucumarioside A$_7$ (117)	*E. fraudatrix*	[67]	Cucumarioside A$_{11}$ (118)	*E. fraudatrix*	[67]
Cucumarioside A$_{12}$ (119)	*E. fraudatrix*	[66]	Cucumarioside A$_{13}$ (120)	*E. fraudatrix*	[67]
Cucumarioside A$_{14}$ (121)	*E. fraudatrix*	[67]	Cucumarioside A$_{15}$ (122)	*E. fraudatrix*	[66]
Cucumarioside G$_1$ (123)	*C. fraudatrix*	[68]	Cucumarioside G$_3$ (124)	*E. fraudatrix*	[69]
Cucumarioside G$_4$ (125)	*E. fraudatrix*	[70]	Pentactaside B (126)	*P. quadrangularis*	[71]
Pentactaside C (127)	*P. quadrangularis*	[71]	Pseudostichoposide B (128)	*P. trachus*	[72]
Variegatuside A (129)	*S. variegates*	[73]	Variegatuside C (130)	*S. variegates*	[21]
Synallactoside A$_1$ (131)	*S. nozawai*	[16]	Thelenotoside A (132)	*Thelenota ananas*	[74]
Thelenotoside B (133)	*T. ananas*	[74]	Cucumechinoside A (134)	*C. echinata*	[75]
Cucumechinoside B (135)	*C. echinata*	[75]	Cucumechinoside C (136)	*C. echinata*	[75]
Cucumechinoside D (137)	*C. echinata*	[75]	Cucumechinoside E (138)	*C. echinata*	[75]
Cucumechinoside F (139)	*C. echinata*	[75]	Lefevreoside A$_1$ (140)	*C. lefevrei*	[76]
Lefevreoside A$_2$ (141)	*C. lefevrei*	[76]	Lefevreoside C (142)	*C. lefevrei*	[76]
Lefevreoside D (143)	*C. lefevrei*	[76]			

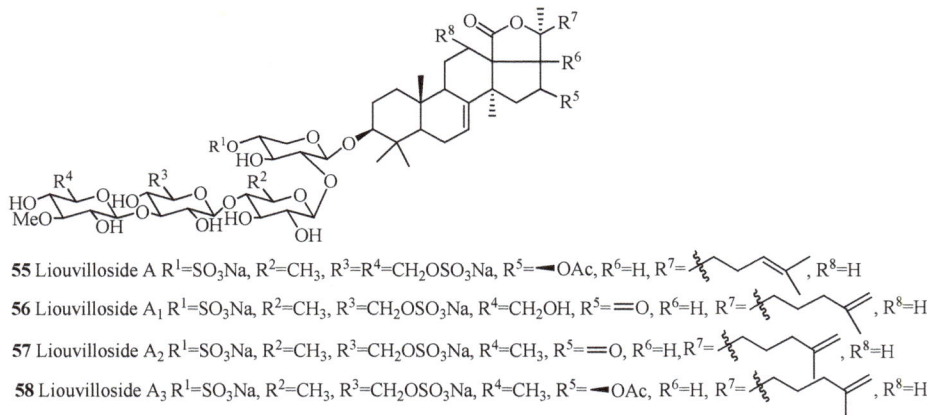

55 Liouvilloside A R^1=SO$_3$Na, R^2=CH$_3$, R^3=R^4=CH$_2$OSO$_3$Na, R^5=◄OAc, R^6=H, R^7= [structure] , R^8=H

56 Liouvilloside A$_1$ R^1=SO$_3$Na, R^2=CH$_3$, R^3=CH$_2$OSO$_3$Na, R^4=CH$_2$OH, R^5==O, R^6=H, R^7= [structure] , R^8=H

57 Liouvilloside A$_2$ R^1=SO$_3$Na, R^2=CH$_3$, R^3=CH$_2$OSO$_3$Na, R^4=CH$_3$, R^5==O, R^6=H,R^7= [structure] , R^8=H

58 Liouvilloside A$_3$ R^1=SO$_3$Na, R^2=CH$_3$, R^3=CH$_2$OSO$_3$Na, R^4=CH$_3$, R^5=◄OAc, R^6=H, R^7= [structure]

Figure 7. *Cont.*

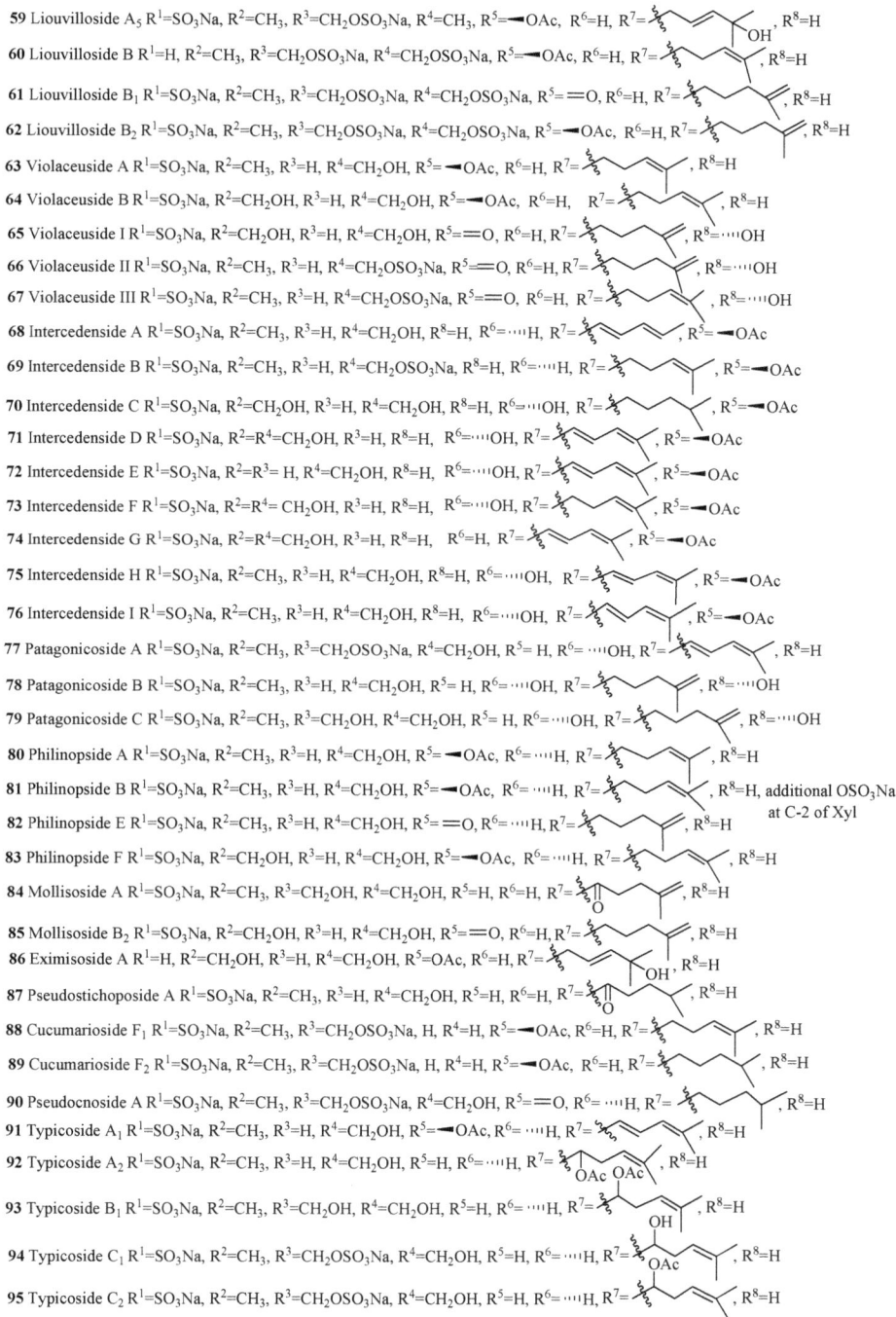

59 Liouvilloside A_5 R^1=SO$_3$Na, R^2=CH$_3$, R^3=CH$_2$OSO$_3$Na, R^4=CH$_3$, R^5=⬤OAc, R^6=H, R^7= [structure] , R^8=H

60 Liouvilloside B R^1=H, R^2=CH$_3$, R^3=CH$_2$OSO$_3$Na, R^4=CH$_2$OSO$_3$Na, R^5=⬤OAc, R^6=H, R^7= [structure] , R^8=H

61 Liouvilloside B_1 R^1=SO$_3$Na, R^2=CH$_3$, R^3=CH$_2$OSO$_3$Na, R^4=CH$_2$OSO$_3$Na, R^5==O, R^6=H, R^7= [structure] , R^8=H

62 Liouvilloside B_2 R^1=SO$_3$Na, R^2=CH$_3$, R^3=CH$_2$OSO$_3$Na, R^4=CH$_2$OSO$_3$Na, R^5=⬤OAc, R^6=H, R^7= [structure] , R^8=H

63 Violaceuside A R^1=SO$_3$Na, R^2=CH$_3$, R^3=H, R^4=CH$_2$OH, R^5=⬤OAc, R^6=H, R^7= [structure] , R^8=H

64 Violaceuside B R^1=SO$_3$Na, R^2=CH$_2$OH, R^3=H, R^4=CH$_2$OH, R^5=⬤OAc, R^6=H, R^7= [structure] , R^8=H

65 Violaceuside I R^1=SO$_3$Na, R^2=CH$_2$OH, R^3=H, R^4=CH$_2$OH, R^5==O, R^6=H, R^7= [structure] , R^8=''''OH

66 Violaceuside II R^1=SO$_3$Na, R^2=CH$_3$, R^3=H, R^4=CH$_2$OSO$_3$Na, R^5==O, R^6=H, R^7= [structure] , R^8=''''OH

67 Violaceuside III R^1=SO$_3$Na, R^2=CH$_3$, R^3=H, R^4=CH$_2$OSO$_3$Na, R^5==O, R^6=H, R^7= [structure] , R^8=''''OH

68 Intercedenside A R^1=SO$_3$Na, R^2=CH$_3$, R^3=H, R^4=CH$_2$OH, R^8=H, R^6=''''H, R^7= [structure] , R^5=⬤OAc

69 Intercedenside B R^1=SO$_3$Na, R^2=CH$_3$, R^3=H, R^4=CH$_2$OSO$_3$Na, R^8=H, R^6=''''H, R^7= [structure] , R^5=⬤OAc

70 Intercedenside C R^1=SO$_3$Na, R^2=CH$_2$OH, R^3=H, R^4=CH$_2$OH, R^8=H, R^6=''''OH, R^7= [structure] , R^5=⬤OAc

71 Intercedenside D R^1=SO$_3$Na, R^2=R^4=CH$_2$OH, R^3=H, R^8=H, R^6=''''OH, R^7= [structure] , R^5=⬤OAc

72 Intercedenside E R^1=SO$_3$Na, R^2=R^3= H, R^4=CH$_2$OH, R^8=H, R^6=''''OH, R^7= [structure] , R^5=⬤OAc

73 Intercedenside F R^1=SO$_3$Na, R^2=R^4= CH$_2$OH, R^3=H, R^8=H, R^6=''''OH, R^7= [structure] , R^5=⬤OAc

74 Intercedenside G R^1=SO$_3$Na, R^2=R^4=CH$_2$OH, R^3=H, R^8=H, R^6=H, R^7= [structure] , R^5=⬤OAc

75 Intercedenside H R^1=SO$_3$Na, R^2=CH$_3$, R^3=H, R^4=CH$_2$OH, R^8=H, R^6=''''OH, R^7= [structure] , R^5=⬤OAc

76 Intercedenside I R^1=SO$_3$Na, R^2=CH$_3$, R^3=H, R^4=CH$_2$OH, R^8=H, R^6=''''OH, R^7= [structure] , R^5=⬤OAc

77 Patagonicoside A R^1=SO$_3$Na, R^2=CH$_3$, R^3=CH$_2$OSO$_3$Na, R^4=CH$_2$OH, R^5= H, R^6= ''''OH, R^7= [structure] , R^8=H

78 Patagonicoside B R^1=SO$_3$Na, R^2=CH$_3$, R^3=H, R^4=CH$_2$OH, R^5= H, R^6= ''''OH, R^7= [structure] , R^8=''''OH

79 Patagonicoside C R^1=SO$_3$Na, R^2=CH$_3$, R^3=CH$_2$OH, R^4=CH$_2$OH, R^5= H, R^6= ''''OH, R^7= [structure] , R^8=''''OH

80 Philinopside A R^1=SO$_3$Na, R^2=CH$_3$, R^3=H, R^4=CH$_2$OH, R^5= ⬤OAc, R^6= ''''H, R^7= [structure] , R^8=H

81 Philinopside B R^1=SO$_3$Na, R^2=CH$_3$, R^3=H, R^4=CH$_2$OH, R^5= ⬤OAc, R^6= ''''H, R^7= [structure] , R^8=H, additional OSO$_3$Na at C-2 of Xyl

82 Philinopside E R^1=SO$_3$Na, R^2=CH$_3$, R^3=H, R^4=CH$_2$OH, R^5= ==O, R^6= ''''H, R^7= [structure] , R^8=H

83 Philinopside F R^1=SO$_3$Na, R^2=CH$_2$OH, R^3=H, R^4=CH$_2$OH, R^5=⬤OAc, R^6= ''''H, R^7= [structure] , R^8=H

84 Mollisoside A R^1=SO$_3$Na, R^2=CH$_3$, R^3=CH$_2$OH, R^4=CH$_2$OH, R^5=H, R^6=H, R^7= [structure] , R^8=H

85 Mollisoside B_2 R^1=SO$_3$Na, R^2=CH$_2$OH, R^3=H, R^4=CH$_2$OH, R^5===O, R^6=H, R^7= [structure] , R^8=H

86 Eximisoside A R^1=H, R^2=CH$_2$OH, R^3=H, R^4=CH$_2$OH, R^5=OAc, R^6=H, R^7= [structure] , R^8=H

87 Pseudostichoposide A R^1=SO$_3$Na, R^2=CH$_3$, R^3=H, R^4=CH$_2$OH, R^5=H, R^6=H, R^7= [structure] , R^8=H

88 Cucumarioside F_1 R^1=SO$_3$Na, R^2=CH$_3$, R^3=CH$_2$OSO$_3$Na, H, R^4=H, R^5=⬤OAc, R^6=H, R^7= [structure] , R^8=H

89 Cucumarioside F_2 R^1=SO$_3$Na, R^2=CH$_3$, R^3=CH$_2$OSO$_3$Na, H, R^4=H, R^5=⬤OAc, R^6=H, R^7= [structure] , R^8=H

90 Pseudocnoside A R^1=SO$_3$Na, R^2=CH$_3$, R^3=CH$_2$OSO$_3$Na, R^4=CH$_2$OH, R^5===O, R^6= ''''H, R^7= [structure] , R^8=H

91 Typicoside A_1 R^1=SO$_3$Na, R^2=CH$_3$, R^3=H, R^4=CH$_2$OH, R^5=⬤OAc, R^6= ''''H, R^7= [structure] , R^8=H

92 Typicoside A_2 R^1=SO$_3$Na, R^2=CH$_3$, R^3=H, R^4=CH$_2$OH, R^5=H, R^6= ''''H, R^7= [structure] , R^8=H

93 Typicoside B_1 R^1=SO$_3$Na, R^2=CH$_3$, R^3=CH$_2$OH, R^4=CH$_2$OH, R^5=H, R^6= ''''H, R^7= [structure] , R^8=H

94 Typicoside C_1 R^1=SO$_3$Na, R^2=CH$_3$, R^3=CH$_2$OSO$_3$Na, R^4=CH$_2$OH, R^5=H, R^6= ''''H, R^7= [structure] , R^8=H

95 Typicoside C_2 R^1=SO$_3$Na, R^2=CH$_3$, R^3=CH$_2$OSO$_3$Na, R^4=CH$_2$OH, R^5=H, R^6= ''''H, R^7= [structure] , R^8=H

Figure 7. *Cont.*

96 Frondoside A$_1$ R^1=SO$_3$Na, R^2=CH$_3$, R^3=R^6=H, R^4=CH$_2$OH, R^5=—OAc, R^7= , R^8=H

97 Okhotoside A$_1$-1 R^1=SO$_3$Na, R^2=CH$_3$, R^3=R^6=H, R^4=CH$_2$OH, R^5=—OAc, R^7= , R^8=H

98 Okhotoside B$_1$ R^1=SO$_3$Na, R^2=R^3=R^4=CH$_2$OH, R^6=H, R^5= —OAc, R^7= , R^8=H

99 Okhotoside B$_2$ R^1=SO$_3$Na, R^2=R^4=CH$_2$OH, R^3=CH$_2$OSO$_3$Na, R^6=H, R^5= —OAc, R^7= , R^8=H

100 Okhotoside B$_3$ R^1=OH, R^2=CH$_2$OH, R^3=R^4=CH$_2$OSO$_3$Na, R^6=H, R^5=—OAc, R^7= , R^8=H

101 Colochiroside A$_1$ R^1=SO$_3$Na, R^2=R^4=CH$_2$OH, R^3=H, R^5= —OAc, R^6=····H, R^7= , R^8=H

102 Colochiroside A$_2$ R^1=SO$_3$Na, R^2=R^4=CH$_2$OH, R^3= R^5=H, R^6=····H, R^7= , R^8=H

103 Colochiroside A$_3$ R^1=SO$_3$Na, R^2=R^4=CH$_2$OH, R^3= R^5=H, R^6=····H,R^7= , R^8=H

104 Colochiroside B$_1$ R^1=SO$_3$Na, R^2=CH$_3$, R^3=H, R^4=CH$_2$OH, R^5= —OAc, R^6=····H, R^7= , R^8=H

105 Colochiroside B$_2$ R^1=SO$_3$Na, R^2=CH$_3$, R^3=H, R^4=CH$_2$OH, R^5= —OAc, R^6=····H, R^7= , R^8=H

106 Cloochiroside B$_3$ R^1=SO$_3$Na, R^2=CH$_3$, R^3=H, R^4=CH$_2$OH, R^5= —OAc, R^6=····H, R^7= , R^8=H

107 Violaceusoside C R^1=SO$_3$Na, R^2=CH$_3$, R^3=H, R^4=CH$_2$OH, R^5==O, R^6=····H, R^7= , R^8=H

108 Violaceusoside D R^1=SO$_3$Na, R^2=CH$_3$, R^3=CH$_2$OSO$_3$Na, R^4=CH$_2$OH, R^5=—OAc, R^6=····H, R^7= , R^8=H

109 Violaceusoside E R^1=SO$_3$Na, R^2=CH$_3$, R^3=H, R^4=CH$_2$OH, R^5==O, R^6= ····H, R^7= , R^8=H
(additional OSO$_3$Na at C-3 of Qui)

110 Violaceusoside G R^1=SO$_3$Na, R^2=CH$_3$, R^3=H, R^4=CH$_2$OSO$_3$Na, R^5=—OAc, R^6= ····H, R^7= , R^8=H
(additional OSO$_3$Na at C-3 of Qui)

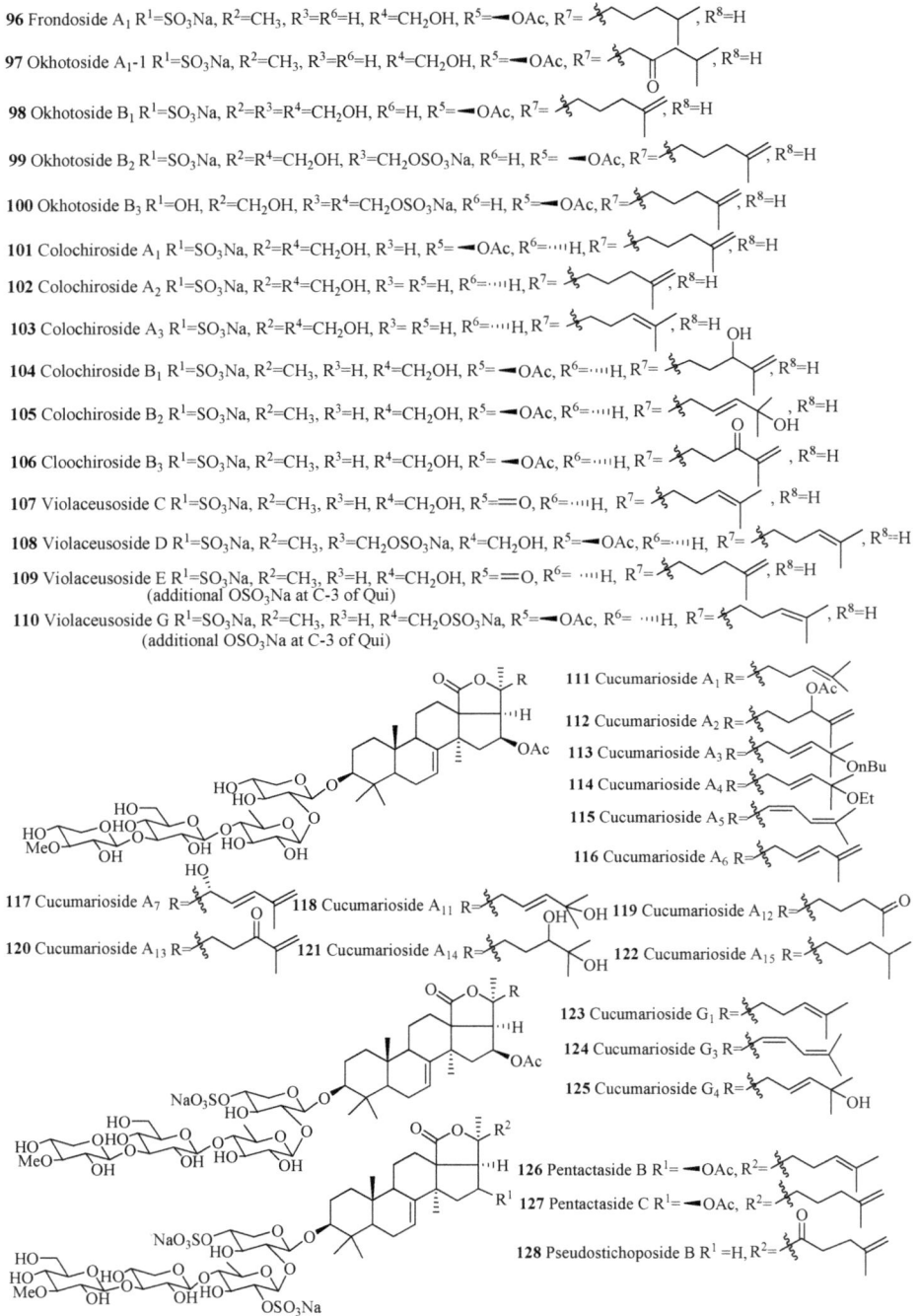

111 Cucumarioside A$_1$ R=

112 Cucumarioside A$_2$ R=

113 Cucumarioside A$_3$ R=

114 Cucumarioside A$_4$ R=

115 Cucumarioside A$_5$ R=

116 Cucumarioside A$_6$ R=

117 Cucumarioside A$_7$ R=

118 Cucumarioside A$_{11}$ R=

119 Cucumarioside A$_{12}$ R=

120 Cucumarioside A$_{13}$ R=

121 Cucumarioside A$_{14}$ R=

122 Cucumarioside A$_{15}$ R=

123 Cucumarioside G$_1$ R=

124 Cucumarioside G$_3$ R=

125 Cucumarioside G$_4$ R=

126 Pentactaside B R^1= —OAc, R^2=

127 Pentactaside C R^1= —OAc, R^2=

128 Pseudostichoposide B R^1 =H, R^2=

Figure 7. *Cont.*

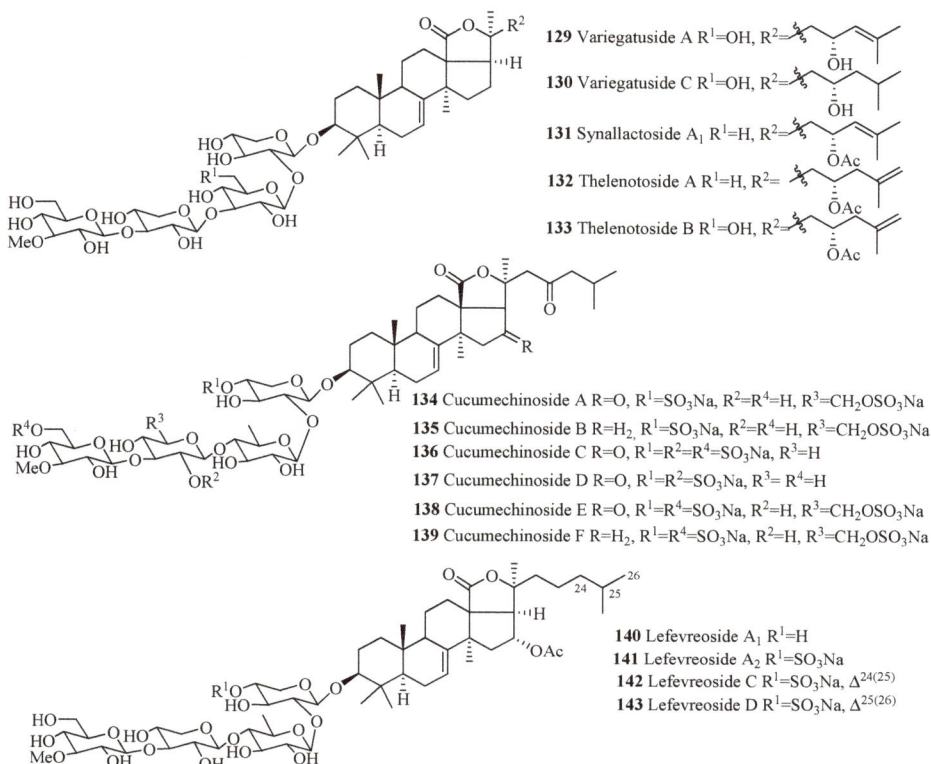

129 Variegatuside A R^1=OH, R^2=

130 Variegatuside C R^1=OH, R^2=

131 Synallactoside A$_1$ R^1=H, R^2=

132 Thelenotoside A R^1=H, R^2=

133 Thelenotoside B R^1=OH, R^2=

134 Cucumechinoside A R=O, R^1=SO$_3$Na, R^2=R^4=H, R^3=CH$_2$OSO$_3$Na

135 Cucumechinoside B R=H$_2$, R^1=SO$_3$Na, R^2=R^4=H, R^3=CH$_2$OSO$_3$Na

136 Cucumechinoside C R=O, R^1=R^2=R^4=SO$_3$Na, R^3=H

137 Cucumechinoside D R=O, R^1=R^2=SO$_3$Na, R^3= R^4=H

138 Cucumechinoside E R=O, R^1=R^4=SO$_3$Na, R^2=H, R^3=CH$_2$OSO$_3$Na

139 Cucumechinoside F R=H$_2$, R^1=R^4=SO$_3$Na, R^2=H, R^3=CH$_2$OSO$_3$Na

140 Lefevreoside A$_1$ R^1=H

141 Lefevreoside A$_2$ R^1=SO$_3$Na

142 Lefevreoside C R^1=SO$_3$Na, $\Delta^{24(25)}$

143 Lefevreoside D R^1=SO$_3$Na, $\Delta^{25(26)}$

Figure 7. Chemical structures of holostane glycosides with 3β-hydroxyholost-7(8)-ene and four sugar units.

Holostane Glycosides with 3β-Hydroxyholost-7(8)-ene Skeleton and 1–3 Sugar Units

The name of the compounds in this group, their producing species, chemical structures and references are summarized in Table 4 and Figure 8. The most common feature of triterpene glycosides is the presence of double bond at C-25(26). Cucumarioside B$_1$ (146) is the geometric isomer of cucumarioside B$_2$ (142) and pentactaside III (148) is the positional isomer of stichoposide A (153).

Table 4. Name and producing species of glycosides with 3β-hydroxyholost-7(8)-ene and 1–3 sugar units.

Compound Name	Producing Species	Reference	Compound Name	Producing Species	Reference
Pentactaside I (144)	*Pentacta quadrangularis*	[77]	Pentactaside II (145)	*P. quadrangularis*	[77]
Cucumarioside B$_1$ (146)	*E. fraudatrix*	[78]	Cucumarioside B$_2$ (147)	*E. fraudatrix*	[78]
Pentactaside III (148)	*P. quadrangularis*	[77]	Stichoposide A (149)	*S. cloronotus*	[79]
Stichoposide B (150)	*Stichopus cloronotus*	[79]	Stichorrenoside A (151)	*Stichopus horrens*	[80]
Stichorrenoside B (152)	*S. horrens*	[80]	Stichorrenoside C (153)	*S. horrens*	[80]
Stichorrenoside D (154)	*S. horrens*	[80]	Hillaside A (155)	*H. hilla*	[81]

144 Pentactaside I R =SO$_3$Na, Δ^{24}
145 Pentactaside II R =SO$_3$Na, $\Delta^{25(26)}$
146 Cucumarioside B$_1$ R =H, $\Delta^{22Z,25(26)}$
147 Cucumarioside B$_2$ R =H, $\Delta^{22E,25(26)}$

148 Pentactaside III R^1=SO$_3$Na, R^2=R^4=H, R^3=OAc, Δ^{24}
149 Stichoposide A R^1=SO$_3$Na, R^2=R^3=H, R^4=OAc, $\Delta^{25(26)}$
150 Stichoposide B R^1=R^3=H, R^2=OH, R^4=OAc, $\Delta^{25(26)}$

151 Stichorrenoside A R^1=CH$_2$OH, R^2=R^4=H, R^3=OH
152 Stichorrenoside B R^1=CH$_2$OH, R^2=SO$_3$Na, R^3=OH, R^4=H
153 Stichorrenoside C R^1=CH$_2$OH, R^2=R^3=H, R^4=OAc, $\Delta^{25(26)}$
154 Stichorrenoside D R^1=R^2=R^3=H, R^4=OAc, $\Delta^{25(26)}$

155 Hillaside A

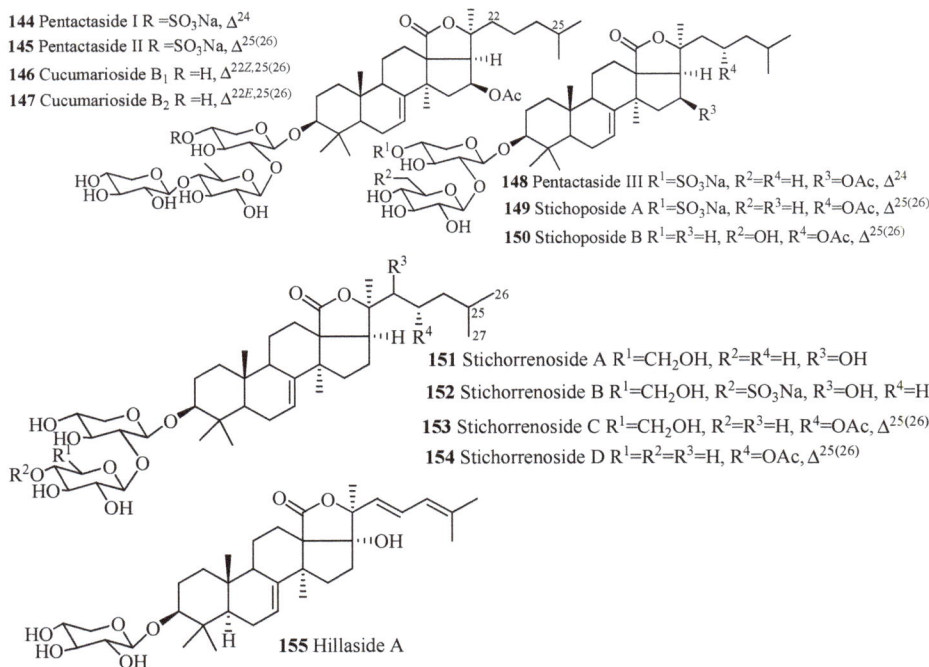

Figure 8. Chemical structures of holostane glycosides with 3β-hydroxyholost-7(8)-ene and 1–3 sugar units.

4.1.2. 3β-Hydroxyholost-9(11)-ene Skeleton Containing Holostane Glycosides

The species *Holothuria lessoni, Bohadschia marmorata and Bohadschia bivittata* produce most of the compounds in this group. For convenience, the large number of compounds in this category can also be further subdivided into four groups depending on the number of sugar units

Holostane Glycosides with 3β-Hydroxyholost-9(11)-ene Skeleton and Six Sugar Units

Similar to 3β-hydroxyholost-7(8)-ene skeleton with six sugar units (Figure 5), 3β-hydroxyholost-9(11)-ene skeleton with six sugar units glycosides also do not have any sulfate group in their carbohydrate chain (Figure 9 and Table 5) except cladolosides K$_1$, K$_2$ and L$_1$ (**197–199**). The most common structural feature of triterpene glycosides in this category is the presence of 3-*O*-methyl-D-glucose at the both end of the straight carbohydrate chain. Holotoxin and parvimoside series (**156–166**) of compounds have a keto group at position C-16. Double bond at C-25(26) among holotoxins (**156–163**) is common, except 26-nor-25-oxo-holotoxin A$_1$ (**159**), where the double bond is replaced by a keto group. The α-hydroxy groups at C-12 and C-17 are commonly found in the aglycone part of lessonioside series of glycosides (**175–177**). The α-hydroxy group at C-12 and C-17, and 22,25-epoxy are common structural characteristics of holothurinosides (**183–188**). Acetoxy group at C-16 and C-22 are frequently observed in cladoloside glycosides (**189–199**).

Table 5. Name and producing species of glycosides with 3β-hydroxyholost-9(11)-ene and six sugar units.

Compound Name	Producing Species	Reference	Compound Name	Pro. Species	Reference
Holotoxin A (**156**)	*Stichopus japonicus*	[82]	Holotoxin A₁ (**157**)	*S. japonicus*	[22]
25,26-dihydroxyholotoxin A₁ (**158**)	*Apostichopus japonicus*	[83]	Oxo-holotoxin A₁ (**159**)	*A. japonicus*	[22]
Holotoxin B (**160**)	*S. japonicus*	[22]	Holotoxin B₁ (**161**)	*S. japonicus*	[22]
Holotoxin D (**162**)	*S. japonicus*	[22]	Holotoxin D₁ (**163**)	*A. japonicus*	[83]
Parvimoside A (**164**)	*Stichopus parvimensis*	[84]	Parvimoside B (**165**)	*S. parvimensis*	[84]
Bivittoside C (**166**)	*Bohadschia bivittata*	[85]	Bivittoside D (**167**)	*B. bivittata*	[85]
25-acetoxybivittoside D (**168**)	*Bohadschia marmorata*	[86]	Arguside B (**169**)	*B. argus*	[87]
Arguside C (**170**)	*B. argus*	[87]	Marmoratoside A (**171**)	*B. marmorata*	[86]
Marmoratoside B (**172**)	*B. marmorata*	[86]	Impatienside A (**173**)	*H. impatiens*	[86]
17α-hydroxyimpatienside A (**174**)	*B. marmorata*	[86]	Lessonioside A (**175**)	*H. lessoni*	[88]
Lessonioside B (**176**)	*Holothuria lessoni*	[88]	Lessonioside D (**177**)	*H. lessoni*	[88]
Variegatuside E (**178**)	*S. variegates*	[21]	Lessonioside C (**179**)	*H. lessoni*	[88]
Lessonioside E (**180**)	*Holothuria lessoni*	[88]	Lessonioside F (**181**)	*H. lessoni*	[88]
Lessonioside G (**182**)	*H. lessoni*	[88]	Holothurinoside F (**183**)	*B. subrubra*	[89]
Holothurinoside H (**184**)	*B. subrubra*	[89]	Holothurinoside H₁ (**185**)	*B. subrubra*	[89]
Holothurinoside I (**186**)	*B. subrubra*	[89]	Holothurinoside I₁ (**187**)	*B. subrubra*	[89]
Holothurinoside K₁ (**188**)	*B. subrubra*	[89]	Cladoloside C (**189**)	*C. schmeltzii*	[90]
Cladoloside C₁ (**190**)	*Cladolabes schmeltzii*	[90]	Cladoloside C₂ (**191**)	*C. schmeltzii*	[90]
Cladoloside C₃ (**192**)	*C. schmeltzii*	[91]	Cladoloside D (**193**)	*C. schmeltzii*	[90]
Cladoloside G (**194**)	*C. schmeltzii*	[91]	Cladoloside H₁ (**195**)	*C. schmeltzii*	[91]
Cladoloside H₂ (**196**)	*C. schmeltzii*	[91]	Cladoloside K₁ (**197**)	*C. schmeltzii*	[92]
Cladoloside K₂ (**198**)	*C. schmeltzii*	[92]	Cladoloside L₁ (**199**)	*C. schmeltzii*	[92]

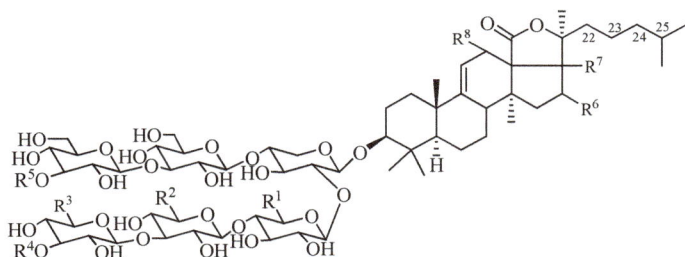

156 Holotoxin A $R^1=R^4=R^5=CH_3$, $R^2=R^3=CH_2OH$, $R^6===O$, $R^7=$ ''''H, $R^8=$H, $\Delta^{25(26)}$

157 Holotoxin A₁ $R^1=R^4=R^5=CH_3$, $R^2=$H, $R^3=CH_2OH$, $R^6===O$, $R^7=$ ''''H, $R^8=$H, $\Delta^{25(26)}$

158 25,26-dihydroxyholotoxin A₁ $R^1=R^4=R^5=CH_3$, $R^2=R^7=R^8=$H, $R^3=CH_2OH$, $R^6===O$,25-OH, 26-OH

159 26-nor-25-oxo-holotoxin A₁ $R^1=R^2=R^4=R^5=CH_3$, $R^3=CH_2OH$, $R^6===O$, $R^7=$ ''''H, $R^8=$H, 25–$==O$

160 Holotoxin B $R^1=R^4=CH_3$, $R^2=R^3=CH_2OH$, $R^5=$H, $R^6===O$, $R^7=$ ''''H, $R^8=$H, $\Delta^{25(26)}$

161 Holotoxin B₁ $R^1=R^4=CH_3$, $R^2=R^5=$H, $R^3=CH_2OH$, $R^6===O$, $R^7=$ ''''H, $R^8=$H, $\Delta^{25(26)}$

162 Holotoxin D $R^1=R^3=CH_2OH$, $R^2=$H, $R^4=R^5=CH_3$, $R^6===O$, $R^7=$ ''''H, $R^8=$H, $\Delta^{25(26)}$

163 Holotoxin D₁ $R^1=R^3=CH_2OH$, $R^2=R^5=R^7=R^8=$H, $R^4=CH_3$, $R^6===O$, $\Delta^{25(26)}$

164 Parvimoside A $R^1=R^4=CH_3$, $R^2=R^3=CH_2OH$, $R^5=$H, $R^6===O$, $R^7=$ ''''H, $R^8=$H

165 Parvimoside B $R^1=R^4=CH_3$, $R^2=R^5=$H, $R^3=CH_2OH$, $R^6===O$, $R^7=$ ''''H, $R^8=$H

166 Bivittoside C $R^1=R^4=R^5=CH_3$, $R^2=R^3=CH_2OH$, $R^6=$H, $R^7=$ ''''H, $R^8=$H

Figure 9. *Cont.*

167 Bivittoside D $R^1=R^4=R^5=CH_3$, $R^2=R^3=CH_2OH$, $R^6=H$, $R^7=$ ''''H, $R^8=$ ''''OH

168 25-acetoxy bivittoside D $R^1=R^4=R^5=CH_3$, $R^2=R^3=CH_2OH$, $R^6=H$, $R^7=$ ''''H, $R^8=$ ''''OH, 25-OAc

169 Arguside B $R^1=R^4=R^5=CH_3$, $R^2=R^3=CH_2OH$, $R^6=H$, $R^7=$ ''''OH, $R^8=$ ''''OH

170 Arguside C $R^1=R^2=R^3=CH_2OH$, $R^4=R^5=CH_3$, $R^6=H$, $R^7=$ ''''H, $R^8=$ ''''OH

171 Marmoratoside A $R^1=R^4=R^5=CH_3$, $R^2=R^3=CH_2OH$, $R^6=H$, $R^7=H$, $R^8=$ ''''OH, $\Delta^{25(26)}$

172 Marmoratoside B $R^1=R^4=R^5=CH_3$, $R^2=R^3=CH_2OH$, $R^6=H$, $R^7=H$, $R^8=$ ''''OH, 25-OH, Δ^{23}

173 Impatienside A $R^1=R^4=R^5=CH_3$, $R^2=R^3=CH_2OH$, $R^6=H$, $R^7=H$, $R^8=$ ''''OH, Δ^{24}

174 17α-hydroxy impatienside A $R^1=R^4=R^5=CH_3$, $R^2=R^3=CH_2OH$, $R^6=H$, $R^7=$ ''''OH, $R^8=$ ''''OH, Δ^{24}

175 Lessonioside A $R^1=R^4=R^5=CH_3$, $R^2=H$, $R^3=CH_2OH$, $R^6=OAc$, $R^7=$ ''''OH, $R^8=$ ''''OH

176 Lessonioside B $R^1=R^3=R^5=CH_3$, $R^2=CH_2OH$, $R^4=H$, $R^6=OAc$, $R^7=$ ''''OH, $R^8=$ ''''OH

177 Lessonioside D $R^1=R^4=R^5=CH_3$, $R^2=CH_2OH$, $R^3=H$, $R^6=OAc$, $R^7=$ ''''OH, $R^8=$ ''''OH

178 Variegatuside E $R^1=R^3=CH_2OH$, $R^2=R^6=R^8=H$, $R^4=R^5=Me$, $R^7=$ ''''H, 23- ''''OH

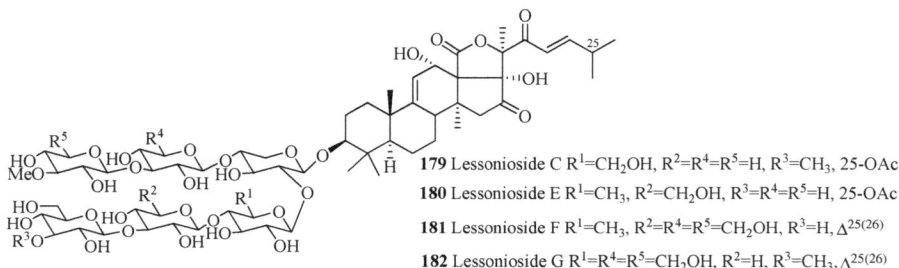

179 Lessonioside C $R^1=CH_2OH$, $R^2=R^4=R^5=H$, $R^3=CH_3$, 25-OAc

180 Lessonioside E $R^1=CH_3$, $R^2=CH_2OH$, $R^3=R^4=R^5=H$, 25-OAc

181 Lessonioside F $R^1=CH_3$, $R^2=R^4=R^5=CH_2OH$, $R^3=H$, $\Delta^{25(26)}$

182 Lessonioside G $R^1=R^4=R^5=CH_2OH$, $R^2=H$, $R^3=CH_3$, $\Delta^{25(26)}$

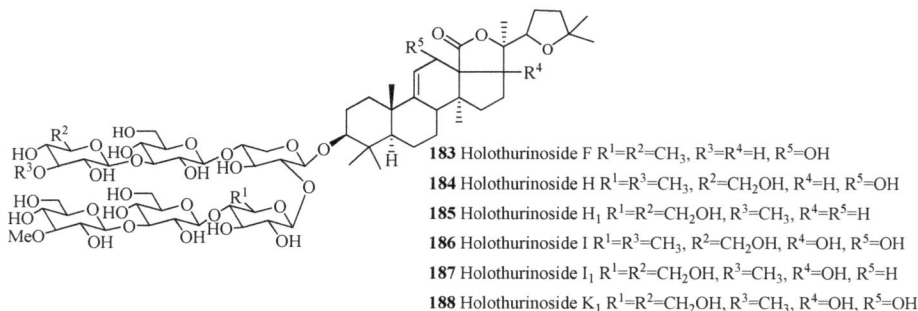

183 Holothurinoside F $R^1=R^2=CH_3$, $R^3=R^4=H$, $R^5=OH$

184 Holothurinoside H $R^1=R^3=CH_3$, $R^2=CH_2OH$, $R^4=H$, $R^5=OH$

185 Holothurinoside H_1 $R^1=R^2=CH_2OH$, $R^3=CH_3$, $R^4=R^5=H$

186 Holothurinoside I $R^1=R^3=CH_3$, $R^2=CH_2OH$, $R^4=OH$, $R^5=OH$

187 Holothurinoside I_1 $R^1=R^2=CH_2OH$, $R^3=CH_3$, $R^4=OH$, $R^5=H$

188 Holothurinoside K_1 $R^1=R^2=CH_2OH$, $R^3=CH_3$, $R^4=OH$, $R^5=OH$

Figure 9. *Cont.*

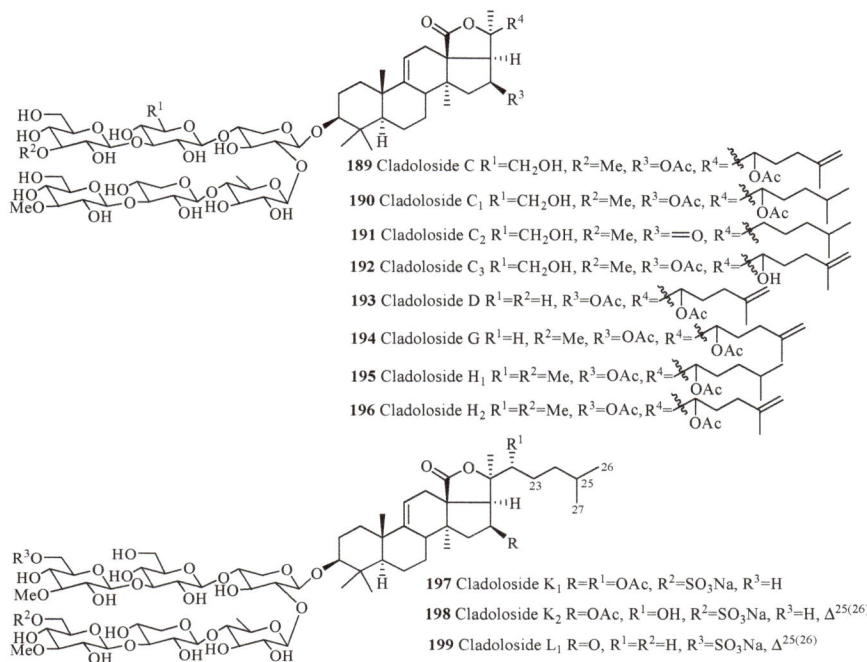

Figure 9. Chemical structures of holostane glycosides with 3β-hydroxyholost-9(11)-ene and six sugar units.

Holostane Glycosides with 3β-Hydroxyholost-9(11)-ene Skeleton and Five Sugar Units

The carbohydrate chains of glycosides in this group are either straight (**200–218** and **223–229**) or branched (**219–222**) (Figure 10 and Table 6). The 22,25-epoxy (**200–202**, **213–215**) and two acetoxy groups, one at C-16 and another at C-22 (**211**, **212**, **223–228**), are common in holothurinosides and cladolosides, respectively. Kolgaosides (**204** and **205**) and achlioniceosides (**216–218**) within their own groups have the same carbohydrate chains and the only difference is in their respective aglycone side chains.

Table 6. Name and producing species of glycosides with 3β-hydroxyholost-9(11)-ene and five sugar units.

Compound Name	Producing Species	Reference	Compound Name	Producing Species	Reference
Holothurinoside A (**200**)	*Holothuria forskalii*	[93]	17-dehydroxyholothurinoside A (**201**)	*Holothuria grisea*	[94]
Holothurinoside A$_1$ (**202**)	*H.lessoni*	[95]	Holothurinoside B (**203**)	*H. forskalii*	[93]
Kolgaoside A (**204**)	*Kolga hyalina*	[96]	Kolgaoside B (**205**)	*K. hyalina*	[96]
Griseaside A (**206**)	*H. grisea*	[94]	Impatienside B (**207**)	*H. axiloga*	[97]
Arguside F (**208**)	*Holothuria axiloga*	[97]	Pervicoside D (**209**)	*H. axiloga*	[97]
Cladoloside B (**210**)	*A. japonicus*	[22]	Cladoloside B$_1$ (**211**)	*C. schmeltzii*	[90]
Cladoloside B$_2$ (**212**)	*C. schmeltzii*	[90]	Holothurinoside E (**213**)	*H. lessoni*	[95]
Holothurinoside E$_1$ (**214**)	*H. lessoni*	[95]	Hclothurinoside M (**215**)	*H. lessoni*	[95]
Achlioniceoside A$_1$ (**216**)	*A. violaecuspidata*	[98]	Achlioniceoside A$_2$ (**217**)	*A. violaecuspidata*	[98]
Achlioniceoside A$_3$ (**218**)	*A. violaecuspidata*	[98]	Ds-penaustroside C (**219**)	*P. australis*	[99]
Ds-penaustroside D (**220**)	*Pentacta australis*	[99]	Frondoside A$_2$-6 (**221**)	*C. frondosa*	[35]
Cladoloside E$_1$ (**222**)	*C. schmeltzii*	[91]	Cladoloside E$_2$ (**223**)	*C. schmeltzii*	[91]
Cladoloside F$_1$ (**224**)	*C. schmeltzii*	[91]	Cladoloside F$_2$ (**225**)	*C. schmeltzii*	[91]
Cercodemasoide A (**226**)	*C. anceps*	[100]	Cladoloside I$_1$ (**227**)	*C. schmeltzii*	[92]
Cladoloside I$_2$ (**228**)	*C. schmeltzii*	[92]	Cladoloside J$_1$ (**229**)	*C. schmeltzii*	[92]

200 Holothurinoside A R^1=R^3=R^4=R^5=H, R^2=CH$_2$OH, R^6=R^7=OH, R^8=

201 17-dehydroxy holothurinoside A R^1=R^3=R^5=R^6=H, R^2=CH$_2$OH, R^4=CH$_3$, R^7=OH, R^8=

202 Holothurinoside A$_1$ R^1=R^7=OH, R^2=CH$_2$OH, R^3=R^4=R^5=R^6=H, R^8=

203 Holothurinoside B R^1=R^3=R^4=R^5=H, R^2=CH$_2$OH, R^6=R^7=OH, R^8=

204 Kolgaoside A R^1=R^3=R^4=R^5=H, R^2=CH$_2$OH, R^6=R^7=OH, R^8=

205 Kolgaoside B R^1=R^3=R^4=R^5=H, R^2=CH$_2$OH, R^6=R^7=OH, R^8=

206 Griseaside A R^1=R^3=R^4=R^5=R^6=H, R^2=CH$_2$OH, R^7=OH, R^8=

207 Impatienside B R^1=R^3=R^4=R^5=R^6=H, R^2=CH$_2$OH, R^7=OH, R^8=

208 Arguside F R^1=R^3=R^4=R^6=H, R^2=CH$_2$OH, R^5=◀OAc, R^7=OH, R^8=

209 Pervicoside D R^1=R^3=R^4=R^5=R^6=H, R^2=CH$_2$OH, R^7=OH, R^8=

210 Cladoloside B R^1=R^2=R^3=R^4=R^6=R^7=H, R^5===O, R^8=

211 Cladoloside B$_1$ R^1=R^2=R^3=R^4=R^6=R^7=H, R^5= ◀OAc, R^8=

212 Cladoloside B$_2$ R^1=R^2=R^3=R^4=R^6=R^7=H, R^5= ◀OAc, R^8=

213 Holothurinoside E R^1=R^3=R^4=R^5=R^6=H, R^2=CH$_2$OH, R^7=OH, R^8=

214 Holothurinoside E$_1$ R^1=OH, R^3=R^4=R^5=R^6=R^7=H, R^2=CH$_2$OH, R^8=

215 Holothurinoside M R^1=R^3=R^5=R^6=H, R^2=CH$_2$OH, R^4=CH$_3$, R^7=OH, R^8=

216 Achlioniceoside A$_1$ R^1=R^4=R^5=R^6=H, R^2=CH$_2$OSO$_3$Na, R^3=SO$_3$Na, R^4=CH$_3$, R^7=OH, R^8=

217 Achlioniceoside A$_2$ R^1=R^4=R^5=R^6=H, R^2=CH$_2$OSO$_3$Na, R^3=SO$_3$Na, R^4=CH$_3$, R^7=OH, R^8=

218 Achlioniceoside A$_3$ R^1=R^4=R^5=R^6=H, R^2=CH$_2$OSO$_3$Na, R^3=SO$_3$Na, R^4=CH$_3$, R^7=OH, R^8=

219 Ds-penaustroside C R^1=R^2=H, $\Delta^{25(26)}$
220 Ds-penaustroside D R^1=R^2=H
221 Frondoside A$_2$-6 R^1=SO$_3$Na, R^2=H, $\Delta^{25(26)}$
222 Cercodemasoide A R^1=R^2=SO$_3$Na, $\Delta^{25(26)}$

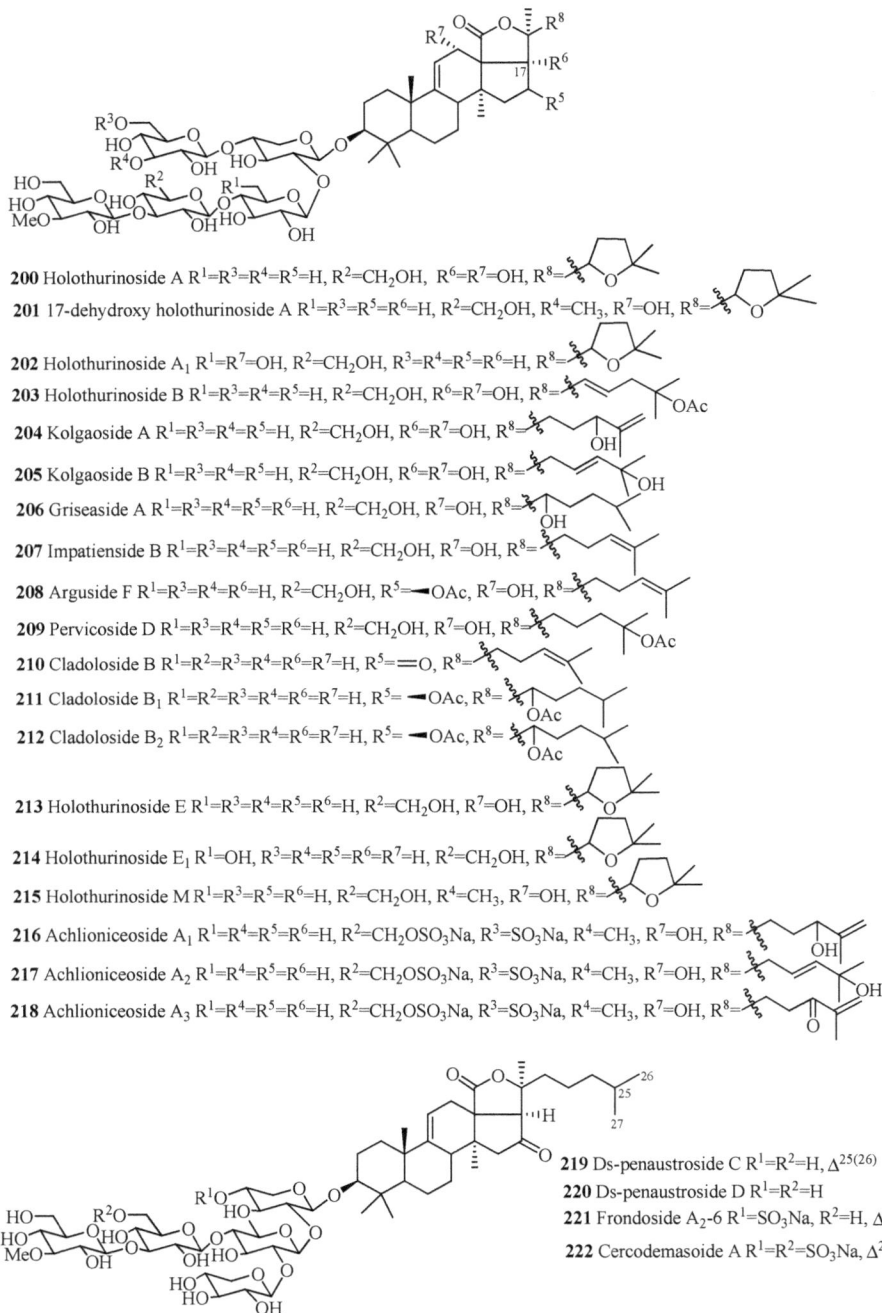

Figure 10. *Cont.*

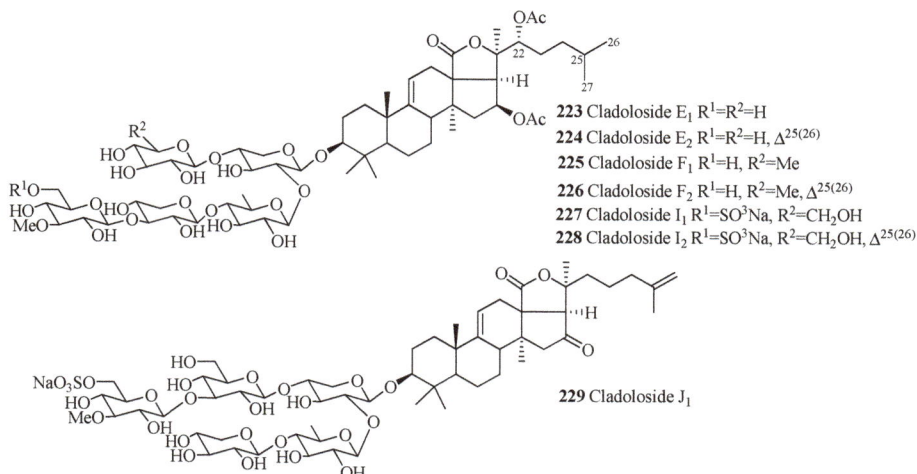

Figure 10. Chemical structures of holostane glycosides with 3β-hydroxyholost-9(11)-ene and five sugar units.

Holostane Glycosides with 3β-Hydroxyholost-9(11)-ene Skeleton and Four Sugar Units

The names and structures of the glycosides belonging to this group are summarized in the Table 7 and Figure 11. Almost all the saponins in this group contain sulfate group at C-4 of xylose sugar. The most common features of holothurins (**230–233**), scabrasides (**235–237**) and echinosides (**243–249**) are the presence of hydroxy groups at C-12 and C-17 (Figure 11). Among the cladoloside series of compounds (**266–271**), either keto or acetoxy group is commonly found at position C-16 and 22. The uncommon linear sugar chain [3-O-MeGlc (1→3)-Glc (1→4)-Xyl (2→1)-Qui] is observed in bivittoside B (**262**). Another exceptional feature has been found in this category of compounds is the presence of three consecutive glucose unit in the linear carbohydrate chain (**258** and **259**).

Table 7. Name and producing species of glycosides with 3β-hydroxyholost-9(11)-ene and four sugar units.

Compound Name	Producing Species	Reference	Compound Name	Producing Species	Reference
Holothurin A (230)	*Actinopyga agassizi*	[101]	Holothurin A₁ (231)	*H. grisea*	[102]
Holothurin A₃ (232)	*Holothuria scabra*	[103]	Holothurin A₄ (233)	*H. scabra*	[103]
Holothurinoside C (234)	*H. forskalii*	[93]	Scabraside A (235)	*H. scabra*	[104]
Scabraside B (236)	*H. scabra*	[104]	Scabraside D (237)	*H. scabra*	[105]
Fuscocineroside A (238)	*H. fuscocinerea*	[106]	Fuscocineroside B (239)	*H. fuscocinerea*	[106]
17-hydroxy fuscocineroside B (240)	*B. marmorata*	[107]	25-hydroxy-fuscocineroside B (241)	*B. marmorata*	[107]
Fuscocineroside C (242)	*H. fuscocinerea*	[106]	Echinoside A (243)	*A. echinites*	[108]
Ds-echinoside A (244)	*P. graeffei*	[109]	24-dehydroechinoside A (245)	*H. scabra*	[105]
22-hydroxy-24-dehydroechinoside A (246)	*Actinopyga flammea*	[110]	24-hydroxy-25-dehydroechinoside A (247)	*A. flammea*	[110]
25-hydroxydehydroechinoside A (248)	*A. flammea*	[110]	22-acetoxyechinoside A (249)	*A. flammea*	[110]
Desholothurin A (250)	*P. graeffei*	[93]	Pervicoside A (251)	*H. pervicax*	[111]
Pervicoside B (252)	*H. pervicax*	[111]	Pervicoside C (253)	*H. pervicax*	[111]
Arguside A (254)	*Bohadschia argus*	[112]	Holothurinoside J₁ (255)	*P. graeffei*	[95]
Hemoiedemoside A (256)	*H. spectabilis*	[113]	Hemoiedemoside B (257)	*H. spectabilis*	[113]
Arguside D (258)	*B. argus*	[114]	Arguside E (259)	*B. argus*	[114]
Psolusoside A (260)	*Psolus fabricii*	[115]	Liouvilloside A₄ (261)	*S. liouvillei*	[46]
Bivittoside B (262)	*Bohadschia bivitta*	[85]	Holothurinoside X (263)	*H. lessoni*	[116]
Holothurinoside Y (264)	*H.lessoni*	[116]	Holothurinoside Z (265)	*H. lessoni*	[116]
Cladoloside A₁ (266)	*Cladolabes chmeltzii*	[117]	Cladoloside A₂ (267)	*C. chmeltzii*	[117]
Cladoloside A₃ (268)	*C. chmeltzii*	[117]	Cladoloside A₄ (269)	*C. chmeltzii*	[117]
Cladoloside A₅ (270)	*C. chmeltzii*	[117]	Cladoloside A₆ (271)	*C. chmeltzii*	[117]
Colochiroside C (272)	*C. chmeltzii*	[64]	Colochiroside D (273)	*C. robustus*	[63]
Mollisoside B₁ (274)	*A. mollis*	[55]	Neothyonidioside (275)	*A. mollis*	[118]

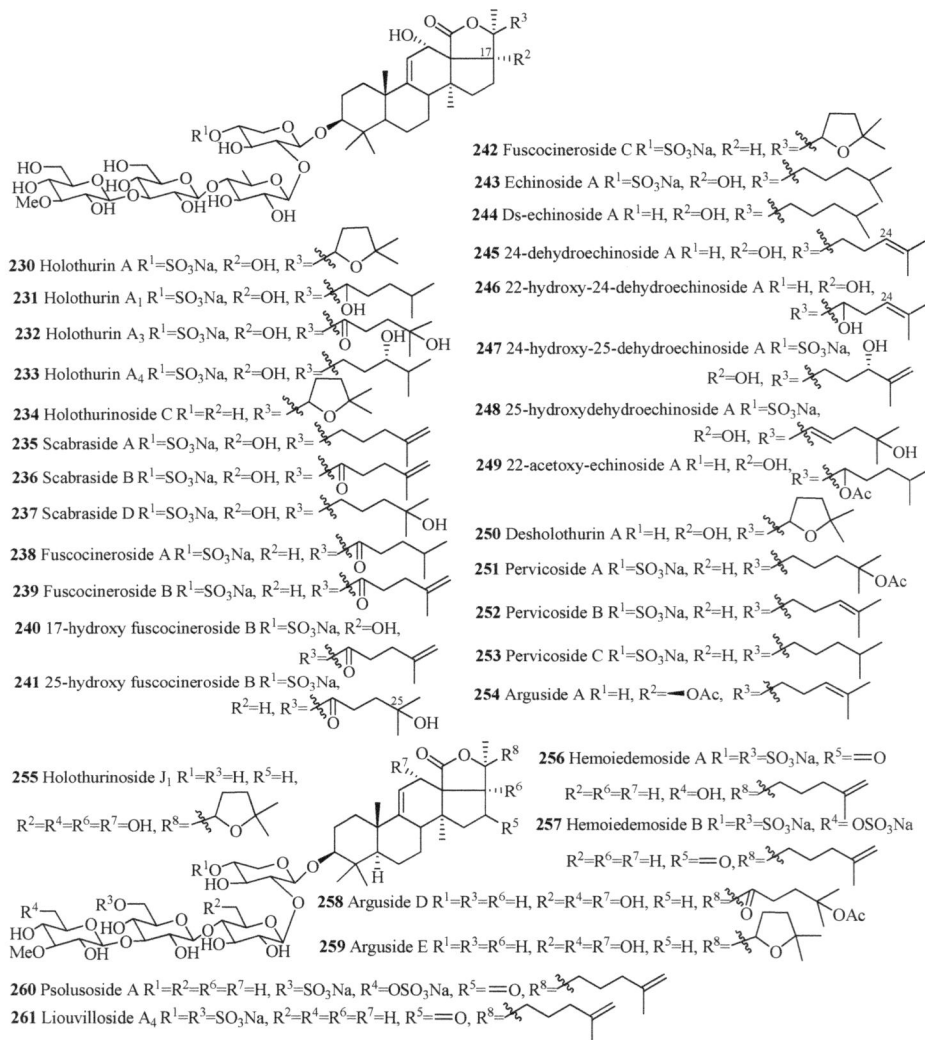

230 Holothurin A R^1=SO$_3$Na, R^2=OH, R^3=

231 Holothurin A$_1$ R^1=SO$_3$Na, R^2=OH, R^3=

232 Holothurin A$_3$ R^1=SO$_3$Na, R^2=OH, R^3=

233 Holothurin A$_4$ R^1=SO$_3$Na, R^2=OH, R^3=

234 Holothurinoside C R^1=R^2=H, R^3=

235 Scabraside A R^1=SO$_3$Na, R^2=OH, R^3=

236 Scabraside B R^1=SO$_3$Na, R^2=OH, R^3=

237 Scabraside D R^1=SO$_3$Na, R^2=OH, R^3=

238 Fuscocineroside A R^1=SO$_3$Na, R^2=H, R^3=

239 Fuscocineroside B R^1=SO$_3$Na, R^2=H, R^3=

240 17-hydroxy fuscocineroside B R^1=SO$_3$Na, R^2=OH,
R^3=

241 25-hydroxy fuscocineroside B R^1=SO$_3$Na,
R^2=H, R^3=

242 Fuscocineroside C R^1=SO$_3$Na, R^2=H, R^3=

243 Echinoside A R^1=SO$_3$Na, R^2=OH, R^3=

244 Ds-echinoside A R^1=H, R^2=OH, R^3=

245 24-dehydroechinoside A R^1=H, R^2=OH, R^3=

246 22-hydroxy-24-dehydroechinoside A R^1=H, R^2=OH,
R^3=

247 24-hydroxy-25-dehydroechinoside A R^1=SO$_3$Na,
R^2=OH, R^3=

248 25-hydroxydehydroechinoside A R^1=SO$_3$Na,
R^2=OH, R^3=

249 22-acetoxy-echinoside A R^1=H, R^2=OH,
R^3=

250 Desholothurin A R^1=H, R^2=OH, R^3=

251 Pervicoside A R^1=SO$_3$Na, R^2=H, R^3=

252 Pervicoside B R^1=SO$_3$Na, R^2=H, R^3=

253 Pervicoside C R^1=SO$_3$Na, R^2=H, R^3=

254 Arguside A R^1=H, R^2=—OAc, R^3=

255 Holothurinoside J$_1$ R^1=R^3=H, R^5=H,
R^2=R^4=R^6=R^7=OH, R^8=

256 Hemoiedemoside A R^1=R^3=SO$_3$Na, R^5===O
R^2=R^6=R^7=H, R^4=OH, R^8=

257 Hemoiedemoside B R^1=R^3=SO$_3$Na, R^4= OSO$_3$Na
R^2=R^6=R^7=H, R^5===O, R^8=

258 Arguside D R^1=R^3=R^6=H, R^2=R^4=R^7=OH, R^5=H, R^8=

259 Arguside E R^1=R^3=R^6=H, R^2=R^4=R^7=OH, R^5=H, R^8=

260 Psolusoside A R^1=R^2=R^6=R^7=H, R^3=SO$_3$Na, R^4=OSO$_3$Na, R^5===O, R^8=

261 Liouvilloside A$_4$ R^1=R^3=SO$_3$Na, R^2=R^4=R^6=R^7=H, R^5===O, R^8=

Figure 11. *Cont.*

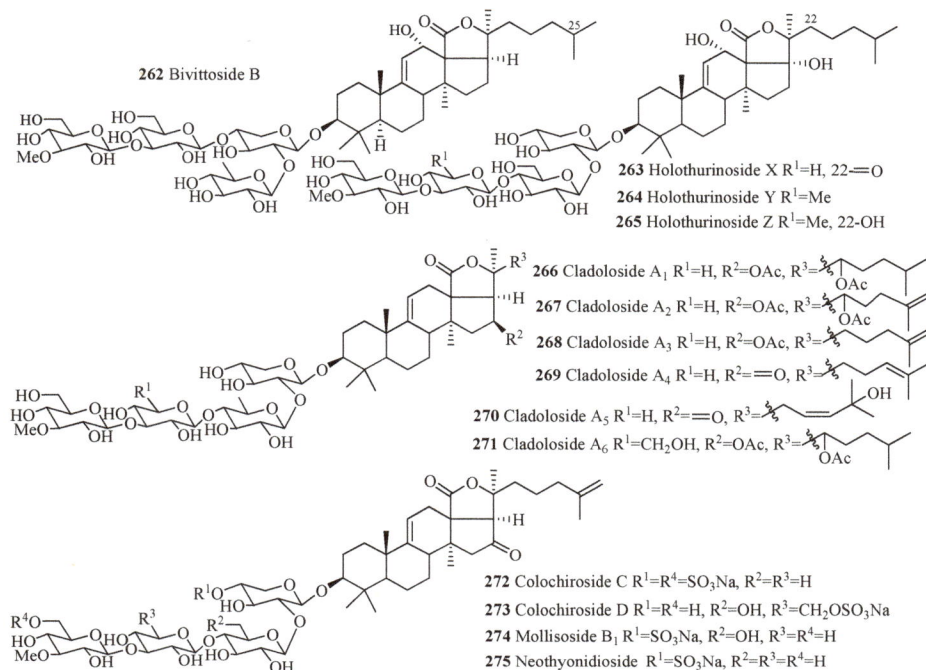

262 Bivittoside B

263 Holothurinoside X R^1=H, 22=O
264 Holothurinoside Y R^1=Me
265 Holothurinoside Z R^1=Me, 22-OH

266 Cladoloside A_1 R^1=H, R^2=OAc, R^3=
267 Cladoloside A_2 R^1=H, R^2=OAc, R^3=
268 Cladoloside A_3 R^1=H, R^2=OAc, R^3=
269 Cladoloside A_4 R^1=H, R^2==O, R^3=
270 Cladoloside A_5 R^1=H, R^2==O, R^3=
271 Cladoloside A_6 R^1=CH$_2$OH, R^2=OAc, R^3=

272 Colochiroside C R^1=R^4=SO$_3$Na, R^2=R^3=H
273 Colochiroside D R^1=R^4=H, R^2=OH, R^3=CH$_2$OSO$_3$Na
274 Mollisoside B$_1$ R^1=SO$_3$Na, R^2=OH, R^3=R^4=H
275 Neothyonidioside R^1=SO$_3$Na, R^2=R^3=R^4=H

Figure 11. Chemical structures of holostane glycosides with 3β-hydroxyholost-9(11)-ene and fours ugar units.

Holostane Glycosides with 3β-Hydroxyholost-9(11)-ene Skeleton and 1–3 Sugar Units

Only one type of carbohydrate chain, D-xylose-D-quinovose, is found in all glycosides in this group having two monosaccharide units (**278–290**), except **291** where carbohydrate chain is D-xylose-D-xylose (Figure 12 and Table 8); sulfate groups at C-4 of xylose units are also commonly found as well, except **285**, **288** and **291**. Hydroxy groups at either C-12 or C-17, or both positions, are observed in all the compounds in this category (Figure 12), except cercodemasoides (**276–279**).

Table 8. Name and producing species of glycosides with 3β-hydroxyholost-9(11)-ene and 1–3sugar units.

Compound Name	Producing Species	Reference	Compound Name	Producing Species	Reference
Cercodemasoide B (**276**)	*Cercodemas anceps*	[100]	Cercodemasoide C (**277**)	*C. anceps*	[100]
Cercodemasoide D (**278**)	*C. anceps*	[100]	Cercodemasoide E (**279**)	*C. anceps*	[100]
Holothurin B (**280**)	*Holothuria lessoni*	[119]	Holothurin B$_1$ (**281**)	*H. lessoni*	[120]
Holothurin B$_2$ (**282**)	*H. polii*	[121]	Holothurin B$_3$ (**283**)	*H. polii*	[121]
Holothurin B$_4$ (**284**)	*H. polii*	[121]	Holothurinoside D (**285**)	*H. forskalii*	[93]
Leucospilotaside A (**286**)	*H. leucospilota*	[122]	Leucospilotaside B (**287**)	*H. leucospilota*	[122]
Bivittoside A (**288**)	*Bohadschia bivittata*	[85]	Echinoside B (**289**)	*A. echinites*	[108]
24-dehydroechinoside B (**290**)	*Actinopyga mauritiana*	[123]	Hillaside C (**291**)	*Holothuria hilla*	[124]
Hillaside B (**292**)	*H. hilla*	[81]			

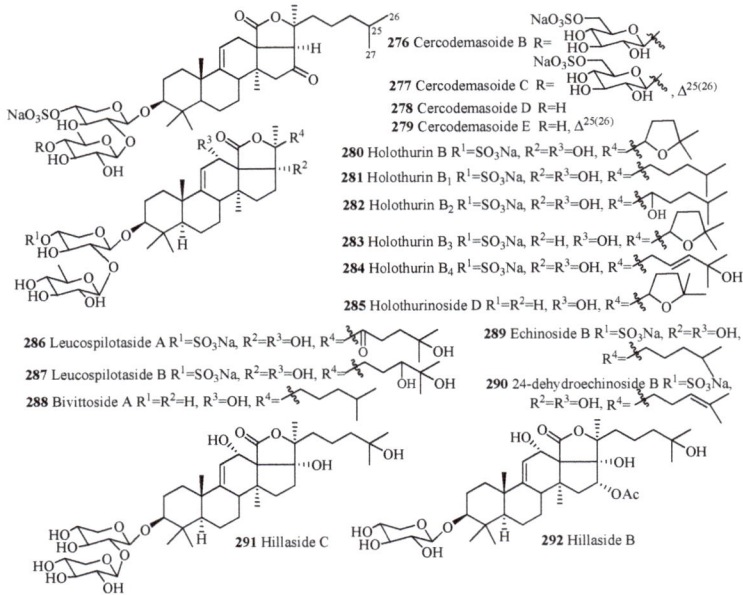

Figure 12. Chemical structure of holostane glycosides with 3β-hydroxyholost-9(11)-ene and 1–3 sugar units.

4.1.3. Holostane Glycosides with 3β-Hydroxyholost-8(9)-ene Skeleton

Only three glycosides belong to this group with carbohydrate chain consisting of 4–5 monosaccharide units (Table 9 and Figure 13). Among holostane sea cucumber glycosides, only one glycoside, synaptoside A_1 (**293**), contains keto group at C-7.

Table 9. Name and producing species of holostane glycosides with 3β-hydroxyholost-8(9)-ene skeleton.

Compound Name	Producing Species	Reference	Compound Name	Producing Species	Reference
Synaptoside A_1 (**293**)	*Synapta maculata*	[41]	Variegatuside B (**294**)	*Stichopus variegates*	[73]
Variegatuside D (**295**)	*Stichopus variegates*	[21]			

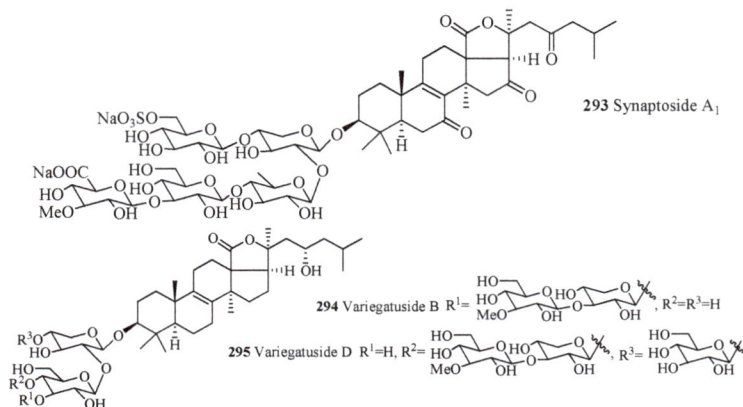

Figure 13. Chemical structures of holostane glycosides with 3β-hydroxyholost-8(9)-ene skeleton.

4.2. Nonholostane Glycosides

As mention earlier, like holostane glycosides, nonholostane glycosides do not have $\gamma(18,20)$-lactone structural unit (Figures 14 and 15, Table 10). There are six different structural units (Figure 14) present in D- and E rings of aglycone in nonholostane glycosides. The aglycone side chain can be long or short, and may contain keto, methylene, hydroxy and acetoxy functional groups (Figure 15). Instead of $\gamma(18,20)$-lactone, some glycosides in this group contain $\gamma(16,18)$-lactone (**296–300**, **314**, **322**, **332–340** and **341**). Cucumariosides A_8 (**305**) and A_9 (**306**) contain uncommon hydroxy group at C-18. Fallaxosides B_1 (**322**) and D_3 (**327**) are novel glycosides with unprecedented skeletons of aglycones. Psolusoside B (**314**) and Kuriloside C (**316**) have four members sugar architecture which are uncommon in both holostane and nonholostane glycosides. Another uncommon feature of this group of compounds is the presence of keto group at C-11 (**323** and **325**). Sulfate group is commonly found at C-4 of first xylose unit (Figure 15). Most of the nonholostane glycosides have branched five members carbohydrate chain (Figure 15).

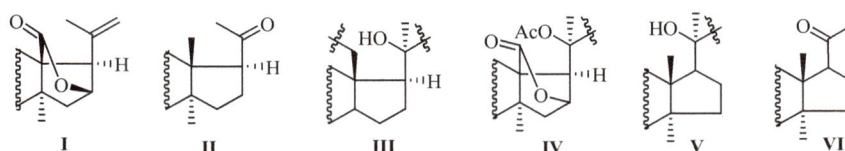

Figure 14. D- and E-ring structural architectures present in nonholotane glycosides.

Table 10. Name and producing species of nonholostane glycosides.

Compound Name	Producing Species	Reference	Compound Name	Producing Species	Reference
Cucumarioside G_2 (**296**)	*E. fraudatrix*	[125]	Cucumarioside A_{10} (**297**)	*E. fraudatrix*	[67]
Calcigeroside B (**298**)	*P. calcigera*	[37]	Calcigeroside C_1 (**299**)	*P. calcigera*	[37]
Cucumarioside H_3 (**300**)	*E. fraudatrix*	[30]	Cucumarioside A_3-2 (**301**)	*C. conicospermium*	[26]
Cucumarioside A_3-3 (**302**)	*C. conicospermium*	[26]	Koreoside A (**303**)	*C. koraiensis*	[126]
Isokoreoside A (**304**)	*C. conicospermium*	[26]	Cucumarioside A_8 (**305**)	*E. fraudatrix*	[67]
Cucumarioside A_9 (**306**)	*E. fraudatrix*	[67]	Holotoxin F (**307**)	*A. japonicus*	[22]
Holotoxin G (**308**)	*A. japonicus*	[22]	Holotoxin H (**309**)	*S. japonicus*	[127]
Holotoxin I (**310**)	*S. japonicus*	[127]	Ds-penaustroside A (**311**)	*P. australis*	[99]
Ds-penaustroside B (**312**)	*P. australis*	[99]	Frondoside C (**313**)	*C. frondosa*	[128]
Psolusoside B (**314**)	*Psolus fabricii*	[129]	Kuriloside A (**315**)	*D. kurilensi*	[130]
Kuriloside C (**316**)	*D. kurilensi*	[130]	Frondoside A_2-7 (**317**)	*C. frondosa*	[36]
Frondoside A_2-8 (**318**)	*C. frondosa*	[36]	Frondoside A_7-3 (**319**)	*C. frondosa*	[43]
Frondoside A_7-4 (**320**)	*C. frondosa*	[43]	Isofrondoside C (**321**)	*C. frondosa*	[43]
Fallaxoside B_1 (**322**)	*C. fallax*	[131]	Fallaxoside C_1 (**323**)	*C. fallax*	[132]
Fallaxoside C_2 (**324**)	*C. fallax*	[132]	Fallaxoside D_1 (**325**)	*C. fallax*	[132]
Fallaxoside D_2 (**326**)	*C. fallax*	[132]	Fallaxoside D_3 (**327**)	*C. fallax*	[131]
Fallaxoside D_4 (**328**)	*C. fallax*	[133]	Fallaxoside D_5 (**329**)	*C. fallax*	[133]
Fallaxoside D_6 (**330**)	*C. fallax*	[133]	Fallaxoside D_7 (**331**)	*C. fallax*	[133]
Magnumoside A_1 (**332**)	*Massinium magnum*	[134]	Magnumoside A_2 (**333**)	*M. magnum*	[134]
Magnumoside A_3 (**334**)	*M. magnum*	[134]	Magnumoside A_4 (**335**)	*M. magnum*	[134]
Magnumoside B_1 (**336**)	*M. magnum*	[134]	Magnumoside B_2 (**337**)	*M. magnum*	[134]
Magnumoside C_1 (**338**)	*M. magnum*	[134]	Magnumoside C_2 (**339**)	*M. magnum*	[134]
Magnumoside C_4 (**340**)	*M. magnum*	[134]	Colochiroside E (**341**)	*C. robustus*	[135]

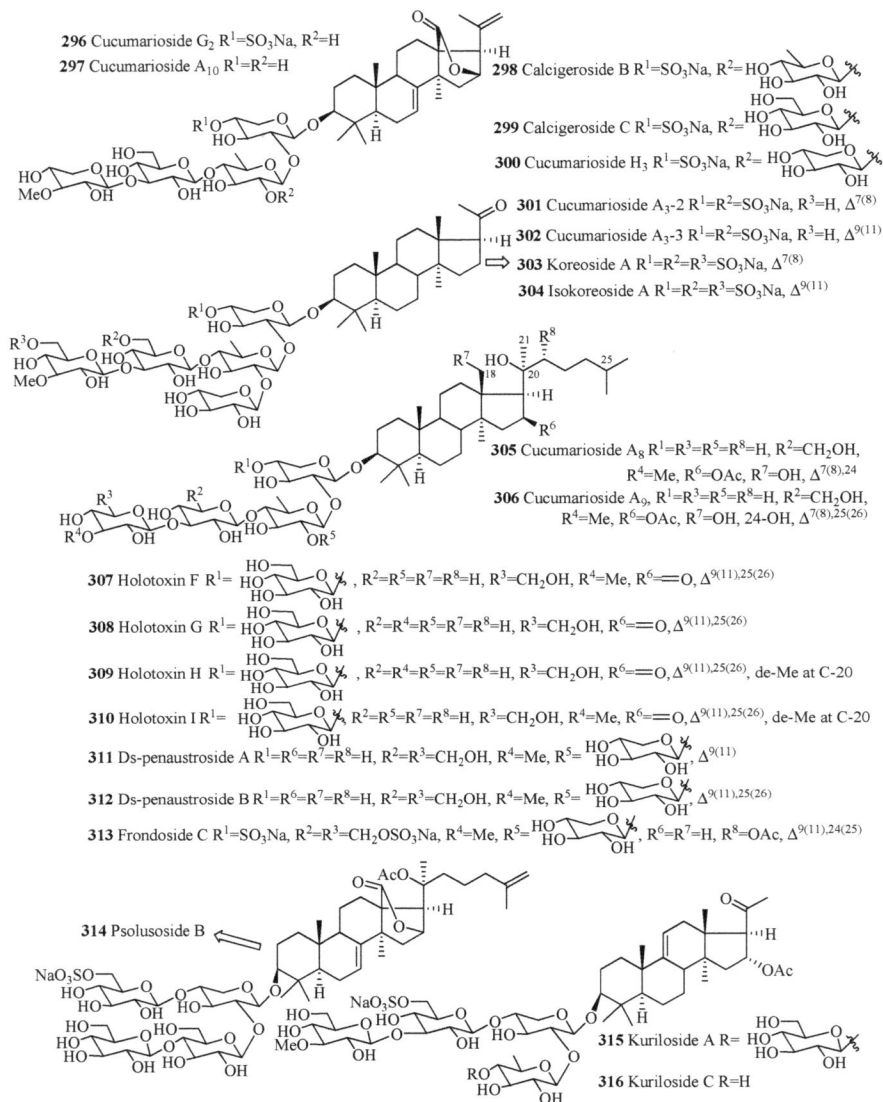

296 Cucumarioside G_2 R^1=SO$_3$Na, R^2=H
297 Cucumarioside A_{10} R^1=R^2=H

298 Calcigeroside B R^1=SO$_3$Na, R^2=H
299 Calcigeroside C R^1=SO$_3$Na, R^2=H
300 Cucumarioside H_3 R^1=SO$_3$Na, R^2=H

301 Cucumarioside A_3-2 R^1=R^2=SO$_3$Na, R^3=H, $\Delta^{7(8)}$
302 Cucumarioside A_3-3 R^1=R^2=SO$_3$Na, R^3=H, $\Delta^{9(11)}$
303 Koreoside A R^1=R^2=R^3=SO$_3$Na, $\Delta^{7(8)}$
304 Isokoreoside A R^1=R^2=R^3=SO$_3$Na, $\Delta^{9(11)}$

305 Cucumarioside A_8 R^1=R^3=R^5=R^8=H, R^2=CH$_2$OH, R^4=Me, R^6=OAc, R^7=OH, $\Delta^{7(8),24}$
306 Cucumarioside A_9, R^1=R^3=R^5=R^8=H, R^2=CH$_2$OH, R^4=Me, R^6=OAc, R^7=OH, 24-OH, $\Delta^{7(8),25(26)}$

307 Holotoxin F R^1= , R^2=R^5=R^7=R^8=H, R^3=CH$_2$OH, R^4=Me, R^6=$=$O, $\Delta^{9(11),25(26)}$

308 Holotoxin G R^1= , R^2=R^4=R^5=R^7=R^8=H, R^3=CH$_2$OH, R^6=$=$O, $\Delta^{9(11),25(26)}$

309 Holotoxin H R^1= , R^2=R^4=R^5=R^7=R^8=H, R^3=CH$_2$OH, R^6=$=$O, $\Delta^{9(11),25(26)}$, de-Me at C-20

310 Holotoxin I R^1= , R^2=R^5=R^7=R^8=H, R^3=CH$_2$OH, R^4=Me, R^6=$=$O, $\Delta^{9(11),25(26)}$, de-Me at C-20

311 Ds-penaustroside A R^1=R^6=R^7=R^8=H, R^2=R^3=CH$_2$OH, R^4=Me, R^5= , $\Delta^{9(11)}$

312 Ds-penaustroside B R^1=R^6=R^7=R^8=H, R^2=R^3=CH$_2$OH, R^4=Me, R^5= , $\Delta^{9(11),25(26)}$

313 Frondoside C R^1=SO$_3$Na, R^2=R^3=CH$_2$OSO$_3$Na, R^4=Me, R^5= , R^6=R^7=H, R^8=OAc, $\Delta^{9(11),24(25)}$

314 Psolusoside B

315 Kuriloside A R=
316 Kuriloside C R=H

Figure 15. *Cont.*

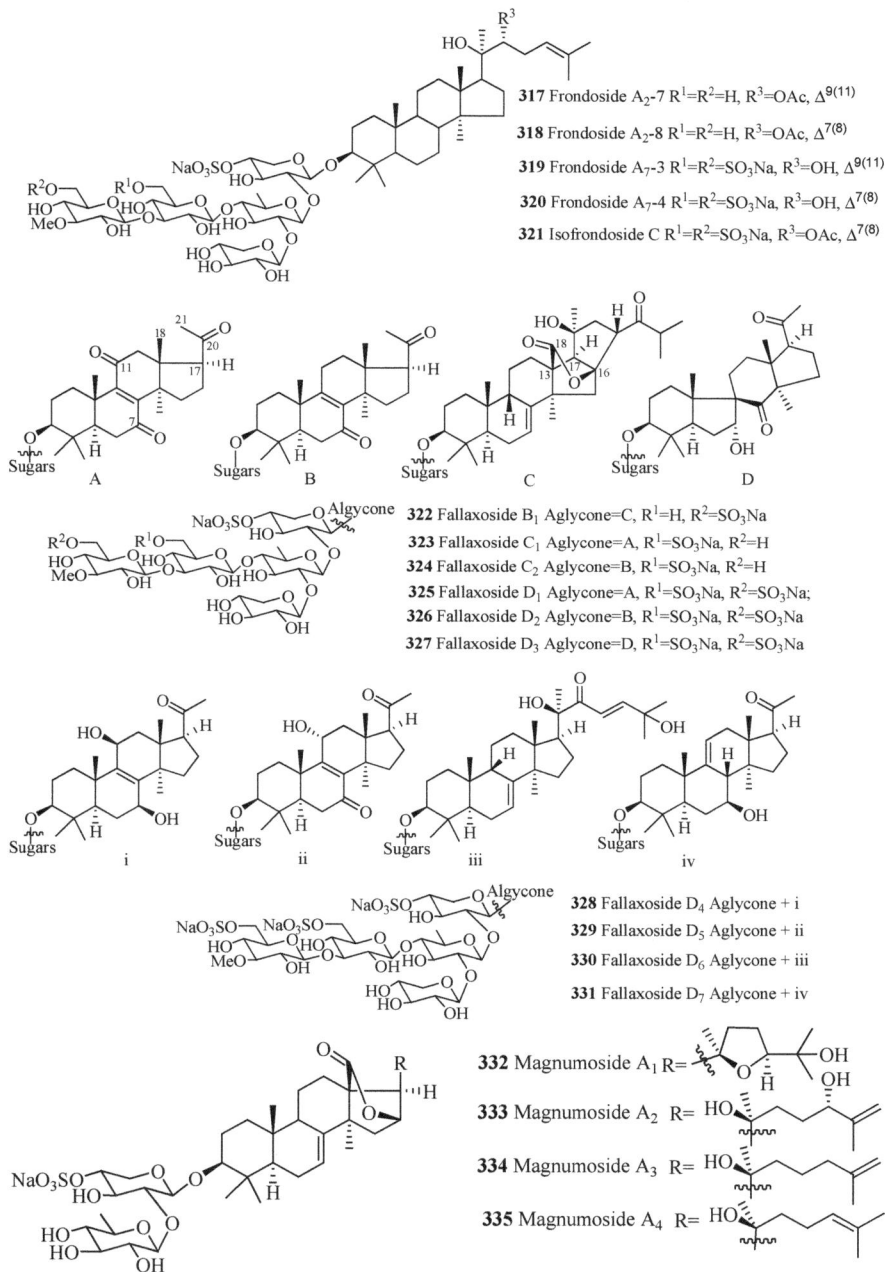

317 Frondoside A$_2$-7 R^1=R^2=H, R^3=OAc, $\Delta^{9(11)}$

318 Frondoside A$_2$-8 R^1=R^2=H, R^3=OAc, $\Delta^{7(8)}$

319 Frondoside A$_7$-3 R^1=R^2=SO$_3$Na, R^3=OH, $\Delta^{9(11)}$

320 Frondoside A$_7$-4 R^1=R^2=SO$_3$Na, R^3=OH, $\Delta^{7(8)}$

321 Isofrondoside C R^1=R^2=SO$_3$Na, R^3=OAc, $\Delta^{7(8)}$

322 Fallaxoside B$_1$ Aglycone=C, R^1=H, R^2=SO$_3$Na

323 Fallaxoside C$_1$ Aglycone=A, R^1=SO$_3$Na, R^2=H

324 Fallaxoside C$_2$ Aglycone=B, R^1=SO$_3$Na, R^2=H

325 Fallaxoside D$_1$ Aglycone=A, R^1=SO$_3$Na, R^2=SO$_3$Na;

326 Fallaxoside D$_2$ Aglycone=B, R^1=SO$_3$Na, R^2=SO$_3$Na

327 Fallaxoside D$_3$ Aglycone=D, R^1=SO$_3$Na, R^2=SO$_3$Na

328 Fallaxoside D$_4$ Aglycone + i

329 Fallaxoside D$_5$ Aglycone + ii

330 Fallaxoside D$_6$ Aglycone + iii

331 Fallaxoside D$_7$ Aglycone + iv

332 Magnumoside A$_1$ R=

333 Magnumoside A$_2$ R=

334 Magnumoside A$_3$ R=

335 Magnumoside A$_4$ R=

Figure 15. *Cont.*

75

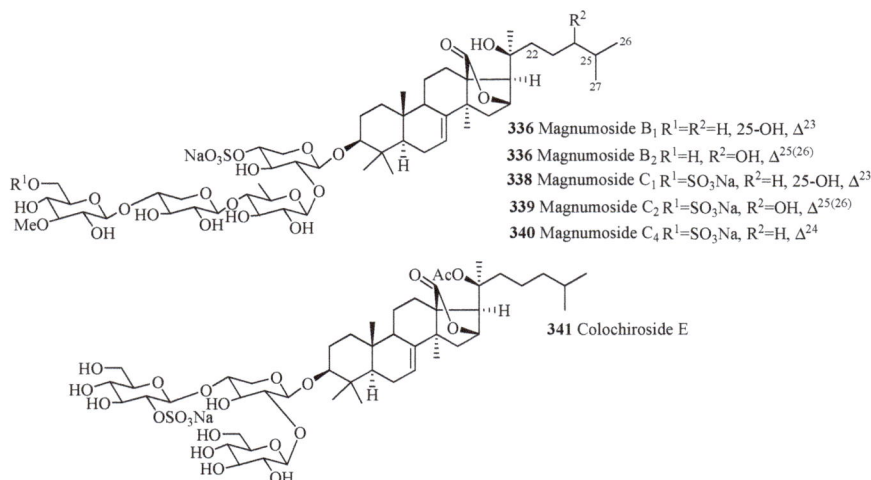

336 Magnumoside B$_1$ R^1=R^2=H, 25-OH, Δ^{23}
336 Magnumoside B$_2$ R^1=H, R^2=OH, $\Delta^{25(26)}$
338 Magnumoside C$_1$ R^1=SO$_3$Na, R^2=H, 25-OH, Δ^{23}
339 Magnumoside C$_2$ R^1=SO$_3$Na, R^2=OH, $\Delta^{25(26)}$
340 Magnumoside C$_4$ R^1=SO$_3$Na, R^2=H, Δ^{24}

341 Colochiroside E

Figure 15. Chemical structures of nonholostane glycosides.

5. The Important Biological Properties of Sea Cucumber Glycosides

Triterpene glycosides are the prime bioactive metabolites of sea cucumbers, and are commonly known as toxins of sea cucumbers to eukaryotic cells. These glycosides showed a wide range of biological activities including cytotoxic, antifungal, antiviral, hemolytic, antiprotozoal and immunomodulatory activities. Sea cucumbers produce some major glycosides in sufficient amount to carry out a wide range of biological activity tests [37,94]. Besides major glycosides, they also produce minor glycosides insufficient to test a range of biological activities [66,67]. The point to be noted here is that sea cucumber glycosides are able to exhibit biological activities in both in vitro and in vivo models [5]. The remarkable biological properties showed by some triterpene glycosides are summarized in Table 11. Triterpene glycosides do not exhibit antibacterial activity, indicating that these glycosides are probably produced by sea cucumbers for defence against eukaryotic predators.

Table 11. Remarkable biological activities exhibited by some sea cucumber glycosides.

Compound	Activity	Against/For	Activity Result	Reference
Hillaside C (**285**)	Cytotoxic	Human tumor cell lines	IC$_{50}$: 0.15–3.20 µg/mL	[124]
Hemoiedemoside A (**251**)	Antifungal	*C. cucumerinum*	20 µg/disc: 23 mm zone	[113]
Fuscocineroside C (**237**)	Cytotoxic	Human tumor cell lines	IC$_{50}$: 0.88 and 0.58 µg/mL	[106]
Intercedenside A (**66**)	Cytotoxic	Human tumor cell lines	ED$_{50}$: 0.96–4.0 µg/mL	[49]
Intercedenside B (**67**)	Cytotoxic	Human tumor cell lines	ED$_{50}$: 0.61–2.0 µg/mL	[49]
Intercedenside C (**68**)	Cytotoxic	Human tumor cell lines	ED$_{50}$: 0.96–4.0 µg/mL	[49]
Holothurinoside A (**195**)	Cytotoxic	Human tumor cell lines	IC$_{50}$: 0.33–0.71 µg/mL	[93]
Holothurinoside C (**229**)	Cytotoxic	Human tumor cell lines	IC$_{50}$: 0.16–0.93 µg/mL	[93]
Liouvilloside A (**53**)	Virucidal	Herpes simplex virus	<10 µg/mL	[44]
Leucospilotaside B (**281**)	Cytotoxic	Human tumor cell lines	IC$_{50}$: 0.44–2.62 µg/mL	[122]
Arguside B (**164**)	Cytotoxic	Human tumor cell lines	IC$_{50}$: 0.38–2.60 µg/mL	[87]
Arguside C (**165**)	Cytotoxic	Human tumor cell lines	IC$_{50}$: 0.38–2.60 µg/mL	[87]
Philinopside A (**78**)	Cytotoxic	Human tumor cell lines	IC$_{50}$: 1.70–3.50 µg/mL	[52]
Philinopside B (**79**)	Cytotoxic	Human tumor cell lines	IC$_{50}$: 0.75–3.0 µg/mL	[53]
Cucumarioside A$_2$-2 (**18**)	Hemolytic	Erythrocyte of mouse	ED50: 0.87 at 10^{-6} M	[136]
Holothurin B (**274**)	Antifungal	*T. mentagrophytes*	MIC-1.5 µg/mL	[137]
Holothurin A$_3$ (**227**)	Cytotoxic	Human tumor cell lines	IC$_{50}$ = 0.32–0.87 µg/mL	[103]
Holothurin A$_4$ (**228**)	Cytotoxic	Human tumor cell lines	IC$_{50}$ = 0.57–1.12 µg/mL	[103]
Scabraside A (**230**)	Antifungal	Eight pathogenic fungal strains	MIC$_{80}$: 2–8 µg/mL	[138]
Echinoside A (**238**)	Antifungal	Eight pathogenic fungal strains	MIC$_{80}$: 1–8 µg/mL	[108]
Cucumarioside A$_2$-2 (**18**)	immunomodulatory	Increased lysosomal activity	0.2–20 ng/mouse	[139]
Frondoside A (**37**)	immunomodulatory	Enhanced phagocytosis	0.001 µg/mL	[140]
Philinopside E (**80**)	Cytotoxicity	Ten tumor cell lines	ED$_{50}$: 0.75–3.50 µg/mL	[54]
Holotoxin A$_1$ (**152**)	Antifungal	Five pathogenic fungi	MIC: 0.5–1.0 µg/mL	[22]
Cucumarioside A$_1$ (**106**)	Hemolytic	Mouse erythrocytes	MEC$_{100}$: 0.7 ± 0.1 µg/mL	[66]

6. Mechanisms of Action

Natural products derived from marine organisms have incredible structural and functional diversity. The mechanism by which triterpene glycosides exhibit anticancer activity primarily involve induction of tumor cell apoptosis through the activation of intracellular caspase cell death pathways, arrest of the cell cycle at S or G_2/M phases and increase of the sub-G_0/G_1 cell population; regulation of nuclear factor NF-κB expression; reduction in cancer cell adhesion; suppression of cell migration and tube formation; suppression of angiogenesis; inhibition of cell proliferation, colony formation, and tumor invasion [141]. However, the detailed mechanism(s) of the anticancer activities of these glycosides remains largely unclear.

Marked membranolytic effects such as increased membrane permeability, loss of barrier function, and the rupture of cell membrane are considered the basic mechanisms underlying a variety of biological activities exerted by triterpene glycosides of sea cucumbers. The glycosides form complex with $\Delta^{5(6)}$-sterols of cellular membrane especially cholesterol. This interaction induces significant changes in the physicochemical properties of cell membranes, such as variations in their stability, microviscosity, and permeability. Saponins form complexes with membrane sterols, leading to cell disruption by the formation of pores. Due to this irreversible interaction, the selective permeability of cell membranes is impaired and cell compounds are transferred into the extracellular matrix, ultimately resulting in cell death [142,143].

7. Structure–Activity Relationships (SARs)

Both glycone and aglycone parts are important for biological activities of sea cucumber glycosides. The structure–activity relationships among sea cucumber glycosides are presumably more complicated. The most important structural characteristics of glycosides that probably contribute in biological activities are mentioned below.

The cytotoxicity not only depends on the chemical structures of the glycosides but also cell types [144]. The presence of 12α-hydroxy and 9(11)-ene structural units in holostane aglycone play key role in cytotoxicity [144]. Number of monosaccharide units in sugar chains and the substitution in side chain of aglycone could affect cytotoxicity. The presence of hydroxy groups in the side chains of glycosides significantly reduces cytotoxicity of the glycosides with increasing distance of hydroxy group from the 18(20)-lactone [30,31]. Linear tetraoside unit plays important role in different biological activities of sea cucumber glycosides [144]. Hexaoside chain containing glycosides show stronger cytotoxic activity than pentaoside chain containing glycosides. Glycosides with hexaosides residue with xylose or quinovose in the fifth position are the most active cytotoxins [144]. Different activities test result indicates that the number of sulfate groups and their position in the carbohydrate chains affect cytotoxicity [144]. It has been shown that the sulfate group attached to C-6 of terminal 3-*O*-methylglucose unit greatly decrease and attached to C-6 of glucose (the third monosaccharide unit) generally increase membranotropic activity [145].

8. Conclusions

Sea cucumbers (or holothurians), a class of marine invertebrates, are used as human food and traditional medicine, especially in some parts of Asia. The majority of the sea cucumbers synthesize glycosides with a polycyclic aglycone that contain either 7(8)- or 9(11)-double bond with up to six monosaccharide residues containing carbohydrate chain. A few of them are known to synthesize aglycone with 8(9)-ene. Sea cucumber glycosides are cytotoxic to eukaryotes; probably produce for escaping from predation by marine eukaryotic organisms. These cucumber metabolites have shown profound cytotoxic and hemolytic activities against eukaryotic organisms but not prokaryotic organisms. Due to significant cytotoxic and antifungal activities, extensive differential SAR studies of these glycosides can be helpful to develop new drugs and agrochemicals.

Acknowledgments: We are also thankful to the World Bank for partial funding of this work through a subproject of Higher Education Quality Enhancement Project (HEQEP), Supplementary Complete Proposal #2071. This research was also supported in part by the Ministry of Oceans and Fisheries (Grant PM60300), Korea. Sincere thanks are due to Prodip Kumar Roy of OIST, Okinawa, Japan for help in literature collection.

Conflicts of Interest: The authors declare no conflict of interest.

References

1. Gomes, A.R.; Freitas, A.C.; Rocha-Santos, T.A.P.; Duarte, A.C. Bioactive compounds derived from echinoderms. *RSC Adv.* **2014**, *4*, 29365–29382. [CrossRef]
2. Brusca, R.C.; Brusca, G.J. *Invertebrates*, 2nd ed.; Sinauer: Sunderland, MA, USA, 2003; pp. 808–826.
3. Leal, M.C.; Madeira, C.; Brandão, C.A.; Puga, J.; Calado, R. Bioprospecting of marine invertebrates for new natural products-A chemical and zoogeographical perspective. *Molecules* **2012**, *17*, 9842–9854. [CrossRef] [PubMed]
4. Shixiu, L.; Nina, A.; Yongjun, M.; Shujuan, S.; Wenjing, F.; Song, H. Bioactive compounds of sea cucumbers and their therapeutic effects. *Chin. J. Oceanol. Limnol.* **2016**, *34*, 549–558. [CrossRef]
5. Janakiram, N.B.; Mohammed, A.; Rao, C.V. Sea cucumbers metabolites as potent anti-cancer agents. *Mar. Drugs* **2015**, *13*, 2909–2923. [CrossRef] [PubMed]
6. Caulier, G.; Dyck, S.; Gerbaux, P.; Eeckhaut, I.; Flammang, P. Review of saponin diversity in sea cucumbers belonging to the family Holothuriidae. *SPC Beche-de-mer Inf. Bull.* **2011**, *31*, 48–54.
7. Hyman, L.H. The Invertebrates. In *Echinodermata*; McGraw Hill: New York, NY, USA, 1955; Volume 4.
8. Bruckner, A.W.; Johnson, K.; Field, J. Conservation strategies for sea cucumbers: Can a CITES Appendix II listing promote sustainable international trade? *SPC Beche-de-mer Inf. Bull.* **2003**, *18*, 24–33.
9. Lawrence, J. *A Functional Biology of Echinoderms = Functional Biology Series 6*; Calow, P., Ed.; Croom Helm Ltd.: London, UK, 1987; p. 340; ISBN 0-7099-1642-6.
10. Higgins, M. Sea cucumbers in a deep pickle. *Environmental News Network*, 30 August 2000.
11. Purcell, S.W.; Samyn, Y.; Conand, C. Commercially important sea cucumbers of the world. In *FAO Species Catalogue for Fishery Purposes*; FAO: Rome, Italy, 2012; Volume 6, p. 150.
12. Weici, T. Chinese medicinal materials from the sea. *Abstr. Chin. Med.* **1987**, *4*, 571–600.
13. Yaacob, H.B.; Kim, K.H.; Shahimi, M.; Aziz, N.S.; Sahil, S.M. Malaysian sea cucumber (Gamat): A prospect in health food and therapeutic. In Proceedings of the Asian Food Technology Seminar, Kuala Lumpur, Malaysia, 6–7 October 1997; p. 6.
14. Bordbar, S.; Anwar, F.; Saari, N. High-value components and bioactives from sea cucumbers for functional foods—A review. *Mar. Drugs* **2011**, *9*, 1761–1805. [CrossRef] [PubMed]
15. Wen, J.; Hu, C.; Fan, S. Chemical composition and nutritional quality of sea cucumbers. *J. Sci. Food Agric.* **2010**, *90*, 2469–2474. [CrossRef] [PubMed]
16. Silchenko, A.S.; Avilov, S.A.; Antonov, A.A.; Kalinin, V.I.; Kalinovsky, A.I.; Smirnov, A.V.; Riguera, R.; Jimenez, C. Triterpene Glycosides from the deep-water North-Pacific sea cucumber *Synallactes nozawai* Mitsukuri. *J. Nat. Prod.* **2002**, *65*, 1802–1808. [CrossRef] [PubMed]
17. Yun, S.H.; Park, E.S.; Shin, S.W.; Na, Y.W.; Han, J.Y.; Jeong, J.S.; Shastina, V.V.; Stonik, V.A.; Park, J.I.; Kwak, J.Y. Stichoposide C induces apoptosis through the generation of ceramide in leukemia and colorectal cancer cells and shows in vivo antitumor activity. *Clin. Cancer Res.* **2012**, *18*, 5934–5948. [CrossRef] [PubMed]
18. Stonik, V.A.; Maltsev, I.I.; Kalinovsky, A.I.; Conde, K.; Elyakov, G.B. Glycosides of marine-invertebrates. XI. Two novel triterpene glycosides from holothurians of Stichopodidae family. *Chem. Nat. Prod.* **1982**, *2*, 194–199.
19. Mal'tsev, I.I.; Stonik, V.A.; Kalinovskii, A.I. Stichoposide E-A new triterpene glycoside from holothurians of the family Stichopodidae. *Chem. Nat. Prod.* **1983**, *19*, 292–295. [CrossRef]
20. Kitagawa, I.; Kobuyashi, M.; Inamoto, T.; Yusuzawa, T.; Kyogoku, Y.; Kido, M. The structures of six antifungal oligoglycosides, stichlorosides A_1, A_2, B_1, B_2, C_1 and C_2 from the sea cucumber *Stichopus chloronotus* (Brandt). *Chem. Pharm. Bull.* **1981**, *29*, 2387–2391. [CrossRef]
21. Wang, X.-H.; Zou, Z.-R.; Yi, Y.-H.; Han, H.; Li, L.; Pan, M.-X. Variegatusides: New non-sulphated triterpene glycosides from the sea cucumber *Stichopus variegates*. *Mar. Drugs* **2014**, *12*, 2004–2018. [CrossRef] [PubMed]

22. Wang, Z.; Zhang, H.; Yuan, W.; Gong, W.; Tang, H.; Liu, B.; Krohn, K.; Li, L.; Yi, Y.; Zhang, W. Antifungal nortriterpene and triterpene glycosides from the sea cucumber Apostichopus japonicas Selenka. *Food Chem.* **2012**, *1*, 295–300. [CrossRef] [PubMed]
23. Drozdova, O.A.; Avilov, S.A.; Kalinovskii, A.I.; Stonik, V.A.; Mil'grom, Y.M.; Rashkes, Y.V. New glycosides from the holothurian *Cucumaria japonica*. *Chem. Nat. Compd.* **1993**, *29*, 200–205. [CrossRef]
24. Avilov, S.A.; Stonik, V.A.; Kalinovskii, A.I. Structures of four new triterpene glycosides from the holothurian *Cucumaria japonica*. *Chem. Nat. Compd.* **1990**, *26*, 670–675. [CrossRef]
25. Avilov, S.; Tishchenko, L.Y.; Stonik, V.A. Structure of cucumarioside A_2-2-A triterpene glycoside from the holothurian *Cucumaria japonica*. *Chem. Nat. Compd.* **1984**, *20*, 759–760. [CrossRef]
26. Avilov, S.A.; Antonov, A.S.; Silchenko, A.S.; Kalinin, V.I.; Kalinovsky, A.I.; Dmitrenok, P.S.; Stonik, V.A.; Riguera, R.; Jimenez, C. Triterpene Glycosides from the Far Eastern sea cucumber *Cucumaria conicospermium*. *J. Nat. Prod.* **2003**, *66*, 910–916. [CrossRef] [PubMed]
27. Drozdova, O.A.; Avilov, S.A.; Kalinin, V.I.; Kalinovsky, A.I.; Stonik, V.A.; Riguera, R.; Jiméne, C. Cytotoxic triterpene glycosides from Far-Eastern sea cucumbers belonging to the genus Cucumaria. *Liebigs Ann. Chem.* **1997**, *11*, 2351–2356. [CrossRef]
28. Drozdova, O.A.; Avilov, S.A.; Kalinovskii, A.I.; Stonik, V.A.; Mil'grom, Y.M.; Rashkes, Y.V. Trisulfated glycosides from the holothurians *Cucumaria japonica*. *Chem. Nat. Compd.* **1993**, *29*, 309–313. [CrossRef]
29. Silchenko, A.S.; Kalinovsky, A.I.; Avilov, S.A.; Andryjaschenko, P.V.; Dmitrenok, P.S.; Yurchenko, E.A.; Kalinin, V.I. Structure of cucumariosides H_5, H_6, H_7 and H_8, triterpene glycosides from the sea cucumber *Eupentacta fraudatrix* and unprecedented aglycone with 16,22-epoxy-group. *Nat. Prod. Commun.* **2011**, *6*, 1075–1082. [PubMed]
30. Silchenko, A.S.; Kalinovsky, A.I.; Avilov, S.A.; Andryjaschenko, P.V.; Dmitrenok, P.S.; Yurchenko, E.A.; Kalinin, V.I. Structures and cytotoxic properties of cucumariosides H_2, H_3 and H_4 from the sea cucumber *Eupentacta fraudatrix*. *Nat. Prod. Res.* **2012**, *26*, 1765–1774. [CrossRef] [PubMed]
31. Silchenko, A.S.; Kalinovsky, A.I.; Avilov, S.A.; Andryjaschenko, P.V.; Dmitrenok, P.S.; Martyyas, E.A.; Kalinin, V.I. Triterpene glycosides from the sea cucumber *Eupentacta fraudatrix*. Structure and biological action of cucumariosides I_1, I_3, I_4, three new minor disulfated pentaosides. *Nat. Prod. Commun.* **2013**, *8*, 1053–1058. [PubMed]
32. Silchenko, A.S.; Kalinovsky, A.I.; Avilov, S.A.; Andryjaschenko, P.V.; Dmitrenok, P.S.; Menchinskaya, E.S.; Aminin, D.L.; Kalinin, V.I. Structure of cucumarioside I_2 from the sea cucumber *Eupentacta fraudatrix* (Djakonov et Baranova) and cytotoxic and immunostimulatory activities of this saponin and relative compounds. *Nat. Prod. Res.* **2013**, *27*, 1776–1783. [CrossRef] [PubMed]
33. Girard, M.; Bélanger, J.; ApSimon, J.W.; Garneau, F.X.; Harvey, C.; Brisson, J.R. Frondoside A, a novel triterpene glycoside from the holothurians *Cucumaria frondosa*. *Can. J. Chem.* **1990**, *68*, 11–18. [CrossRef]
34. Findlay, J.A.; Yayli, N.; Radics, L. Novel sulfated oligosaccharides from the sea cucumber *Cucumaria frondosa*. *J. Nat. Prod.* **1992**, *55*, 93–101. [CrossRef] [PubMed]
35. Silchenko, A.S.; Avilov, S.A.; Antonov, A.S.; Kalinovsky, A.I.; Dmitrenok, P.S.; Kalinin, V.I.; Stonik, V.A.; Woodward, C.; Collin, P.D. Glycosides from the sea cucumber *Cucumaria frondosa*. III. Structure of frondosides A_2-1, A_2-2, A_2-3, and A_2-6, four new minor monosulfated triterpene glycosides. *Can. J. Chem.* **2005**, *83*, 21–27. [CrossRef]
36. Silchenko, A.S.; Avilov, S.A.; Antonov, A.S.; Kalinovsky, A.I.; Dmitrenok, P.S.; Kalinin, V.I.; Stonik, V.A.; Woodward, C.; Collin, P.D. Glycosides from the sea cucumber *Cucumaria frondosa*. IV. Structure of frondosides A_2-4, A_2-7, and A_2-8, three new minor monosulfated triterpene glycosides. *Can. J. Chem.* **2005**, *83*, 2120–2126. [CrossRef]
37. Avilov, S.A.; Antonov, A.S.; Drozdova, O.A.; Kalinin, V.I.; Kalinovsky, A.I.; Stonik, V.A.; Riguera, R.; Lenis, L.A.; Jiménez, C. Triterpene glycosides from the Far-Eastern sea cucumber *Pentamera calcigera*. 1. Monosulfated glycosides and cytotoxicity of their unsulfated derivatives. *J. Nat. Prod.* **2000**, *63*, 65–71. [CrossRef] [PubMed]
38. Avilov, S.A.; Antonov, A.S.; Drozdova, O.A.; Kalinin, V.I.; Kalinovsky, A.I.; Riguera, R.; Lenis, L.A.; Jiménez, C. Triterpene Glycosides from the far eastern sea cucumber *Pentamera calcigera* II: Disulfated glycosides. *J. Nat. Prod.* **2000**, *63*, 1349–1355. [CrossRef] [PubMed]
39. Yong-Juan, Z.; Yang-Hua, Y. Antitumor activities in vitro of the triterpene glycoside colochiroside A from sea cucumber *Colochirus anceps*. *J. Mod. Oncol.* **2011**, *2*, 205–207.

40. Afiyatullov, S.S.; Kalinovskii, A.I.; Stonik, V.A. Structures of cucumariosides C_1 and C_2-Two new triterpene glycosides from the holothurians *Eupentacta fraudatrix*. *Chem. Nat. Compd.* **1987**, *23*, 691–696. [CrossRef]

41. Avilov, S.A.; Silchenko, A.S.; Antonov, A.S.; Kalinin, V.I.; Kalinovsky, A.I.; Smirnov, A.V.; Dmitrenok, P.S.; Evtushenko, E.V.; Fedorov, S.N.; Savina, A.S.; et al. Synaptosides A and A_1, triterpene glycosides from the sea cucumber *Synapta maculata* containing 3-*O*-methylglucuronic acid and their cytotoxic activity against tumor cells. *J. Nat. Prod.* **2008**, *71*, 525–531. [CrossRef] [PubMed]

42. Silchenko, A.S.; Avilov, S.A.; Kalinin, V.I.; Stonik, V.A.; Kalinovskiĭ, A.I.; Dmitrenok, P.S.; Stepanov, V.G. Monosulfated triterpene glycosides from *Cucumaria okhotensis* Levin et Stepanov, a new species of sea cucumbers from sea of Okhotsk. *Russ. J. Bioorg. Chem.* **2007**, *33*, 73–82. [CrossRef]

43. Silchenko, A.S.; Avilov, S.A.; Kalinovsky, A.I.; Dmitrenok, P.S.; Kalinin, V.I.; Morre, J.; Deinzer, M.L.; Woodward, C.; Collin, P.D. Glycosides from the North Atlantic sea cucumber *Cucumaria frondosa* V-Structures of five new minor trisulfated triterpene oligoglycosides, frondosides A_7-1, A_7-2, A_7-3, A_7-4, and isofrondoside C. *Can. J. Chem.* **2007**, *85*, 626–636. [CrossRef]

44. Maier, M.S.; Roccatagliata, A.J.; Kuriss, A.; Chludil, H.; Seldes, A.M.; Pujol, C.A.; Damonte, E.B. Two new cytotoxic and virucidal trisulfated triterpene glycosides from the Antarctic sea cucumber *Staurocucumis liouvillei*. *J. Nat. Prod.* **2001**, *64*, 732–736. [CrossRef] [PubMed]

45. Antonov, A.S.; Avilov, S.A.; Kalinovsky, A.I.; Anastyuk, S.D.; Dmitrenok, P.S.; Evtushenko, E.V.; Kalinin, V.I.; Smirnov, A.V.; Taboada, S.; Ballesteros, M.; et al. Triterpene glycosides from Antarctic sea cucumbers. 1. Structure of liouvillosides A_1, A_2, A_3, B_1, and B_2 from the sea cucumber *Staurocucumis liouvillei*: New procedure for separation of highly polar glycoside fractions and taxonomic revision. *J. Nat. Prod.* **2008**, *71*, 1677–1685. [CrossRef] [PubMed]

46. Antonov, A.S.; Avilov, S.A.; Kalinovsky, A.I.; Dmitrenok, P.S.; Kalinin, V.I.; Taboada, S.; Ballesteros, M.; Avila, C. Triterpene glycosides from Antarctic sea cucumbers III. Structures of liouvillosides A_4 and A_5, two minor disulphated tetraosides containing 3-*O*-methylquinovose as terminal monosaccharide units from the sea cucumber *Staurocucumis liouvillei* (Vaney). *Nat. Prod. Res.* **2011**, *25*, 1324–1333. [CrossRef] [PubMed]

47. Zhang, S.Y.; Yi, Y.H.; Tang, H.F.; Li, L.; Sun, P.; Wu, J. Two new bioactive triterpene glycosides from the sea cucumber Pseudocolochirus violaceus. *J. Asian Nat. Prod. Res.* **2006**, *8*, 1–8. [CrossRef] [PubMed]

48. Zhang, S.Y.; Yi, Y.H.; Tang, H.F. Cytotoxic sulfated triterpene glycosides from the sea cucumber *Pseudocolochirus violaceus*. *Chem. Biodivers.* **2006**, *3*, 807–817. [CrossRef] [PubMed]

49. Zou, Z.-R.; Yi, Y.-H.; Wu, H.-M.; Wu, J.-H.; Liaw, C.C.; Lee, K.H. Intercedensides A–C, three new cytotoxic triterpene glycosides from the sea cucumber *Mensamaria intercedens* Lampert. *J. Nat. Prod.* **2003**, *66*, 1055–1060. [CrossRef] [PubMed]

50. Zou, Z.; Yi, Y.; Wu, H.; Yao, X.; Du, L.; Jiuhong, W.; Liaw, C.C.; Lee, K.H. Intercedensides D–I, cytotoxic triterpene glycosides from the sea cucumber *Mensamaria intercedens* Lampert. *J. Nat. Prod.* **2005**, *68*, 540–546. [CrossRef] [PubMed]

51. Murray, A.P.; Muniaín, C.; Seldes, A.M.; Maier, M.S. Patagonicoside A: A novel antifungal disulfated triterpene glycoside from the sea cucumber *Psolus patagonicus*. *Tetrahedron* **2001**, *57*, 9563–9568. [CrossRef]

52. Careaga, V.P.; Muniain, C.; Maier, M.S. Patagonicosides B and C, two antifungal sulfated triterpene glycosides from the sea cucumber *Psolus patagonicus*. *Chem. Biodivers.* **2011**, *8*, 467–475. [CrossRef] [PubMed]

53. Yi, Y.H.; Xu, Q.Z.; Li, L.; Zhang, S.L.; Wu, H.M.; Ding, J.; Tong, Y.G.; Tan, W.F.; Li, M.H.; Tian, F.; et al. Philinopsides A and B, two new sulfated triterpene glycosides from the sea cucumber *Pentacta quadrangularis*. *Helv. Chim. Acta* **2006**, *9*, 54–63. [CrossRef]

54. Zhang, S.L.; Li, L.; Yi, Y.H.; Sun, P. Philinopsides E and F, two new sulfated triterpene glycosides from the sea cucumber *Pentacta quadrangularis*. *Nat. Prod. Res.* **2006**, *20*, 399–407. [CrossRef] [PubMed]

55. Moraes, G.; Northcote, P.T.; Silchenko, A.S.; Antonov, A.S.; Kalinovsky, A.I.; Dmitrenok, P.S.; Avilov, S.A.; Kalinin, V.I.; Stonik, V.A. Mollisosides A, B_1, and B_2: Minor triterpene glycosides from the New Zealand and South Australian sea cucumber *Australostichopus mollis*. *J. Nat. Prod.* **2005**, *68*, 842–847. [CrossRef] [PubMed]

56. Kalinin, V.I.; Avilov, S.A.; Kalinina, E.Y.; Korolkova, O.G.; Kalinovsky, A.I.; Stonik, V.A.; Riguera, R.; Jiménez, C. Structure of eximisoside A, a novel triterpene glycoside from the far-eastern sea cucumber Psolus eximius. *J. Nat. Prod.* **1997**, *60*, 817–819. [CrossRef] [PubMed]

57. Kalinin, V.I.; Stonik, V.A.; Kalinovskii, A.I.; Isakov, V.V. Structure of pseudostichoposide A-The main triterpene glycoside from the holothurian *Pseudostichopus trachus*. *Chem. Nat. Compd.* **1989**, *25*, 577–582. [CrossRef]

58. Popov, R.S.; Avilov, S.A.; Silchenko, A.S.; Kalinovsky, A.I.; Dmitrenok, P.S.; Grebnev, B.B.; Ivanchina, N.V.; Kalinin, V.I. Cucumariosides F_1 and F_2, two new triterpene glycosides from the sea cucumber *Eupentacta fraudatrix* and their LC-ESI MS/MS identification in the starfish *Patiria pectinifera*, a predator of the sea cucumber. *Biochem. Syst. Ecol.* **2014**, *57*, 191–197. [CrossRef]
59. Careaga, V.P.; Bueno, C.; Muniain, C.; Alché, L.; Maier, M.S. Pseudocnoside A, a new cytotoxic and antiproliferative triterpene glycoside from the sea cucumber *Pseudocnus dubiosus leoninus*. *Nat. Prod. Res.* **2014**, *28*, 213–220. [CrossRef] [PubMed]
60. Silchenko, A.S.; Kalinovsky, A.I.; Avilov, S.A.; Andryjaschenko, P.V.; Dmitrenok, P.S.; Martyyas, E.A.; Kalinin, V.I.; Jayasandhya, P.; Rajan, G.C.; Padmakumar, K.P. Structures and biological activities of typicosides A_1, A_2, B_1, C_1 and C_2, triterpene glycosides from the sea cucumber *Actinocucumis typica*. *Nat. Prod. Commun.* **2013**, *8*, 301–310. [PubMed]
61. Aminin, D.L.; Silchenko, A.S.; Avilov, S.A.; Stepanov, V.G.; Kalinin, V.I. Immunomodulatory action of monosulfated triterpene glycosides from the sea cucumber *Cucumaria okhotensis*: Stimulation of activity of mouse peritoneal macrophages. *Nat. Prod. Commun.* **2010**, *5*, 1877–1880. [PubMed]
62. Silchenko, A.S.; Avilov, S.A.; Kalinin, V.I.; Kalinovsky, A.I.; Dmitrenok, P.S.; Fedorov, S.N.; Stepanov, V.G.; Dong, Z.; Stonik, V.A. Constituents of the sea cucumber *Cucumaria okhotensis*. Structures of okhotosides B_1–B_3 and cytotoxic activities of some glycosides from this species. *J. Nat. Prod.* **2008**, *71*, 351–356. [CrossRef] [PubMed]
63. Silchenkoa, A.S.; Kalinovskya, A.I.; Avilova, S.A.; Andryjaschenko, P.V.; Dmitrenok, P.S.; Yurchenko, E.A.; Kalinin, V.I.; Dolmatov, I.Y. Colochirosides A_1, A_2, A_3, and D, four novel sulfated triterpene glycosides from the sea cucumber *Colochirus robustus* (Cucumariidae, Dendrochirotida). *Nat. Prod. Commun.* **2016**, *11*, 381–386.
64. Silchenkoa, A.S.; Kalinovskya, A.I.; Avilova, S.A.; Andryjaschenko, P.V.; Dmitrenok, P.S.; Yurchenko, E.A.; Kalinin, V.I.; Dolmatov, I.Y. Colochirosides B_1, B_2, B_3 and C, novel sulfated triterpene glycosides from the sea cucumber *Colochirus robustus* (Cucumariidae, Dendrochirotida). *Nat. Prod. Commun.* **2015**, *10*, 687–694.
65. Silchenko, A.S.; Kalinovsky, A.I.; Avilov, S.A.; Andryjaschenko, P.V.; Dmitrenok, P.S.; Kalinin, V.I.; Yurchenko, E.A.; Dautov, S.S. Structures of violaceusosides C, D, E and G, sulfated triterpene glycosides from the sea cucumber *Pseudocolochirus violaceus* (Cucumariidae, Dendrochirotida). *Nat. Prod. Commun.* **2014**, *9*, 391–399. [PubMed]
66. Silchenko, A.S.; Kalinovsky, A.I.; Avilov, S.A.; Andryjaschenko, P.V.; Dmitrenok, P.S.; Martyyas, E.A.; Kalinin, V.I. Triterpene glycosides from the sea cucumber *Eupentacta fraudatrix*. Structure and biological action of cucumariosides A_1, A_3, A_4, A_5, A_6, A_{12} and A_{15}, seven new minor non-sulfated tetraosides and unprecedented 25-keto, 27-norholostane aglycone. *Nat. Prod. Commun.* **2012**, *7*, 517–525. [PubMed]
67. Silchenko, A.S.; Kalinovsky, A.I.; Avilov, S.A.; Andryjaschenko, P.V.; Dmitrenok, P.S.; Martyyas, E.A.; Kalinin, V.I. Triterpene glycosides from the sea cucumber *Eupentacta fraudatrix*. Structure and cytotoxic action of cucumariosides A_2, A_7, A_9, A_{10}, A_{11}, A_{13} and A_{14}, seven new minor non-sulfated tetraosides and an aglycone with an uncommon 18-hydroxy group. *Nat. Prod. Commun.* **2012**, *7*, 845–852. [PubMed]
68. Afiyatullov, S.S.; Tishchenko, L.Y.; Stonik, V.A.; Kalinovskii, A.I.; Elyakov, G.B. Structure of cucumarioside G_1-A new triterpene glycoside from the holothurians *Cucumaria fraudatrix*. *Chem. Nat. Compd.* **1985**, *21*, 228–232. [CrossRef]
69. Kalinin, V.I.; Avilov, S.A.; Kalinovskii, A.I.; Stonik, V.A. Cucumarioside G_3-A minor triterpene glycoside from the holothurian *Eupentacta fraudatrix*. *Chem. Nat. Compd.* **1992**, *28*, 635–636. [CrossRef]
70. Kalinin, V.I.; Avilov, S.A.; Kalinovskii, A.I.; Stonik, V.A.; Mil'grom, Y.M.; Rashkes, Y.V. Cucumarioside G_4-A new triterpenglycoside from the holothurian *Eupentacta fraudatrix*. *Chem. Nat. Compd.* **1992**, *28*, 600–603. [CrossRef]
71. Han, H.; Xu, Q.Z.; Yi, Y.H.; Gong, W.; Jiao, B.H. Two new cytotoxic disulfated holostane glycosides from the sea cucumber *Pentacta quadrangularis*. *Chem. Biodivers.* **2010**, *7*, 158–167. [CrossRef] [PubMed]
72. Silchenko, A.S.; Avilov, S.A.; Kalinin, V.I.; Kalinovsky, A.I.; Stonik, V.A.; Smirnov, A.V. Pseudostichoposide B-New triterpene glycoside with unprecedent type of sulfatation from the deep-water North-Pacific Sea cucumber *Pseudostichopus trachus*. *Nat. Prod. Res.* **2004**, *18*, 565–570. [CrossRef] [PubMed]
73. Wang, X.-H.; Li, L.; Yi, Y.-H.; Sun, P.; Yan, B.; Pan, M.-X.; Han, H.; Wang, X.-D. Two new triterpene glycosides from sea cucumber *Stichopus variegatus*. *Chin. J. Nat. Med.* **2006**, *4*, 177–180.

74. Stonik, V.A.; Mal'tsev, I.I.; Elyakov, G.B. The structure of thelenotosides A and B from the holothurians *Thelenota ananas*. *Chem. Nat. Compd.* **1982**, *18*, 590–593. [CrossRef]
75. Miyamoto, T.; Togawa, K.; Higuchi, R.; Komori, T.; Sasaki, T. Constituents of holothuroidea, II. Six newly identified biologically active triterpenoid glycoside sulfates from the sea cucumber *Cucumaria echinata*. *Liebigs Ann. Chem.* **1990**, *5*, 453–460. [CrossRef]
76. Rodriguez, J.; Riguera, R. Lefevreiosides: Four new triterpene glycosides from the sea cucumber *Cucumaria lefevrei*. *J. Chem. Res.* **1989**, *11*, 342–343.
77. Han, H.; Xu, Q.Z.; Tang, H.F.; Yi, Y.H.; Gong, W. Cytotoxic holostane-type triterpene glycosides from the sea cucumber *Pentacta quadrangularis*. *Planta Med.* **2010**, *76*, 1900–1904. [CrossRef] [PubMed]
78. Silchenko, A.S.; Kalinovsky, A.I.; Avilov, S.A.; Andryjaschenko, P.V.; Dmitrenok, P.S.; Martyyas, E.A.; Kalinin, V.I. Triterpene glycosides from the sea cucumber *Eupentacta fraudatrix*. Structure and biological activity of cucumariosides B_1 and B_2, two new minor non-sulfated unprecedented triosides. *Nat. Prod. Commun.* **2012**, *7*, 1157–1162. [PubMed]
79. Sharypov, V.F.; Chumak, A.D.; Stonik, V.A.; Elyakov, G.B. Glycosides of marine invertebrates. X. The structure of stichoposides A and B from the holothurians *Stichopus cloronotus*. *Chem. Nat. Compd.* **1981**, *17*, 139–142. [CrossRef]
80. Cuong, N.X.; Vien, L.T.; Hoang, L.; Hanh, T.T.H.; Thao, D.T.; Thanh, N.V.; Nam, N.H.; Thung, D.C.; Kiem, P.V.; Minh, C.V. Cytotoxic triterpene diglycosides from the sea cucumber *Stichopus horrens*. *Bioorg. Med. Chem. Lett.* **2017**, *27*, 2939–2942. [CrossRef] [PubMed]
81. Wu, J.; Yi, Y.H.; Tang, H.F.; Wu, H.M.; Zhou, Z.R. Hillasides A and B, two new cytotoxic triterpene glycosides from the sea cucumber *Holothuria hilla* Lesson. *J. Asian Nat. Prod. Res.* **2007**, *9*, 609–615. [CrossRef] [PubMed]
82. Dong, P.; Xue, C.-H.; Yu, L.-F.; Xu, J.; Chen, S.-G. Determination of triterpene glycosides in sea cucumber (*Stichopus japonicus*) and its related products by high-performance liquid chromatography. *J. Agric. Food Chem.* **2008**, *56*, 4937–4942. [CrossRef] [PubMed]
83. Wang, Z.; Gong, W.; Sun, G.; Tang, H.; Liu, B.; Li, L.; Yi, Y.; Zhang, W. New holostan-type triterpene glycosides from the sea cucumber Apostichopus japonicus. *Nat. Prod. Commun.* **2012**, *7*, 1431–1434. [PubMed]
84. Iñiguez-Martinez, A.M.; Guerra-Rivas, G.; Rios, T.; Quijano, L. Triterpenoid oligoglycosides from the sea cucumber *Stichopus parvimensis*. *J. Nat. Prod.* **2005**, *68*, 1669–1673. [CrossRef] [PubMed]
85. Ohta, T.; Hikino, H. Structures of four new triterpenoidal oligosides, bivittosides A, B, C and D from the sea cucumber *Bohadschia bivittata* Mitsukuri. *Chem. Pharm. Bull.* **1981**, *29*, 282–285.
86. Yuan, W.H.; Yi, Y.H.; Tang, H.F.; Liu, B.S.; Wang, Z.L.; Sun, G.Q.; Zhang, W.; Li, L.; Sun, P. Antifungal triterpene glycosides from the sea cucumber *Bohadschia marmorata*. *Planta Med.* **2009**, *75*, 168–173. [CrossRef] [PubMed]
87. Liu, B.S.; Yi, Y.H.; Li, L.; Sun, P.; Yuan, W.H.; Sun, G.Q.; Han, H.; Xue, M. Argusides B and C, two new cytotoxic triterpene glycosides from the sea cucumber *Bohadschia argus*. *Chem. Biodivers.* **2008**, *5*, 1288–1297. [CrossRef] [PubMed]
88. Bahrami, Y.; Franco, C.M.M. Structure elucidation of new acetylated saponins, lessoniosides A, B, C, D, and E, and non-acetylated saponins, lessoniosides F and G, from the viscera of the sea cucumber *Holothuria lessoni*. *Mar. Drugs* **2015**, *13*, 597–617. [CrossRef] [PubMed]
89. Dyck, S.V.; Gerbaux, P.; Flammang, P. Qualitative and quantitative saponin contents in five sea cucumbers from the Indian Ocean. *Mar. Drugs* **2010**, *8*, 173–189. [CrossRef] [PubMed]
90. Silchenko, A.S.; Kalinovsky, A.I.; Avilov, S.A.; Andryjaschenko, P.V.; Dmitrenok, P.S.; Yurchenko, E.A.; Dolmatov, I.Y.; Kalinin, V.I.; Stonik, V.A. Structure and biological action of cladolosides B_1, B_2, C, C_1, C_2 and D, six new triterpene glycosides from the sea cucumber *Cladolabes schmeltzii*. *Nat. Prod. Commun.* **2013**, *8*, 1527–1534. [PubMed]
91. Silchenko, A.S.; Kalinovsky, A.I.; Avilov, S.A.; Andryjaschenko, P.V.; Dmitrenok, P.S.; Yurchenko, E.A.; Dolmatov, I.Y.; Kalinin, V.I. Structures and biological activities of cladolosides C_3, E_1, E_2, F_1, F_2, G, H_1 and H_2, eight triterpene glycosides from the sea cucumber *Cladolabes schmeltzii* with one known and four new carbohydrate chains. *Carbohydr. Res.* **2015**, *23*, 22–31. [CrossRef] [PubMed]
92. Silchenko, A.S.; Kalinovsky, A.I.; Avilov, S.A.; Andryjaschenko, P.V.; Dmitrenok, P.S.; Chingizova, E.A.; Dolmatov, I.Y.; Kalinin, V.I. Cladolosides I_1, I_2, J_1, K_1, K_2 and L_1, monosulfated triterpene glycosides with new carbohydrate chains from the sea cucumber *Cladolabes schmeltzii*. *Carbohydr. Res.* **2017**, *5*, 80–87. [CrossRef] [PubMed]

93. Rodriguez, J.; Castro, R.; Riguera, R. Holothurinosides: New antitumour non sulphated triterpenoid glycosides from the sea cucumber *Holothuria forskalii*. *Tetrahedron* **1991**, *47*, 4753–4762. [CrossRef]

94. Sun, G.-Q.; Li, L.; Yi, Y.-H.; Yuan, W.-H.; Liu, B.-S.; Weng, Y.-Y.; Zhang, S.-L.; Sun, P.; Wang, Z.-L. Two new cytotoxic nonsulfated pentasaccharide holostane (=20-hydroxylanostan-18-oic acid gamma-lactone) glycosides from the sea cucumber *Holothuria grisea*. *Helv. Chim. Acta* **2008**, *9*, 1453–1460. [CrossRef]

95. Bahrami, Y.; Zhang, W.; Franco, C. Discovery of novel saponins from the viscera of the sea cucumber *Holothuria lessoni*. *Mar. Drugs* **2014**, *12*, 2633–2667. [CrossRef] [PubMed]

96. Silchenko, A.S.; Kalinovsky, A.I.; Avilov, S.A.; Andryjashchenko, P.V.; Fedorov, S.N.; Dmitrenok, P.S.; Yurchenko, E.A.; Kalinin, V.I.; Rogacheva, A.V.; Gebruk, A.V. Kolgaosides A and B, two new triterpene glycosides from the Arctic deep water sea cucumber *Kolga hyalina* (Elasipodida: Elpidiidae). *Nat. Prod. Commun.* **2014**, *9*, 1259–1264. [PubMed]

97. Yuan, W.H.; Yi, Y.H.; Tan, R.X.; Wang, Z.L.; Sun, G.Q.; Xue, M.; Zhang, H.W.; Tang, H.F. Antifungal triterpene glycosides from the sea cucumber *Holothuria* (Microthele) *axiloga*. *Planta Med.* **2009**, *75*, 647–653. [CrossRef] [PubMed]

98. Antonov, A.S.; Avilov, S.A.; Kalinovsky, A.I.; Anastyuk, S.D.; Dmitrenok, P.S.; Kalinin, V.I.; Taboada, S.; Bosh, A.; Avila, C.; Stonik, V.A. Triterpene glycosides from Antarctic sea cucumbers. 2. Structure of achlioniceosides A_1, A_2, and A_3 from the sea cucumber *Achlionice violaecuspidata* (=*Rhipidothuria racowitzai*). *J. Nat. Prod.* **2009**, *72*, 33–38. [CrossRef] [PubMed]

99. Miyamoto, T.; Togawa, K.; Higuchi, R.; Komori, T.; Sasaki, T. Structures of four new triterpenoid oligoglycosides: D_S-Penaustrosides A, B, C, and D from the sea cucumber *Pentacta australis*. *J. Nat. Prod.* **1992**, *55*, 940–946. [CrossRef] [PubMed]

100. Cuong, N.X.; Vien, L.T.; Hanh, T.T.; Thao, N.P.; Thaodo, T.; Thanh, N.V.; Nam, N.H.; Thungdo, C.; Kiem, P.V.; Minh, C.V. Cytotoxic triterpene saponins from *Cercodemas anceps*. *Bioorg. Med. Chem. Lett.* **2015**, *15*, 3151–3156. [CrossRef] [PubMed]

101. Chanley, J.D.; Ledeen, R.; Wax, J.; Nigrelli, R.F.; Sobotka, H. Holothurin I. The isolation, properties and sugar components of holothurin A. *J. Am. Chem. Soc.* **1959**, *81*, 5180–5183. [CrossRef]

102. Oleinikova, G.K.; Kuznetsova, T.A.; Ivanova, N.S.; Kalinovskii, A.I.; Rovnykh, N.V.; Elyakov, G.B. Glycosides of marine invertebrates. XV. A new triterpene glycoside-Holothurin A_1-from Caribbean holothurians of the family Holothuriidae. *Chem. Nat. Compd.* **1982**, *18*, 430–434. [CrossRef]

103. Dang, N.H.; Thanh, N.V.; Kiem, P.V.; Huong, M.; Minh, C.V.; Kim, Y.H. Two new triterpene glycosides from the Vietnamese sea cucumber *Holothuria scabra*. *Arch. Pharm. Res.* **2007**, *30*, 1387–1391. [CrossRef] [PubMed]

104. Han, H.; Yi, Y.; Xu, Q.; La, M.; Zhang, H. Two new cytotoxic triterpene glycosides from the sea cucumber *Holothuria scabra*. *Planta Med.* **2009**, *75*, 1608–1612. [CrossRef] [PubMed]

105. Han, H.; Li, L.; Yi, Y.-H.; Wang, X.-H.; Pan, M.-X. Triterpene glycosides from sea cucumber *Holothuria scabra* with cytotoxic activity. *Chin. Herb. Med.* **2012**, *4*, 183–188. [CrossRef]

106. Zhang, S.-Y.; Yi, Y.-H.; Tang, H.-F. Bioactive Triterpene glycosides from the sea cucumber *Holothuria fuscocinerea*. *J. Nat. Prod.* **2006**, *69*, 1492–1495. [CrossRef] [PubMed]

107. Yuan, W.; Yi, Y.; Tang, H.; Xue, M.; Wang, Z.; Sun, G.; Zhang, W.; Liu, B.; Li, L.; Sun, P. Two new holostan-type triterpene glycosides from the sea cucumber *Bohadschia marmorata*. *Chem. Pharm. Bull.* **2008**, *56*, 1207–1211. [CrossRef] [PubMed]

108. Kitagawa, I.; Inamoto, T.; Fuchida, M.; Okada, S.; Kobayashi, M.; Nishino, T.; Kyogoku, Y. Structures of echinosides A and B, two antifungal oligoglycosides from the sea cucumber *Actinopyga echinites*. *Chem. Pharm. Bull.* **1980**, *28*, 1651–1653. [CrossRef]

109. Zhao, Q.; Liu, Z.-D.; Xue, Y.; Wang, J.F.; Li, H.; Tang, Q.J.; Wang, Y.M.; Dong, P.; Xue, C.H. Ds-echinoside A, a new triterpene glycoside derived from sea cucumber, exhibits antimetastatic activity via the inhibition of NF-κB-dependent MMP-9 and VEGF expressions. *J. Zhejiang Univ. Sci. B* **2011**, *12*, 534–544. [CrossRef] [PubMed]

110. Bhatnagar, S.; Dudouet, B.; Ahond, A.; Poupat, C.; Thoison, O.; Clastres, A.; Laurent, D.; Potier, P. Invertébrés marins du lagon néocalédonien. IV: Saponines et sapogénines d'une holothurie, Actinopyga flammea. *Bull. Soc. Chim. Fr.* **1985**, *1*, 124–129. (In French)

111. Kitagawa, I.; Kobayashi, M.; Son, B.W.; Siuzukia, S.; Kyogokub, Y. Marine Natural Products. XIX. Pervicosides A, B, and C, lanostane-type triterpene-oligoglycoside sulfates from the sea cucumber *Holothuria pervicax*. *Chem. Pharm. Bull.* **1989**, *37*, 1230–1234. [CrossRef]

112. Liu, B.-S.; Yi, Y.-H.; Li, L.; Zhang, S.L.; Han, H.; Weng, Y.Y.; Pan, M. Arguside A: A new cytotoxic triterpene glycoside from the sea cucumber *Bohadschia argus. Chem. Biodivers.* **2007**, *4*, 2845–2851. [CrossRef] [PubMed]

113. Chludil, H.D.; Muniain, C.C.; Seldes, A.M.; Maier, M.S. Cytotoxic and antifungal triterpene glycosides from the patagonian sea cucumber *Hemoiedema spectabilis. J. Nat. Prod.* **2002**, *65*, 860–865. [CrossRef] [PubMed]

114. Liu, B.-S.; Yi, Y.-H.; Li, L.; Sun, P.; Han, H.; Sun, G.Q.; Wang, X.H.; Wang, Z.L. Argusides D and E, two new cytotoxic triterpene glycosides from the sea cucumber *Bohadschia argus. Chem. Biodivers.* **2008**, *5*, 1425–1433. [CrossRef] [PubMed]

115. Kalinin, V.I.; Kalinovsky, A.I.; Stonik, V.A. Structure of psolusoside A-the major triterpene glycoside from holothurian *Psolus fabricii. Chem. Nat. Compd.* **1985**, *21*, 197–202. [CrossRef]

116. Bahrami, Y.; Zhang, W.; Chataway, T.; Franco, C. Structural elucidation of novel saponins in the sea cucumber *Holothuria lessoni. Mar. Drugs* **2014**, *12*, 4439–4473. [CrossRef] [PubMed]

117. Silchenko, A.S.; Kalinovsky, A.I.; Avilov, S.A.; Andryjaschenko, P.V.; Dmitrenok, P.S.; Yurchenko, E.A.; Dolmatov, I.Y.; Savchenko, A.M.; Kalinin, V.I. Triterpene glycosides from the sea cucumber *Cladolabes schmeltzii*. II. Structure and biological action of cladolosides A_1–A_6. *Nat. Prod. Commun.* **2014**, *9*, 1421–1428. [PubMed]

118. Yibmantasiri, P.; Leahy, D.C.; Busby, B.P.; Angermayr, S.A.; Sorgo, A.G.; Boeger, K.; Heathcott, R.; Barber, J.M.; Moraes, G.; Matthews, J.H.; et al. Molecular basis for fungicidal action of neothyonidioside, a triterpene glycoside from the sea cucumber, *Australostichopus mollis. Mol. Biosyst.* **2012**, *8*, 902–912. [CrossRef] [PubMed]

119. Kitagawa, I.; Nishino, T.; Matsuno, T.; Akutsu, H.; Kyogoku, Y. Structure of holothurin B-a pharmacologically active triterpene-oligoglycoside from the sea cucumber *holothuria leucospilota* (Brandt). *Tetrahedron Lett.* **1978**, *19*, 985–988. [CrossRef]

120. Kuznetsova, T.A.; Kalinovskaya, N.I.; Kalinovskii, A.I.; Oleinikova, G.K.; Rovnykh, N.V.; Elyakov, G.V. Glycosides of marine invertebrates. XIV. Structure of holothurin B_1 from the holothurians *Holothuria floridana. Chem. Nat. Compd.* **1982**, *18*, 449–451. [CrossRef]

121. Silchenko, A.S.; Stonik, V.A.; Avilov, S.A.; Kalinin, V.I.; Kalinovsky, A.I.; Zaharenko, A.M.; Smirnov, A.V.; Mollo, E.; Cimino, G. Holothurins B_2, B_3, and B_4, new triterpene glycosides from mediterranean sea cucumbers of the genus Holothuria. *J. Nat. Prod.* **2005**, *68*, 564–567. [CrossRef] [PubMed]

122. Hua, H.; Yi, Y.-H.; Li, L.; Liu, B.-S.; Pan, M.-X.; Yan, B.; Wang, X.-H. Triterpene glycosides from sea cucumber *Holothuria leucospilota. Chin. J. Nat. Med.* **2009**, *7*, 346–350. [CrossRef]

123. Kobayashi, M.; Hori, M.; Kan, K.; Yasuzawa, T.; Matsui, M.; Shigeki, S.; Kitagawa, I. Marine Natural Products. XXVII. Distribution of lanostane-type triterpene oligoglycosides in ten kinds of okinawan sea cucumbers. *Chem. Pharm. Bull.* **1991**, *39*, 2282–2287. [CrossRef]

124. Wu, J.; Yi, Y.H.; Tang, H.F.; Zou, Z.R.; Wu, H.M. Structure and cytotoxicity of a new lanostane-type triterpene glycoside from the sea cucumber *Holothuria hilla. Chem. Biodivers.* **2006**, *3*, 1249–1254. [CrossRef] [PubMed]

125. Avilov, S.A.; Kalinin, V.I.; Makarieva, T.N.; Stonik, V.A.; Kalinovsky, A.I.; Rashkes, Y.W.; Milgrom, Y.M. Structure of cucumarioside G_2, a novel nonholostane glycoside from the sea cucumber *Eupentacta fraudatrix. J. Nat. Prod.* **1994**, *57*, 1166–1171. [CrossRef] [PubMed]

126. Avilov, S.A.; Kalinovsky, A.I.; Kalinin, V.I.; Stonik, V.A.; Riguera, R.; Jiménez, C. Koreoside A, a new nonholostane triterpene glycoside from the sea cucumber *Cucumaria koraiensis. J. Nat. Prod.* **1997**, *60*, 808–810. [CrossRef] [PubMed]

127. Liu, B.-S.; Zhang, H.-W.; Zhang, W.; Yi, Y.H.; Li, L.; Tang, H.; Wang, Z.-L.; Yuan, W.-H. Triterpene Glycosides-Antifungal Compounds of Sea Cucumber Holotoxins D-I and Preparation Method Thereof. Chinese Patent CN101671385 B, 30 May 2012.

128. Avilov, S.A.; Drozdova, O.A.; Kalinin, V.I.; Kalinovsky, A.I.; Stonik, V.A.; Gudimova, E.N.; Riguera, R.; Jimenez, C. Frondoside C, a new nonholostane triterpene glycoside from the sea cucumber *Cucumaria frondosa*: Structure and cytotoxicity of its desulfated derivative. *Can. J. Chem.* **1998**, *76*, 137–141. [CrossRef]

129. Kalinin, V.I.; Kalinovskii, A.I.; Stonik, V.A.; Dmitrenok, P.S.; El'kin, Y.N. Structure of psolusoside B-a nonholostane triterpene glycoside of the holothurian genus Psolus. *Chem. Nat. Compd.* **1989**, *25*, 311–317. [CrossRef]

130. Avilov, S.A.; Kalinovskii, A.I.; Stonik, V.A. Two new triterpene glycosides from the holothurian *Duasmodactyla kurilensis. Chem. Nat. Compd.* **1991**, *27*, 188–192. [CrossRef]

131. Silchenkoa, A.S.; Kalinovsky, A.I.; Avilov, S.A.; Dmitrenok, P.S.; Kalinin, V.I.; Berdyshev, D.V.; Chingizova, E.A.; Andryjaschenko, P.V.; Minin, K.V.; Stonika, V. Fallaxosides B$_1$ and D$_3$, triterpene glycosides with novel skeleton types of aglycones from the sea cucumber *Cucumaria fallax*. *Tetrahedron* **2017**, *73*, 2335–2341. [CrossRef]

132. Silchenko, A.S.; Kalinovskya, A.I.; Avilov, S.A.; Andryjaschenko, P.V.; Dmitrenok, P.S.; Kalinin, V.I.; Martyyas, E.A.; Minin, K.V. Fallaxosides C$_1$, C$_2$, D$_1$ and D$_2$, unusual oligosulfated triterpene glycosides from the sea cucumber *Cucumaria fallax* (Cucumariidae, Dendrochirotida, Holothurioidea) and taxonomic status of this animal. *Nat. Prod. Commun.* **2016**, *11*, 939–945.

133. Silchenko, A.S.; Kalinovskya, A.I.; Avilov, S.A.; Andryjaschenko, P.V.; Dmitrenok, P.S.; Kalinin, V.I.; Chingizova, E.A.; Minin, K.V.; Stonik, V.A. Structures and biogenesis of fallaxosides D$_4$, D$_5$, D$_6$ and D$_7$, trisulfated non-holostane triterpene glycosides from the sea cucumber *Cucumaria fallax*. *Molecules* **2016**, *21*, 939. [CrossRef] [PubMed]

134. Silchenko, A.S.; Kalinovsky, A.I.; Avilov, S.A.; Kalinin, V.I.; Andrijaschenko, P.V.; Dmitrenok, P.S.; Chingizova, E.A.; Ermakova, S.P.; Malyarenko, O.S.; Dautova, T.N. Nine new triterpene glycosides, magnumosides A$_1$–A$_4$, B$_1$, B$_2$, C$_1$, C$_2$ and C$_4$, from the Vietnamese sea cucumber *Neothyonidium* (=*Massinium*) *magnum*: Structures and activities against tumor cells independently and in synergy with radioactive irradiation. *Mar. Drugs* **2017**, *16*, 256. [CrossRef] [PubMed]

135. Silchenko, A.S.; Kalinovsky, A.I.; Avilov, S.A.; Andryjaschenko, P.V.; Dmitrenok, P.S.; Yurchenko, E.A.; Dolmatov, I.Y.; Dautov, S.S.; Stonik, V.A.; Kalinin, V.I. Colochiroside E, an unusual non-holostane triterpene sulfated trioside from the sea cucumber *Colochirus robustus* and evidence of the impossibility of a 7(8)-double bond migration in lanostane derivatives having an 18(16)-lactone. *Nat. Prod. Commun.* **2016**, *11*, 741–746. [PubMed]

136. Kalinin, V.I.; Prkofieva, N.G.; Likhatskaya, G.N. Hemolytic activities of triterpene glycosides from the holothurian order Dendrochirotida: Some trends in the evolution of this group of toxins. *Toxicon* **1996**, *34*, 475–483. [CrossRef]

137. Kumar, R.; Chaturvedi, A.K.; Shukla, P.K.; Lakshmi, V. Antifungal activity in triterpene glycosides from the sea cucumber *Actinopyga lecanora*. *Bioorg. Med. Chem. Lett.* **2007**, *17*, 4387–4391. [CrossRef] [PubMed]

138. Hua, H.; Yang-hua, Y.; Li, L.; Liu, B.S.; La, M.P.; Zhang, H.W. Antifungal active triterpene glycosides from sea cucumber *Holothuria scabra*. *Acta Pharm. Sin.* **2009**, *44*, 620–624.

139. Aminin, D.L.; Pislyagin, E.A.; Menchinskaya, E.S.; Silchenko, A.S.; Avilov, S.A.; Kalinin, V.I. Immunomodulatory and anticancer activity of sea cucumber triterpene glycosides. In *Studies in Natural Products Chemistry*; Atta-ur-Rahman, Ed.; Elsevier Science: Amsterdam, The Netherlands, 2013; Volume 41, pp. 75–94.

140. Aminin, D.L.; Agafonova, I.G.; Kalinin, V.I.; Silchenko, A.S.; Avilov, S.A.; Stonik, V.A.; Collin, P.D.; Woodward, C. Immunomodulatory properties of frondoside A, a major triterpene glycoside from the North Atlantic commercially harvested sea cucumber *Cucumaria frondosa*. *J. Med. Food* **2008**, *11*, 443–453. [CrossRef] [PubMed]

141. Wang, J.; Han, H.; Chen, X.; Yi, Y.; Sun, H. Cytotoxic and apoptosis-inducing activity of triterpene glycosides from Holothuria scabra and Cucumaria frondosa against HepG2 cells. *Mar. Drugs* **2014**, *24*, 4274–4290. [CrossRef] [PubMed]

142. Popov, A.; Kalinovskaia, N.; Kuznetsova, T.; Agafonova, I.; Anisimov, M. Role of sterols in the membranotropic activity of triterpene glycosides. *Antibiotiki* **1983**, *28*, 656–659. [PubMed]

143. Segal, R.; Schlosser, E. Role of glycosides in the membranlytic, antifungal action of saponins. *Arch. Microbiol.* **1975**, *104*, 147–150. [CrossRef] [PubMed]

144. Aminin, D.L.; Menchinskaya, E.S.; Pislyagin, E.A.; Silchenko, A.S.; Avilov, S.A.; Kalinin, V.I. Sea cucumber triterpene glycosides as anticancer agents. In *Studies in Natural Products Chemistry*, 1st ed.; Atta-ur-Rahman, Ed.; Elsevier Science: Amsterdam, The Netherlands, 2016; Volume 49, pp. 55–105; ISBN 978-0-444-63601-0.
145. Kalinin, V.I.; Aminin, D.L.; Avilov, S.A.; Silchenko, A.S.; Stonik, V.A. Triterpene glycosides from sea cucumbers (Holothurioidae, Echinodermata), biological activities and functions. In *Studies in Natural Product Chemistry (Bioactive Natural Products)*; Atta-ur-Rahman, Ed.; Elsevier Science: Amsterdam, The Netherlands, 2008; Volume 35, pp. 135–196.

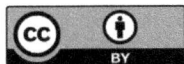

© 2017 by the authors. Licensee MDPI, Basel, Switzerland. This article is an open access article distributed under the terms and conditions of the Creative Commons Attribution (CC BY) license (http://creativecommons.org/licenses/by/4.0/).

marine drugs

MDPI

Article

Three New Cytotoxic Steroidal Glycosides Isolated from *Conus pulicarius* Collected in Kosrae, Micronesia

Yeon-Ju Lee [1,2,*], Saem Han [1], Su Hyun Kim [1,2], Hyi-Seung Lee [1,2], Hee Jae Shin [1,2], Jong Seok Lee [1,2] and Jihoon Lee [1,2]

[1]   Marine Nautral Product Chemistry Laboratory, Korea Institute of Ocean Science and Technology, Ansan 15627, Korea; gkstoa1126@naver.com (S.H.); tngus173@kiost.ac.kr (S.H.K.); hslee@kiost.ac.kr (H.-S.L.); shinhj@kiost.ac.kr (H.J.S.); jslee@kiost.ac.kr (J.S.L.); jihoonlee@kiost.ac.kr (J.L.)
[2]   Department of Marine Biotechnology, University of Science and Technology, Daejeon 34113, Korea
*   Correspondence: yjlee@kiost.ac.kr; Tel.: +82-31-400-6171

Received: 23 October 2017; Accepted: 23 November 2017; Published: 4 December 2017

Abstract: Three new sulfated steroidal glycosides (**3–5**), along with known cholesterol derivatives (**1,2**), were isolated from the visceral extract of the cone snail *Conus pulicarius*. The structure of each new compound was elucidated by nuclear magnetic resonance spectroscopy and high-resolution mass spectrometry. The three new compounds exhibited significant in vitro cytotoxicity (GI_{50} values down to 0.49 µM) against the K562 human leukemia cell line.

Keywords: *Conus pulicarius*; steroidal glycoside; cholesterol sulfate; cytotoxicity; leukemia

1. Introduction

Cone snails are predatory marine molluscs that secrete venom to capture prey, such as marine worms, small fish, molluscs, and other cone snails. The venom that produced by cone snails is composed of various modified peptides, such as conotoxin, which is produced by the Conus species. Conotoxins have generated tremendous interest in the fields of biology and pharmacology, as these peptides cause neurophysiological responses by modulating the activity of ion channels. Over 100,000 neuroactive conotoxins have been discovered from cone snails, which now comprise over 1000 species in the tropical and subtropical areas [1], since the first conotoxins were isolated and characterized [2,3]. During these investigations, ziconotide, the conotoxin peptide that is derived from *Conus magus*, has gained approval from the Food and Drugs Administration (FDA) as an analgesic for severe and chronic pain, and several other conotoxins are now under investigation in clinical trials as medical agents for the same purpose [4,5].

Small molecules that are produced by the Conus species have gained much less attention as compared to conotoxins, presumably based upon the assumption that the predatory or protective mechanism of the Conus species is mainly dependent on the production and secretion of conotoxins. Despite a thorough literature search, only two publications on the small molecule metabolite that is isolated from the Conus species could be found. One publication describes the isolation of cholesterol and the epidioxysterol **1** from the three species of Conus cone snails (*Conus ebraeus*, *C. leopardus*, and *C. tessulatus*) [6], and the other describes the isolation of a guanine derivative that causes paralysis in mice [7]. Additionally, there is one publication that reported the isolation of thiazoline metabolites (pulicatins) from the cultivation of bacteria *Streptomyces* sp. CP32 associated with *Conus pulicarius* [8]. These findings led us to investigate the metabolites that contained in the Conus species, as marine invertebrates are considered to have diverse and complex symbiotic relationships and chemical defense mechanisms. In this work, we investigated the visceral extract of *Conus pulicarius* collected off the coast of Kosrae, the Federated States of Micronesia (Figure 1), in search for novel toxic metabolites. Herein, five cholesterol derivatives (**1–5**, Figure 2), which were isolated from this organism, have been described. While compounds **1** and **2** were the previously identified epidioxysterol and cholesterol sulfate, respectively, compounds **3–5** were new steroidal glycosides. In vitro cytotoxicity tests revealed that these new steroidal glycosides were extremely cytotoxic against the human leukemia cell line K562.

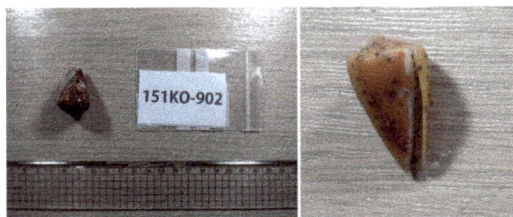

Figure 1. Specimen of *Conus pulicarius* collected in Kosrae.

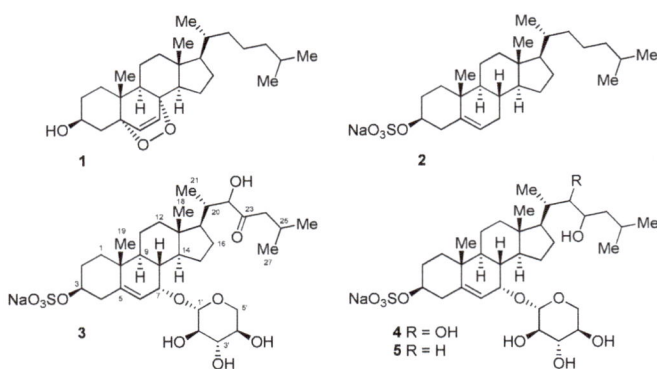

Figure 2. Structures of the isolated cholesterol derivatives.

2. Results

2.1. Isolation of Cholesterol Derivatives from the Conus Pulicarius Cone Snails

The grinded and lyophilized whole-body tissue of *Conus pulicarius* specimens were extracted with methanol and dichloromethane. The combined extracts were partitioned between *n*-butanol and water, and the *n*-butanol fraction was subsequently partitioned between 15% aqueous methanol and *n*-hexane. The 15% aqueous methanol fraction was subjected to reverse-phase flash column chromatography using the ODS resin with aqueous methanol gradient elution (50% aqueous methanol to 100% methanol) to afford six fractions. The growth inhibitory activity of each fraction against the human leukemia cell line K562 was evaluated to trace the cytotoxic metabolites in the extract. The second and third fractions eluted with 40% (GI_{50} 3.4 µg/mL) and 30% aqueous methanol (GI_{50} 0.9 µg/mL), respectively, demonstrated high levels of cytotoxicity. These fractions were further purified by size-exclusion column chromatography on the Sephadex LH-20 column, and reverse-phase HPLC, using the YMC-Pack Pro C18 ODS column. Compounds **3** and **4** were obtained from the 40% aqueous methanol fraction, and **5** was obtained from the 30% aqueous methanol fraction. Known compounds **1** and **2** were obtained from the fractions that did not exhibit cytotoxicity at the concentration of 100 µg/mL (100% methanol and 10% aqueous methanol fractions, respectively).

2.2. Structure Elucidation of the Isolated Compounds

A comparison of nuclear magnetic resonance (NMR), mass spectrometry (MS), and optical rotation data with those reported previously confirmed that compounds **1** and **2** were 5α,8α-epidioxysterol and cholesterol sulfate [6,9–11] (Figure 2).

Compounds **3–5** were found to share the same tetracyclic carbon framework, with the only difference between these compounds being the substitution at C-17, as judged by ^{1}H and ^{13}C NMR (Table 1) and high-resolution mass spectrometry data.

Table 1. ^{1}H and ^{13}C NMR data (500 and 125 MHz) for compounds **3–5** [a,b].

Postion	3		4		5	
	δ_C	δ_H (J in Hz)	δ_C	δ_H (J in Hz)	δ_C	δ_H (J in Hz)
1α	37.6	1.23 (m)	37.7	1.22 (m)	37.7	1.22 (m)
1β		1.88 (m)		1.86 (m)		1.88 (m)
2α	29.7	2.07 (br d, 12.9)	29.7	2.07 (br d, 12.0)	29.8	2.07 (br d, 12.4)
2β		1.65 (m)		1.65 (m)		1.64 (m)
3	79.3	4.21 (dddd, 16.0, 13.0, 4.8, 4.8)	79.3	4.20 (dddd, 15.0, 13.1, 5.5, 5.2)	79.3	4.20 (dddd, 16.0, 13.1, 4.5, 4.5)
4α	40.4	2.61 (dd, 13.0, 4.8)	40.4	2.61 (dd, 13.1, 5.2)	40.4	2.61 (dd, 13.1, 4.5)
4β		2.40 (dd, 13.0, 13.0)		2.42 (dd, 13.1, 13.1)		2.42 (dd, 13.1, 13.1)
5	148.2		148.1		148.2	
6	122.0	5.74 (dd, 5.5, 1.5)	122.1	5.74 (dd, 5.0, 1.3)	122.1	5.73 (dd, 4.9, 1.3)
7	70.1	3.98 (br s)	70.1	4.00 (br s)	70.2	3.96 (br s)
8	38.5	1.55 (ovl)	38.7	1.53 (ovl)	38.4	1.53 (ovl)
9	43.0	1.54 (ovl)	43.0	1.54 (ovl)	43.0	1.54 (ovl)
10	38.7		38.4		38.7	
11α	21.8	1.54 (ovl)	21.8	1.54 (ovl)	21.8	1.54 (ovl)
11β		1.21 (ovl)		1.29 (ovl)		1.29 (ovl)
12α	40.0	1.23 (ovl)	40.5	1.22 (ovl)	40.4	1.21 (ovl)
12β		1.93 (m)		1.98 (br d, 12.4)		2.00 (br d, 12.4)
13	43.0		43.0		43.3	
14	49.8	1.72 (m)	49.8	1.68 (m)	49.7	1.63 (m)
15α	24.6	1.97 (ovl)	24.7	1.95 (ovl)	24.8	1.92 (ovl)
15β		1.10 (m)		1.09 (m)		1.05 (m)
16α	29.0	1.98 (ovl)	28.9	1.95 (m)	29.6	2.05 (m)
16β		1.44 (m)		1.25 (ovl)		1.21 (ovl)
17	53.3	1.57 (ovl)	53.4	1.56 (ovl)	58.2	1.15 (m)
18	11.9	0.75 (s)	11.8	0.71 (s)	11.9	0.70 (s)
19	18.5	1.03 (s)	18.6	1.02 (s)	18.6	1.02 (s)
20	40.1	1.97 (m)	38.9	1.53 (m)	35.2	1.44 (m)
21	13.3	0.76 (d, 6.8)	12.6	0.91 (d 6.4)	20.0	0.98 (d, 6.4)
22	80.8	4.12 (br s)	78.2	3.31 (ovl)	46.3	1.44 (ovl)
						1.54 (ovl)
23	215.0		72.2	3.55 (ddd, 10.5, 8.2, 2.6)	69.1	3.69 (m)
24	48.5	2.38 (dd, 18.3, 6.8)	43.3	1.14 (ddd, 13.6, 10.5, 2.6)	47.5	1.22 (ovl)
		1.96 (ovl)		1.24 (ovl)		1.25 (ovl)
25	25.4	2.12 (m)	25.3	1.86 (m)	25.5	1.84 (m)
26	22.9	0.91 (d, 6.6)	21.7	0.92 (d, 6.6)	22.0	0.90 (d, 6.7)
27	23.0	0.93 (d, 6.8)	24.5	0.94(d, 6.7)	22.0	0.92 (d, 6.7)
1'	101.3	4.40 (d, 7.4)	101.3	4.40 (d, 7.4)	101.3	4.40 (d, 7.5)
2'	75.2	3.10 (dd, 8.9, 7.4)	75.2	3.10 (dd, 8.9, 7.4)	75.2	3.10 (dd, 8.9, 7.5)
3'	77.9	3.31 (ovl)	77.8	3.33 (ovl)	77.9	3.32 (ovl)
4'	71.4	3.46 (ddd, 10.0, 9.0, 5.3)	71.4	3.46 (ddd, 10.2, 9.4, 5.3)	71.4	3.47 (ddd, 9.9, 8.9, 5.3)
5'α	66.8	3.83 (dd, 11.4, 5.3)	66.8	3.83 (dd, 11.4, 5.3)	66.8	3.83 (dd, 11.4, 5.3)
5'β		3.19 (dd, 11.4, 10.0)		3.19 (dd, 11.4, 10.2)		3.19 (dd, 11.4, 9.9)

[a] Data were obtained in CD$_3$OD. [b] These assignments are based on HSQC, COSY, and HMBC results.

Compound **3** was obtained as a colorless oil. Its molecular formula was determined as $C_{32}H_{51}NaO_{11}S$ by HRFABMS and ESIMS, which showed pseudomolecular ion peaks that were corresponding to $[M - Na]^-$ and $[M + Na]^+$, respectively. The tetracyclic carbon framework was analogous to that of cholesterol sulfate **2**, except for the presence of the oxymethine group at the C-7 position (δ_H 3.98, δ_C 70.1), as judged by the COSY correlation between the proton NMR signals at δ_H 5.74 (H-6), and 3.98 (H-7), in addition to the HMBC correlations between H-7 and the carbon signals at δ_C 148.2 (C-5), 122.0 (C-6), and 43.0 (C-9) (Table 1, Figure 3).

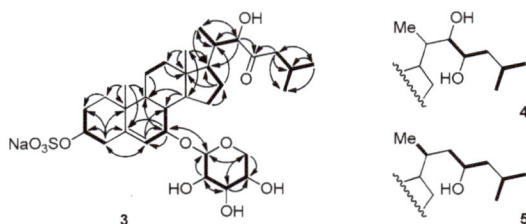

Figure 3. Selected COSY and HMBC correlations for compounds 3–5.

The relative configuration of the tetracyclic core was confirmed on the basis of coupling constants and correlations observed in the NOESY spectrum (Figure 4). Especially, the NOESY correlation between the proton signals at δ_H 4.21 (H-3) and 1.23 (H-1α), and the trans diaxial coupling (J = 13.0 Hz) of H-3 with an axial proton at C-4 (H-4β, δ 2.40), both supported the α orientation of H-3. The relative stereochemistry at C-7, where the additional oxygen is attached, was confirmed by a NOESY correlation between H-7 and H-15β (δ 1.10), which suggested that H-7 had the β-pseudoequatorial orientation. This assignment is in accordance with the previous reports, which describe compounds with similar structures as that of **1**. In the case of 3β,7β-dihydroxy-5-chole-24-oic acid, which was sulfated at C-3 and *N*-acetylglucosaminidated at C-7, the H-7 of the α-orientation appeared at δ 3.80 ppm, with a coupling constant of 7.8 to 8.4 Hz [12]. In other reports, comparative data are provided for the C-7 epimers of the synthesized 5-androstene-3,7,17-triol derivative. In the NMR spectra, the H-7 of the 7β-derivative oriented to the α-face appeared as a doublet with J = 7.9 Hz, whereas that of the 7α-derivative appeared as a broad singlet [13]. The same tendency has been observed in the case of 24-methylene-cholest-5-ene-3β,7α-diol and its C-7 epimer [14]. As the H-7 of compound **3** appeared as a broad singlet, this proton was confirmed to have an β-orientation.

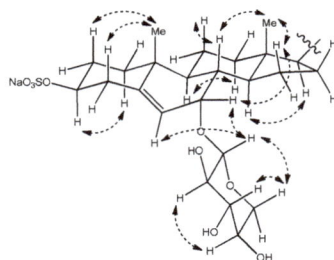

Figure 4. Selected NOESY correlations for compound **3**.

The following proton signals were common in the ^{1}H NMR spectra of all three compounds—a dioxymethine signal at δ 4.40 (H-1′), three hydroxymethine signals at δ 3.10 (H-2′), 3.31 (H-3′), and 3.46 (H-4′), and the signals of the two protons that were attached to the same oxymethylene carbon (C-5′, δ_C 66.8) at δ 3.83 (H-5′α) and 3.19 (H-5′β). This consistency in signals indicated the presence of the sugar moiety, which was identified as β-D-xylose based upon the interpretation of the coupling constants and NOESY correlations between the signals in this region. In detail, a proton signal at the anomeric position (H-1′) was coupled to a signal of H-2′ with J = 7.4 Hz, and H-2′ was again coupled to H-3′ with J = 8.9 Hz. NOESY correlations were also observed between H-1′, H-3′, and H-5′β (Figures 3 and 4). These observations hinted at a diaxial relationship existing between these protons, and thus the sugar moiety was identified as β-D-xylose. This assignment was in accordance with the result that was obtained by the treatment of compound **3** with 2N HCl, which showed that the ^{1}H NMR data and optical rotation value of the hydrolysis product coincided with those of D-xylose.

The xylose moiety was connected to C-7 of the tetracyclic carbon framework, as judged by the HMBC correlations between the anomeric proton and the C-7 oxymethine carbon.

The remaining oxymethine proton signal appearing at δ_H 4.12 (H-22) showed HMBC correlations with the carbon signals at δ_C 53.3 (C-17), 40.1 (C-20), and 13.3 (C-21), and the signal of the ketone carbon at δ_C 215.0 (C-23). The two signals of the protons attached to the α-carbon with the chemical shift of δ_C 48.5 (C-24) appeared at δ_H 2.38 and 1.96 (H-24), and these signals showed COSY and HMBC correlations with the proton and carbon signals of isopropyl methine (C-25, δ_C 25.4). Based on these observations, the side branch attached at C-17 could be established, as depicted in Figures 2 and 3.

Compound **4** was obtained as a pale-yellow amorphous solid. The ^{1}H NMR data for **4** was quite similar to that of **3**, except for the additional oxymethine proton signal at δ_H 3.55 (H-23). In the ^{13}C NMR spectra, the corresponding carbon signal at δ_C 72.2 (C-23) was observed and the signal corresponding to the carbonyl carbon was absent. Based upon these observations, **4** was identified as the 22,23-dihydroxy derivative, i.e., the reduced form of **3**. This assignment is in accordance with the molecular formula of $C_{32}H_{53}NaO_{11}S$ that were derived from (−)-HRFABMS, the COSY, and HMBC correlations (Figure 3).

Compound **5** had one less oxymethine signal in its ^{1}H and ^{13}C NMR spectra as compared to **2**. Instead, a carbon signal was observed at δ_C 46.3 (C-22), which was correlated to the two protons that appeared at δ_H 1.44 and 1.54 (H-22) in the HSQC spectra. The molecular formula of $C_{32}H_{53}NaO_{10}S$ obtained by (−)-HRFABMS also suggests that **5** has one less hydroxy group as compared to **4**. Consequently, the structure of **5** established from the COSY and HMBC correlations was as depicted in Figures 2 and 3.

For the establishment of absolute stereochemistry at C-22 of **3**, C-22 and C-23 of **4**, and C-23 of **5**, we have tried to prepare the MTPA ester derivatives of the aglycon. Disappointingly, attempts to obtain the desulfated aglycon under various conditions, such as using an acid (2N HCl, *p*-toluenesulfonic acid) or a base (pyridine, potassium carbonate) only resulted in the decomposition of the starting material with the formation of products whose ^{1}H NMR spectrum had few assignable signals. The direct acylation of the obtained compounds using MTPA chloride and the acetonide formation of **2** also failed because of the decomposition of the starting material. No valid method for establishing the absolute configuration of the oxymethine stereogenic center of the side branch in the new compounds could be found up to now.

The relative stereochemistry of C-20 in compounds **3**–**5** was established to be the same as that of cholesterol sulfate **2** based on the comparison of ^{1}H and ^{13}C NMR data of **2** and **5**. In detail, the carbon signal of C-17 appeared at δ_C 58.2, and the signal of the attached proton appeared at δ_H 1.15 in the NMR spectra of **5**, whereas these signals were observed at δ_C 57.5 and δ_H 1.09 in the spectra of **2**. The signals of C-20, C-21 and the attached proton were also similar; δ_{c-20} 37.1, δ_{c-21} 19.2, and δ_{H-21} 1.40, δ_{H-21} 0.95 in the NMR data of **2**, δ_{c-20} 35.2, δ_{c-21} 20.0, and δ_{H-20} 1.44, δ_{H-21} 0.98 in those of **5** (see Supplementary Materials).

All of the isolated compounds were tested for in vitro cytotoxicity against the human leukemia cell line K562. While compounds **1** and **2** did not exhibit any cytotoxicity (GI_{50} > 60.00 μM), the new sulfated steroidal glycosides **3**–**5** demonstrated potent cytotoxicities with GI_{50} values of 1.50 ± 0.25 μM, 1.39 ± 0.05 μM, and 0.49 ± 0.03 μM, respectively. Staurosporine, used as a positive control, showed an GI_{50} value of 2.29 ± 0.02 μM with in the same 96 well-plate.

3. Discussion

Five cholesterol derivatives (**1**–**5**), including three new sulfated steroidal glycosides (**3**–**5**), were isolated from the *Conus pulicarius* that were collected in Kosrae, Micronesia. The characteristic structural features of the new compounds include the sulfate group at the C-3 position and the xylose linked to C-7, which is different from those of known steroidal glycosides. Sulfated steroidal glycosides have been primarily isolated from marine organisms, such as algae and invertebrates [15,16]. Especially, the starfishes of various species are frequently found to contain sulfated steroidal glycosides, called asterosaponins, which have a sulfate group at the C-3 position and various sugar moieties linked to C-6. Compounds (**3–5**) were named as Conusaponin A-C, as these are the first example of steroidal glycosides isolated from Conus species.

The new compounds showed potent growth inhibitory activity against the human leukemia cell line K562. This finding, combined with those regarding the previously reported steroidal glycosides with potent activities against various cancer cell lines [16–22], would provide new insights into the structure-activity relationships of cytotoxic sulfated steroidal glycosides.

4. Materials and Methods

4.1. General Procedures

The optical rotations were measured using a JASCO digital polarimeter in a 5 cm long cell. Fourier transform infra-red (FTIR) spectra were recorded on a JASCO FT/IR-4100 spectrometer (JASCO, Tokyo, Japan). ^{1}H and ^{13}C NMR spectra were recorded on Varian Unity 500 500 MHz and 125 MHz spectrometers, respectively. The chemical shifts have been reported in ppm and referenced to the solvent resonances, resulting from incomplete deuteration as the internal references (CD$_3$OD: δ_H 3.31 ppm, δ_C 49.00 ppm). HPLC was performed with YMC-Pack Pro C18 columns using a Shodex RI-101 detector (Shoko Science, Yokohama, Japan).

4.2. Biological Material Collection, Extraction, and Isolation

Twenty specimens of *Conus pulicarius* (3–4 cm) were collected by hand at 1–3 m depth offshore of Kosrae, the Federated States of Micronesia, in January, 2015. The collected specimens (300 g, wet wt.) were immediately freeze-dried and kept at −20 °C until the time of our investigation. The specimens were thawed at room temperature in a fume hood for 3 h, and then the shell was removed from the viscera. The viscera were then grinded in a blender and lyophilized to yield the 17.7 g of a sticky solid. This solid was extracted using methanol (300 mL × 2) and dichloromethane (300 mL × 1) at room temperature. The combined extract (2.8 g) was partitioned between *n*-butanol and water, and the organic layer (820 mg) was further partitioned between 15% aqueous methanol and *n*-hexane. Subsequently, the aqueous methanol fraction (430 mg) was subjected to reverse-phase column chromatography (YMC Gel ODS-A, 60 Å, 230 mesh) with a stepped gradient solvent system of 50, 40, 30, 20, and 10% aqueous methanol, and 100% methanol. The fraction eluted with 40% aqueous methanol (34.0 mg) was then subjected to size-exclusion column chromatography (LH-20), followed by further purification by reverse-phase HPLC (YMC-Pack Pro C18) to afford **3** (3.2 mg) and **4** (5.0 mg). The 30% aqueous methanol fraction (59.0 mg) was also subjected to size-exclusion chromatography and reverse-phase HPLC to afford **5** (3.1 mg). The 10% aqueous methanol and 100% methanol fractions were purified by reverse-phase HPLC to afford **1** (2.8 mg) and **2** (0.8 mg), respectively.

Compound **3**: pale yellow amorphous solid; $[\alpha]_D^{25}$ −73.1 (*c* 0.5, CH$_3$OH); UV λ_{max} (log ε) 285 (4.5), 211 (3.4) nm; IR (KBr) ν_{max} 3337, 2921, 2885, 1055, 1033, 1014 cm^{-1}; ^{1}H and ^{13}C NMR (CD$_3$OD, 500 and 125 MHz), see Table 1 and Supplementary Materials; (+)-LRESIMS *m/z* 689.84 [M + Na]$^+$; (−)-HRFABMS *m/z* 643.3156 [M − Na]$^-$ (calcd. for C$_{32}$H$_{51}$O$_{11}$S, *m/z* 643.3152).

Compound **4**: pale yellow amorphous solid; $[\alpha]_D^{25}$ −59.1 (*c* 0.5, CH$_3$OH); UV λ_{max} (log ε) 286 (3.2), 235 (3.5), 211 (4.5) nm; IR (KBr) ν_{max} 3726, 2866, 1055, 1032, 1012 cm^{-1}; ^{1}H and ^{13}C NMR (CD$_3$OD, 500 and 125 MHz), see Table 1 and Supplementary Materials; (+)-LRESIMS *m/z* 691.67 [M + Na]$^+$; (−)-HRFABMS *m/z* 645.3307 [M − Na]$^-$ (calcd. for C$_{32}$H$_{53}$O$_{11}$S, *m/z* 645.3309).

Compound **5**: pale yellow amorphous solid; $[\alpha]_D^{25}$ −40.7 (*c* 0.5, CH$_3$OH); UV λ_{max} (log ε) 277 (3.9), 236 (4.2), 211 (4.5) nm; IR (KBr) ν_{max} 3725, 2865, 1055, 1033, 1055 cm^{-1}; ^{1}H and ^{13}C NMR (CD$_3$OD, 500 and 125 MHz), see Table 1 and Supplementary Materials; (+)-LRESIMS *m/z* 675.70 [M + Na]$^+$; (−)-HRFABMS *m/z* 629.3363 [M − Na]$^-$ (calcd. for C$_{32}$H$_{53}$O$_{10}$S, *m/z* 629.3359).

4.3. Cytotoxicity Assay

The growth inhibition assay against human leukemia cell line K562 was performed according to a published protocol [23,24]. In brief, the cells were added to a 96-well plate containing either a control (staurosprine) or the test compounds. After incubation for 48 h, 10 μL of the WST-1 solution was added to each well of the culture plate (containing 100 μL of the RPMI medium). After incubation for 2 h at 37 °C, the optical density (OD) of the assay solution was measured at 450 nm by using the ELISA plate reader. Cell viability was calculated as a percentage, with the following equation: % cell viability = (OD$_{sample}$/OD$_{control}$) × 100. The GI$_{50}$ values were determined by plotting cell viability versus the concentration of compound. Results were reported as the average values and standard deviations of triplicate samples.

Supplementary Materials: The following are available online at www.mdpi.com/1660-3397/15/12/379/s1, ^{1}H and ^{13}C NMR spectra of **1–5**, and 2D (HMBC, HSQC, COSY, NOESY) NMR spectra of **3–5**.

Acknowledgments: This work was supported by a grant of the Korea Institute of Ocean Science and Technology and the Ministry of Oceans and Fisheries, Republic of Korea. We thank the Kosrae State Government, the Federated States of Micronesia, for allowing marine organism research.

Author Contributions: Collection of the *Conus pulicarius*, isolation and purification of the secondary metabolites, and structure elucidation of isolated compounds were carried out by Yeon-Ju Lee, Saem Han, Hyi-Seung Lee, Hee Jae Shin, Jong Seok Lee, and Jihoon Lee. Evaluation of the cytotoxicity against human leukemia cell line (K562) of the isolated compounds was carried out by Su-Hyun Kim. Yeon-Ju Lee wrote the manuscript and the manuscript was finalized through contributions from all authors.

Conflicts of Interest: The authors declare no conflict of interest.

References

1. Franco, A.; Pisarewicz, K.; Moller, C.; Mora, D.; Fields, G.B.; Mari, F. Hyperhydroxylation: A new strategy for neuronal targeting by venomous marine molluscs. In *Molluscs: From Chemo-Ecological Study to Biotechnological Application*, 1st ed.; Cimino, G., Gavagnin, M., Eds.; Springer: Berlin/Heidelberg, Germany, 2006; pp. 83–103.

2. Cruz, L.J.; Gray, W.R.; Oliviera, B.M. Purification and properties of a myotoxin from *Conus geographus* venom. *Arch. Biochem. Biophys.* **1978**, *190*, 539–548. [CrossRef]

3. Olivera, B.M.; Gray, W.R.; Zeikus, R.; McIntosh, J.M.; Varga, J.; Rivier, J.; de Santos, V.; Cruz, L.J. Peptide neurotoxins from fish-hunting cone snails. *Science* **1985**, *230*, 1338–1343. [CrossRef] [PubMed]

4. Brady, R.M.; Baell, J.B.; Norton, R.S. Strategies for the development of conotoxins as new therapeutic leads. *Mar. Drugs* **2013**, *11*, 2293–2313. [CrossRef] [PubMed]

5. Munasinghe, N.R.; Christie, M.J. Conotoxins that could provide analgesia through voltage gated sodium channel inhibition. *Toxins* **2015**, *7*, 5386–5407. [CrossRef] [PubMed]

6. Aknin, M.; Faure, I.V.; Gaydou, E.M. 5α,8α-Epidioxycholest-6-en-3-β-ol from three cone snails of the Indian Ocean. *J. Am. Oil Chem. Soc.* **1998**, *75*, 1679–1681. [CrossRef]

7. Neves, J.L.B.; Lin, Z.; Imperial, J.S.; Antunes, A.; Vasconcelos, V.; Oliviera, B.M.; Schmidt, E.W. Small molecules in the cone snail arsenal. *Org. Lett.* **2015**, *17*, 4933–4935. [CrossRef] [PubMed]

8. Lin, Z.; Antemano, R.R.; Hughen, R.W.; Tianero, M.D.B.; Peraud, O.; Haygood, M.G.; Concepcion, G.P.; Oliviera, B.M.; Light, A.; Schmidt, E.W. Pulicatins A–E, neuroactive thiazoline metabolites from cone snail-associated bacteria. *J. Nat. Prod.* **2010**, *73*, 1922–1926. [CrossRef] [PubMed]

9. Gunatilaka, A.A.L.; Gopichand, Y.; Schmitz, F.J.; Djerassi, C. Minor and trace sterols in marine invertebrates. 26. Isolation and structure elucidation of nine new 5α,8α-epidoxy sterols from four marine organisms. *J. Org. Chem.* **1981**, *46*, 3860–3866. [CrossRef]

10. Miyamoto, T.; Honda, M.; Sugiyama, S.; Higuchi, R.; Komori, T. Isolation and structure of two 5,8α-epidioxysterols and a cholesteryl ester mixture from the albumen gland of *Aplysia juliana*. *Liebigs Ann. Chem.* **1988**, *1988*, 589–592. [CrossRef]

11. Minn, C.V.; Kiem, P.V.; Huong, L.M.; Kim, Y.H. Cytotoxic constituents of *Diadema setosum*. *Arch. Pharm. Res.* **2004**, *27*, 734–737. [CrossRef]

12. Kakiyama, G.; Ogawa, S.; Iida, T.; Fujimoto, Y.; Mushiake, K.; Goto, T.; Mano, N.; Goto, J.; Nambara, T. Nuclear magnetic resonance spectroscopy of 3β,7β-dihydroxy-5-cholen-24-oic acid multi-conjugates: Unusual bile acid metabolites in human urine. *Chem. Phys. Lipids* **2006**, *140*, 48–54. [CrossRef] [PubMed]

13. Li, H.-P.; Yu, P.; Zhang, H.-J.; Liu, H.-M. Synthesis of 5-androstene-3β,7α,17β-triol and 5-androstene-3β,7β,17β-triol. *Chin. J. Chem.* **2008**, *26*, 1666–1668. [CrossRef]

14. De Riccardis, F.; Minale, L.; Iorizzi, M.; Debitus, C.; Lévi, C. Marine Sterols. Side-chain-oxygenated sterols, possibly of abiotic origin, from the New Caledonian sponge *Stelodoryx chlorophylla*. *J. Nat. Prod.* **1993**, *56*, 282–287. [CrossRef]

15. D'Auria, M.V.; Minale, L.; Riccio, R. Polyoxygenated steroids of marine origin. *Chem. Rev.* **1993**, *93*, 1839–1895. [CrossRef]

16. Ivanchina, N.V.; Kicha, A.A.; Stonik, V.A. Steroid glycosides from marine organisms. *Steroids* **2011**, *76*, 425–454. [CrossRef] [PubMed]

17. Malyarenko, T.V.; Kicha, A.A.; Ivanchina, N.V.; Kalinovsky, A.I.; Popov, R.S.; Vishchuk, O.S.; Stonik, V.A. Asterosaponins from the Far Eastern starfish *Leptasterias ochotensis* and their anticancer activity. *Steroids* **2014**, *87*, 119–127. [CrossRef] [PubMed]

18. Nguyen, P.T.; Luyen, B.T.T.; Kim, E.-J.; Kang, H.-K.; Kim, S.; Cuong, N.X.; Nam, N.H.; Kiem, P.V.; Minh, C.V.; Kim, Y.H. Asterosaponins from the starfish *Astropecten monacanthus* suppress growth and induce apoptosis in HL-60, PC-3, and SNU-C5 human cancer cell lines. *Biol. Pharm. Bull.* **2014**, *37*, 315–321.

19. Ngoan, B.T.; Hanh, T.T.H.; Vien, L.T.; Diep, C.N.; Thao, N.P.; Thao, D.T.; Thanh, N.V.; Cuong, N.X.; Nam, N.H.; Thung, D.C.; et al. Asterosaponins and glycosylated polyhydroxysteroids from the starfish *Culcita novaeguineae* and their cytotoxic activities. *J. Asian Nat. Prod. Res.* **2015**, *17*, 1010–1017. [CrossRef] [PubMed]

20. Kang, J.-X.; Kang, Y.-F.; Han, H. Three new cytotoxic polyhydroxysteroidal glycosides from starfish *Craspidaster hesperus*. *Mar. Drugs* **2016**, *14*, 189. [CrossRef] [PubMed]

21. Calabro, K.; Kalahroodi, E.L.; Rodrigues, D.; Díaz, C.; de la Cruz, M.; Cautain, B.; Laville, R.; Reyes, F.; Pérez, T.; Soussi, B.; et al. Poecillastrosides, steroidal saponins from the Mediterranean deep-sea sponge *Poecillastra compressa* (Bowerbank, 1866). *Mar. Drugs* **2017**, *15*, 199. [CrossRef] [PubMed]

22. Kicha, A.A.; Kalinovsky, A.I.; Ivanchina, N.V.; Malyarenko, T.V.; Dmitrenok, P.S.; Kuzmich, A.S.; Sokolova, E.V.; Stonik, V.A. Furostane series asterosaponins and other unusual steroid oligoglycosides from the tropical starfish *Pentaceraster regulus*. *J. Nat. Prod.* **2017**, *80*, 2761–2770. [CrossRef] [PubMed]

23. Ishiyama, M.; Shiga, M.; Sasamoto, K.; Mizoguchi, M.; He, P.-G. A new sulfonated tetrazolium salt that produces a highly water-soluble formazan dye. *Chem. Pharm. Bull.* **1993**, *41*, 1118–1122. [CrossRef]

24. Wang, X.-D.; Li, C.-Y.; Jiang, M.-M.; Li, D.; Wen, P.; Song, X.; Chen, J.-D.; Guo, L.-X.; Hu, X.-P.; Li, G.-Q.; et al. Induction of apoptosis in human leukemia cells through an intrinsic pathway by cathachunine, a unique alkaloid isolated from *Catharanthus roseus*. *Phytomedicine* **2016**, *23*, 641–653. [CrossRef] [PubMed]

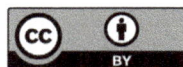

© 2017 by the authors. Licensee MDPI, Basel, Switzerland. This article is an open access article distributed under the terms and conditions of the Creative Commons Attribution (CC BY) license (http://creativecommons.org/licenses/by/4.0/).

marine drugs

MDPI

Review

The Anti-Cancer Effects of Frondoside A

Thomas E. Adrian [1],* and Peter Collin [2]

[1] Department of Physiology, Faculty of Medicine and Health Sciences, United Arab Emirates University, P.O. Box 17666 Al Ain, United Arab Emirates

[2] Coastside Bio Resources, Deer Isle, ME 04627, USA; pcollin48@gmail.com

* Correspondence: tadrian@uaeu.ac.ae; Tel.: +971-3-713-7551; Fax: +971-3-767-1966

Received: 31 January 2018; Accepted: 16 February 2018; Published: 19 February 2018

Abstract: Frondoside A is a triterpenoid glycoside from the Atlantic Sea Cucumber, *Cucumaria frondosa*. Frondoside A has a broad spectrum of anti-cancer effects, including induction of cellular apoptosis, inhibition of cancer cell growth, migration, invasion, formation of metastases, and angiogenesis. In cell lines and animal models studied to date, the anti-cancer effects of the compound are seen in all solid cancers, lymphomas, and leukemias studied to date. These effects appear to be due to potent inhibition of p21-activated kinase 1 (PAK1), which is up-regulated in many cancers. In mouse models, frondoside A has synergistic effects with conventional chemotherapeutic agents, such as gemcitabine, paclitaxel, and cisplatin. Frondoside A administration is well-tolerated. No side effects have been reported and the compound has no significant effects on body weight, blood cells, or on hepatic and renal function tests after long-term administration. Frondoside A may be valuable in the treatment of malignancies, either as a single agent or in combination with other therapeutic modalities.

Keywords: cancer; frondoside A; tumor growth; metastases; apoptosis; invasion; angiogenesis

1. Background

There is a desperate need for new and effective therapeutic agents for the treatment of cancer. It is particularly important to target growth, survival, migration, and metastases pathways in cancer with agents that have little or no toxicity towards normal cells. Over the years, there has been a search for such novel drugs in natural products. Many plant-derived compounds have been developed and used for treating cancer. Examples include doxorubicin, bleomycin, mitomycin, vincristine, and vinblastine. Marine organisms represent a vast untapped potential source of anti-cancer compounds and considerable effort has been invested in this area in recent years [1,2]. To date, there has been limited success in terms of marine-derived compounds or direct synthetic analogs of marine-derived compounds reaching the market for treatment of cancer and other disorders. The four notable exceptions for the treatment of cancer include cytarabine, trabectedin, eribulin mesylate, and monomethyl auristatin E (MMAE). Cytarabine, the pyrimidine nucleoside, 3-β-D-arabinofuranosylcytosine was synthesized following the discovery of arabinose-containing spongonucleosides from the sponge, *Cryptotethia crypta*. Cytarabine becomes incorporated into DNA in the place of a cytosine residue and halts DNA synthesis in the S phase of the cell cycle. It is used in the treatment of acute lymphocytic and myeloid leukemias, as well as chronic myeloid leukemia and non-Hodgkin's lymphoma [1,2]. Gemcitabine, which is important in the treatment of pancreatic and non-small cell lung cancer, is a fluorinated analog of cytarabine. Trabectidine is a tetrahydroisoquinoline alkaloid produced synthetically. Trabectidine was originally isolated from the mangrove sea squirt *Ecteinascidia turbinata* but was subsequently shown to be produced by *Candidatus Endoecteinascidia frumentensis*, a microbial symbiont of the tunicate. Trabectidin inhibits activated transcription, notably of the drug resistance proteins, which are recognized to be the major pathways of resistance to chemotherapeutic drugs, such as doxorubicin and the taxanes [1,2]. Eribulin mesylate is a synthetic analogue of halichondrin B, a mitotic inhibitor from *Halichondria* sponges, which is used to treat patients with metastatic breast cancer or inoperable liposarcoma [2]. Monomethyl auristatin E (MMAE) is a synthetic highly potent antimitotic drug that is derived from peptides occurring in the marine shell-less mollusk, *Dolabella auricularia* called dolastatins. Because MMAE is highly toxic it is linked to a monoclonal antibody (MAB) that targets a membrane protein, CD30 found on anaplastic large cell lymphoma and Hodgkin's lymphoma cells [2].

The search for anti-cancer compounds across different marine phyla has so far revealed several thousands of active compounds [2]. Of particular interest are echinoderms, which are phyla only found in the marine environment, which includes sea stars, sea urchins, sand dollars, sea cucumbers, and sea lilies. Sea cucumbers have been used in traditional Chinese medicine for treatment of cancer, inflammation, and other conditions for hundreds of years [3,4].

Triterpenoid glycosides from various sea cucumber species are known to have anti-cancer activity [5–10]. One particular triterpenoid glycoside, frondoside A has received particular attention, since it has shown potent anti-cancer effects in a broad spectrum of solid malignancies as well as in leukemias. Here, we will review the nature of frondoside A, its effects on cancer cell growth, cell cycle, apoptosis, angiogenesis, migration, invasion, and formation of metastases [11–24]. We will also review the pharmacokinetics, toxicity, interactions with other anti-cancer therapeutics, effects on the immune system, and possible mechanisms of action of this compound [13,16,21–37].

2. Structure of Frondoside A

Frondoside A is a triterpenoid glycoside with an acetoxy group at C-16 in the aglycone, which is a lanostane derivative. Frondoside A is a pentaoside with xylose as the third monosaccharide residue and 3-O-methylglucose as the terminal monosaccharide residue. It has a sulphate group on the first sugar residue. For the structure of frondoside A see Figure 1. Frondoside A differs from its closest cousin cucumarioside A$_2$-2 (from *Cucumaria japonica*) in the functional group at C-16 of the aglycone (a keto group in cucumarioside A$_2$-2) and the third carbohydrate group in the carbohydrate chain (glucose in cucumarioside A$_2$-2). Frondosides B and C, also derived from *Cucumaria frondosa*, are found at slightly higher concentrations and have two and three sulphate groups, respectively, and some other minor structural differences compared with one in frondoside A (see Figure 1). Frondoside A has a molecular mass of 1334 Da.

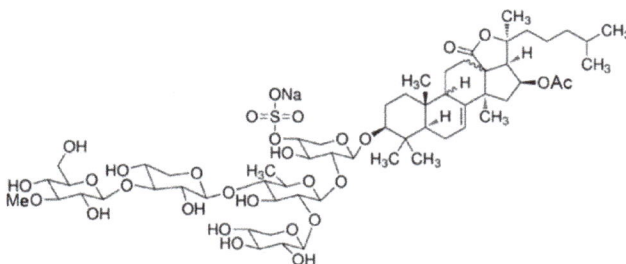

Figure 1. The structure of frondoside A.

The frondosides (A, B and C) can be readily isolated and purified, as previously described [28]. The resulting compounds have been shown to have high purity [11]. Frondoside A is extracted from either the freeze-dried cooking water from the sea cucumber processing plant or from freeze dried skin of the animal [28]. Briefly, the freeze dried powders are dissolved in chloroform/methanol [28]. Following evaporation, the extract is dissolved in water and mixed with ethyl acetate. After phase separation, the water phase is then loaded onto a Teflon column (DuPont 9B, Wilmington, DE, USA). The column is then washed with water to remove salts and pigments and the crude glycoside fraction eluted with 65% acetone. The glycosides are then purified on a Si 40 L 2632-2 flash column (Biotage, Charlotte, NC, USA) with the mobile phase mixture of chloroform/ethanol/water (100:100:17) as solvent. Purification is monitored by thin layer chromatography with 100:100:17 chloroform/ethanol/water as the solvent system. The frondoside A yield is approximately 0.1% of either starting material [28].

The ability of frondoside A to form supramolecular complexes with cholesterol was investigated using transmission electron microscopy [34]. The tubular nanoparticles that were detected were comprised of frondoside with cholesterol [34].

3. Effects of Frondoside A on Cancer Cell Proliferation and Viability

The effects of frondoside A on cell viability or proliferation has been tested using multiple different methods in many different cancers. This has included studies on pancreatic ductal adenocarcinoma, breast, non-small cell lung, colon, prostate, cervix, bladder (transitional cell), Burkitt lymphoma, malignant germ cell, and acute leukemias [11–14,16,18–21,23–27]. Methods employed have included cell counts, thymidine incorporation, MTT assay, and CellTiterGlo (Promega, Madison, WI, USA) assays. The results summarized as approximate IC_{50} are shown in Table 1. The IC_{50} for the effect of frondoside A from these studies across different cancer cell lines varies only between 0.1 and 3.0 μM. In the instances where the effect of frondoside A has been tested on immortalized non-malignant cell lines, these are much less responsive than the malignant cells, particularly when compared under identical conditions.

Table 1. Effect of frondoside A on viability of different cancer cell lines reported in the literature.

Cell Line	Cancer Origin	Approximate IC_{50} μM	Hours Treated	Notes	Ref.
MiaPaca-2	Pancreas	0.5	24		[23]
AsPC-1	Pancreas	1.0	24		[25]
S2013	Pancreas	1.0	24		[25]
MDA-MB-231	Breast	1.2	48	Triple receptor negative	[13]
MCF-10A	Breast	5.0	48	Non-Malignant	[13]
66.1	Breast	0.5	24		[14]
MDA-MB-231	Breast	0.3	24	Three-dimensional culture	[17]
MDA-MB-435	Breast	2.5	24		[16]
MCF-7	Breast	2.0	24		[16]
LNM35	Lung	1.5	24	Met Sub-line of NCI-H460	[16]
A549	Lung	2.5	24		[16]
NCI-H460	Lung	2.5	24	Luciferase expressing cells	[16]
LNM35	Lung	0.6	72		[34]
HepG2	Liver	1.5	24		[16]
DLD-1	Colon	1.2	48		[23]
PC-1	Prostate	0.3	48		[23]
PC-3	Prostate	1.3	48		[18]
DU145	Prostate	1.0	48		[18]
LNCaP	Prostate	0.3	48		[18]
22Rv1	Prostate	0.1	48		[18]
VCaP	Prostate	0.2	48		[18]
MRC-9	Fibroblast	4.5	48	Non-Malignant	[18]

Table 1. *Cont.*

Cell Line	Cancer Origin	Approximate IC$_{50}$ μM	Hours Treated	Notes	Ref.
HEK293	Embryonic Kidney	1.9	48	Non-Malignant	[18]
HUVEC	Umbilical Vascular Endothelial	1.6	48	Non-Malignant	[18]
HT-1197	Bladder	2.3	48		[19]
486p	Bladder	1.1	48		[19]
RT4	Bladder	0.6	48		[19]
RT112	Bladder	0.5	48		[19]
T24	Bladder	1.5	48		[19]
TCC-SUP	Bladder	1.1	48		[19]
BL-2	Burkitt Lymphoma	0.2	48		[20]
CA46	Burkitt Lymphoma	0.2	48		[20]
Daudi	Burkitt Lymphoma	0.2	48		[20]
Raji	Burkitt Lymphoma	0.5	48		[20]
DG-75	Burkitt Lymphoma	0.2	48		[20]
EB1	Burkitt Lymphoma	0.6	48		[20]
Namalwa	Burkitt Lymphoma	0.2	48		[20]
Ramos	Burkitt Lymphoma	0.1	48		[20]
HL-60	Promyelocytic Leukemia	0.5	24		[12]
CCRF-CEM	T-Lymphoblastic Leukemia	1.5	48		[21]
THP-1	Monocytic Leukemia	3.0	48		[21]
HL-60	Promyelocytic Leukemia	2.5	48		[21]
NNCIT	Metastatic Germ Cell Tumor	0.5	Not reported	Cisplatin-resistant sublines equally sensitive	[24]
2102EP	Metastatic Germ Cell Tumor	0.5			[24]

As mentioned above, several other sea cucumber-derived glycosylated triterpenoids have anti-cancer effects [5–10]. The activity of frondoside A was compared with frondosides B and C. In AsPC-1 and S2103 human pancreatic cancer cells studied in culture, frondoside A more potently reduced the number of viable cells than its disulphated cousin, frondoside B [26]. The trisulphated frondoside C and the parent aglycone had no effect on cell viability [26].

Frondoside A was submitted to the National Cancer Institute Developmental Therapeutics Program and was run twice through the NCI-60 cancer cell line screen. This screen includes leukemia and non-small cell lung, colon, CNS, melanoma, ovarian, renal, prostate, and breast cancer cell lines. Out of 57 cell lines investigated, frondoside A inhibited growth with ED_{50} below 1 μM for all but four cell lines (two melanoma, one renal, and one ovarian) (Coastside Bio Resources—unpublished data).

4. Effects of Frondoside A on Cancer Growth

The results of studies of frondoside A undertaken in mice are summarized in Table 2. Frondoside A at an intraperitoneal (IP) dose of 10 μg/kg/day significantly reduced growth of AsPC-1 pancreatic cancer subcutaneous xenografts in athymic mice over a 32-day period [11]. No significant changes in body weights between frondoside A and vehicle control-treated animals were seen in these experiments [11].

Table 2. Effects of frondoside A *in vivo* in different mouse cancer models.

Cell Line	Cancer Origin	Dose	Outcome	Ref.
AsPC-1	Pancreas	10 μg/kg/day	Tumor size 56% of control at 32 days	[11]
AsPC-1	Pancreas	100 μg/kg/day + gemcitabine	Tumor size 13% of control at 30 days and combination had greater effect than either drug alone	[23]
S2013	Pancreas	100 μg/kg/day + gemcitabine	Tumor size 21% of control at 30 days and combination had greater effect than either drug alone	[23]
MDA-MB-231	Breast	100 μg/kg/day	Tumor size 4% of control at 27 days	[13]
LNM35	Lung	10 μg/kg/day	Tumor size 56% of control at 25 days	[16]
LNM35	Lung	1000 μg/kg/day	Tumor size 55% of control at 25 days	[16]
LNM35	Lung	100 μg/kg/day + cisplatin	Tumor size 32% of control at 10 days and combination had greater effect than either drug alone	[16]
PC-3	Prostate	100 μg/kg/day	Tumor size 58% of control at 30 days and reduced number of lung metastases	[18]
DU145	Prostate	800 μg/kg/day	Tumor size 47% of control at 25 days, abolished lung metastases and reduced circulating tumor cells	[18]

In xenografts of MDA-MB-231 breast cancer cells the effect of frondoside A at 100 μg/kg/day IP was more effective than in the pancreatic cancer model [13]. Treatment began when the tumors averaged 200 mm^3 in size. While tumors in the control group continued to grow exponentially, tumors in the frondoside A-treated group were reduced to almost nothing after treatment for 24 days [13]. Tumor weight was similarly dramatically decreased by frondoside A [13]. Again, there was no difference in body weight between treated and control animals.

Subcutaneous frondoside A also inhibited the growth of LNM35 lung cancer cell xenografts [16]. By the end of a 10-day treatment period, frondoside A at a dose of 10 μg/kg/day IP had reduced tumor growth by more than 40% [16]. Increasing the IP frondoside A dose to 1000 μg/kg/day IP did not improve the efficacy of the compound, suggesting a narrow therapeutic window [16].

Frondoside A caused similar reductions in size of prostate cancer xenografts, using both PC-3 and DU145 prostate cancer cells [18]. For PC-3 cells treated with 100 μg/kg/day IP frondoside A, there was a modest inhibition of tumor growth over the 30-day treatment period [18]. Because they were less sensitive to the drug *in vitro*, animals with DU145 cells xenografts were treated with a higher dose (800 μg/kg/day IP) of frondoside A. This caused a more substantial reduction in tumor growth [18].

5. Effects of Frondoside A on Cell Cycle

In prostate cancer cells, the effects of frondoside A appear to be cell line dependent. In cultured PC-3 cells, frondoside A caused a dose-responsive increase in cells arrested in the G2/M phase of the cell cycle and a reduction in the proportion in the G0/G1 phase [18]. In contrast, in DU145 and LNCaP cells no changes in the proportions of cells in the different phases were seen [18]. Similarly, there was no significant effect of frondoside A on cell cycle phase distribution in prostate cancer cells [19]. In four Burkitt lymphoma cell lines (BL-2, CA46, Namalwa, and Ramos) frondoside A caused a dose-responsive increase of cells in the G1 phase, with no significant changes in other phases [20].

6. Effects of Frondoside A on Programmed Cell Death

In cultured AsPC-1 pancreatic cancer cells, frondoside A was shown to induce apoptosis, as indicated by morphological changes, including cytoplasmic shrinkage, membrane blebbing, nuclear condensation, and loss of adhesion [11]. The induction of early and late apoptosis was confirmed by annexin V binding, which indicates the externalization of phosphatidylserine and by terminal deoxynucleotidyl triphosphate nick-end labeling (TUNEL) assay, indicating DNA fragmentation, respectively [11]. The apoptosis was associated with an increased expression of the pro-apoptosis protein, Bax, decrease in expression of the anti-apoptosis proteins, Bcl-2 and Mcl-1, and activation of caspase 3, 7, and 9 by cleavage [11]. In pancreatic cancer cells, frondoside A also resulted in a time-dependent increase in expression of the cyclin-dependent kinase inhibitor, p21. The increased expression of p21 is not a response to increased p53 activity, as p53 is mutated and inactive in the pancreatic cancer cells studied [11]. These findings indicate that in pancreatic cancer, frondoside A induces apoptosis via the mitochondrial pathway, while effects via death receptors were not investigated.

In cultured MDA-MB-231 breast cancer cells, frondoside A induced apoptosis, as indicated by an increase in proportion of cells in the sub-G1 fraction in fluorescence-activated cell sorting analysis and by increased activity of caspase 3/7, as well as caspase 8 and caspase 9 [13]. Activation of caspase 3/7 was blocked by the caspase inhibitor, Z-DEVD-FMK [13]. In studies by the same group, frondoside A induced a similar increase in caspase 3/7 activity in LNM35 lung cancer cells [16].

In cultured PC-3, DU145 and LNCaP prostate cancer cells, frondoside A was shown to induce apoptosis by both the sub-G1 fraction during cell cycle analysis and increase in annexin V binding [18]. The pan-caspase inhibitor, Z-VAD-FMK significantly decreased induction of apoptosis in DU145 cells, but not in PC-3 of LNCaP cells [18]. The apoptosis induced by frondoside A was accompanied by induction of caspase 3 and poly (ADP-ribose) polymerase (PARP) cleavage and activation, upregulation of the pro-apoptosis factors Bax and PTEN or Bad and downregulation of the anti-apoptosis protein Bcl-2 [18]. In PC-3 and DU145 cells, frondoside A increased the level of phosphor-mTOR and expression of p21. In contrast, expression of p21 was decreased in frondoside A-treated LNCaP cells [18]. In addition, frondoside A also inhibited pro-survival autophagy in prostate cancer cells [18].

In the bladder urothelial carcinoma cell line, RT112 frondoside A induced caspase-independent apoptosis. Frondoside A induced a concentration-dependent increase in expression of Bax and p21, activation of caspases 3, 8, and 9, PARP cleavage, and DNA fragmentation [19]. The induction of apoptosis was not affected by pre-treatment with the pan-caspase inhibitor, Z-VAD-FMK [19]. As in pancreatic cancer, the increase in p21 expression was not driven by a change in p53 and inhibition of p53 activity did not suppress frondoside A induced cell death [19]. As in prostate cancer cells, frondoside A inhibited pro-survival autophagy in RT112 cells with time and concentration-dependent accumulation of the autophagy-related proteins, LC3B-II and p62 and accumulation of cellular autophagosomes [19].

In Burkitt lymphoma cell lines, CA46, Namalwa, Ramos, and BL-2, frondoside A induced phosphatidyl serine externalization, caspase-3 activation, decreased expression of BCl-2 and survivin, increased the cytoplasmic content of cytochrome C and apoptosis-inducing factor (AIF), as well as DNA fragmentation, indicating apoptosis [20]. However, again the pan-caspase inhibitor, Z-VAD-FMK did not diminish frondoside A-induced apoptosis in any of the tested cell lines, indicating that the induction of apoptosis was not caspase-dependent [20]. Similarly, frondoside A inhibited pro-survival autophagy in RT112 cells with time-dependent accumulation of the autophagy-related proteins, LC3B-II and SQSTM1/p62 [20]. Furthermore, the effects of frondoside A were independent of p53 status and the apoptosis induction was not antagonized by p53 inhibition [20].

In vitro treatment of NCCIT and 2102EP germ cell tumor lines resulted in caspase-independent apoptosis and the use of the caspase inhibitor, Z-VAD-FMK confirmed that extensive apoptosis occurred despite caspase inhibition [24]. As in the Burkitt lymphoma cells, the apoptosis was associated with increased accumulation of AIF, and again frondoside A inhibited pro-survival autophagy [24].

In HL60, THP-1, and NB4 human leukemia cells, frondoside A induced time and concentration-dependent apoptosis, as indicated by annexin V binding [12]. In HL60 cells, apoptosis was not associated with a change in mitochondrial permeability or cytochrome C release into the cytoplasm. However, after six hours of frondoside A treatment there was an increase in the activation of caspases 3, 7, 8, and 9, and cleavage of PARP [12]. Depending on the time point or concentration of frondoside A, pretreatment of HL60 cells with caspase inhibitors, Z-DEVD-FMK or Z-VAD-FMK had little or no effect on the induction of apoptosis, indicating once again that the apoptosis in leukemia cells was caspase-independent [12].

For many years, caspase-dependent apoptosis was considered synonymous with programmed cell death, however it has become evident in recent years that there are caspase-independent forms of programmed cell death. It is likely that alternate or backup pathways evolved as the caspase-dependent pathway could be circumvented by viruses or cell transformation. A classification of different pathways of programmed cell death was proposed by Leist and Jäättelä [37]. Their classification was based on both morphological and biochemical criteria and included three forms of programmed cell death in addition to classical necrosis. The first was the classical, caspase-dependent apoptosis with cell shrinkage, membrane blebbing, chromatin condensation, phosphatidylserine relocation to the outer cell membrane, activation of the caspase cascade, and internucleosomal DNA cleavage [37]. The second was apoptosis-like cell death with less compact chromatin condensation, phosphatidylserine translocation, but without activation of the caspase cascade [37]. The third was necrosis-like cell death occurring in the absence of either chromatin condensation or caspase activation [37]. In addition, it is now clear that there are other specialized forms of programmed cell death not fitting into the above models, including paraptosis and dark cell death [38,39]. Finally, another form of programmed cell death is autophagy, characterized by marked cytoplasmic vacuolization, where cellular components are destroyed through an autophagosomic-lysosomal pathway [40].

Activation of the death receptor pathway by the binding of tumor necrosis factor-α associated ligands or the Fas ligand to their respective receptors can induce either classical apoptosis or necrosis-like cell death, depending on the experimental conditions [41,42]. In addition, knockout studies have revealed that necrosis-like cell death triggered through the death receptor pathway requires Fas-associated death domain (FADD)-mediated activation of the protein kinase receptor interacting protein (RIP), which activates nuclear factor kB (NF-κB) [41]. The molecular mechanisms of death receptor-mediated cell death have not been completely characterized, but mitochondrial dysfunction and non-caspase-proteases appear to be involved in this process [43–45]. In the presence of caspase inhibitors, death receptor-mediated necrosis requires a mitochondrial step, but Bid cleavage and mitochondrial cytochrome c release are not involved [43,44]. In contrast, necrosis-like cell death is associated with the increased production of mitochondrial reactive oxygen species and antioxidants can block this form of cell death [41–43,46]. Thus, there are several possible mechanisms to account for the observed caspase-independent programmed cell death that is seen in several of the frondoside A-treated cell lines.

Extensive studies have been carried out using caspase inhibitors, particularly the broad-spectrum caspase inhibitor, Z-VAD-FMK. These studies have revealed that apoptosis can be slowed but never completely prevented by the inhibitor, suggesting that caspase-dependent and independent apoptosis pathways may be triggered simultaneously [47]. Indeed, it has been proposed that no experimental system exists where Z-VAD-FMK can prevent cell death [48]. This has been tested with many different apoptosis triggers and induction of apoptosis through both the death receptor-mediated and intrinsic mitochondrial pathways [47–51]. It is also possible that pan-caspase inhibitors, such as Z-VAD-FMK do not completely inhibit activity of all pro-apoptotic caspases. Furthermore, their inhibition of other proteases, such as calpains and cathepsins may add to the difficulty in interpreting experimental data. Caspase-independent apoptosis pathways are likely to involve other mitochondrial proteins, such as apoptosis-inducing factor (AIF), as well as other cellular proteases [52]. AIF is found in the slime mold, *Dicostelium discoideum*, which predates the evolutionary development of caspases [53]. Non-caspase proteases that appear to be involved in programmed cell death include granzymes A and B, HtrA2, which is released from mitochondria, cathepsins B and D, and calpains [48].

7. Anti-Angiogenic Effects of Frondoside A

Frondoside A has been shown to have antiangiogenic effects in the chick chorioallentoic membrane (CAM) assay, inhibition of vascular tube formation in cultured human umbilical vein endothelial cells (HUVEC), and in xenografts of human lung tumors [16]. In the CAM assay, frondoside A caused concentration-dependent inhibition of basal angiogenesis at concentrations as low as 100 and 500 nM [16]. Furthermore, frondoside A (500 nM) completely abolished the increased angiogenesis that was triggered by basic fibroblast growth factor (bFGF, 2 μg/L [16]. When cultured on Matrigel-coated plates, HUVEC cells spontaneously form vascular tube-like structures. Frondoside A (500 nM) almost completely abolished vascular tube formation at a concentration of (500 nM), but had no significant effect on the viability of the HUVEC cells at this concentration, indicating a lack of cytotoxicity on the HUVEC cells [16]. Microvessel density, measured by CD31 immunohistochemical staining in the periphery of xenografted tumors, was markedly reduced by frondoside A in animals treated with a dose of 10 μg/kg/day IP [16].

8. Effects of Frondoside A on Migration and Invasion

Progression of cancer is associated with loss of the normal constraints on cellular migration and invasion. Frondoside A has been shown to inhibit migration and invasion of both breast and lung cancer cells [13,16]. Migration is measured microscopically in the wound-healing model, where a 1 mm scrape is made with pipette tip though a confluent monolayer of cells, as cells move in to fill the gap. Frondoside A caused concentration and time-dependent inhibition of migration of MBA-MD-231 breast cancer cells and LNM35 lung cancer cells at concentrations (0.1–1.0 μM) that have no effect on viability during the time interval of the wounding assay [13,16]. The effect of frondoside A on invasion was measured using the Matrigel invasion assay in the same cell lines. Frondoside A caused concentration-dependent inhibition of invasion over a 24-hour period [13,16]. Marked inhibition of invasion was seen at frondoside A concentrations (0.1–0.5 μM) that had little or no effect on cell viability [13].

In a separate study in MDA-MB-231 cells, frondoside A inhibited TPA-induced colony formation, migration, and invasion associated with reduction in the expression, secretion, and enzymatic activity of matrix metalloproteinase-9 (MMP-9), enhanced expression of tissue inhibitors of metalloproteinases 1 and 2 (TIMP-1 and TIMP-2), as well as reduced activation of activator protein-1 (AP-1, a heterodimer of c-Fos and c-Jun) and nuclear factor kappa B (NF-κB) transcription factors [15]. These findings suggest that the inhibition of invasion is mediated via the changes in these factors [15].

Frondoside A has been shown to inhibit formation of metastases in breast, lung, and prostate cancers [14,16,18]. For example, breast cancer metastases were investigated after 66.1 mouse mammary cancer cells, pretreated with frondoside A, or control vehicle, for 30 minutes, were injected into the tail vein of mice and the spontaneous development of lung metastases counted after three weeks. In this model, pretreatment with 5 μM frondoside A IP reduced the number of lung tumor colonies by 45% [14]. In a separate experiment, 1 μM frondoside A IP also markedly reduced the formation of metastases, while exposure to 0.1 μM frondoside A was ineffective [14]. In a more clinically relevant model, the 66.1 cells were implanted subcutaneously proximal to the right mammary gland of mice and frondoside A treatment was administered IP each day for 10 days. Formation of spontaneous metastases was significantly inhibited by frondoside A at 50 μg/kg/day and even at 10 μg/kg/day the inhibition almost reached statistical significance ($p < 0.06$) [14].

A separate study investigated the effect of frondoside A on development of axillary lymph node metastases after subcutaneous implantation of LNM35 lung cancer cells [16]. Frondoside A at a dose of 10 µg/kg/day IP significantly reduced the average weight of the lymph nodes by more than 50%; however, a higher dose of 1 mg/kg/day was no more effective [16].

In xenografts comprised of PC-3 prostate cancer cells, frondoside A markedly reduced the number of lung metastases and caused a similar decrease in the presence of cancer cells detected using a human DNA detection method [18]. With DU145 cell xenografts, there were no lung metastases detected by microscopy and there was a marked reduction in the tumor cell detection in lung using the human DNA detection method; furthermore, frondoside A significantly reduced the detection of tumor cells in the blood using this method [18].

9. Effects of Frondoside A on Multidrug Resistance

Development of resistance of cancer cells to antitumor drugs with completely different mechanisms of action is a well-known phenomenon, known as multidrug resistance (MDR) [35]. The major mechanism of multidrug resistance is through the upregulation of transmembrane transport proteins that efflux drugs from the cells, lowering the intracellular concentrations of drugs and rendering them ineffective. The major drug efflux protein is known as permeability glycoprotein (P-glycoprotein). Activity of P-glycoprotein can be measured by efflux of fluorescein dyes, which enter the cells by diffusion through the cell membrane. Frondoside A, or nanoparticle complexes of frondoside A with cholesterol can block P-glycoprotein activity [35]. Inhibition of MDR was seen with a frondoside A concentration of only 750 pM (1 ng/mL) and no greater effect was seen when concentrations were increased to 7.5 or 75 nM. On a molar basis, frondoside A was more effective than verapamil, the most effective concentration of which was 26.4 nM (12 ng/mL) [35].

10. Interactions with Other Anticancer Drugs

The results of the following studies are summarized in Table 2. In MDA-MB-231 cells in culture, frondoside A enhanced the anti-proliferative effects of paclitaxel, a drug that targets tubulin and prevents microtubule formation, in an apparently additive manner [13]. The combination of frondoside A with cisplatin, a drug which inhibits DNA replication, was tested in the mouse xenograft model with LMN35 lung cancer cells [16]. When administered daily, each of these drugs alone inhibited tumor growth and by the tenth day tumor size was about 40% lower in the treated groups. The combination of the two, however, suppressed tumor growth by 68% ($p < 0.05$) [16]. Combinations of frondoside A with both cisplatin and gemcitabine (another drug that impairs DNA synthesis) were tested in RT112 urothelial cancer cells [19]. Both drug combinations had marked synergistic effects in these cells [19]. Because frondoside A has similar growth inhibitory effects in cancer cells regardless of their p53 status, a study was conducted to investigate the effects of frondoside A and cisplatin after pretreating cells with pifithrin-α (Pif-α), which is a chemical inhibitor of p53 transcriptional activity in wild-type p53 BL-2 Burkitt lymphoma cells [20]. There was a clear additive effect of frondoside A and Pif-α in these experiments, while the effect of cisplatin was antagonized by Pif-α [20]. These findings indicate that while cisplatin activity is p53-dependent, functional p53 is not required for the anti-cancer activity of frondoside A [20].

Studies in AsPC-1 and S2013 pancreatic cancer cells revealed marked synergistic effects of low concentrations of frondoside A with gemcitabine in cell culture [25]. Furthermore, the combination also showed enhanced effects compared with either drug alone in the xenograft model of pancreatic cancer using either cell line [25].

Frondoside A also potentiates the actions of several conventional therapeutic agents in acute leukemia cell lines [21]. Frondoside A enhanced the anti-leukemic effects of vincristine, asparaginase, and prednisolone in CCRF-CEM, THP-1, and HL-60 cells [21]. Synergistic effects were seen with frondoside A in combination with each of the three other drugs in CCRF-CEM and THP-1 cells [21].

11. Effects of Frondoside A on the Immune System

Frondoside A exhibits a range of very potent immunomodulatory effects *in vitro* and in animals. While the observed effects of frondoside A in the human xenograft models in athymic mice are clearly not related to effects on the immune system, such immunological effects may contribute to the anti-cancer effects of the compound in other animal tumor models and could potentially contribute an additive effect if frondoside A becomes used as a drug in humans.

Frondoside A potently stimulates lysosomal activity in mouse macrophages *in vivo* [28]. The maximal stimulatory effect was seen with 0.2 µg/mouse and the effect was maintained for 10 days [28]. This dose is similar to the lowest dose (10 µg/kg/day) that has shown anti-cancer activity in athymic mice [16], but it is intriguing that the effect lasts for ten days after a single dose [28]. Frondoside A also stimulates an increase in the number of antibody plaque-forming B-cells in the spleen of mice in immunized with sheep erythrocytes, again with a maximal effect seen at a dose of 0.2 µg/mouse [28]. Frondoside A also had a weak effect on IgM production in response to immunization with sheep erythrocytes. However, frondoside A had no effect on immunoglobulin production in mice immunized with ovalbumin [28]. Frondoside A stimulated lysosomal activity in mouse macrophages by 30% *in vitro* at concentrations of 75–285 nM (0.1–0.38 µg/mL) [28]. Frondoside A very potently enhances macrophage phagocytosis of the bacterium Staphylococcus aureus and stimulates production of reactive oxygen species *in vitro* at a maximal effective concentration of 750 pM (1 ng/mL) [28]. Hence, frondoside A is an immunostimulant of cell-based immunity including phagocytosis without significant amplification of humoral immune activity or adjuvant properties and may be valuable in treating disorders where depleted immune status contributes to the pathological process [28].

One study investigated the protein changes that occurred in frondoside A stimulated splenocyte cultures using proteomics [29]. Thirty proteins were differentially expressed, including down-regulation of Septin-2, a protein that hetero-oligomerizes with other septins to form filaments. Loss of Septin-2 causes actin stress fibers to disintegrate and cells to lose polarity. Other down-regulated proteins include NADH dehydrogenase iron-sulfur protein 3 (an enzyme which is a component of mitochondrial NADH: ubiquinone oxidoreductase), and GRB2-related adaptor protein 2 (an adaptor-like protein involved in leukocyte-specific protein-tyrosine kinase signaling) [29]. Up-regulated proteins include N-ethylmaleimide-sensitive factor-like 1 cofactor p47 (a protein necessary for the fragmentation of Golgi stacks during mitosis and for their reassembly after mitosis), and heterogeneous nuclear ribonucleoprotein K (a nucleic acid-binding protein that serves as a docking platform integrating transduction pathways to nucleic acid -directed processes) [29]. Together with the results of proliferation and adhesion assays, these changes suggest that in addition to stimulating splenocyte proliferation, frondoside A has immunostimulatory effects that enhance the cellular defense mechanism necessary to fight pathogens for which lymphocytes and splenocytes need to be recruited [29].

Another study revealed that frondoside A inhibits the non-specific esterase of mouse spleen lymphocytes, but the concentrations for this inhibitory effect was higher than required for the immunomodulatory effects [30].

In macrophages, frondoside A stimulates spreading, lysosomal activity, and the formation of reactive oxygen species [31].

Prostaglandin E_2 (PGE$_2$) from tumor cells inhibits natural killer (NK) cell functions. Indeed, several functions of these cells, including lysis, migration, and cytokine production, are compromised in tumor bearing mice. Similarly, PGE$_2$ prevents migration, the cytotoxic effects, and interferon γ (IFNγ) production in cultured NK cells. Frondoside A, which acts as a blocker for EP$_4$ prostaglandin receptors, inhibits breast cancer metastases in an NK cell-dependent manner and protects IFNγ production from NK cells from PGE$_2$ mediated suppression [32].

12. Pharmacokinetics of Frondoside A and Route of Administration

The pharmacokinetics of frondoside A were investigated in mice following intravenous (IV) and intraperitoneal (IP) administration at a bolus dose of 100 μg/kg. Plasma frondoside A concentrations were measured using a liquid chromatography mass spectrometry (LC-MS/MS) method [26]. The mean C_{max} following IV administration of frondoside A was 129nM, while that following IP administration was 18.3 nM at 45 min, which is about seven-fold lower than with IV administration at the same dose [26]. The calculated bioavailability after IP administration was approximately 20%. Following IV administration, plasma concentrations of frondoside A remained above 7.5 nM for 17 h, while for IP administration, plasma levels remained above this level for only 4 h [26]. In contrast, oral dosing resulted in very low and variable plasma concentrations of frondoside A near to or below the detection limit of the assay. The half-life of IV administered frondoside A was 8.5 h [26].

The low plasma concentrations of frondoside A after oral administration were confirmed when the effect on growth of AsPC-1 xenografts was compared with IP administration in athymic mice. While IP administration resulted in near to complete inhibition of tumor growth, oral administration was completely ineffective with the time course being almost identical to the vehicle control. These findings suggest very low bioavailability from the oral administration of frondoside A, which is likely to reflect either poor absorption or rapid digestion in the intestine. Indeed, since the aglycone showed no anti-cancer effect, it is likely that the glycosyl groups are cleaved by digestive enzymes, resulting in an inactive aglycone [26].

13. Toxicity of Frondoside A

The reported studies of frondoside A *in vivo* have failed to show any hint of a toxic effect at the studied doses, which are up to 1000 μg/kg/day [11,13,14,16,18,25]. There are no apparent side effects and body weight, liver function, and hematological parameters are not adversely affected by the drug. In a study of athymic mice with MDA-MB-231 cell xenografts, frondoside A administered at 100 μg/kg/day had absolutely no effect on numbers of white blood cells, red blood cells, platelets, or hemoglobin, or on plasma concentrations of blood urea nitrogen, creatinine, aspartate aminotransferase, or alanine aminotransferase [13]. A study in mice with xenografts of PC-3 prostate cancer cells revealed no significant changes in hemoglobin, WBC, lymphocyte, monocyte, neutrophil, or platelet counts with frondoside A at a dose of 100 μg/kg/day [18]. At a higher dose of 800 μg/kg/day, frondoside A caused non-significant increases in WBC, lymphocyte, and neutrophil counts, but a significant ($p < 0.01$) increase in monocyte count in mice with DU145 prostate cancer xenografts [18]. A formal study of the toxicity of frondoside A revealed that the LD_{50} in mice was 9.9 mg/kg, which is 100-fold greater than the dose used in most of the *in vivo* experiments testing efficacy [28].

14. Mechanisms of Action

Up until now, the mechanism by which frondoside A triggers its anti-cancer and other effects has been somewhat of a mystery and several possible mechanisms have been proposed, however new evidence reveals a unifying hypothesis that can account for most, if not all, of the observed biological mechanisms.

Acting as potent inhibitor of the multi-drug resistance, G-glycoprotein would certainly be valuable in the treatment of cancer, regardless of the mechanisms that mediate the effects of frondoside A on proliferation, cell cycle, apoptosis, migration, invasion and angiogenesis [35].

Because of the steroid backbone of the molecule, an early study investigated whether frondoside A had estrogenic activity using a yeast two-hybrid system [33]. No appreciable estrogenic activity was detected [33].

In a study that showed marked effects of frondoside A on the inhibition of 66.1 mouse mammary cancer cell growth and the development of metastases revealed that the compound also blocked binding and activation of the EP_4, and to a lesser extent, EP_2 prostaglandin receptors [14].

Frondoside A caused inhibition of tritiated PGE_2 from binding to EP_4 receptors with an IC_{50} of approximately 3.7 μM and EP2 receptors with an IC_{50} of approximately 16.5 μM [14]. Frondoside A was also able to cause concentration-dependent inhibition of PGE_2-stimulated intracellular cyclic AMP concentrations [14]. Complete inhibition of PGE_2-stimulated intracellular cyclic AMP was seen at a frondoside A concentration of 5 μM [14]. Curiously, in the absence of PGE_2, frondoside A at a concentration of 1 μM caused an increase in intracellular cAMP levels, almost rivalling that of PGE_2 [14]. Furthermore, it is notable that the IC_{50} for the effect of frondoside A on cell proliferation was 0.5 μM, almost eight-fold lower than that for inhibition of PGE_2 binding to EP_4 receptors and 33-fold lower for EP_2 receptor binding [14]. These findings suggest that even if prostaglandin receptor blockade contributes to the anti-cancer effects of frondoside A, other more potent mechanisms are likely to be involved.

Another study, which was designed to investigate the mechanism of action, employed microarray using a human oligonucleotide expression array library coupled with real-time RT-PCR to study the transcriptome of S2013 pancreatic cancer cells treated with 2μM frondoside A for 6h as compared with that of untreated cells [52]. Expression of genes showing the greatest changes were confirmed by real-time RT-PCR and time-courses of gene expression were investigated in seven cancer cell lines. Marked changes were seen in expression of several genes involved in growth regulation. Downregulated genes included E2F1, cyclin A2, cdc20, cdc21, cdc45, and cdc47, all of which play important roles in DNA replication and cell cycle control [54]. Upregulated genes included fatty acid binding protein 3 (FABP3), growth and development factor 15 (GDF15), p21^{WAF-1} (which has been shown to be upregulated in multiple studies as outlined above), repressor of E1A, dual-specificity phosphatase, and death-associated protein kinase-1 [54]. Attention was focused on GDF15 and FABP3 [54]. GDF15 belongs to the transforming growth factor superfamily that plays a role in regulating inflammatory and apoptotic pathways during tissue injury, and mediates apoptosis induction in response to NSAIDS. FABP3 is a candidate tumor-suppressor that arrests growth of mammary epithelial cells. Knockdown of expression of either GDF15 or FABP3 using specific siRNA in AsPC-1 cells reversed the growth inhibitory effects of frondoside A. These findings suggest that both GDF15 and FABP3 are involved in the growth inhibitory effects of frondoside A in pancreatic cancer. Since this mechanism appears unique, it explains the synergistic anti-cancer effects seen when combined with other agents, such as cisplatin, paclitaxel, and gemcitabine.

In a study investigating the effects of frondoside A in migration and invasion of breast cancer cells, it was revealed that frondoside A could inhibit TPA-induced activation of MMP-9 via pathways involving inhibition of activation of two transcription factors, AP-1 and NF-κB [15]. Furthermore, frondoside A reduced the ATP-stimulated phosphorylation of several kinase pathways, including phosphoinositide 3 kinase/protein kinase B pathway (PI3K/Akt), the extracellular signal-regulated kinases (ERK1/2), and p38 mitogen activated protein kinase (p38 MAPK), which are all involved in growth stimulatory and cell survival pathways [15]. This study provided valuable insight into how frondoside A could be having widespread effects in the inhibition of cell growth, cell survival, migration, invasion, metastasis, and angiogenesis.

A breakthrough in our understanding of the mechanisms by which frondoside A has such widespread effects came recently when a paper revealed that it was a potent inhibitor (IC50 1.2 μM) of RAC/CDC42-activated kinase (PAK1), with an IC_{50} around 1.2 μM *in vitro* (not in cell culture) [36]. Furthermore, its direct action is highly specific for PAK1, because IC_{50} for other kinases such as LIM kinase and AKT is around 60 μM [36]. This potency is in line with the anticancer effects of frondoside A, which from multiple studies is approximately 1 μM (see Table 1). The discovery that frondoside A inhibits PAK1 is unifying since this kinase is upstream of several other transduction mechanisms, including Ap-1 and NF-κB, already implicated in the actions of the compound [15]. Furthermore, PAK1 is involved in stimulating cancer cell growth, invasion, and metastasis [55,56]. PAK1 activation also potently increases angiogenesis and tumor cell-survival autophagy [36,57]. So being a PAK1 inhibitor may explain the broad spectrum of biological actions on tumors, including inhibition of growth, migration, invasion, metastasis, angiogenesis, and pro-survival autophagy, as well as the induction of apoptosis. Expression of the p21 gene is suppressed by PAK-1 and is increased by frondoside A [36,58].

The major aspect of the biological effects of frondoside A that cannot be readily explained by PAK-1 inhibition are the immunomodulatory effects of the compound [28–30]. PAK1 appears to act as an immuno-suppressor, and either PAK1 si-RNA or chemical PAK1-inhibition boosts the immune response in mice [59]. However, the *in vitro* effects are seen at concentrations that are much lower than those that have either anti-cancer or PAK-1 inhibitory effects and the *in vivo* effects are seen with very low doses of the compound [28,29]. One possible explanation is that the immunomodulatory effects are mediated by a metabolite of frondoside A, perhaps its aglycone, which is likely to be absorbed intact from the gut. Alternatively, perhaps the immune modulatory effects are mediated by action in the gut and do not require absorption of the compound. A recent study demonstrated that curcumin, another compound with poor oral availability but potent effects on the attenuating arthritis, was mediated by increasing neuroexcitability of the vagus nerve [60]. It is interesting to speculate that frondoside A might also activate a similar gut/brain axis.

15. Conclusions

Frondoside A has potent anti-cancer effects in all solid malignancy, lymphoma, and leukemia cell types investigated to date. Frondoside A causes growth inhibition, induction of apoptosis inhibition of migration, invasion and metastases, and blocks angiogenesis. The effects of frondoside A are mediated by inhibition of PAK1 and perhaps other mechanisms. Frondoside A potentiates the effects of conventional therapeutic agents, such as paclitaxel, cisplatin, and gemcitabine in several different cancer types. Over a fairly broad therapeutic range in experimental animals, frondoside A is well tolerated and appears to have no toxicity on bone marrow, liver, kidney, or other tissues, and does not affect body weight. Frondoside A can be readily produced from the waste-stream of certain sea cucumber processing; however, it could also be produced from cell culture of the skin from the source organism or conceivably by chemical synthesis [61]. Frondoside A may be valuable in the treatment of a wide range of malignancies either as a single agent or in combination with other therapeutics.

Acknowledgments: The authors thank Binh C Nguyen for preparation of the figure showing the structure of frondoside A. The authors are also grateful for the NCI60 cell line screen performed by the Developmental Therapeutics Program, National Cancer Institute, Bethesda, MD, USA. The studies undertaken by the authors on frondoside A were partially funded by a pre-clinical development RAID grant (#259) from the National Cancer Institute, Bethesda, MD, USA; by a grant from the Terry Fox Cancer Fund for Research in Cancer Therapy. Coastside Bio Resources received funding from the Maine Technology Institute, Brunswick, ME, USA.

Author Contributions: TEA and PC reviewed all available literature on the anti-cancer effects of frondoside A, prepared and reviewed the manuscript.

Conflicts of Interest: T.E.A. and P.C. are holders of patents: WO2005072528 and US 7144867 B2, concerning the use of frondoside A in cancer therapy.

References

1. Adrian, T.E. Novel marine-derived anti-cancer agents. *Curr. Pharm. Des.* **2007**, *13*, 3417–3426. [CrossRef] [PubMed]
2. Correia-da-Silva, M.; Sousa, E.; Pinto, M.M.M.; Kijjoa, A. Anticancer and cancer preventive compounds from edible marine organisms. *Semin. Cancer Biol.* **2017**, *66*, 55–64. [CrossRef] [PubMed]
3. Tang, W. Chinese medicinal materials from the sea. *Abstr. Chin. Med.* **1987**, *1*, 571–600.
4. Pangestuti, R.; Arifin, Z. Medicinal and health benefit effects of functional sea cucumbers. *J. Trad. Complim. Med.* **2017**. [CrossRef]
5. Guo, Y.; Ding, Y.; Xu, F.; Liu, B.; Kou, Z.; Xiao, W.; Zhu, J. Systems pharmacology-based drug discovery for marine resources: An example using sea cucumber (Holothurians). *J. Ethnopharmacol.* **2015**, *165*, 61–72. [CrossRef] [PubMed]
6. Li, Y.X.; Himaya, S.W.; Kim, S.K. Triterpenoids of marine origin as anti-cancer agents. *Molecules* **2013**, *18*, 7886–7909. [CrossRef] [PubMed]

7. Wargasetia, T.L.; Widodo. Mechanisms of cancer cell killing by sea cucumber-derived compounds. *Investig. New Drugs.* **2017**, *35*, 820–826. [CrossRef] [PubMed]
8. Janakiram, N.B.; Mohammed, A.; Rao, C.V. Sea Cucumbers Metabolites as Potent Anti-Cancer Agents. *Mar. Drugs.* **2015**, *13*, 2909–2923. [CrossRef] [PubMed]
9. Park, J.I.; Bae, H.R.; Kim, C.G.; Stonik, V.A.; Kwak, J.Y. Relationships between chemical structures and functions of triterpene glycosides isolated from sea cucumbers. *Front. Chem.* **2014**, *2*, 77. [CrossRef] [PubMed]
10. Yu, S.; Ye, X.; Huang, H.; Peng, R.; Su, Z.; Lian, X.Y.; Zhang, Z. Bioactive sulfated saponins from sea cucumber *Holothuria moebii*. *Planta Med.* **2015**, *81*, 152–159. [CrossRef] [PubMed]
11. Li, X.; Roginsky, A.B.; Ding, X.Z.; Woodward, C.; Collin, P.; Newman, R.A.; Bell, R.H.; Adrian, T.E. Review of the apoptosis pathways in pancreatic cancer and the anti-apoptotic effects of the novel sea cucumber compound, Frondoside A. *Ann. N. Y. Acad. Sci.* **2008**, *1138*, 181–198. [CrossRef] [PubMed]
12. Jin, J.O.; Shastina, V.V.; Shin, S.W.; Xu, Q.; Park, J.I.; Rasskazov, V.A.; Avilov, S.A.; Fedorov, S.N.; Stonik, V.A.; Kwak, J.Y. Differential effects of triterpene glycosides, frondoside A and cucumarioside A2-2 isolated from sea cucumbers on caspase activation and apoptosis of human leukemia cells. *FEBS Lett.* **2009**, *583*, 697–702. [CrossRef] [PubMed]
13. Al Marzouqi, N.; Iratni, R.; Nemmar, A.; Arafat, K.; Al Sultan, M.A.; Yasin, J.; Collin, P.; Mester, J.; Adrian, T.E.; Attoub, S. Frondoside A inhibits human breast cancer cell survival, migration, invasion and the growth of breast tumor xenografts. *Eur. J. Pharmacol.* **2011**, *668*, 25–34. [CrossRef] [PubMed]
14. Ma, X.; Kundu, N.; Collin, P.D.; Goloubeva, O.; Fulton, A.M. Frondoside A inhibits breast cancer metastasis and antagonizes prostaglandin E receptors EP4 and EP2. *Breast Cancer Res. Treat.* **2012**, *132*, 1001–1008. [CrossRef] [PubMed]
15. Park, S.Y.; Kim, Y.H.; Kim, Y.; Lee, S.J. Frondoside A has an anti-invasive effect by inhibiting TPA-induced MMP-9 activation via NF-κB and AP-1 signaling in human breast cancer cells. *Int. J. Oncol.* **2012**, *41*, 933–940. [CrossRef] [PubMed]
16. Attoub, S.; Arafat, K.; Gélaude, A.; Al Sultan, M.A.; Bracke, M.; Collin, P.; Takahashi, T.; Adrian, T.E.; De Wever, O. Frondoside A suppressive effects on lung cancer survival, tumor growth, angiogenesis, invasion, and metastasis. *PLoS ONE* **2013**, *8*, e53087. [CrossRef] [PubMed]
17. Kundu, N.; Ma, X.; Kochel, T.; Goloubeva, O.; Staats, P.; Thompson, K.; Martin, S.; Reader, J.; Take, Y.; Collin, P.; Fulton, A. Prostaglandin E receptor EP4 is a therapeutic target in breast cancer cells with stem-like properties. *Breast Cancer Res. Treat.* **2014**, *143*, 19–31. [CrossRef] [PubMed]
18. Dyshlovoy, S.A.; Menchinskaya, E.S.; Venz, S.; Rast, S.; Amann, K.; Hauschild, J.; Otte, K.; Kalinin, V.I.; Silchenko, A.S.; Avilov, S.A.; et al. The marine triterpene glycoside frondoside A exhibits activity *in vitro* and *in vivo* in prostate cancer. *Int. J. Cancer.* **2016**, *138*, 2450–2465. [CrossRef] [PubMed]
19. Dyshlovoy, S.A.; Madanchi, R.; Hauschild, J.; Otte, K.; Alsdorf, W.H.; Schumacher, U.; Kalinin, V.I.; Silchenko, A.S.; Avilov, S.A.; Honecker, F.; et al. The marine triterpene glycoside frondoside A induces p53-independent apoptosis and inhibits autophagy in urothelial carcinoma cells. *BMC Cancer* **2017**, *17*, 93. [CrossRef] [PubMed]
20. Dyshlovoy, S.A.; Rast, S.; Hauschild, J.; Otte, K.; Alsdorf, W.H.; Madanchi, R.; Kalinin, V.I.; Silchenko, A.S.; Avilov, S.A.; Dierlamm, J.; et al. Frondoside A induces AIF-associated caspase-independent apoptosis in Burkitt lymphoma cells. *Leuk. Lymphoma* **2017**, *58*, 2905–2915. [CrossRef] [PubMed]
21. Sajwani, F.H.; Collin, P.; Adrian, T.E. Frondoside A potentiates the effects of conventional therapeutic agents in acute leukemia. *Leukem. Res.* **2017**, *63*, 98–108. [CrossRef] [PubMed]
22. Aminin, D.L.; Menchinskaya, E.S.; Pisliagin, E.A.; Silchenko, A.S.; Avilov, S.A.; Kalinin, V.I. Anticancer activity of sea cucumber triterpene glycosides. *Mar. Drugs* **2015**, *13*, 1202–1223. [CrossRef] [PubMed]
23. Adrian, T.E.; Collin, P. Anticancer Glycoside Compounds. U.S. Patent 7144867, 5 December 2005.
24. Alsdorf, W.H.; Dyshlovoy, S.; Otte, K.; Haussschild, J.; Bokemeyer, C.; Honecker, F.; von Amsberg, G. Cytotoxic activity and molecular mechanisms of action of the marine triterpene glycoside frondoside A in germ cell tumors. *Oncol. Res. Treat.* **2016**, *39* (Suppl. 3), 214.
25. Al Shemaili, J.; Mensah-Brown, E.; Parekh, K.; Thomas, S.A.; Attoub, S.; Hellman, B.; Nyberg, F.; Adem, A.; Collin, P.; Adrian, T.E. Frondoside A enhances the antiproliferative effects of gemcitabine in pancreatic cancer. *Eur. J. Cancer* **2014**, *50*, 1391–1398. [CrossRef] [PubMed]

26. Al Shemaili, J.; Parekh, K.A.; Newman, R.A.; Hellman, B.; Woodward, C.; Adem, A.; Collin, P.; Adrian, T.E. Pharmacokinetics in Mouse and Comparative Effects of Frondosides in Pancreatic Cancer. *Mar. Drugs* **2016**, *14*, 6. [CrossRef] [PubMed]

27. Silchenko, A.S.; Avilov, S.A.; Kalinin, V.I.; Kalinovsky, A.I.; Dmitrenok, P.S.; Fedorov, S.N.; Stepanov, V.G.; Dong, Z.; Stonik, V.A. Constituents of the sea cucumber Cucumaria okhotensis. Structures of okhotosides B1-B3 and cytotoxic activities of some glycosides from this species. *J. Nat. Prod.* **2008**, *71*, 351–356. [CrossRef] [PubMed]

28. Aminin, D.L.; Agafonova, I.G.; Kalinin, V.I.; Silchenko, A.S.; Avilov, S.A.; Stonik, V.A.; Collin, P.D.; Woodward, C. Immunomodulatory properties of frondoside A, a major triterpene glycoside from the North Atlantic commercially harvested sea cucumber Cucumaria frondosa. *J. Med. Food* **2008**, *11*, 443–453. [CrossRef] [PubMed]

29. Aminin, D.L.; Koy, C.; Dmitrenok, P.S.; Müller-Hilke, B.; Koczan, D.; Arbogast, B.; Silchenko, A.A.; Kalinin, V.I.; Avilov, S.A.; Stonik, V.A.; et al. Immunomodulatory effects of holothurian triterpene glycosides on mammalian splenocytes determined by mass spectrometric proteome analysis. *J. Proteomics* **2009**, *72*, 886–906. [CrossRef] [PubMed]

30. Aminin, D.L.; Silchenko, A.S.; Avilov, S.A.; Stepanov, V.G.; Kalinin, V.I. Cytotoxic action of triterpene glycosides from sea cucumbers from the genus Cucumaria on mouse spleen lymphocytes. Inhibition of nonspecific esterase. *Nat. Prod. Commun.* **2009**, *4*, 773–776. [PubMed]

31. Aminin, D.L.; Silchenko, A.S.; Avilov, S.A.; Stepanov, V.G.; Kalinin, V.I. Immunomodulatory action of monosulfated triterpene glycosides from the sea cucumber *Cucumaria okhotensis*: Stimulation of activity of mouse peritoneal macrophages. *Nat. Prod. Commun.* **2010**, *5*, 1877–1880. [PubMed]

32. Holt, D.M.; Ma, X.; Kundu, N.; Collin, P.D.; Fulton, A.M. Modulation of host natural killer cell functions in breast cancer via prostaglandin E2 receptors EP2 and EP4. *J. Immunother.* **2012**, *35*, 179–188. [CrossRef] [PubMed]

33. Kovalchuk, S.N.; Kozhemyako, V.B.; Atopkina, L.N.; Silchenko, A.S.; Avilov, S.A.; Kalinin, V.I.; Rasskazov, V.A.; Aminin, D.L. activity of triterpene glycosides in yeast two-hybrid assay. *J. Steroid Biochem. Mol. Biol.* **2006**, *101*, 226–231. [CrossRef] [PubMed]

34. Mazeĭka, A.N.; Popov, A.M.; Kalinin, V.I.; Avilov, S.A.; Sil'chenko, A.S.; Kostetskiĭ, E. Complexation between triterpene glycosides of holothurians and cholesterol is the basis of lipid-saponin carriers of subunit protein antigens. *Biofizika* **2008**, *53*, 826–835. [PubMed]

35. Menchinskaya, E.S.; Aminin, D.L.; Avilov, S.A.; Silchenko, A.S.; Andryjashchenko, P.V.; Kalinin, V.I.; Stonik, V.A. Inhibition of tumor cells multidrug resistance by cucumarioside A2-2, frondoside A and their complexes with cholesterol. *Nat. Prod. Commun.* **2013**, *8*, 1377–1380. [PubMed]

36. Nguyen, B.C.Q.; Yoshimura, K.; Kumazawa, S.; Tawata, S.; Maruta, H. Frondoside A from sea cucumber and nymphaeols from *Okinawa propolis*: Natural anti-cancer agents that selectively inhibit PAK1 *in vitro*. *Drug Discov. Ther.* **2017**, *11*, 110–114. [CrossRef] [PubMed]

37. Leist, M.; Jaattela, M. Four deaths and a funeral: From caspases to alternative mechanisms. *Nat. Rev. Mol. Cell. Biol.* **2001**, *2*, 589–598. [CrossRef] [PubMed]

38. Sperandio, S.; de Belle, I.; Bredesen, D.E. An alternative, nonapoptotic form of programmed cell death. *Proc. Natl. Acad. Sci. USA* **2000**, *97*, 14376–14381. [CrossRef] [PubMed]

39. Turmaine, M.; Raza, A.; Mahal, A.; Mangiarini, L.; Bates, G.P.; Davies, S.W. Nonapoptotic neurodegeneration in a transgenic mouse model of Huntington's disease. *Proc. Natl. Acad. Sci. USA* **2000**, *97*, 8093–8097. [CrossRef] [PubMed]

40. Lee, C.Y.; Baehrecke, E.H. Steroid regulation of autophagic programmed cell death during development. *Development* **2001**, *128*, 1443–1455. [PubMed]

41. Holler, N.; Zaru, R.; Micheau, O.; Thome, M.; Attinger, A.; Valitutti, S.; Bodmer, J.L.; Schneider, P.; Seed, B.; Tschopp, J. Fas triggers an alternative, caspase-8-independent cell death pathway using the kinase RIP as effector molecule. *Nat. Immunol.* **2000**, *1*, 489–495. [CrossRef] [PubMed]

42. Los, M.; Mozoluk, M.; Ferrari, D.; Stepczynska, A.; Stroh, C.; Renz, A.; Herceg, Z.; Wang, Z.Q.; Schulze-Osthoff, K. Activation and caspase-mediated inhibition of PARP: A molecular switch between fibroblast necrosis and apoptosis in death receptor signaling. *Mol. Biol. Cell* **2002**, *13*, 978–988. [CrossRef] [PubMed]

43. Vercammen, D.; Brouckaert, G.; Denecker, G.; Van de Craen, M.; Declercq, W.; Fiers, W.; Vandenabeele, P. Dual signaling of the Fas receptor: Initiation of both apoptotic and necrotic cell death pathways. *J. Exp. Med.* **1998**, *188*, 919–930. [CrossRef] [PubMed]

44. Denecker, G.; Vercammen, D.; Steemans, M.; Vanden Berghe, T.; Brouckaert, G.; Van Loo, G.; Zhivotovsky, B.; Fiers, W.; Grooten, J.; Declercq, W.; Vandenabeele, P. Death receptor-induced apoptotic and necrotic cell death: Differential role of caspases and mitochondria. *Cell Death Differ.* **2001**, *8*, 829–840. [CrossRef] [PubMed]

45. Foghsgaard, L.; Wissing, D.; Mauch, D.; Lademann, U.; Bastholm, L.; Boes, M.; Elling, F.; Leist, M.; Jäättelä, M. Cathepsin B acts as a dominant execution protease in tumor cell apoptosis induced by tumor necrosis factor. *J. Cell Biol.* **2001**, *153*, 999–1010. [CrossRef] [PubMed]

46. Schulze-Osthoff, K.; Bakker, A.C.; Vanhaesebroeck, B.; Schulze-Osthoff, K.; Bakker, A.C.; Vanhaesebroeck, B.; Beyaert, R.; Jacob, W.A.; Fiers, W. Cytotoxic activity of tumor necrosis factor is mediated by early damage of mitochondrial functions. Evidence for the involvement of mitochondrial radical generation. *J. Biol. Chem.* **1992**, *267*, 5317–5323. [PubMed]

47. McCarthy, N.J.; Whyte, M.K.; Gilbert, C.S.; Evan, G.I. Inhibition of Ced3/ICE-related proteases does not prevent cell death induced by oncogenes, DNA damage, or the Bcl-2 homologue Bak. *J. Cell Biol.* **1997**, *136*, 215–227. [CrossRef] [PubMed]

48. Borner, C.; Monney, L. Apoptosis without caspases: An inefficient molecular guillotine? *Cell Death Differ.* **1999**, *6*, 497–507. [CrossRef] [PubMed]

49. Déas, O.; Dumont, C.; MacFarlane, M.; Rouleau, M.; Hebib, C.; Harper, F.; Hirsch, F.; Charpentier, B.; Cohen, G.M.; Senik, A. Caspase-independent cell death induced by antiCD2 or staurosporine in activated human peripheral T lymphocytes. *J. Immunol.* **1998**, *161*, 3375–3383. [PubMed]

50. Miller, T.M.; Moulder, K.L.; Knudson, C.M.; Creedon, D.J.; Deshmukh, M.; Korsmeyer, S.J.; Johnson, E.M. Bax deletion further orders the cell death pathway in cerebellar granule cells and suggests a caspase-independent pathway to cell death. *J. Cell Biol.* **1997**, *139*, 205–217. [CrossRef] [PubMed]

51. Xiang, J.; Chao, D.T.; Korsmeyer, S.J. BAX-induced cell death may not require interleukin 1 beta-converting enzyme-like proteases. *Proc. Natl. Acad. Sci. USA* **1996**, *93*, 14559–14563. [CrossRef] [PubMed]

52. Daugas, E.; Susin, S.A.; Zamzami, N.; Ferri, K.F.; Irinopoulou, T.; Larochette, N.; Prévost, M.C.; Leber, B.; Andrews, D.; Penninger, J.; Kroeme, G. Mitochondrionuclear translocation of AIF in apoptosis and necrosis. *FASEB J.* **2000**, *14*, 729–739. [CrossRef] [PubMed]

53. Arnoult, D.; Tatischeff, I.; Estaquier, J.; Girard, M.; Sureau, F.; Tissier, J.P.; Grodet, A.; Dellinger, M.; Traincard, F.; Kahn, A.; et al. On the evolutionary conservation of the cell death pathway: Mitochondrial release of an apoptosis-inducing factor during *Dictyostelium discoideum* cell death. *Mol. Biol. Cell* **2001**, *12*, 3016–3030. [CrossRef] [PubMed]

54. Al Shemaili, J.; Parekh, K.; Thomas, S.A.; Kelly, D.L.; Ding, X.Z.; Attoub, S.; Collin, S.P.; Adrian, T.E. Studies on the Mechanism of Action of Frondoside A in Pancreatic Cancer. *Pancreatology* **2013**. [CrossRef]

55. Kumar, R.; Gururaj, A.E.; Barnes, C.J. p21-Activated kinases in cancer. *Nat. Rev. Cancer* **2006**, *6*, 459–471. [CrossRef] [PubMed]

56. Rane, C.; Minden, A. P21 activated kinases: Structure, regulation, and functions. *Small GTPases* **2014**, *5*, e28003. [CrossRef] [PubMed]

57. Wang, Z.; Jia, G.; Li, Y.; Liu, J.; Luo, J.; Zhang, J.; Xu, G.; Chen, G. Clinicopathological signature of p21-activated kinase 1 in prostate cancer and its regulation of proliferation and autophagy via the mTOR signaling pathway. *Oncotarget* **2017**, *8*, 22563–22580. [CrossRef] [PubMed]

58. Nheu, T.; He, H.; Hirokawa, Y.; Walker, F.; Wood, J.; Maruta, H. PAK is essential for RAS-induced upregulation of cyclin D1 during the G1 to S phase transition. *Cell Cycle* **2004**, *3*, 71–74. [CrossRef] [PubMed]

59. Huynh, N.; Wang, K.; Yim, M.; Dumesny, C.J.; Sandrin, M.S.; Baldwin, G.S.; Nikfarjam, M.; He, H. Depletion of p21-ctivated kinase 1 up-regulates the immune system of APCΔ14/+ mice and inhibits intestinal tumorigenesis. *BMC Cancer* **2017**, *17*, 431. [CrossRef] [PubMed]

60. Dou, Y.; Luo, J.; Wu, X.; Wei, Z.; Tong, B.; Yu, J.; Wang, T.; Zhang, X.; Yang, Y.; Yuan, X.; et al. Curcumin attenuates collagen-induced inflammatory response through the "gut-brain axis". *J. Neuroinflamm.* **2018**, *15*, 6. [CrossRef] [PubMed]

61. Gomes, N.G.; Dasari, R.; Chandra, S.; Kiss, R.; Kornienko, A. Marine Invertebrate Metabolites with Anticancer Activities: Solutions to the "Supply Problem". *Mar. Drugs* **2016**, *14*, 5. [CrossRef] [PubMed]

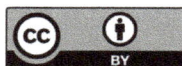

© 2018 by the authors. Licensee MDPI, Basel, Switzerland. This article is an open access article distributed under the terms and conditions of the Creative Commons Attribution (CC BY) license (http://creativecommons.org/licenses/by/4.0/).

marine drugs

MDPI

Article

Cytotoxic Polyhydroxysteroidal Glycosides from Starfish *Culcita novaeguineae*

Yunyang Lu [1], Hu Li [1,2], Minchang Wang [3], Yang Liu [1], Yingda Feng [1], Ke Liu [3] and Haifeng Tang [1,*]

[1] Institute of Materia Medica, School of Pharmacy, Fourth Military Medical University, Xi'an 710032, China; luyunyanggq@163.com (Y.L.); pharm_lihu@163.com (H.L.); so870823@163.com (Y.L.); fyd1991@sina.com (Y.F.)

[2] First Motorized Detachment of Shanghai Armed Police Corps, Shanghai 200126, China

[3] Nuclear Magnetic Resonance Center, Xi'an Modern Chemistry Research Institute, Xi'an 710065, China; wmc204@163.com (M.W.); happycoco5133@163.com (K.L.)

* Correspondence: tanghaifeng71@163.com; Tel.: +86-29-8477-4748

Received: 7 February 2018; Accepted: 10 March 2018; Published: 13 March 2018

Abstract: Four new polyhydroxysteroidal glycosides—culcinosides A–D (**1**, **2**, **4**, and **7**)—along with three known compounds—echinasteroside C (**3**), linckoside F (**5**), and linckoside L3 (**6**)—were isolated from the ethanol extract of starfish *Culcita novaeguineae* collected from the Xisha Islands of the South China Sea. The structures of new compounds were elucidated through extensive spectroscopic studies and chemical evidence, especially two-dimensional (2D) NMR techniques. The cytotoxicity of the new compounds against human glioblastoma cell lines U87, U251, and SHG44 were evaluated.

Keywords: *Culcita novaeguineae*; starfish; polyhydroxysteroidal glycoside; cytotoxicity

1. Introduction

The starfish is a sea animal belonging to Asteroidea: Echinodermata that is distributed worldwide; there are approximately 1900 species grouped into 370 genera [1]. Steroidal glycosides are the predominant metabolites of starfish, and are responsible for their general toxicity. Based on structural characteristics, they have been subdivided into three groups: asterosaponins, polyhydroxysteroidal glycosides, and cyclic steroidal glycosides [2]. Polyhydroxysteroidal glycosides are abundant in the metabolism of starfish; more than 500 have been identified in total [3]. In general, polyhydroxysteroidal glycosides consist of an oxygenated steroidal aglycone with more than three hydroxy groups, and one or two (rarely three) monosaccharide residues attached to the steroidal nucleus or side chain. Polyhydroxysteroidal glycosides have been reported to show a broad spectrum of biological activities, including hemolytic, cytotoxic, immunoregulatory, anti-bacterial, neuritogenic, anti-inflammatory, and anti-biofouling effects [4–12]. *Culcita novaeguineae* is plentiful in the South China Sea; it is used as a folk medicine for the treatment of rheumatism, and as a tonic in China [13]. The chemical constituent investigation of this starfish has led to the isolation of several polyhydroxysteroid glycosides and asterosaponins by scientists around the world [14,15]. The previous work that our team carried out on *Culcita novaeguineae* led to the isolation of a series of novel asterosaponins. Some of these have shown significant cytotoxicity against several human cancer cell lines, such as asterosaponin 1, through suppressing the proliferation of human glioblastoma cell line U87 with an IC$_{50}$ of 4.3 μg/mL [2,6,16–19]. However, no polyhydroxysteroidal glycosides, as a large class of bioactive metabolites of starfish, were found in our previous work. Therefore, as part of a continuous search for bioactive steroidal glycosides from starfish, we aimed for the polyhydroxysteroidal glycosides in *Culcita novaeguineae*. Herein, we report the isolation, structural elucidation, and biological activity screening of four new polyhydroxysteroidal glycosides, culcinosides A–D (**1**, **2**, **4**, and **7**), together with three known compounds, which were identified as echinasteroside C (**3**), linckoside F (**5**), and linckoside L3 (**6**), through a comparison of the physical and spectra data with literature values (Figure 1) [10,12,20].

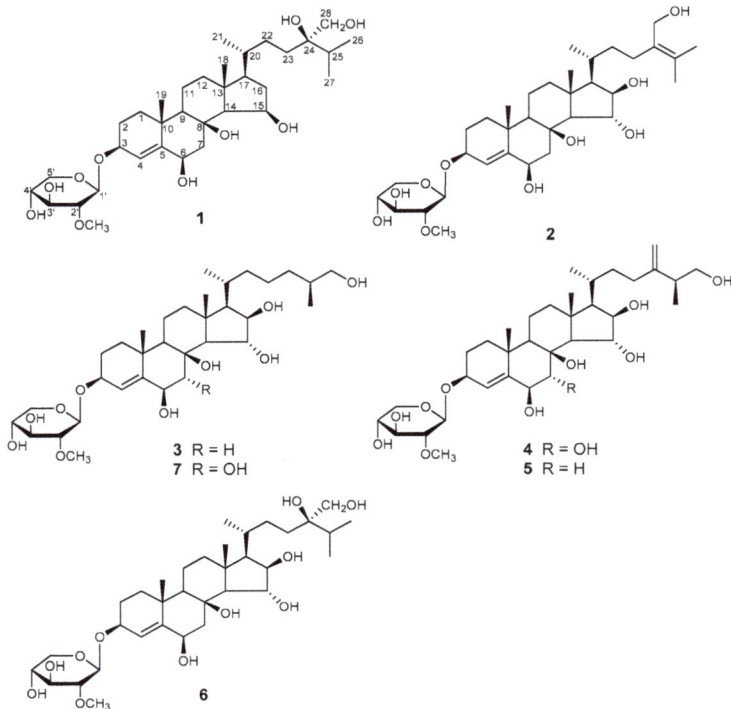

Figure 1. The structures of compounds **1–7** isolated from starfish *Culcita novaeguineae*.

2. Results and Discussion

2.1. Structure Elucidation

Culcinoside A (**1**) was isolated as a colorless powder, and was positive for the Liebermann–Burchard and Molisch tests, which indicated that it might be a steroidal glycoside. The molecular formula of compound **1** was determined as $C_{34}H_{58}O_{10}$ by ESIMS at m/z 649 [M + Na]$^+$ and HRESIMS at m/z 649.3942 [M + Na]$^+$ (calculated for $C_{34}H_{58}O_{10}Na$, 649.3928). The ^{1}H-NMR, ^{13}C-NMR, and DEPT spectra suggested the existence of a trisubstituted double bond (δ_C 126.5, δ_H 5.94; δ_C 148.9), two angular methyls (δ_C 16.0, C-18; δ_C 23.1, C-19) with singlets (δ_H 1.30, H-18; δ_H 1.66, H-19), three doublets (δ_H 1.07, δ_C 19.4, C-21; δ_H 1.22, δ_C 18.0, C-26; δ_H 1.20, δ_C 18.1, C-27), three oxidized methines (δ_C 69.5, δ_H 4.90; δ_C 75.9, δ_H 4.77; δ_C 76.6, δ_H 4.48), and two oxygenated quaternary carbon (δ_C 76.0, δ_C 76.2). A comprehensive analysis and comparison of the above data with that of co-isolated linckoside L3 (**6**) indicated that they may share the same steroidal aglycone and side chain (Table 1). A difference was recognized in ring D, where a secondary alcohol (δ_C 83.1, δ_H 4.04) in compound **6** was replaced by one methylene (δ_H 2.15 and 2.27, δ_C 42.3, CH$_2$-16) of compound **1**. Furthermore, this substitution was witnessed by the upfield shift of C-15 (δ_C 69.5, δ_H 4.90) in compound **1** when compared with that of **6** (δ_C 80.6, δ_H 4.17). The position of the double bond was determined by HMBC correlations for H-4 to C-2, C-6, and C-10; H-3 and H-5 to C-4 and C-5; and H-19 to C-5. This connection was further confirmed by the ^{1}H-^{1}H COSY correlations for H-3 to H-4. The assignment of the NMR signals associated with the aglycone moiety and side chain

(Table 1) was derived from HSQC, ^{1}H-^{1}H COSY, HMBC, and TOCSY experiments. The normally occurring 2-*O*-methyl-β-D-xylopyranose (2-OMe-Xyl) moiety in the polyhydroxysteroidal glycosides was detected in compound **1** by analyzing the one-dimensional (1D) and two-dimensional (2D) NMR spectra, and by comparing the monosaccharide signals with those co-isolated known compounds and the literature values [21–23]. This was further confirmed by the demethylation and acid hydrolysis of compound **1** with 2 M trifluoroacetic acid, followed by derivatization with 1-(trimethylsily)-imidazole, gas chromatography (GC) analysis sequentially, and a comparison with the corresponding derivatives of a standard monosaccharide [6,8]. The attachment of the monosaccharide to C-3 was confirmed by HMBC correlation for H-3 to C-1′ (δ_C 104.8) of the Xyl, and H-1′ (δ_H 4.84) of the Xyl to C-3 of the aglycone (Figure 2). The NOESY correlations of H-3 to H-1b, H-1b to H-9, H-6 to H-7b, and H-7b to H-9, and the lack of correlation between H-1 and H-6 indicated the α-orientation of H-3 and H-6 (Figure 3). The β-orientation of the hydroxy at C-15 was determined by the NOESY correlation of H-16b to H-15 and H-17, and the lack of correlation between H-14 and H-15. The 20*R* configuration was deduced from the NOESY correlation of H-20 to H-18, and the large coupling constant of H-17 (J = 9.1) [10]. It has been reported that small but important differences in the signals for the HC(28), H′C(28), and C(28) atoms in the NMR spectra of the synthetic 24*R* and 24*S* epimers of 24-hydroxymethyl-24-hydroxycholesterol (24*R*: $\Delta\delta_H$ = 0.04, δ_C = 66.0; 24*S*: $\Delta\delta_H$ = 0.06, δ_C = 66.3) [12]. The NMR spectroscopic data of compound **1** at CH$_2$-28 ($\Delta\delta_H$ = 0.04, δ_C = 66.1) coincided with that of the 24*R* epimer. Thus, the absolute configuration of C-24 was determined as *R*. Therefore, the structure of compound **1** was established as (24*R*)-3-*O*-(2-*O*-methyl-β-D-xylopyranosyl)-cholesta-4-ene-3β,6β,8,15β,24,28-hexaol.

Table 1. The ^{1}H-NMR and ^{13}C-NMR data of compounds **1**, **2**, **4**, and **7** (δ in ppm, *J* in Hz).

Position	1 c,e		2 d,e		4 c,f		7 c,e	
	δ_C	δ_H	δ_C	δ_H	δ_C	δ_H	δ_C	δ_H
1a	39.4	1.85 m	39.4	1.86 m	39.6	1.77 m	39.4	1.90 m
1b		1.39 m		1.40 m		1.32 m		1.57 m
2a	28.2	2.28 m	28.2	2.28 m	28	1.99 m	28.3	2.28 m
2b		2.09 m		2.09 m		1.76 m		2.12 m
3	76.6	4.48 brt (7.2)	76.7	4.48 m	77.5	4.24 brt (8.2)	76.6	4.51 m
4	126.5	5.94 s	126.5	5.94 s	130.3	5.70 s	129.8	6.17 s
5	148.9	-	149	-	145.4	-	146.2	-
6	75.9	4.77 d (2.5)	76	4.76 d (2.3)	79.9	4.12 d(3.1)	80	4.87 d(2.7)
7a	44.9	3.40 dd (14.8, 2.5)	44.9	3.49 dd (14.7, 2.3)	73.9	3.96 d(3.1)	74.5	4.84 d(2.7)
7b		2.07 m		2.08 m				
8	76	-	76	-	78	-	78.1	-
9	57.6	1.24 m	60.8	1.55 m	51.5	1.34 m	51.3	1.91 m
10	37.6	-	37.7	-	37.4	-	37.3	-
11a	19.7	2.10 m	19.6	2.15 m	19.4	1.89 m	19.5	2.27 m
11b		1.55 m		1.57 m		1.53 m		1.67 m
12a	42.5	2.07 m	43	2.14 m	43.1	1.98 m	43	2.16 m
12b		1.28 m		1.32 m		1.22 m		1.40 m
13	45	-	45	-	45.5	-	45.3	-
14	66.6	1.56 m	64.1	1.51 m	59.5	1.42 d (10.6)	59.7	2.05 d (10.5)
15	69.5	4.90 m	80.8	5.08 m	80.1	4.20 dd (10.6, 1.8)	80.4	5.11 brd (10.5)
16a	42.3	2.27 m	83	4.78 m	82.6	4.03 dd (7.4, 1.8)	82.5	4.72 dd (7.1, 1.2)
16b		2.15 m						
17	55.8	1.61 brd (9.1)	60.8	1.55 m	61.4	1.29 dd (10.8, 7.4)	61.6	1.54 m
18	16	1.30 s	17.5	1.74 s	17	1.16 s	17.6	1.77 s
19	23.1	1.66 s	23.1	1.67 s	23.2	1.34 s	23.6	1.68 s
20	36.6	1.54 m	30.6	2.42 m	30.7	1.90 m	30.5	2.40 m
21	19.4	1.07 d (6.2)	19.1	1.21 d (6.7)	18.5	0.96 d (6.7)	18.8	1.14 d (6.7)
22a	30.6	1.92 m	35.7	2.20 m	35.4	1.74 m	37.1	1.96 m
22b		1.41 m		1.54 m		1.23 m		1.33 m
23a	32	2.03 m	29.2	2.55 t (7.3)	33	2.15 m	25	1.69 m
23b		1.85 m		1.52 m		1.97 m		1.44 m
24a	76.2	-	135	-	154	-	35	1.64 m
24b								1.23 m

Table 1. *Cont.*

Position	1 [c,e]		2 [d,e]		4 [c,f]		7 [c,e]	
	δ_C	δ_H	δ_C	δ_H	δ_C	δ_H	δ_C	δ_H
25	34	2.26 m	128.1	-	43.5	2.31 m	37.3	1.82 m
26a	18	1.20 d (6.8)	20.7	1.75 s	67.6	3.58 m	68	3.76 dd (10.4, 5.6)
26b						3.37 m		3.64 m
27	18.1	1.22 d (6.8)	21.1	1.77 s	17.4	1.07 d (6.5)	18	1.08 d (6.7)
28a	66.1	4.03 m	62.4	4.51 m	109.4	4.84 s	-	-
28b		3.97 m		4.42 m		4.77 s		
2-OMe-Xyl								
1'	104.8	4.84 d (7.6)	104.8	4.84 d (7.6)	104.7	4.44 d (7.6)	104.7	4.76 d (7.6)
2'	85.6	3.46 dd (8.8, 7.6)	85.6	3.46 dd (8.8, 7.6)	85	2.85 dd (9.0, 7.6)	85.5	3.44 dd (8.9, 7.6)
3'	78.2	4.08 m	78.2	4.08 br.t(8.8)	77.6	3.33 m	78.1	4.04 br.t (8.9)
4'	71.6	4.23 m	71.6	4.23 m	71.4	3.50 m	71.6	4.20 m
5'a	67.5	4.35 dd (11.3, 5.4)	67.5	4.34 dd (11.4, 5.4)	66.9	3.84 dd (11.5, 5.4)	67.5	4.32 dd (11.3, 5.3)
5'b		3.67 m		3.67 t (11.4)		3.18dd (11.5, 10.4)		3.62 m
2-OMe	61.2	3.72 s	61.2	3.72 s	61.3	3.59 s	61.1	3.68 s

[c] The NMR data were recorded at 500 MHz for δ_H and 125 MHz for δ_C; [d] the NMR data were recorded at 800 MHz for δ_H and 200 MHz for δ_C; [e] in C_5D_5N; [f] in CD_3OD.

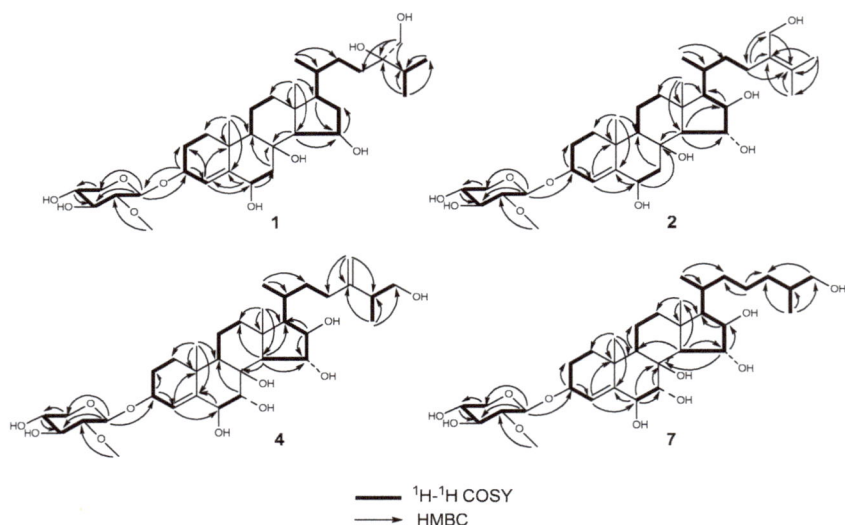

Figure 2. The key ^{1}H-^{1}H COSY and HMBC correlations of the new compounds culcinosides A–D (1, 2, 4, and 7).

Culcinoside B (**2**), a colorless powder, was positive for the Liebermann–Burchard and Molisch tests, which indicated that it might be a steroidal glycoside. The molecular formula of compound **2** ($C_{34}H_{56}O_{10}$) was deduced from HRESIMS at m/z 647.3795 [M + Na]$^+$ (calculated for $C_{34}H_{56}O_{10}Na$, 647.3771). The ^{1}H, ^{13}C, and DEPT NMR spectra signals belonging to the tetracyclic moiety of the aglycone of compound **2** revealed the presence of two angular methyls (δ_C 17.5, δ_H 1.74 s, CH$_3$-18; δ_C 23.1, δ_H 1.67 s, CH$_3$-19), one trisubstituted double bond 4(5) (δ_C 126.5, δ_H 5.94, C-4; δ_C 149.0, C-5), three oxygenated methines (δ_C 76.0, δ_H 4.76, CH-6; δ_C 80.8, δ_H 5.08, CH-15; δ_C 83.0, δ_H 4.78, CH-16), one oxygenated methine (CH-3) bearing a monosaccharide residue (δ_C 76.7, δ_H 4.48), and one quaternary oxygenated carbon C-8 (δ_C 76.0). All of the above data were similar to the known compounds echinasteroside C (**3**) and linckoside A, which possessed the same Δ^4-3β,6β,8,15α,16β-pentahydroxycholestane aglycone [11,20]. The chemical shift of the anomeric proton at δ_H 4.84 (J = 7.6) associated with the anomeric carbon at δ_C 104.8 in the HSQC spectrum and the carbon signals at δ_C 61.2, 67.5, 71.6, 78.16, and 85.6 suggested the presence of the 2-*O*-methyl-β-D-xylopyranose monosaccharide residue, and this was further confirmed by acid hydrolysis followed by GC analysis. The connection of the monosaccharide to C-3 was deduced from the HMBC correlation for H-1' of Xyl to C-3 of the aglycone (Figure 2). All of the H and C signals of compound **2** were assigned by the 2D NMR spectra, including HSQC, ^{1}H-^{1}H COSY, and HMBC (Table 1). The structure of the side chain for compound **2** was elucidated on the basis of 2D NMR spectra. The tetrasubstituted double bond at C-24 and C-25, and the C-28 hydroxymethyl were determined by HMBC correlations for H-23 (2H) to C-24, C-25 and C-28; H-26 and H-27 to C-24 and C-25; and H-28 (2H) to C-23, C-24, and C-25. The 3β, 6β, 15α, and 16β orientations for the aglycone of **2** were confirmed by the cross-peaks of the NOESY spectrum (Figure 3). The 20*R* configuration was deduced from the NOESY correlation of H-20 to H-18, and Hα-13 to H-21. According to the data above, the structure of compound **2** was elucidated as 3-*O*-(2-*O*-methyl-β-D-xylopyranosyl)-cholesta-4,24-diene-3β,6β,8,15α,16β,28-hexaol.

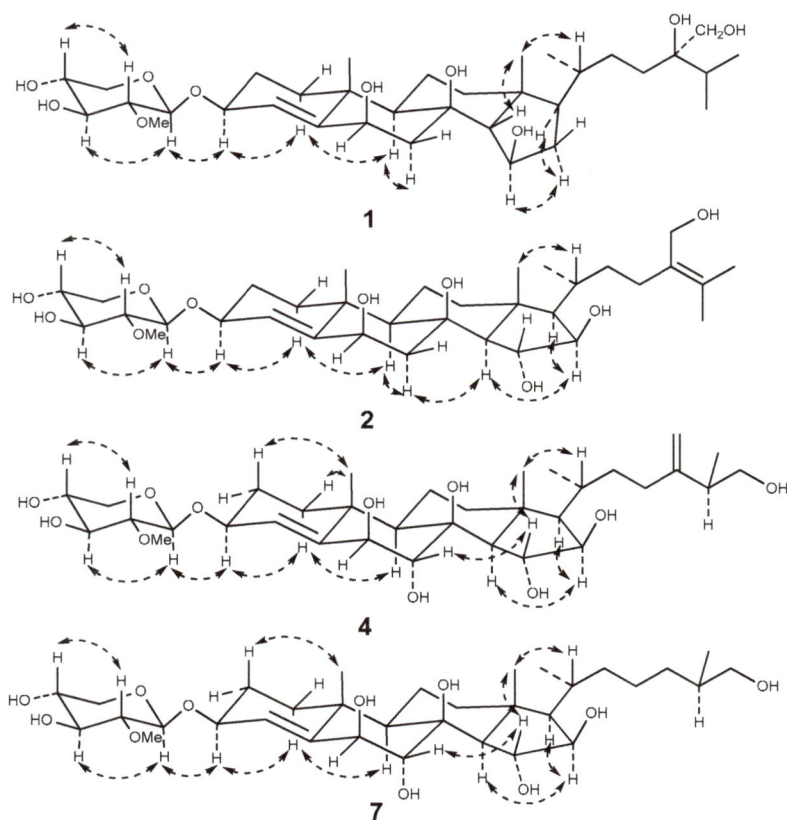

Figure 3. The key NOESY correlations of the new compounds culcinosides A-D (**1**, **2**, **4**, and **7**).

Culcinoside C (**4**), a colorless powder, was positive for the Liebermann–Burchard and Molisch tests, which indicated that it might be a steroidal glycoside. The HRESIMS at m/z 663.3696 [M + Na]$^+$ (calculated for $C_{34}H_{56}O_{11}Na$, 663.3720) indicated that the molecular formula of **4** was $C_{34}H_{56}O_{11}$. The ^{1}H, ^{13}C, and DEPT NMR spectra revealed two double bonds, including one trisubstituted double bond (δ_C 130.3, δ_H 5.70, C-4; δ_C 145.4, C-5) and one terminal double bond (δ_C 154.0, C-28; δ_C 109.4, δ_H 4.77, 4.84), one anomeric carbon (δ_C 104.7 with δ_H 4.44), two angular methyl (δ_C 17.0, δ_H 1.16 s, CH$_3$-18; δ_C 23.2, δ_H 1.34 s, CH$_3$-19), one hydroxymethyl (δ_C 67.6, δ_H 3.38, 3.59), five oxygenated methines (δ_C 77.5, δ_H 4.24, C-3; δ_C 79.9, δ_H 4.13, C-6; δ_C 73.9, δ_H 3.98, C-7; δ_C 80.1, δ_H 4.20, C-15; and δ_C 82.6, δ_H 4.03, C-16), and one oxygenated quaternary carbon (δ_C 78.0, C-8). All of the chemical shifts belonging to compound **4** were similar to those of the known compound linckoside F (**5**) from the starfish *Linckia laevigata* [10]. A detailed comparison of the NMR spectra for compounds **4** and **5** indicated that the only difference was that one methylene (δ_C 44.6, δ_H 2.04, 3.39, CH$_2$-7) in **5** was replaced by an oxygenated methine in **4** (δ_C 73.9, δ_H 3.98, CH-7). The assignments of the NMR signals associated with compound **4** were derived from the HSQC, ^{1}H-^{1}H COSY, HMBC, and TOCSY experiments (Table 1). The NOESY correlation for H-7 to H-15 and H-18 to H-15 suggested the α orientation of C-7 (Figure 3). The 20*R* configuration was deduced from the NOESY correlation of H-18 to H-20, and the chemical shift of H-21 δ_H 0.96 (δ_H 0.90–0.96 for 20*R* steroid). The stereochemistry at C-25 was expected as *S* by analogy with co-occurring compound **5**, and on the basis of the comparison of their NMR spectra. Thus, the structure of **4** was established as (25*S*)-3-*O*-(2-*O*-methyl-β-D-xylopyranosyl)-cholesta-4,24(28)-diene-3β,6β,7α,8,15α,16β,26-heptaol.

Culcinoside D (**7**) was obtained as a colorless powder. The positive results of the Liebermann–Burchard and Molisch tests suggested that it might be a steroidal glycoside. The molecular formula was determined as C$_{33}$H$_{56}$O$_{11}$ by HRESIMS at *m/z* 651.3740 [M + Na]$^+$ (calculated for C$_{33}$H$_{56}$O$_{11}$Na, 651.3720). The ^{1}H-NMR, ^{13}C-NMR, and DEPT spectra of compound **7** revealed the presence of a steroidal aglycone with two angular methyls (δ_C 17.6, δ_H 1.77, CH$_3$-18; δ_C 23.6, δ_H 1.68, CH$_3$-19), one 4(5) double bond (δ_C 129.8, δ_H 6.17, C-4; δ_C 146.2, C-5), five oxygenated methine groups (δ_C 76.6, δ_H 4.51, C-3; δ_C 80.0, δ_H 4.87, C-6; δ_C 74.5, δ_H 4.84, C-7; δ_C 80.4, δ_H 5.11, C-15; δ_C 82.5, δ_H 4.72, C-16), and a quaternary carbon (δ_C 78.1, C-8) bearing a hydroxy group. The anomeric carbon (δ_C 104.7) with δ_H at 4.76 (d, 7.6) indicated the presence of the common 2-*O*-methyl-β-D-xylopyranosyl moiety, and their ^{1}H and ^{13}C signals were assigned by the 2D NMR data (Table 1). The only difference between compounds **7** and **3**, which was elucidated as echinasteroside C isolated from the starfish *Echinaster brasiliensis*, was that a methylene (δ_C 45.0, δ_H 2.10 and 3.45, CH$_2$-7) in compound **3** was substituted by one oxygenated methine (δ_C 74.5, δ_H 4.84, CH-7) in compound **7** [20]. Therefore, the structure of **7** was elucidated as (25*S*)-3-*O*-(2-*O*-methyl-β-D-xylopyranosyl)-cholesta-4-ene-3β,6β,7α,8,15α,16β,26-heptaol.

2.2. Cytotoxic Activities

The cytotoxic activity of the new compounds **1**, **2**, **4**, and **7** against human glioblastoma cell lines U87, U251, and SHG44 were evaluated using the 3-(4,5-dimethylthiazol-2-yl)-2,5-diphenyltetrazolium bromide (MTT) colorimetric assay method in vitro [24]. Compound **1** exhibited cytotoxicity against the three cancer cell lines, and compounds **2**, **4**, and **7** showed moderate activity (Table 2). Doxorubicin was used as the positive control.

Table 2. Cytotoxic activity of the new compounds in vitro (mean ± SD, *n* = 3).

Compounds	Cytotoxic Activity (IC$_{50}$, μM)		
	U87	U251	SHG44
1	9.35 ± 0.46	11.28 ± 0.65	8.04 ± 0.32
2	33.52 ± 1.23	40.76 ± 1.58	36.54 ± 1.44
4	26.33 ± 1.16	22.66 ± 1.28	35.26 ± 1.51
7	43.25 ± 1.73	28.93 ± 1.83	26.22 ± 1.64
Doxorubicin	0.33 ± 0.02	0.24 ± 0.01	0.15 ± 0.01

3. Experimental Section

3.1. General Experimental Procedures

Optical rotations were measured with a Perkin-Elmer 343 polarimeter (German Perkin-Elmer Corporation, Boelingen, Germany). 1D and 2D NMR spectra were recorded on a Bruker AVANCE III 500 and 800 MHz spectrometer with TMS (Tetramethylsilane) as the internal standard. ESIMS and HRESIMS were carried out on a Micromass Quattro mass spectrometer (Waters, Shanghai, China). HPLC was carried out on a Dionex P680 liquid chromatograph (Dionex, Germering, Germany) equipped with a UV 170 UV/Vis detector using a YMC-Pack C18 column (20 × 250 mm i.d., 5 μm, YMC Co., Ltd., Kyoto, Japan) and monitored at 206 nm, 225 nm, 275 nm, and 300 nm, simultaneously. GC was performed on a Finnigan Voyager apparatus using an l-Chirasil-Val column (25 m × 0.32 mm i.d.) for the analyses of the trimethylsilyated hydrolysates. Column chromatographies were performed on silica gel (200–300 mesh and 300–400 mesh; Qingdao Marine Chemical Inc., Qingdao, China), reversed phase silica gel (Lichroprep RP-18, 40–63 μm, Merck Inc., New York, NY, USA), and Sephadex LH-20 (40–70 μm, GE-Healthcare, Uppsala, Sweden). Chemical reagents for isolation were of analytical grade, and purchased from Tianjin Fuyu Chemical Co. Ltd. (Tianjin, China).

3.2. Animal Material

The starfish were collected from the South China Sea (Xisha Islands, Sansha, Hainan Province, China) in August 2015. The organisms were identified as *Culcita novaeguineae* by Dr. Ning Xiao (Institute of Oceanology, Chinese Academy of Science, Qingdao, China). A voucher specimen (No. HX201508) was deposited in the Institute of Materia Medica, School of Pharmacy, Fourth Military Medical University (Xi'an, China).

3.3. Extraction and Isolation

The starfish (80.0 kg, wet weight) were cut into pieces, and then extracted with 75% ethanol three times, each time for 2 h under reflux. The extract was combined and dried in vacuo to leave a residue, which was suspended in water and then partitioned with petroleum ether and *n*-butanol sequentially. The *n*-butanol part (320.0 g) was subjected to silica gel column chromatography eluting with a $CHCl_3/CH_3OH/H_2O$ (50:1:0 to 6:3.5:1) gradient to give 16 major fractions, which were obtained based on TLC analysis. Fraction 10 was subjected to size exclusion chromatography on a Sephadex LH-20 column eluting with $CHCl_3/CH_3OH$ (1:1) to remove the impurities, then was further purified by HPLC to give compounds **1** (3.4 mg, t_R = 35.5 min) and **2** (1.6 mg, t_R = 57.6 min), eluting with CH_3CN/H_2O (2:3) at a flow rate of 6 mL/min. RP-C_{18} column chromatography eluted with $CH_3OH:H_2O$ (1:1 to 1:0) and Sephadex LH-20 column chromatography equilibrated with $CHCl_3/CH_3OH$ (1:1) were used successively on the purification of fraction 11 to obtain the subfraction fr.11-2-4. Finally, fraction 11-2-4 was subjected to HPLC eluting with CH_3CN/H_2O (1:1.5) to afford compounds **3** (57.1 mg, t_R = 25.6 min), **4** (57.2 mg, t_R = 27.3 min), and **5** (141.3 mg, t_R = 29.3 min). Fraction 12 (6.1 g) was subjected to size exclusion chromatography on a Sephadex LH-20 column equilibrated with $CHCl_3/CH_3OH$ (1:1) to remove impurities and give three subfractions (Fr.12-1 to Fr.12-3). The subfraction 12-2 (2.2 g) was purified by a RP-C_{18} column chromatography eluting with $CH_3OH:H_2O$ (3:2 to 1:0) to give 10 subfractions. Then, fraction 12-2-8 (150.0 mg) was purified by semi-preparative HPLC eluting with CH_3CN/H_2O (2:3) at a flow rate of 6 mL/min to yield compound **6** (54.0 mg, t_R = 27.2 min). Compound **7** (26.6 mg, t_R = 33.0 min) was obtained from fraction 12-2-9 by HPLC eluting with CH_3CN/H_2O (2:3) at a flow rate of 6 mL/min.

3.4. Spectral and Physicochemical Data of New Compounds

Culcinoside A (**1**): $C_{34}H_{58}O_{10}$, colorless powder, $[\alpha]_D^{22}$ −13.6 (*c* 0.03, MeOH), ^{1}H- and ^{13}C-NMR data are shown in Table 1; ESIMS *m/z* 649 [M + Na]$^+$; HRESIMS *m/z* 649.3942 [M + Na]$^+$ (calculated for $C_{34}H_{58}O_{10}Na$, 649.3928).

Culcinoside B (**2**): $C_{34}H_{56}O_{10}$, colorless powder, $[\alpha]_D^{22}$ −10.3 (*c* 0.04, MeOH), ^{1}H- and ^{13}C-NMR data are shown in Table 1; ESIMS *m/z* 647 [M + Na]$^+$; HRESIMS *m/z* 647.3795 [M + Na]$^+$ (calculated for $C_{34}H_{56}O_{10}Na$ 647.3771).

Culcinoside C (**4**): $C_{34}H_{56}O_{11}$, colorless powder, $[\alpha]_D^{22}$ −28.4 (*c* 0.21, MeOH), ^{1}H- and ^{13}C-NMR data are shown in Table 1; ESIMS *m/z* 663 [M + Na]$^+$; HRESIMS *m/z* 663.3696 [M + Na]$^+$ (calculated for $C_{34}H_{56}O_{11}Na$ 663.3720).

Culcinoside D (**7**): $C_{33}H_{56}O_{11}$, colorless powder, $[\alpha]_D^{22}$ −16.5 (*c* 0.11, MeOH), ^{1}H- and ^{13}C-NMR data are shown in Table 1; ESIMS *m/z* 651 [M + Na]$^+$; HRESIMS *m/z* 651.3740 [M + Na]$^+$ (calculated for $C_{33}H_{56}O_{11}Na$, 651.3720).

3.5. Demethylation and Acid Hydrolysis of the New Compounds

The new compounds (each 1.5 mg) were mixed with 1 mL of dry dichloromethane and 0.01 mL of boron tribromide at −80 °C for 30 min, and then stood overnight at 10 °C under anhydrous conditions. The solvent and reagent were evaporated to dryness in vacuo at room temperature. The demethylated derivative of the new compound was heated with 1.0 mL of trifluoroacetic acid (TFA) at 120 °C for 2 h. The reaction mixture was evaporated in vacuo, and the residue was partitioned between CH_2Cl_2 and H_2O. The aqueous phase was concentrated and dissolved in 1-(trimethylsilyl)imidazole and anhydrous pyridine (0.1 mL). Then, the solution was stirred at 60 °C for 5 min, and dried with a stream of N_2. The residue was partitioned between CH_2Cl_2 and H_2O. The CH_2Cl_2 layer was analyzed by GC with an initial temperature of 100 °C for 1 min, and then temperature programmed to 180 °C at a rate of 5 °C/min. The peak of the derivative of the sample was detected at 11.25 and 12.46 min for compound **1**, 11.25 and 12.45 min for compound **2**, 11.23 and 12.45 for compound **4**, and 11.24 and 12.26 min for compound **7**. The retention time of the authentic samples after being treated simultaneously with 1-(trimethylsily)imidazole in pyridine were 11.23 and 12.44 min (D-xylose), and 11.34 and 12.40 min (L-xylose), respectively [6].

3.6. Assays for In Vitro Cytotoxicity

The cytotoxicity of new compounds **1**, **2**, **4**, and **7** against human glioblastoma cell lines U87, U251, and SHG44 were evaluated by the 3-(4,5-dimethylthiazol-2-yl)-2,5-diphenyltetrazolium bromide (MTT) colorimetric assay method in vitro. All of the cells were cultured in RPMI-1640 medium supplemented with 10% fetal bovine serum, 100 U/mL benzyl penicillin, and 100 U/mL streptomycin at 37 °C in a humidified atmosphere with 5% CO_2. The logarithmic phase cells were seeded on 96-well plates at a concentration of 4×10^3 cell/mL, and incubated with various concentrations (100 μM, 80 μM, 60 μM, 40 μM, 20 μM, 10 μM, 1 μM, and 0.25 μM in medium containing less than 0.1% DMSO) of test compounds in triple wells for 48 h, and doxorubicin was used as the positive control. Next, 20 μL MTT (5 mg/mL) was added to each well, and incubated for another 4 h. The water-insoluble dark blue formazan crystals formed during MTT cleavage in actively metabolizing cells were dissolved in DMSO. The optical density of each well was measured with a Bio-Rad 680 microplate reader at 570 nm. Cytotoxicity was expressed as the concentration of drug inhibiting cell growth by 50% (IC_{50}).

Supplementary Materials: The NMR and HRESIMS data of the new compounds and the ^{13}C-NMR data of the known compounds are available online at www.mdpi.com/1660-3397/16/3/92/s1.

Acknowledgments: This research was financially supported by the National Nature Science Foundation of China (No. 81473132).

Author Contributions: The listed authors contributed to this work as described in the following. Y.L., H.L., and Y.L. carried out the extraction and isolation. Y.L. also collected the organism of *Culcita novaeguineae* and participated in the structural elucidation. M.W. and K.L. participated in the structural elucidation. Y.F. conducted the MTT colorimetric assay and helped interpret the results. Corresponding author H.T. organized the study and participated in the structural elucidation. All authors helped prepare the manuscript and approved the final version.

Conflicts of Interest: The authors declare no conflict of interest.

Abbreviations

The following abbreviations are used in this paper:

DEPT	Distortionless enhancement by polarization transfer
ESIMS	Electron spray ionization mass spectrum
^{1}H-^{1}H COSY	^{1}H-^{1}H Correlation spectroscopy
HMBC	^{1}H-detected heteronuclear multiple bond correlation
HPLC	High performance liquid chromatography
HRESIMS	High resolution electron spray ionization mass spectrum
HSQC	^{1}H-detected heteronuclear single quantum correlation
NMR	Nuclear magnetic resonance
NOESY	Nuclear overhauser enhancement spectroscopy
TLC	Thin layer chromatography
TOCSY	Total correlation spectroscopy

References

1. Mah, C.L.; Blake, D.B. Global diversity and phylogeny of the Asteroidea (Echinodermata). *PLoS ONE* **2012**, *7*, e35644. [CrossRef] [PubMed]
2. Tang, H.; Yi, Y.; Li, L.; Sun, P. Bioactive asterosaponins from the starfish *Culcita novaeguineae*. *J. Nat. Prod.* **2005**, *68*, 337–341. [CrossRef] [PubMed]
3. Kicha, A.A.; Ivanchina, N.V.; Kalinovsky, A.I.; Dmitrenok, P.S.; Stonik, V.A. Steroidal monoglycosides from the Far Eastern starfish *Hippasteria kurilensis* and hypothetic pathways of polyhydroxysteroid biosynthesis in starfish. *Steroids* **2009**, *74*, 238–244. [CrossRef] [PubMed]
4. Blunt, J.W.; Copp, B.R.; Keyzers, R.A.; Munro, M.H.G.; Prinsep, M.R. Marine natural products. *Nat. Prod. Rep.* **2015**, *32*, 116–211. [CrossRef] [PubMed]
5. Mayer, A.M.S.; Rodríguez, A.D.; Taglialatela-Scafati, O.; Fusetani, N. Marine pharmacology in 2009–2011: Marine compounds with antibacterial, antidiabetic, antifungal, anti-inflammatory, antiprotozoal, antituberculosis, and antiviral activities; affecting the immune and nervous systems, and other miscellaneous mechanisms of Action. *Mar. Drugs* **2013**, *11*, 2510–2573. [PubMed]
6. Ma, N.; Tang, H.F.; Qiu, F.; Lin, H.W.; Tian, X.R.; Yao, M.N. Polyhydroxysteroidal glycosides from the starfish *anthenea chinensis*. *J. Nat. Prod.* **2010**, *73*, 590–597. [CrossRef] [PubMed]
7. Ivanchina, N.V.; Kicha, A.A.; Stonik, V.A. Steroid glycosides from marine organisms. *Steroids* **2011**, *76*, 425–454. [CrossRef] [PubMed]
8. Kang, J.X.; Kang, Y.F.; Han, H. Three New Cytotoxic Polyhydroxysteroidal Glycosides from Starfish *Craspidaster hesperus*. *Mar. Drugs* **2016**, *14*, 189. [CrossRef] [PubMed]
9. Malyarenko, T.V.; Kharchenko, S.D.; Kicha, A.A.; Ivanchina, N.V.; Dmitrenok, P.S.; Chingizova, E.A.; Pislyagin, E.A.; Evtushenko, E.V.; Antokhina, T.I.; Van Minh, C.; et al. Anthenosides L–U, Steroidal Glycosides with Unusual Structural Features from the Starfish *Anthenea aspera*. *J. Nat. Prod.* **2016**, *79*, 3047–3056. [CrossRef] [PubMed]
10. Han, C.; Qi, J.; Ojika, M. Structure–activity relationships of novel neuritogenic steroid glycosides from the Okinawan starfish *Linckia laevigata*. *Bioorg. Med. Chem.* **2006**, *14*, 4458–4465. [CrossRef] [PubMed]
11. Qi, J.; Ojika, M.; Sakagami, Y. Linckosides A and B, two new neuritogenic steroid glycosides from the Okinawan starfish *Linckia laevigata*. *Bioorg. Med. Chem.* **2002**, *10*, 1961–1966. [CrossRef]
12. Kicha, A.A.; Ivanchina, N.V.; Kalinovsky, A.I.; Dmitrenok, P.S.; Sokolova, E.V.; Agafonova, I.G.; Morre, J.; Stonik, V.A. Four new steroid glycosides from the Vietnamese starfish *Linckia laevigata*. *Russ. Chem. Bull.* **2007**, *56*, 823–830. [CrossRef]
13. Guan, H.S.; Wang, S.G. *Chinese Marine Herbal*; Shanghai Science and Technology Press: Shanghai, China, 2009; Volume 3, pp. 608–610.

14. Ngoan, B.T.; Hanh, T.T.H.; Vien, L.T.; Diep, C.N.; Thao, N.P.; Thao, D.T.; Van Thanh, N.; Cuong, N.X.; Nam, N.H.; Thung, D.C.; et al. Asterosaponins and glycosylated polyhydroxysteroids from the starfish *Culcita novaeguineae* and their cytotoxic activities. *J. Asian Nat. Prod. Res.* **2015**, *17*, 1010–1017. [CrossRef] [PubMed]

15. Iorizzi, M.; Minale, L.; Riccio, R.; Higa, T.; Tanaka, J. Starfish saponins, Part 46.[1]Steroidal glycosides and polyhydroxysteroids from the starfish *Culcita novaeguineae*. *J. Nat. Prod.* **1991**, *54*, 1254–1264. [CrossRef] [PubMed]

16. Tang, H.F.; Yi, Y.H.; Li, L.; Sun, P.; Zhang, S.Q.; Zhao, Y.P. Asterosaponins from the starfish *Culcita novaeguineae* and their bioactivities. *Fitoterapia* **2006**, *77*, 28–34. [CrossRef] [PubMed]

17. Tang, H.F.; Cheng, G.; Wu, J.; Chen, X.L.; Zhang, S.Y.; Wen, A.D.; Lin, H.W. Cytotoxic asterosaponins capable of promoting polymerization of tubulin from the starfish *Culcita novaeguineae*. *J. Nat. Prod.* **2009**, *72*, 284–289. [CrossRef] [PubMed]

18. Tang, H.F.; Yi, Y.H.; Li, L.; Sun, P.; Zhang, S.Q.; Zhao, Y.P. Three New Asterosaponins from the Starfish *Culcita novaeguineae* and their Bioactivity. *Planta Med.* **2005**, *71*, 458–463. [CrossRef] [PubMed]

19. Cheng, G.; Zhang, X.; Tang, H.F.; Zhang, Y.; Zhang, X.H.; Cao, W.D.; Gao, D.K.; Wang, X.L.; Jin, B.Q. Asterosaponin 1, a cytostatic compound from the starfish *Culcita novaeguineae*, functions by inducing apoptosis in human glioblastoma U87MG cells. *J. Neurooncol.* **2006**, *79*, 235–241. [CrossRef] [PubMed]

20. Iorizzi, M.; de Riccardis, F.; Minale, L.; Riccio, R. Starfish saponins, 52. Chemical constituents from the starfish *echinaster brasiliensis*. *J. Nat. Prod.* **1993**, *56*, 2149–2162. [CrossRef] [PubMed]

21. Kicha, A.A.; Ivanchina, N.V.; Kalinovsky, A.I.; Dmitrenok, P.S.; Smirnov, A.V. Two New Steroid Glycosides from the Far East Starfish *Hippasteria kurilensis*. *Russ. J. Bioorg. Chem.* **2009**, *35*, 504–509. [CrossRef]

22. Zhu, D.; Yu, B. Total Synthesis of Linckosides A and B, the Representative Starfish Polyhydroxysteroid Glycosides with Neuritogenic Activities. *J. Am. Chem. Soc.* **2015**, *137*, 15098–15101. [CrossRef] [PubMed]

23. Malyarenko, T.V.; Kicha, A.A.; Kalinovsky, A.I.; Ivanchina, N.V.; Popov, R.S.; Pislyagin, E.A.; Menchinskaya, E.S.; Padmakumar, K.P.; Stonik, V.A. Four New Steroidal Glycosides, Protolinckiosides A–D, from the Starfish *Protoreaster lincki*. *Chem. Biodivers.* **2016**, 998–1007. [CrossRef] [PubMed]

24. Alley, M.C.; Scudiero, D.A.; Monks, A.; Hursey, M.L.; Czerwinski, M.J.; Fine, D.L.; Abbott, B.J.; Mayo, J.G.; Shoemaker, R.H.; Boyd, M.R. Feasibility of drug screening with panels of human tumor cell lines using a microculture tetrazolium assay. *Cancer Res.* **1988**, *48*, 589–601. [PubMed]

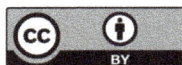

© 2018 by the authors. Licensee MDPI, Basel, Switzerland. This article is an open access article distributed under the terms and conditions of the Creative Commons Attribution (CC BY) license (http://creativecommons.org/licenses/by/4.0/).

marine drugs

MDPI

Communication

Angucycline Glycosides from Mangrove-Derived *Streptomyces diastaticus* subsp. SCSIO GJ056

Chun Gui [1,2], Yena Liu [3], Zhenbin Zhou [1,2], Shanwen Zhang [1,2], Yunfeng Hu [1], Yu-Cheng Gu [4], Hongbo Huang [1,*] and Jianhua Ju [1,2,*]

[1]   CAS Key Laboratory of Tropical Marine Bio-resources and Ecology, Guangdong Key Laboratory of Marine Materia Medica, RNAM Center for Marine Microbiology, South China Sea Institute of Oceanology, Chinese Academy of Sciences, 164 West Xingang Road, Guangzhou 510301, China; guichun1988@sina.com (C.G.); zzb1881396@163.com (Z.Z.); sherry920111@163.com (S.Z.); yunfeng.hu@scsio.ac.cn (Y.H.)

[2]   University of Chinese Academy of Sciences, 19 Yuquan Road, Beijing 110039, China

[3]   State Key Laboratory of Oncology in South China, Collaborative Innovation Center for Cancer Medicine, Sun Yat-Sen University Cancer Center, Guangzhou 510060, China; LIUYN@sysucc.org.cn

[4]   Syngenta Jealott's Hill International Research Centre, Bracknell, Berkshire RG42 6EY, UK; yucheng.gu@syngenta.com

*   Correspondence: huanghb@scsio.ac.cn (H.H.); jju@scsio.ac.cn (J.J.); Tel./Fax: +86-20-3406-6449 (H.H.); Tel./Fax: +86-20-8902-3028 (J.J.)

check for
updates

Received: 15 May 2018; Accepted: 25 May 2018; Published: 28 May 2018

Abstract: Nine new angucycline glycosides designated urdamycins N1–N9 (**1–9**), together with two known congener urdamycins A (**10**) and B (**11**), were obtained from a mangrove-derived *Streptomyces diastaticus* subsp. SCSIO GJ056. The structures of new compounds were elucidated on the basis of extensive spectroscopic data analysis. The absolute configurations of **6–9** were assigned by electronic circular dichroism calculation method. Urdamycins N7 (**7**) and N8 (**8**) represent the first naturally occurring (5*R*, 6*R*)-angucycline glycosides, which are diastereomers of urdamycins N6 (**6**) and N9 (**9**), respectively.

Keywords: mangrove-derived *Streptomyces*; angucycline; urdamycin

1. Introduction

The angucycline group members are type II polyketide derived metabolites obtained exclusively from actinomycetes [1–3]. Angucycline compounds exhibited various bioactivities, including antitumor, cytostatic, enzyme inhibition, antibacterial, antiviral, and inhibition of platelet aggregation function [4–7].

During the course of searching for novel anti-infective and antitumor agents from the marine environment, we found that the chemical profile of strain SCSIO GJ056 cultivated in AM2 medium revealed an array of secondary metabolites showing typical UV/VIS absorptions, which were similar to those of angucyclines/anthracyclines. Subsequent solvent extraction and isolation procedures led to the purification and structure elucidation of nine new angucycline glycosides, named urdamycins N1–N9 (**1–9**), together with two known urdamycins A (**10**) and B (**11**). Urdamycins N7 (**7**) and N8 (**8**) represent the first naturally occurring (5*R*, 6*R*)-angucycline glycosides. Herein, we report the fermentation, isolation, and structure elucidation of these compounds.

2. Results and Discussion

The strain SCSIO GJ056 was fermented (15 L) and the fermentation broth was extracted with butanone. The extract was subjected to repetitive silica gel column chromatography, followed by preparative HPLC purification to yield compounds **1–11** (Figure 1). The known urdamycins A (**10**)

and B (**11**) were identified by comparisons of MS, ^{1}H, and ^{13}C NMR spectroscopic data with those previously reported [8].

Compound **1** was obtained as a yellowish powder. Its molecular formula was determined to be $C_{38}H_{46}O_{14}$ on the basis of HRESIMS peak at m/z 725.2834 $[M - H]^-$, indicating 16 degrees of unsaturation. The ^{13}C and DEPT NMR spectra of **1** displayed 38 carbon resonances, including five methyls, six methylenes, 14 methines, and 13 nonprotonated carbons. The ^{1}H NMR spectrum showed one chelated hydroxy group signal at δ_H 12.55 (1H, br s, 8-OH), a pair of *ortho*-coupled aromatic proton signals at δ_H 7.81 (d, 7.8 Hz, H-10) and 7.59 (d, 7.8 Hz, H-11), and a singlet aromatic proton signal at δ_H 7.65 (s, H-6). The HMBC correlations (Figure 2) from H-6 to C-4a, C-5, C-7, and C-12a, from H-11 to C-7a, C-9, and C-12, and from H-10 to C-8, C-9, and C-11a confirmed the existence of the anthraquinone skeleton (rings B, C, and D). Further HMBC correlations of H_2-2/C-1, C-12b, C-4; H_2-4/C-2, C-4a, C-12b; and H_3-13/C-2, C-3, C-4 allowed the assignment of the angular ring (ring A) with a methyl group (CH$_3$-13) substitution at C-3. A methoxy group (OCH$_3$-14) attached at C-5 in ring B was deduced by the HMBC correlation of H_3-14/C-5. A hydroxy group linked at C-3 in ring A was inferred based on the ^{13}C NMR chemical shift at δ_C 71.8. The absolute configuration of C-3 was tentatively deduced to be *R*, which was identical with that of urdamycinone B and N05WA963D in light of the similar ^{13}C NMR resonances of C-3 and CH$_3$-13, as well as the similar biosynthetic pathway [8,9].

In addition, three anomeric methine signals at δ_H 4.82 and δ_C 71.1 (CH-1'), δ_H 4.96 and δ_C 97.4 (CH-1''), and δ_H 4.45 and δ_C 101.5 (CH-1'''), together with three doublet methyl signals at δ_H 1.37 (CH$_3$-6'), δ_H 1.16 (CH$_3$-6''), and δ_H 1.23 (CH$_3$-6''') revealed the presence of a trisaccharide moiety consisting of three deoxy sugars in **1**. The ^{1}H-^{1}H COSY spectrum allowed the full assignment of the sugar moieties from CH-1' to CH$_3$-6', from CH-1'' to CH$_3$-6'', and from CH-1''' to CH$_3$-6'''. The HMBC correlations of H-3'/C-1'' and H-4''/C-1''' confirmed the existence of a β-olivose-(1→4)-α-rhodinose-(1→3)-β-olivosyl unit. This trisaccharide was connected with the aglycone at C-9 based on the HMBC correlations of H-1'/C-9 and H-9/C-1'. The relative configuration of the trisaccharide moiety was deduced by ^{1}H-^{1}H coupling constants (Table 1) and NOE experiment (Figure 3). Detailed comparisons showed that the ^{1}H and ^{13}C NMR spectroscopic data of the sugar units were almost identical with those in urdamycin A [10,11]. Thus, the structure of **1** was determined and named urdamycin N1.

Compound **2**, isolated as a dark red powder, has the molecular formula of $C_{38}H_{44}O_{13}$ on the basis of HRESIMS peak at m/z 707.2708 $[M - H]^-$, showing 17 degrees of unsaturation and an 18 amu less than that of compound **1**. An obvious red shift on the UV-VIS spectrum of **2** relative to that of **1** indicated an additional conjugated system in **2**. The ^{13}C and DEPT NMR data of **2** displayed 38 carbon signals attributable to five methyls, four methylenes, 16 methines, and 13 nonprotonated carbons. The ^{1}H and HSQC NMR spectra suggested three singlet olefnic proton signals at δ_H 7.58 (H-4), δ_H 7.54 (H-6), and δ_H 6.99 (H-2), and a pair of *ortho*-coupled aromatic proton signals at δ_H 7.82 (d, 7.6 Hz, H-10) and 7.68 (d, 7.6 Hz, H-11). Comparing the ^{1}H and ^{13}C NMR spectroscopic data to those of **1** revealed that **2** possessed a similar core structure with that of **1**. The difference between **2** and **1** was the aromatization of ring A in **2**, which supported by the HMBC correlations from CH$_3$-13 to C-2, C-3, and C-4, from H-2 to C-1, C-4, and C-12b, and from H-4 to C-2, C-4a, and C-12b. Compound **2** possessed the same trisaccharide moiety with **1** according to similar ^{1}H and ^{13}C NMR signals in aliphatic area. The structure of **2** was elucidated as shown in Figure 1 by detailed analysis of 2D NMR spectra data.

Compound **3**, a dark green powder, was isolated as minor component from the extract. Its molecular formula of $C_{26}H_{24}O_8$ was determined by the HRESIMS peak at m/z 463.1409 $[M - H]^-$, indicating 15 degrees of unsaturation. Comprehensive analysis of its ^{1}H and ^{13}C NMR spectroscopic data revealed that **3** had the same aglycone with that of **2**. However, a set of ^{1}H and ^{13}C resonances ascribed to β-olivose-(1→4)-α-rhodinosyl moiety disappeared, indicating the absence of two sugar units in **3**. This is consistent with the HRESIMS data, which showing a $C_{12}H_{20}O_5$ fragment loss relative to **2**. Therefore, the structure of **3** was established and named urdamycin N3.

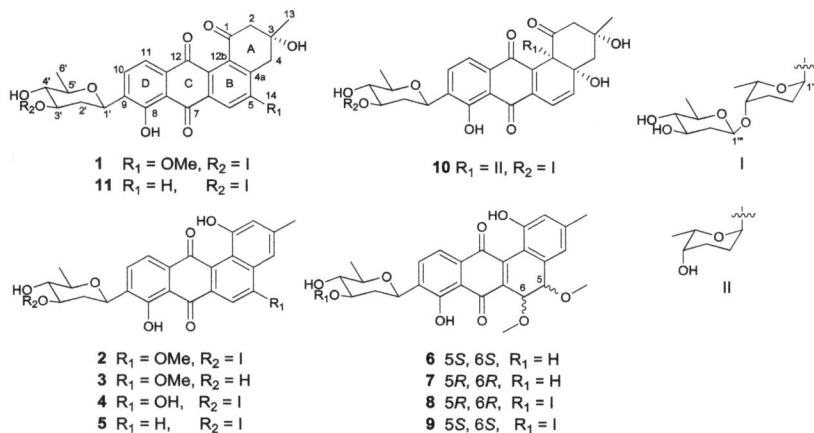

Figure 1. Structures of compounds **1–11**.

Table 1. The ^{1}H and ^{13}C NMR data of compounds **1–3** (δ in ppm, J in Hz).

Position	**1** [a] δ_C	δ_H	**2** [b] δ_C	δ_H	**3** [c] δ_C	δ_H
1	198.4		155.3		155.2	
2	53.2	2.90, dd (14, 1.1); 3.0, m	118.7	6.99, s	118.8	6.98, s
3	71.8		140.8		140.9	
4	37.5	3.18, m; 2.80, d (18.1)	113.0	7.58, s	113.2	7.58, m
4a	137.9		126.0		126.0	
5	160.9		160.3		160.5	
6	108.2	7.65, s	99.8	7.54, s	100.0	7.54, s
6a	135.1		135.8		136.1	
7	187.9		187.5		187.6	
7a	114.8		113.9		114.1	
8	158.0		156.8		157.0	
9	136.6		136.8		137.3	
10	133.9	7.81, d (7.8)	133.4	7.82, d (7.6)	133.3	7.80, m
11	119.5	7.59, d (7.8)	119.9	7.68, d (7.6)	120.0	7.67, m
11a	133.8		133.7		133.8	
12	182.3		185.6		186.0	
12a	128.4		129.8		129.9	
12b	137.4		120.4		120.5	
13	30.1	1.42, s	21.2	2.42, s	21.2	2.41, s
14	56.5	3.99, s	56.6	4.14, s	56.6	4.13, s
1′	71.1	4.82, d (10.6)	70.4	4.8, d (13.7)	70.8	4.78, d (10.9)
2′	37.6	1.41, m	39.7	1.35, m	40.0	1.31, dd (11.4)
		2.42, dd (12.3, 4.2)		2.01, m		2.28, d (10.2)
3′	81.6	3.67, ddd (11.4, 8.4, 5.1)	74.6	3.69, ddd (11.1, 8.9, 4.9)	71.7	3.55, t (11.8)
4′	76.0	3.13, m	74.5	3.06, dd (8.9, 5.4)	77.1	2.90, t (8.8)
5′	76.1	3.45, m	76.2	3.47, q (6.0)	76.3	3.38, m
6′	18.4	1.37, d (6.1)	18.5	1.30, d (6.1)	18.5	1.28, d (6.1)
1″	97.4	4.96, s	91.9	4.90, d (2.3)		
2″	25.1	1.47, m	24.1	1.29, m		
		2.06, m		1.83, m		
3″	24.5	1.9, m	24.1	1.76, m; 1.95, m		
4″	76.2	3.49, m	75.4	3.44, m		
5″	67.5	4.09, m	65.3	4.15, m		
6″	16.9	1.16, d (6.5)	17.0	1.05, d (6.5)		
1‴	101.5	4.45, dd (9.7, 1.5)	101.0	4.48, dd (9.7, 1.6)		
2‴	38.9	2.19, ddd (12.5, 4.8, 1.5)	36.0	1.24, m		
		1.60, td (12.1, 10.0)		2.47, m		
3‴	71.4	3.45, m	70.3	3.33, m		
4‴	77.0	2.95, t (8.9)	76.8	2.72, m		
5‴	71.7	3.16, m	71.6	3.11, dq (9.0, 6.2)		
6‴	17.7	1.23, d (6.2)	18.2	1.14, d (6.2)		

[a] Recorded in CDCl$_3$-CD$_3$OD (9:1); [b] Recorded in DMSO; [c] Recorded in DMSO-CD$_3$OD (9:1).

Compound **4** was obtained as a dark green powder. Its molecular formula was determined to be $C_{37}H_{42}O_{13}$ by the HRESIMS peak at *m/z* 693.2554 [M − H]⁻. The ¹H and ¹³C NMR data of **4** were closely similar to those of **2**, except that the methoxy signals at δ_H 4.14, δ_C 56.6 in **2** were absent. The ¹³C NMR signal of C-5 shifted from δ_C 160.3 in **2** to δ_C 163.6 in **4**, indicating the OMe-5 in **2** was replaced by OH-5 in **4**. Compound **4** was named urdamycin N4.

Compound **5** was obtained as a red powder. The molecular formula of $C_{37}H_{42}O_{12}$, as determined by HRESIMS, which was one oxygen atom less than that of **4**. The ¹H and ¹³C NMR spectroscopic data were similar with those of **4**, except that two pairs of *ortho*-coupled aromatic signals were observed. Additionally, the ¹³C NMR signal at δ_C 163.6 for the oxygen-bearing aromatic C-5 in **4** was replaced by an aromatic methine signal at δ_C 135.4. Thus, the structure of **5** was determined as 5-demethoxy-urdamycin N2, designated as urdamycin N5.

The molecular formulae of compounds **6** and **7** were determined both to be $C_{27}H_{28}O_9$ by HRESIMS, indicating 14 degrees of unsaturation. The ¹H and ¹³C NMR spectroscopic data of **6** were similar with those of **3**, except that two aromatic carbon signals at δ_C 160.5 (C-5) and 100.0 (C-6) in **3** were replaced by two oxygen-bearing methine carbon signals at δ_C 78.1 (C-5) and 70.2 (C-6). Furthermore, two methoxys were attached at C-5 and C-6 based on the HMBC correlations of H_3-14/C-5 and H_3-15/C-6, respectively. Small coupling constants (2.8 Hz) between H-5 and H-6 revealed a *trans* configuration of H-5 and H-6, indicating an (5R, 6R) or (5S, 6S) configuration of **6**. To determine the absolute configurations of **6**, comparisons of the experimental and ECD spectra using a time-dependent density functional theory (TDDFT) were employed. Comparison of the experimental and calculated CD spectra (Figure 4) established the absolute configuration as (5S, 6S) for **6**, which were the same as those of PMO70747, PD116740, and TAN-1085 [12–17]. Compound **7** possessed the same planar structure with that of **6**, as deduced by the COSY and HMBC spectra (Figure 2). However, the experimental and calculated CD spectra of **7** showed cotton effects totally opposite to those of **6**, respectively, inferring the (5R, 6R) configuration for **7** (Figure 4). Compounds **6** and **7** were named urdamycins N6 and N7, respectively.

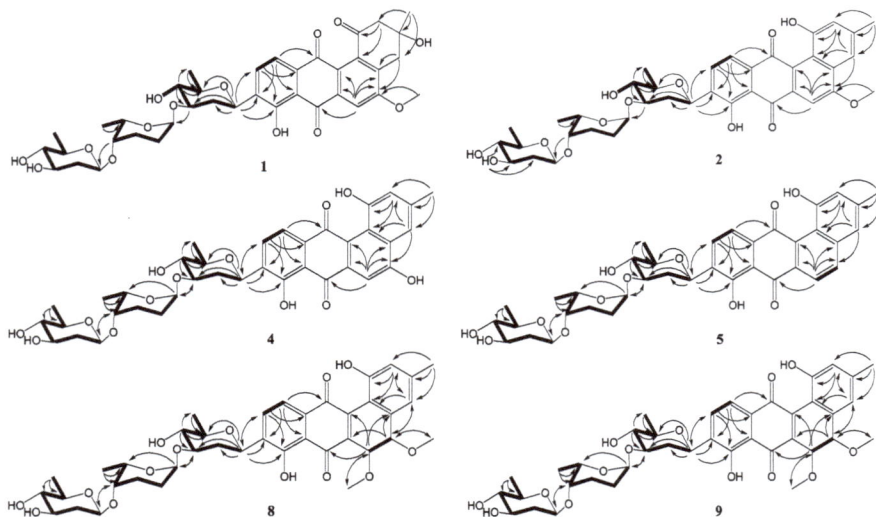

Figure 2. *Cont.*

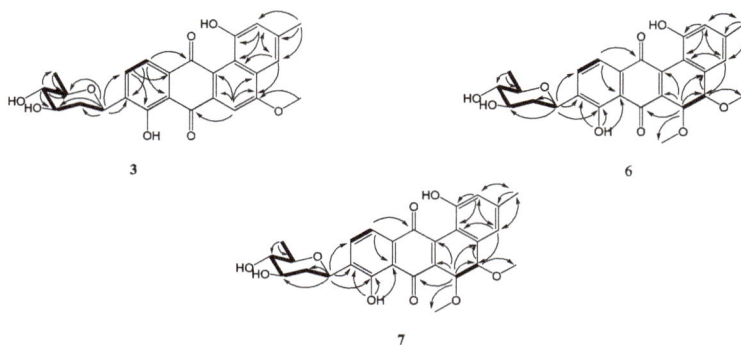

Figure 2. COSY (**bold**) and selected HMBC (**arrow**) correlations for **1–9**.

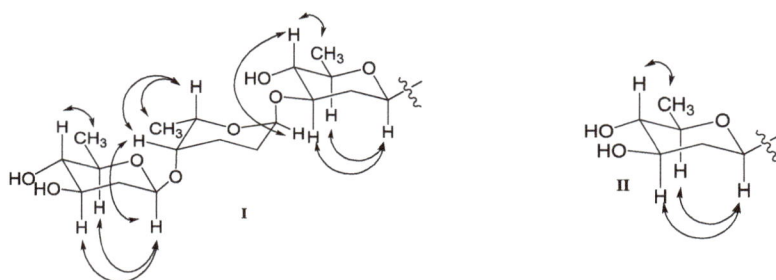

Figure 3. Key NOESY correlations of β-olivose-(1→4)-α-rhodinose-(1→3)-β-olivose in **1**, **2**, **4**, **5**, **8**, and **9** (**I**), and β-olivose in **3**, **6** and **7** (**II**).

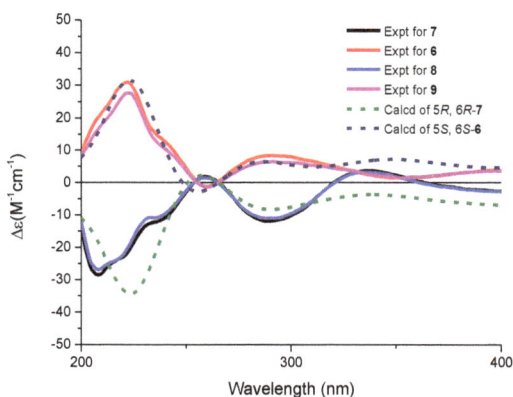

Figure 4. Experimental and calculated ECD spectra of **6–9** in methanol.

Compounds **8** and **9** were isolated as red powder, both had the same molecular formula of $C_{39}H_{48}O_{14}$ as determined by HRESIMS. The ^1H and ^{13}C NMR spectroscopic data of **8** and **9** resembled those of **2**, except that two aromatic carbon signals at δ_C 160.3 (C-5) and 99.8 (C-6) in **2** were replaced by two oxygen-bearing methine carbon signals at δ_C 80.0 (C-5) and 67.4 (C-6) in **8**, and at δ_C 78.1 (C-5) and 70.2 (C-6) in **9**. Two methoxys were attached at C-5 and C-6 in **8** and **9** based on the HMBC correlations of H$_3$-14/C-5 and H$_3$-15/C-6, respectively. Small coupling constants of H5/H6 revealed the both *trans* configurations in compounds **8** and **9**. The absolute configurations were determined to be (5*R*, 6*R*) for **8** and (5*S*, 6*S*) for **9** by comparing their CD curve to those of **7** and **6**, respectively (Figure 4). Finally, compounds **8** and **9** were elucidated and named urdamycin N8 and urdamycin N9, respectively. Compounds **7** and **8** represent the first naturally occurring (5*R*, 6*R*)-angucycline metabolite.

3. Experimental Section

3.1. General Experimental Procedures

Column chromatography (CC) was performed using silica gel (100–200 mesh; Jiangpeng Silica gel development, Inc., Shandong, China). Thin layer chromatography (TLC) was conducted with precoated glass plates (0.1–0.2 mm; silica gel GF$_{254}$, 10–40 nm, Jiangpeng, China). HPLC analyses were performed with a 1260 infinity system (Agilent, Santa Clara, CA, USA) using a Phenomenex Prodigy ODS (2) column (150 × 4.6 mm, 5 μm; USA). Semi-preparative HPLC were performed with a Primaide 1110 solvent delivery module equipped with a 1430 photodiode array detector (Hitachi, Tokyo, Japan), using a YMC-Pack ODS-A column (250 mm × 10 mm, 5 μm; YMC Co., Ltd., Kyoto, Japan). UV spectra were recorded on a U-2910 spectrometer (Shimadzu, Kyoto, Japan); IR spectra were obtained on an IRAffinity-1 spectrophotometer (Shimadzu, Kyoto, Japan). CD spectra were measured on a Chirascan circular dichroism spectrometer (Applied Photophysics, Leatherhead, UK). High-resolution mass spectral data were obtained on a MaXis Q-TOF mass spectrometer (Bruker, Billerica, MA, USA). Optical rotations were recorded with an MCP-500 polarimeter (Anton Paar, Graz, Austria). NMR spectra were recorded on a Bruker Avance 500 or a Bruker Avance 700 spectrometer (Bruker, Billerica, MA, USA). Carbon signals and the residual proton signals of DMSO-d_6 (δ_C 39.52 and δ_H 2.50), CD$_3$OD (δ_C 49.0 and δ_H 4.87), and CDCl$_3$ (δ_C 77.16 and δ_H 7.26) were used for calibration. Coupling constants (*J*) are given in Hz.

3.2. Bacterial Materials

Strain SCSIO GJ056 was isolated from a mangrove-derived sediment sample collected in Yalong bay, China. It was identified as *Streptomyces diastaticus* subsp. on the basis of morphological characteristics and 16S rRNA sequence analysis by comparisons with other sequences in the GenBank database. The DNA sequence has been deposited in GenBank (accession no. MH368281). The strain was preserved at the RNAM Center for Marine Microbiology, South China Sea Institute of Oceanology, Chinese Academy of Sciences and also at the China General Microbiological Culture Collection Center (CGMCC, Beijing, China), CGMCC No. 13648.

3.3. Fermentation, Extraction, and Isolation of the Compounds

A portion of spore and mycelium mixture of SCSIO GJ056 grown on ISP4 medium agar plates were inoculated into 50 mL modified AM2 medium (0.5% soybean flour, 0.5% soluble starch, 0.2% yeast extract, 0.2% peptone, 2.0% glucose, 0.05% KH$_2$PO$_4$, 0.05% MgSO$_4$·7H$_2$O, 0.4% NaCl, 0.2% CaCO$_3$, 3.0% sea salt (Guangdong Province Salt Industry Group, Guangzhou, China), pH 7.2 before sterilization) in 250 mL Erlenmeyer flasks, and were incubated at 28 °C on a rotary shaker at 200 rpm for 1.5 days as the seed culture. Then the 50 mL of culture solution was transferred into a 1 L Erlenmeyer flask and then incubated at 28 °C, 200 rpm for seven days. On the seventh day, the entire culture broth (15 L) was harvested and centrifuged to yield the mycelial cake and liquid broth. The liquid broth was extracted with butanone for three times, and the mycelial cake was extracted using 1 L of acetone for three times. The combined organic layers were dried under vacuum to yield a residue. The residue was subjected to silica gel CC using gradient elution with CHCl$_3$ and MeOH mixtures (100:0, 99:1, 97:3, 95:5, 90:10, 80:20, and 50:50, *v*/*v*) to give seven fractions (Fr.A1–Fr.A7). Fr.A1 and Fr.A2 were combined after HPLC analysis and purified by silica gel CC eluting with petroleum ether and EtOAc mixtures (100:0, 90:10, 80:20, 70:30, 60:40, 40:60, 20:80, 0:100, *v*/*v*) to give eight fractions (Fr.B1–Fr.B8). Fr.B4 was subjected to Sephadex LH-20 CC eluted with CHCl₃/MeOH (1:1) to obtain **1** (6 mg). Fr.B5 and Fr.B6 were combined and further purified by semi-preparative HPLC with an ODS column to afford **10** (220 mg) at t_R 26 min and **11** (70 mg) at t_R 30 min. Fractions B1 and B2 were combined and subjected to preparative TLC using CHCl₃/MeOH (92:8) to obtain six sub-fractions (Fr.C1–Fr.C6). Fr.C1 was purified by preparative HPLC with an ODS column eluted with CH₃CN/H₂O (30:70 to 100:0 over 28 min, then hold 7 min, 9 mL/min) to afford **7** (0.6 mg) and **6** (0.6 mg) at t_R 13.5 min, 14.5 min, respectively. Fr.C2 was purified by preparative HPLC with an ODS column eluted with CH₃CN/H₂O (30:70 to 100:0 over 28 min, then hold 7 min, 9 mL/min) to afford **8** (0.7 mg), **9** (0.6 mg), and **5** (0.6 mg) at t_R 15.5 min, 16.5 min, and 26 min, respectively. Fr.C3 was purified by preparative HPLC with an ODS column eluted with CH₃CN/H₂O (30:70 to 100:0 over 28 min, then hold 7 min, 9 mL/min) to afford **2** (8 mg) and **3** (7 mg) at t_R 32 min, 32.5 min, respectively. Fr.C6 was purified by preparative HPLC eluted with CH₃CN/H₂O (30:70 to 100:0 over 28 min, then held for 7 min, 9 mL/min) to afford **4** (8 mg) at t_R 25 min.

3.4. Spectral Data

Urdamycin N1 (**1**). Dark red powder; $[\alpha]_D^{20}$ + 24 (*c* 0.05, CDCl₃); UV (CDCl₃) λ_{max} (log *ε*) 240 (4.06), 285 (4.27), 411 (3.69); IR ν_{max} 3391, 2932, 1705, 1667, 1632, 1582, 1492, 1364, 1279, 1061, 1011, 754 cm⁻¹; ¹H NMR (500 MHz, CDCl₃/CD₃OD) and ¹³C NMR (125 MHz, CDCl₃/CD₃OD) data, Table 1; (-)-HR-ESI-MS *m/z* 725.2834 ([M − H]⁻, calcd for C₃₈H₄₅O₁₄, 725.2815).

Urdamycin N2 (**2**). Dark green powder; $[\alpha]_D^{20}$ + 235 (*c* 0.06, CDCl₃); UV (CDCl₃) λ_{max} (log *ε*) 241 (4.62), 263 (4.55), 324 (4.71), 434 (4.17), IR ν_{max} 3379, 2926, 1631, 1504, 1435, 1300, 1061, 1011, 758 cm⁻¹; ¹H NMR (700 MHz, DMSO-d_6) and ¹³C NMR (176 MHz, DMSO-d_6) data, Table 1; (-)-HR-ESI-MS *m/z* 707.2708 ([M − H]⁻, calcd for C₃₈H₄₃O₁₃, 707.2709).

Urdamycin N3 (**3**). Dark green powder; $[\alpha]_D^{20}$ − 430 (*c* 0.04, CDCl₃); UV (CDCl₃) λ_{max} (log *ε*) 240 (4.48), 263 (4.39), 324 (4.55), 433 (4.02), IR ν_{max} 3360, 2920, 1630, 1506, 1435, 1229, 1090, 1057, 772 cm⁻¹; ¹H NMR (700 MHz, DMSO-d_6/CD₃OD) and ¹³C NMR (176 MHz, DMSO-d_6/CD₃OD) data, Table 1; (-)-HR-ESI-MS *m/z* 463.1409 ([M − H]⁻, calcd for C₂₆H₂₃O₈, 463.1398).

Urdamycin N4 (**4**). Dark green powder; $[\alpha]_D^{20}$ + 125 (*c* 0.06, CDCl₃); UV (CDCl₃) λ_{max} (log *ε*) 207 (3.92), 240 (4.16), 263 (4.05), 323 (4.18), 434 (3.67), IR ν_{max} 3397, 2930, 1628, 1437, 1298, 1096, 1061, 1013, 852, 786 cm⁻¹; ¹H NMR (500 MHz, DMSO-d_6/CD₃OD) and ¹³C NMR (125MHz, DMSO-d_6/CD₃OD) data, Table 2; (-)-HR-ESI-MS *m/z* 693.2554 ([M − H]⁻, calcd for C₃₇H₄₁O₁₃, 693.2553).

Urdamycin N5 (**5**). Dark green powder; $[\alpha]_D^{20}$ + 250 (*c* 0.01, CDCl₃); UV (CDCl₃) λ_{max} (log *ε*) 240 (4.98), 322 (4.85), 437 (4.46), IR ν_{max} 3392, 2924, 1626, 1435, 1267, 1061, 1013, 773 cm⁻¹; ¹H NMR (700 MHz, DMSO-d_6/CD₃OD) and ¹³C NMR (176 MHz, DMSO-d_6/CD₃OD) data, Table 2; (-)-HR-ESI-MS *m/z* 677.2606 ([M − H]⁻, calcd for C₃₇H₄₁O₁₂, 677.2604).

Urdamycin N6 (**6**). Red powder; $[\alpha]_D^{20}$ + 325 (*c* 0.06, CDCl₃); UV (CDCl₃) λ_{max} (log *ε*) 219 (4.57), 257 (4.19), 291 (4.04), 325 (3.67), 454 (3.90), IR ν_{max} 3379, 2928, 1614, 1435, 1246, 1086, 752 cm⁻¹; ¹H NMR (700 MHz, CDCl₃) and ¹³C NMR (176 MHz, CDCl₃) data, Table 2; (-)-HR-ESI-MS *m/z* 495.1667 ([M − H]⁻, calcd for C₂₇H₂₇O₉, 495.1661).

Urdamycin N7 (**7**). Red powder; $[\alpha]_D^{20}$ + 130 (*c* 0.06, CDCl₃); UV (CDCl₃) λ_{max} (log *ε*) 218 (4.50), 259 (4.13), 284 (4.03), 325 (3.64), 451 (3.85), IR ν_{max} 3360, 2918, 1612, 1435, 1238, 1086, 1060, 756 cm⁻¹; ¹H NMR (700 MHz, CDCl₃) and ¹³C NMR (176 MHz, CDCl₃) data, Table 3; (-)-HR-ESI-MS *m/z* 495.1675 ([M − H]⁻, calcd for C₂₇H₂₇O₉, 495.1661).

Urdamycin N8 (**8**). Red powder; $[\alpha]_D^{20}$ + 75 (*c* 0.04, CDCl₃); UV (CDCl₃) λ_{max} (log *ε*) 240 (4.39), 266 (4.27), 465 (3.91), IR ν_{max} 3379, 2932, 1612, 1435, 1238, 1057, 1009, 748 cm⁻¹; ¹H NMR (700 MHz, CDCl₃) and ¹³C NMR (176 MHz, CDCl₃) data, Table 3; (-)-HR-ESI-MS *m/z* 739.2984 ([M − H]⁻, calcd for C₃₉H₄₇O₁₄, 739.2971).

Urdamycin N9 (**9**). Red powder; $[\alpha]_D^{20}$ + 233 (*c* 0.04, CDCl$_3$); UV (CDCl$_3$) λ_{max} (log ε) 240 (4.31), 265 (4.28), 296 (4.08), 472 (3.94), IR ν_{max} 3395, 2932, 1614, 1435, 1369, 1248, 1088, 1059, 1010.7, 756 cm^{-1}; ^{1}H NMR (700 MHz, CDCl$_3$) and ^{13}C NMR (176 MHz, CDCl$_3$) data, Table 3; (-)-HR-ESI-MS *m/z* 739.2974 ([M − H]$^-$, calcd for C$_{39}$H$_{47}$O$_{14}$, 739.2971).

Table 2. The ^{1}H and ^{13}C NMR data of compounds **4–6** (δ in ppm, *J* in Hz).

Position	4 [a]		5 [a]		6 [b]	
	δ_C	δ_H	δ_C	δ_H	δ_C	δ_H
1	155.4		155.0		157.1	
2	119.6	6.97, m	117.3	7.0, s	126.0	6.73, s
3	139.7		141.5		144.0	
4	114.4	7.63, m	119.5	7.37, s	123.0	6.89, s
4a	121.7		138.6		139.2	
5	163.6		135.4	8.22, d (8.5)	78.1	4.23, d (2.8)
6	105.6	7.54, s	121.5	8.18, d (8.5)	70.2	4.91, d (2.8)
6a	136.5		133.8		141.6	
7	188.7		188.0		189.1	
7a	114.2		114.4		113.7	
8	156.8		156.7		157.6	
9	137.5		136.8		135.9	
10	133.6	7.8, m	133.5	7.86, d (7.8)	133.0	7.88, d (7.9)
11	120.2	7.71, m	118.7	7.67, d (7.8)	121.4	7.80, d (7.9)
11a	134.3		134.5		131.5	
12	184.6		186.8		189.0	
12a	130.4		134.4		143.0	
12b	122.1		119.9		112.9	
13	21.1	2.40, s	21.1	2.45, s	21.4	2.34, s
14					58.5	3.45, s
15					56.7	3.26, s
1'	70.6	4.78, dd (11.1, 3.0)	70.5	4.83, d (11.4)	71.4	4.92, d (11.0)
2'	40.0	1.36, dd (22.4, 11.2) 2.02, dd (12.2, 5.0)	39.5	1.35, td (11.9, 9.9) 2.01, ddd (12.2, 5.0, 1.5)	39.5	1.46, dd (23.8, 11.7) 2.54, dd (12.1, 3.9)
3'	74.9	3.69, ddd (11.2, 9.0, 4.9)	74.9	3.70, ddd (11.1, 8.9, 4.8)	73.2	3.85, m
4'	74.8	3.05, t (9.0)	74.7	3.06, t (8.9)	78.2	3.21, t (8.9)
5'	76.4	3.48, m	76.3	3.48, overlapped	76.0	3.53, dt (15.1, 6.1)
6'	18.6	1.29, d (6.0)	18.5	1.30, d (6.1)	18.2	1.42, d (6.1)
1''	92.4	4.89, m	92.2	4.89, d (2.7)		
2''	24.3	1.27, m 1.84, m	24.2	1.26, m 1.83, m		
3''	24.3	1.77, m; 1.96, m	24.2	1.77, m; 1.95, m		
4''	75.7	3.44, m	75.6	3.44, overlapped		
5''	65.6	4.15, q (6.5)	65.5	4.15, q (6.4)		
6''	17.1	1.05, d (6.5)	17.0	1.04, d (6.4)		
1'''	101.3	4.47, d (9.6)	101.2	4.47, d (9.7)		
2'''	36.3	1.23, m; 2.46, m	36.2	1.24, m; 2.47, m		
3'''	70.6	3.32, m	70.5	3.33, ddd (11.8, 8.7, 5.1)		
4'''	77.0	2.72, t (8.8)	76.9	2.72, t (8.7)		
5'''	71.8	3.1, m	71.7	3.1, m		
6'''	18.3	1.14, d (6.2)	18.2	1.14, d (6.1)		

[a] Recorded in DMSO-CD$_3$OD (9:1); [b] Recorded in CDCl$_3$.

Table 3. ^{1}H and ^{13}C-NMR data of compounds **7–9** in CDCl$_3$ (δ in ppm, *J* in Hz).

Position	7		8		9	
	δ_C	δ_H	δ_C	δ_H	δ_C	δ_H
1	156.5		156.5		157.1	
2	120.6	6.81, s	120.6	6.81, s	126.0	6.73, s
3	145.4		145.4		144.0	
4	119.0	7.17, s	119.0	7.16, s	123.0	6.89, s
4a	138.8		138.8		139.5	
5	80.0	4.27, d (2.2)	80.0	4.27, d (2.5)	78.1	4.23, d (2.9)
6	67.4	4.99, d (3.1)	67.4	4.99, d (3.1)	70.2	4.91, d (2.9)
6a	140.2		140.2		141.6	
7	189.0		188.9		189.1	

Table 3. *Cont.*

Position	7		8		9	
	δ_C	δ_H	δ_C	δ_H	δ_C	δ_H
7a	113.6		113.5		113.7	
8	157.6		157.7		157.7	
9	139.4		139.7		135.9	
10	133.2	7.90, d (7.9)	133.2	7.89, d (7.9)	133.0	7.87, d (7.8)
11	121.5	7.80, d (7.9)	121.5	7.78, d (7.9)	121.4	7.79, d (7.8)
11a	131.3		131.3		131.4	
12	188.7		188.8		189.0	
12a	143.1		143.2		143.0	
12b	112.5		112.5		112.9	
13	21.9	2.36, s	21.9	2.36, s	21.4	2.34, s
14	58.2	3.69, s	58.2	3.69, s	58.5	3.44, s
15	59.3	3.42, s	59.3	3.41, s	56.7	3.26, s
1′	71.4	4.94, d (11.0)	71.3	4.89, dd (9.5, 1.1)	71.4	4.87, d (10.4)
2′	39.4	1.46, d (12.1)	37.7	1.48, d (11.7)	37.7	1.47, m
		2.53, dd (12.7, 3.5)		2.48, m		2.50, ddd (13.0, 4.9, 1.7)
3′	73.2	3.87, m	82.4	3.72, ddd (11.6, 8.3, 5.1)	82.5	3.71, ddd (11.5, 8.3, 5.1)
4′	78.2	3.22, t (8.9)	76.3	3.18, t (8.7)	76.3	3.18, t (8.7)
5′	76.1	3.54, dt (15.1, 6.0)	76.3	3.51, td (12.2, 6.1)	76.3	3.51, q (6.0)
6′	18.2	1.43, d (6.1)	18.6	1.44, d (6.0)	18.6	1.44, d (6.0)
1″			97.9	5.04, s	98.0	5.03, s
2″			25.3	1.55, d (13.9)	25.4	1.54, d (13.8)
				2.15, m		2.13, m
3″			24.7	1.95, m	24.7	1.96, m
				2.13, m		2.13, m
4″			76.1	3.55, m	76.1	3.55, m
5″			67.7	4.13, dd (12.9, 6.4)	67.7	4.13, q (6.0)
6″			17.2	1.24, d (6.5)	17.1	1.23, d (6.5)
1‴			101.5	4.55, dd (9.5, 1.1)	101.5	4.52, dd (9.6, 1.6)
2‴			39.3	1.71, dd (21.9, 12.1)	39.3	1.71, td (12.1, 9.9)
				2.30, dd (12.5, 5.0)		2.29, ddd (12.4, 4.9, 1.5)
3‴			71.7	3.59, m	71.7	3.59, m
4‴			77.7	3.11, t (8.9)	77.7	3.11, t (8.9)
5‴			72.0	3.26, dq (9.1, 6.1)	72.0	3.24, m
6‴			17.9	1.31, d (6.1)	17.9	1.31, d (6.2)

3.5. Electronic Circular Dichroism (ECD) Calculation

Monte Carlo conformational searches were carried out by means of the Spartan's 10 software (Wavefunction, Inc., Irvine, CA, USA) using Merck Molecular Force Field (MMFF). The conformers with Boltzmann-population of over 5% were chosen for electronic circular dichroism (ECD) calculations, and then the conformers were initially optimized at B3LYP/6-31+g (d, p) level in methanol using the conductor-like polarizable continuum model (CPCM). The theoretical calculation of ECD was conducted in methanol using Time-dependent Density functional theory (TD-DFT) at the B3LYP/6-311+g (d, p) level for all conformers of compounds **6** and **7**. Rotatory strengths for a total of 10 excited states were calculated. ECD spectra were generated using the program SpecDis 1.6 (University of Würzburg, Würzburg, Germany) and GraphPad Prism 5 (University of California San Diego, San Diego, CA, USA) from dipole-length rotational strengths by applying Gaussian band shapes with sigma = 0.3 eV.

4. Conclusions

The early report of urdamycin derivatives, urdamycins A–F, were isolated from *Streptomyces fradiae* Tu 2717 by Drautz in 1986. Since then, many urdamycin congeners were discovered. Structurally, urdamycins have different aglycone parts, whereas the sugar moieties are always the same [10]. Most of them were decorated with a trisaccharide chain composed of β-olivose-(1→4)-α-rhodinose-(1→3)-β-olivose via a C-C linkage. Diverse biological activities of these angucycline antibiotics were evaluated, and the most important were their cytotoxicities against the tumor cell lines. At the same time, this potent cytotoxicity also limited their use in the clinic. In this study, nine new angucycline glycosides, urdamycin N1–N9 (**1–9**), together with two known congener urdamycins A (**10**) and B (**11**) were obtained from a mangrove-derived *Streptomyces diastaticus* subsp. SCSIO GJ056. Compounds **7** and **8** are the first naturally occurring (5*R*, 6*R*) angucycline glycosides. We will further investigate the biological activity of these new angucycline compounds.

Supplementary Materials: The following are available online at http://www.mdpi.com/1660-3397/16/6/185/s1. This section includes 1D, 2D NMR spectra for new compounds **1–9**, and computational details of **6** and **7**.

Author Contributions: C.G. performed the experiments and wrote the draft manuscript. Y.L. performed the ECD calculations. Z.Z. and S.Z. contributed to the isolation and identification of compounds. Y.H. provided the strain. H.H. revised the manuscript. Y.-C.G. and J.J. supervised the whole work, and edited the manuscript. All authors read and approved the final manuscript.

Funding: This research was funded by the National Natural Science Foundation of China [grant numbers 41476133, 81425022, and U1501223], the Program of Chinese Academy of Sciences [grant number XDA11030403], and the Natural Science Foundation of Guangdong Province [grant number 2016A030312014].

Acknowledgments: We thank Syngenta Ph.D. Fellowship Awarded to Chun Gui. We are grateful to Zhihui Xiao, Aijun Sun, Yun Zhang and Chuanyun Li in the analytical facility at SCSIO for recording spectroscopic data.

Conflicts of Interest: The authors declare no conflict of interest.

References

1. Rohr, J.; Thiericke, R. Angucycline group antibiotics. *Nat. Prod. Rep.* **1992**, *9*, 103–137. [CrossRef] [PubMed]
2. Kharel, M.K.; Pahari, P.; Shepherd, M.D.; Tibrewal, N.; Nybo, S.E.; Shaaban, K.A.; Rohr, J. Angucyclines: Biosynthesis, mode-of-action, new natural products, and synthesis. *Nat. Prod. Rep.* **2012**, *29*, 264–325. [CrossRef] [PubMed]
3. Zhang, Y.; Huang, H.; Chen, Q.; Luo, M.; Sun, A.; Song, Y.; Ma, J.; Ju, J. Identification of the grincamycin gene cluster unveils divergent roles for GcnQ in different hosts, tailoring the L-rhodinose moiety. *Org. Lett.* **2013**, *15*, 3254–3257. [CrossRef] [PubMed]
4. Hertweck, C.; Luzhetskyy, A.; Rebets, Y.; Bechthold, A. Type II polyketide synthases: Gaining a deeper insight into enzymatic teamwork. *Nat. Prod. Rep.* **2007**, *24*, 162–190. [CrossRef] [PubMed]
5. Song, Y.; Liu, G.; Li, J.; Huang, H.; Zhang, X.; Zhang, H.; Ju, J. Cytotoxic and antibacterial angucycline- and prodigiosin-analogues from the deep-sea derived *Streptomyces* sp. SCSIO 11594. *Mar. Drugs* **2015**, *13*, 1304–1316. [CrossRef] [PubMed]
6. Lai, Z.; Yu, J.; Ling, H.; Song, Y.; Yuan, J.; Ju, J.; Tao, Y.; Huang, H. Grincamycins I–K, cytotoxic angucycline glycosides derived from marine-derived actinomycete *Streptomyces lusitanus* SCSIO LR32. *Planta Med.* **2018**, *84*, 201–207. [CrossRef] [PubMed]
7. Zhu, X.; Duan, Y.; Cui, Z.; Wang, Z.; Li, Z.; Zhang, Y.; Ju, J.; Huang, H. Cytotoxic rearranged angucycline glycosides from deep sea-derived *Streptomyces lusitanus* SCSIO LR32. *J. Antibiot.* **2017**, *70*, 819–822. [CrossRef] [PubMed]
8. Rohr, J.; Zeeck, A. Metabolic products of microorganisms. 240. Urdamycins, new angucycline antibiotics from *Streptomyces fradiae*. II. Structural studies of urdamycins B to F. *J. Antibiot.* **1987**, *40*, 459–467. [CrossRef] [PubMed]
9. Ren, X.; Lu, X.; Ke, A.; Zheng, Z.; Lin, J.; Hao, W.; Zhu, J.; Fan, Y.; Ding, Y.; Jiang, Q.; et al. Three novel members of angucycline group from *Streptomyces* sp. N05WA963. *J. Antibiot.* **2011**, *64*, 339–343. [CrossRef] [PubMed]
10. Drautz, H.; Zähner, H.; Rohr, J.; Zeeck, A. Metabolic products of microorganisms. 234 Urdamycins, new angucycline antibiotics from *Streptomyces fradiae*. *J. Antibiot.* **1986**, *39*, 1657–1669. [CrossRef] [PubMed]
11. Zeeck, A.; Rohr, J.; Sheldrick, G.M.; Jones, P.G.; Paulus, E.F. Structure of a new antibiotic and cytotoxic indicator substance, urdamycin A. *J. Chem. Res.* **1986**, 104–105.
12. Pérez, M.; Schleissner, C.; Rodríguez, P.; Zúñiga, P.; Benedit, G.; Sánchez-Sancho, F.; de la Calle, F. PM070747, a new cytotoxic angucyclinone from the marine-derived *Saccharopolyspora taberi* PEM-06-F23-019B. *J. Antibiot.* **2009**, *62*, 167–169. [CrossRef] [PubMed]
13. Hong, S.T.; Carney, J.R.; Gould, S.J. Cloning and heterologous expression of the entire gene clusters for PD 116740 from *Streptomyces* strain WP 4669 and tetrangulol and tetrangomycin from *Streptomyces rimosus* NRRL 3016. *J. Bacteriol.* **1997**, *179*, 470–476. [CrossRef] [PubMed]

14. Mori, K.; Ohmori, K.; Suzuki, K. Stereochemical relay via axially chiral styrenes: Asymmetric synthesis of the antibiotic TAN-1085. *Angew. Chem. Int. Ed. Engl.* **2009**, *48*, 5633–5637. [CrossRef] [PubMed]
15. Mori, K.; Tanaka, Y.; Ohmori, K.; Suzuki, K. Synthesis and stereochemical assignment of angucycline antibiotic, PD-116740. *Chem. Lett.* **2008**, *37*, 470–471. [CrossRef]
16. Ohmori, K.; Mori, K.; Ishikawa, Y.; Tsuruta, H.; Kuwahara, S.; Harada, N.; Suzuki, K. Concise total synthesis and structure assignment of TAN-1085. *Angew. Chem. Int. Ed. Engl.* **2004**, *43*, 3167–3171. [CrossRef] [PubMed]
17. Hauser, F.M.; Dorsch, W.A.; Mal, D. Total synthesis of (±)-*O*-methyl PD 116740. *Org. Lett.* **2002**, *4*, 2237–2239. [CrossRef] [PubMed]

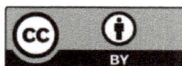

© 2018 by the authors. Licensee MDPI, Basel, Switzerland. This article is an open access article distributed under the terms and conditions of the Creative Commons Attribution (CC BY) license (http://creativecommons.org/licenses/by/4.0/).

marine drugs

MDPI

Review

Marine Carbohydrate-Based Compounds with Medicinal Properties

Ariana A. Vasconcelos [1] and Vitor H. Pomin [1,2,*]

[1]   Program of Glycobiology, Institute of Medical Biochemistry Leopoldo de Meis, and University Hospital Clementino Fraga Filho, Federal University of Rio de Janeiro, Rio de Janeiro, RJ 21941-913, Brazil; arianaavasconcelos@gmail.com

[2]   Department of BioMolecular Sciences, Division of Pharmacognosy, and Research Institute of Pharmaceutical Sciences, School of Pharmacy, University of Mississippi, Oxford, MS 38677-1848, USA

*   Correspondence: pominvh@bioqmed.ufrj.br or vpomin@olemiss.edu; Tel.: +1-(662)-915-3114

check for updates

Received: 5 June 2018; Accepted: 4 July 2018; Published: 9 July 2018

Abstract: The oceans harbor a great diversity of organisms, and have been recognized as an important source of new compounds with nutritional and therapeutic potential. Among these compounds, carbohydrate-based compounds are of particular interest because they exhibit numerous biological functions associated with their chemical diversity. This gives rise to new substances for the development of bioactive products. Many are the known applications of substances with glycosidic domains obtained from marine species. This review covers the structural properties and the current findings on the antioxidant, anti-inflammatory, anticoagulant, antitumor and antimicrobial activities of medium and high molecular-weight carbohydrates or glycosylated compounds extracted from various marine organisms.

Keywords: marine organisms; carbohydrate; glycoside; antioxidant; anticoagulant; anti-inflammatory; antitumor; antimicrobial

1. Introduction

The oceans cover about 70% of the earth's surface, and harbor a great diversity of living beings, ranging from unicellular bacteria to large multicellular mammals [1]. The large biodiversity of the marine environment is also accompanied with great chemical variety, which makes this habitat a promising source of new biomedically active molecules [2,3]. Currently some products obtained from marine sources are in the clinical trials phase for possible use as analgesics [4], anticancer drugs [5], and for treatments against viruses [6–8]. Despite these studies, marine potential remains largely unknown.

Among the promising but poorly explored marine molecules are carbohydrates, which stand out for their varied structural and chemical characteristics. Besides participating in energy storage and as a structural component (especially in exoskeletons of invertebrates), carbohydrates also play many other key biological roles such as fertilization signaling [9–11], pathogen recognition [12], cellular interactions [13], tumor metastasis [14], in addition to important pharmacological activities such as antitumor [15,16], antiviral [17,18], anticoagulants [19], antioxidants [20] and anti-inflammatory [2,21,22].

In this review we will discuss about the structural and biological aspects of the various carbohydrate-based compounds of marine origin endowed with potential biomedical and biotechnological applications. The main goal of this report is to reinforce to the scientific community the great value of marine-derived carbohydrates and glycosylated compounds of medium and high molecular-weight (MW) to drug discovery and development. Although these molecules can present actions on multiple systems, attention is paid more to their antioxidant, anti-inflammatory, anticoagulant, antitumor and antimicrobial properties.

2. Diversity of Carbohydrates from Marine Sources

Carbohydrates are the most abundant biomolecules on earth considering cellulose and chitin as the main representatives. These organic compounds act not only as the main energy source (as seen in starch and glycogen) but also as biologically functional structural players in events of cellular recognition, especially when present at the cell surface [23]. Carbohydrates are also the most complex biomolecules in terms of structure. The enhanced dynamic behavior, large conformational fluctuations, diversity of monomeric units accompanied by various enantiomers, multiple types of glycosidic bonds, and extensive post-polymerization modifications are factors that contribute to increase the structural complexity of these molecules. The carbohydrate classes are also vast. It can include both neutral and negatively charged saccharides with variable lengths. Famous examples are the *N*-linked or *O*-linked oligosaccharides in glycoproteins, glycosaminoglycan (GAG) in proteoglycans, glycolipids, sulfated fucans, sulfated galactans, among many other highly glycosylated products [24].

3. Structure and Function

3.1. Neutral and Acididc Polysaccharides

3.1.1. Laminaran

The main chain of laminarans, also found in brown alga, is mostly consisted of 3-linked β-D-glucose (Glc) residues (Figure 1) with a small proportion (usually less than 10%) of branches of single β-D-Glc residues attached to C-6 of the Glc residues of the backbone [25]. According to the reducing terminal ends, laminarans can be divided in two types: the first type with chains which are terminated by D-Glc residues (type G) (Figure 1A) and the second type with chains ending with D-mannitol (Man) residues (type M) (Figure 1B) [26]. The proportions of the two types of laminaran, and their consequent structures, vary according to the seaweed species. Environmental factors such as seasonal periods, salt concentration and frond age are additional influencing factors on chemical structures of laminaran [27]. Other environmental factors, including water temperature, salinity, waves, sea currents and depth of immersion (maybe pressure) have been also reported to influence on laminaran chemical composition [28]. Laminarans exist in either highly or poorly soluble forms. The first form is characterized by complete solubility in cold water, while the other is only soluble in hot water. The different solubility levels are influenced by the presence and number of branching residues. The higher the branching content, the greater the solubility in cold water [26].

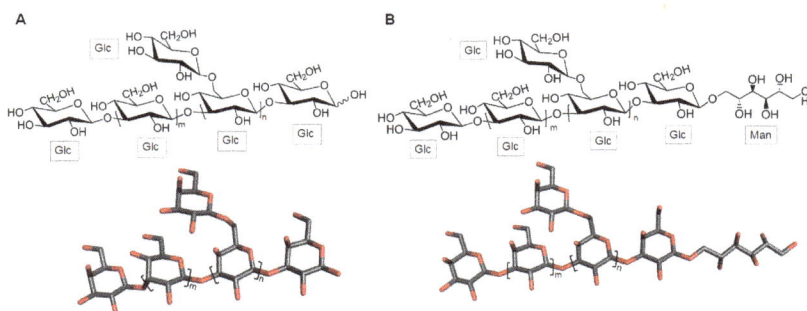

Figure 1. Representative chemical structure of laminaran which is composed of a backbone of 3-linked β-D-glucose (Glc) units with possible 6-linked branches of Glc residues and with reducing terminal ends with (**A**) Glc units (laminaran type G) or (**B**) D-mannitol (Man) residues (laminaran type M).

Laminaran exerts many bioactivities such as anticancer, anti-inflammatory, anticoagulant and antioxidant effects [28]. A recent review was published discussing the anticancer effects of two brown algal polysaccharides and emphasis was given on laminaran [25]. In this review laminaran enhances the therapeutic effects of commercial anticancer drugs [25]. For instance, laminaran can inhibit the in vitro formation of colonies of colon cancer cells DLD-1. This polysaccharide also showed a synergistic effect with X-ray irradiation against this same cancer cell line by decreasing the amounts and size of the colonies [29]. In the study of Malyarenko et al., lamellar sulfates of *Fucus evanescens* showed the capacity to decrease the migration ability of cancer cells in vitro by inhibiting the activity of certain metalloproteinases such as MMP-2 and MMP-9 [30].

According to the publication of Lee et al., laminaran shows also the capacity to enhance the release of some inflammatory mediators [31]. This makes laminaran a potential therapeutic with immunostimulatory and anti-inflammatory properties [31]. With respect to antimicrobial activity, this marine glycan shows also the inhibitory capacity on both Gram-positive and Gram-negative bacteria such as *Salmonella typhimurium*, *Listeria monocytogenes* and *Vibrio parahaemolyticus* to adhere on HT-29-Luc cells of human enterocytes, besides inhibiting the invasion of *S. typhimurium* in this cell line [32]. The literature survey showed that laminaran is able to prevent HIV activity by decreasing (a) the adsorption of the HIV particle in human lymphocytes and (b) the efficiency of the HIV reverse transcriptase, which plays an important role in the proliferation of the virus during the infection cycle [33]. This study suggests that laminaran acts as an efficient inhibitor of HIV replication and proliferation [33].

3.1.2. Alginic Acid

Alginic acid is a polysaccharide obtained from brown algae. It has linear structure and consists of β-D-manuronic acid (ManA) and α-L-guluronic acid (GulA) in repeating building blocks. These building blocks may be composed of consecutive GulA residues [GulA-GulA-GulA-GulA]$_n$, consecutive ManA residues [ManA-ManA-ManA-ManA]$_n$, or alternating ManA and GulA residues [GulA-ManA-GulA-ManA]$_n$ (Figure 2) [34]. This polysaccharide has a wide spectrum of application in medicine, in the food industry, in biotechnology and in other industrial sectors [35].

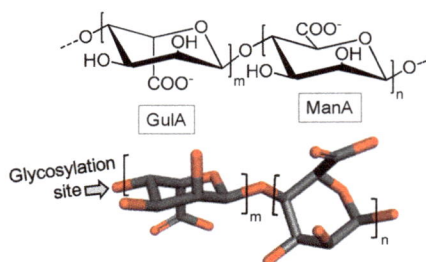

Figure 2. Chemical structure of alginate. It is composed of building blocks of α-L-guluronate (GulA) and β-D-mannuronate (ManA) units.

In the study of So et al., alginic acid was shown to be a promising antioxidant agent against oxidative stress induced by free radicals [36]. In a work published five years later, Sarithakumari et al. investigated the antioxidant and the anti-inflammatory potential of alginic acid, isolated from the brown algal species *Sargassum wightii*, by in vivo assays using rats with induced arthritis [37]. Histopathological analysis of the animal paw tissue showed that treatment with alginic acid was able to decrease the paw edema as well as the inflammatory infiltrates in the studied animal models. This polysaccharide was also able to reduce the activity of various enzymes such as cyclooxygenase, lipoxygenase and myeloperoxidase, besides reducing the levels of C-reactive protein, ceruloplasmin and rheumatoid factor. Reduction of lipid peroxidation and increased antioxidant enzyme activity was also reported [37].

Supportively Endo et al. showed in a separate work two years later that alginic acid is able to eliminate free radicals and reduce the ferrous ion in stored pork [38]. The antioxidant activity of alginic acid was attributed to its capacity to chelate metal, to scavenge free radicals and to reduce ferric ions in the tissue. This last ability is quite useful in light of the elevated levels of ferrous ions in pork meat. The literature also reported the antimicrobial activity of this polysaccharide [38]. For instance, in the work of Neettoo et al., an alginate-based coating was tested in order to increase the microbiological safety in the digestions of cold-smoked salmon. This study demonstrated the efficacy of alginate to control the growth of *Listeria monocytogenes*, a bacterium responsible for serious infections, mainly those caused by salmon uptake [39].

3.2. Sulfated Polysaccharides

3.2.1. Fucoidan

Composed of complex structure, fucoidans are obtained from brown algae. They generally consist of a backbone mostly 3-linked α-L-fucose (Fuc) (Figure 3A) or alternating α-L-Fuc residues with 3- and 4-glycosidic linkages (Figure 3B). Either case can be replaced with sulfate or acetyl groups, and/or side chains containing Fuc or other glycosyl units [40]. In addition to Fuc residues, they may contain small amounts of several other monosaccharides, such as Glc, galactose (Gal), xylose and/or mannose [41].

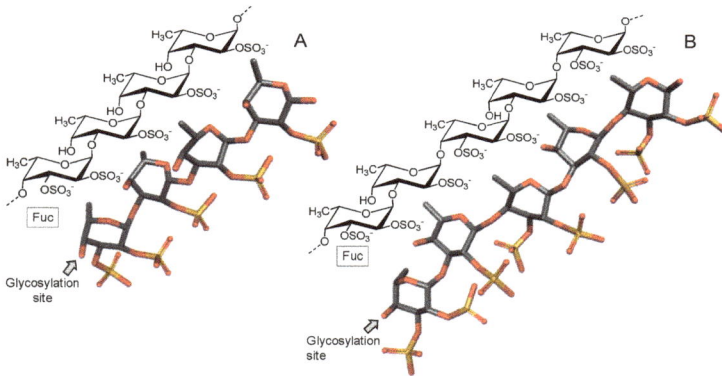

Figure 3. Fucoidans are polymers mostly composed of α-L-fucose (Fuc) residues either (**A**) mostly 3-linked or (**B**) 3- and 4-linked.

One of the first attempts to propose fucoidan structures was made in 1950 by Percival and Ross [42]. They analyzed the fucoidan-containing extract from *Fucus vesiculosus*. In order to understand some of the fucoidan's biological activities, Patankar et al. have revised the fucoidan structure four decades later and described it as a polysaccharide consisted mainly of 3-linked α-L-Fuc units (Figure 3A) [43]. More recent papers stated that Fuc units in the fucoidan backbone can occur in the α-1,2 linkage type besides the α-1,3 and/or α-1,4 bonds [44]. It was also stated that sulfation can occur at C-2, C-3 and/or C-4 as well [44]. Despite the many published works regarding fucoidan, the relationship between structure and biological activities is not clearly and easily established because of the obstacles in full structure determination [45,46]. However, the scientific interest on fucoidan is so appealing because of the large spectrum of its application that intense research is annually carried out in terms of both structure and biomedical properties [47].

The highly cited review of Fitton covered potential applications of fucoidan in several types of therapies in which it was observed that the anti-inflammatory potential of fucoidan lies on its pleiotropic effects. These include selectin inhibition, complement inhibition and enzyme inhibitory activity [48]. In a comparative study of the anticoagulant property of fucoidans, extracted from various species of algae, *Laminaria saccharina* was found to furnish the fucoidan with the highest level of activity [49,50]. In vitro and in vivo assays are capable to evaluate the safety and clinical effects of fucoidan ingestion on homeostasis. Very strong in vitro anticoagulant activity has been observed as opposed to a modest effect on the in vivo assay [51]. Investigations on the antioxidant activity of fucoidan conclude that oral administration of this polysaccharide may lower serum parameters such as triacylglycerides, total cholesterol, low-density lipoprotein cholesterol and plasma Glc levels, and improve the anti-oxidation and innate immunity of catfish *Pelteobagrus fulvidraco* [52].

Other works have reported the anticancer activity of fucoidans extracts. An example is the well-cited paper from Cumashi et al. in which nine different fucoidans have been screened in terms of their multiple biomedical properties [49]. It has been shown that fucoidan from *L. saccharina*, *L. digitata*, *Fucus serratus*, *F. distichus* and *F. vesiculosus* have the capacity to block adhesion of MDA-MB-231 breast carcinoma cells, resulting in potential beneficial therapeutics against tumor metastasis [49]. Following the same rationale, other researchers have demonstrated that fucoidan of other seaweed species such as *Ecklonia cava*, *Sargassum hornery* and *Costaria costata* can present positive effects on human melanoma and colon cancer [53]. Fucoidan from other brown seaweeds like *Saccharina japonicus* and *Undaria pinnatifida* possess high antitumor activity and can inhibit proliferation and colony formation of breast cancer and melanoma cancer cell lines [54]. Fractions of native fucoidan and its derivatives have shown activity against the formation of colonies of two colorectal carcinoma cells, DLD-1 and HCT-116 [55].

The literature also mentions the antimicrobial properties of fucoidan [8,56]. An example of these is the publication of Thuy et al., where the anti-HIV activity of fucoidan, extracted from three brown algae *Sargassum mcclurei*, *S. polycystum* and *Turbinara ornate,* is reported [56]. All these fucoidan types tested in this work exhibited anti-HIV effects. The mechanism of action has been attributed to the capacity of this polysaccharide in blocking the first steps of HIV entry into the target cells [8,56]. A very recent study described the synthesis of silver nanoparticles (AgNPs) using fucoidan extracted from the alga *Padina tetrastromatica* as part of the coating material [57]. The focus of this work was on the increased antibacterial activity of antibiotics coated with AgNPs and fucoidan against antibiotic resistant bacteria. The synergistic effect of the combined antibiotics and the fucoidan in nanoparticles resulted in a two-fold increase of the antibacterial activity as compared to the antibiotic and the sulfated polysaccharide used in separate treatments.

3.2.2. Carrageenan/Agaran

Carrageenans are sulfated galactans found in red seaweeds and composed of linear chains of alternating 3-linked β-D-Gal (conventionally ascribed as A units) and 4-linked α-D-Gal or α-D-3,6-anhydrogalactose (AnGal) (B units), thus forming disaccharide-repeating building blocks [58].

Carrageenans are classified according to the presence of the 3,6-anhydrous bridge at the 4-linked AnGal residues and the positions and numbers of sulfate groups (Figure 4). Carrageenans are traditionally identified by a Greek prefix accordingly to their structures. Structures vary in terms of sulfation patterns and the presence of AnGal units. The International Union of Pure and Applied Chemistry (IUPAC) establishes a nomenclature based on a code for the carrageenans: G = 3-linked β-D-Gal; D = 4-linked α-D-Gal; DA = 4-linked α-D-3,6-AnGal and S = sulfate ester (SO_3^-) [59,60].

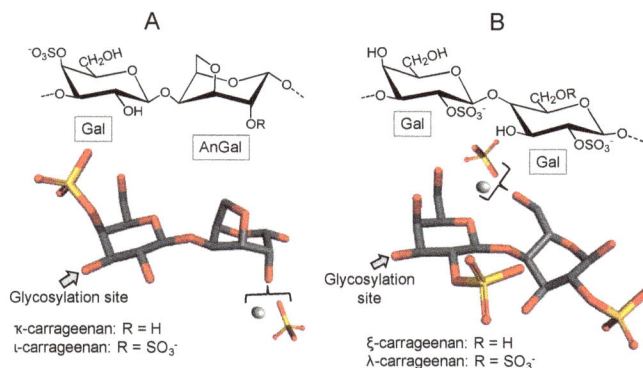

Figure 4. Representative chemical structures of carrageenans. These polymers are made up of alternating 3-linked β-D-galactose (Gal) units and (**A**) 4-linked α-D-anydrogalactose (AnGal) as seen in kappa (κ) and iota (ι) carrageenans or (**B**) α/β-D-Gal units as seen in zeta (ξ) and lambda (λ) carrageenans. These polymers also contain sulfate as their major substituent.

In Figure 4, four illustrative structures are shown: (A) one composed of AnGal units, and (B) other composed of Gal units, both either in their sulfated or non-sulfated forms of occurrence. The three most commercially exploited carrageenans are kappa (κ), iota (ι) and lambda (λ). Their corresponding names, based on the IUPAC nomenclature and on the letter codes, are carrageenan 4-sulfate (DA-G4S), carrageenan 2,4-disulfate (DA2S-G4S), and carrageenan 2,6,2-trisulfate (D2S,6S-G2S), respectively [59, 60]. In addition to these three major types of carrageenans, two other types, called carrageenans ν and μ are frequently found in carrageenan commercial samples. They are the biological precursors of ι- and κ-carrageenans, respectively [60].

In the food industry, carrageenans are widely explored because of their physicochemical properties like emulsifying, thickening, gelling and stabilizing effects. These properties give textural properties and protective effects to a wide range of food products [61]. Carrageenans are also widely used in the pharmaceutical and cosmetic industries [62].

Carrageenan-derived oligosaccharides produced by γ-irradiation exhibited antioxidant property in various assays such as the hydroxyl radical scavenging, the reduction power and the 1,1-diphenyl-2-picrylhydrazyl (DPPH) radical scavenging ability [63]. The effect observed was dose-dependent and the carrageenan types were also observed to have different impact on the antioxidant activity, following the order of λ < ι <κ [63].

Talarico et al. analyzed the action of λ and ι carrageenans against dengue virus serotypes. In this study, both carrageenans were shown to be potent inhibitors of the multiplication of dengue virus type 2 (DENV-2) and 3 (DENV-3) in Vero and HepG2 cells, with effective concentration values of 50% (EC$_{50}$) of 0.14 to 4.1 μg [18].

Still, with respect to antiviral activity, Diogo et al. evaluated the action of λ-carrageenan against two viral pathogens of veterinary interest, bovine herpesvirus type 1 (BoHV-1) and suid herpesvirus type 1 (SuHV-1) [64]. λ-Carrageenan was able to reduce the infectivity of both types of virus. The concentration required to inactivate 50% of the virus, virucidal concentration (VC$_{50}$) was 0.96 ± 0.08 μg/mL for BoHV-1 and 31.10 ± 2.28 μg/mL for SuHV-1. The antiviral activity of λ-carrageenan for BoHV-1, expressed in inhibitory concentration (IC$_{50}$), was 0.52 ± 0.01 μg/mL, whereas for SuHV-1 was 10.42 ± 0.88 μg/mL.

In vitro tests have shown that ι-carrageenan is a potent inhibitor of the influenza A (H1N1) virus infection [65]. From this information Leibbrandt et al. decided to test a commercially available nasal spray containing ι-carrageenan in a model of influenza A infection in mice. Treatment of mice infected with a lethal dose of influenza A PR8/34 H1N1 virus and administered with ι-carrageenan at a concentration of 60 µg/mL repeated twice daily starting within 48 hours post-infection and resulted in strong protection of the mice, in a similar to those treated with oseltamivir [65].

Another study, also related to the antiviral potential of carrageenans, investigated the role of λ-carrageenan in the inhibition of rabies virus (RABV) infection [66]. The λ-carrageenan oligosaccharide (P32) specifically inhibited the replication of several RABV strains, and acted primarily by suppressing viral replication during the early post-adsorption period, thereby preventing viral internalization and viral fusion mediated by viral glycoproteins. The authors suggest that P32 derived from λ-carrageenan is a promising agent for the development of novel anti-RABV drugs [66].

Studies on the cytotoxic effects of κ- and λ-carrageenans on human cervical carcinoma cells (HeLa) and human umbilical vein endothelial cells (HUVEC) showed that both carrageenans had no significant effect on HUVEC (normal cells). However, both carrageenans were cytotoxic to HeLa, although λ-carrageenan has stronger cytotoxicity when compared to κ-carrageena. In addition, λ-carrageenan was shown to have a stronger effect on suppression of tumor cell proliferation and cell division compared to κ-carrageenan [67].

A study by a Russian group which investigated a κ/β-carrageenan extracted from the red alga *Tichocarpus crinitus* for its anti-inflammatory property through in vivo models. The work showed that the dose of 100 mg/kg of κ/β-carrageenan (orally administered) stimulates the induction of anti-inflammatory cytokines, such as interleukin (IL)-10, in mouse blood cells by more than 2.5-fold when compared to control. However, it has no effect on the production of pro-inflammatory cytokines, such as tumor necrosis factor-α (TNF-α). In addition, pre-treatment with carrageenan has been shown to reduce the excessive activation of the inflammatory cells triggered by lipopolysaccharide [68].

Murad et al. reported that the carrageenan (predominantly ι-carrageenan) extracted from the red alga inhibited cell growth, induced apoptosis and promoted DNA damage in a breast cancer cell line (MDA-MB-231) at the concentration of 50 µM [69].

Luo et al. reported the antitumor action of λ-carrageenan on melanoma cells B16-F10 and breast cancer 4T1. This carrageenan, when administered intratumorally at a dose of 50 mg/kg, can inhibit the growth of B16-F10 and 4T1 tumors in mice besides increasing the tumor immune response and increasing the number of immunostimulatory cell infiltrates as well as the production of pro-inflammatory cytokines. In addition, when used as a vaccine adjuvant, λ-carrageenan notably increased the preventive and therapeutic effects of vaccines against cancer [70].

In a recent work, McKim et al. investigated the effects of three commercial forms of carrageenan: λ, κ and ι. The parameters evaluated were intestinal absorption, pro-inflammatory signaling pathways, oxidative stress and cytotoxicity using four cell types (three of intestinal lineage, Caco-2, HT-29 HCT-8 and one hepatic lineage HepG2). None of the carrageenans showed any effect in the tests performed, and did not reproduce any of the in vitro findings already reported in the literature. At the conclusion of the study, the researchers reinforced the importance of further investigations to check reproducibility outside the discoveries of their laboratory, and before risk assessment, regimental decisions, or policy statements take place [71].

Agaran (and agarose) are structurally related polysaccharides of carrageenans. While carrageenans bear the β-D-Gal units in their backbones, agaran and agarose carry the α-L-Gal units. The chemical difference of agaran and agarose is that the latter is composed of the α-L-anGal unit [58]. These polysaccharides are also found in red seaweeds and can show different patterns of sulfation [58]. A recent paper of the group of Prof. Norma Benevides has shown the neuroprotective effects of a sulfated agaran isolated from the red alga *Gracilaria cornea* [72]. The study was developed on rats subjected to 6-hydroxydopamine (6-OHDA) in order to create an in vivo model of the Parkinson's disease. The results have shown that 60 µg of sulfated agaran of *G. cornea* intrastriatally injected can promote neuroprotection in vivo as seen by reduction of the oxidative/nitroactive stress and by alterations of the monoamine contents promoted by 6-OHDA injection. In addition, this agaran was observed to also modulate the transcription of neuroprotection- and inflammation-related genes as well as returning behavioral activities and weight gain to normal conditions [72].

3.2.3. Sulfated Polymannuronate

Sulfated polymannuronate (SPM), also known as sulfated polymannuroguluronate, is a sulfated polysaccharide extracted from brown algae, rich in 4-linked β-D-ManA with a mean MW of 10,000 Da (Figure 5) [73,74]. Sulfation can occur at either C-2 or C-3. The propylene glycol mannuronate sulfate is another version of this polysaccharide also with medical interest.

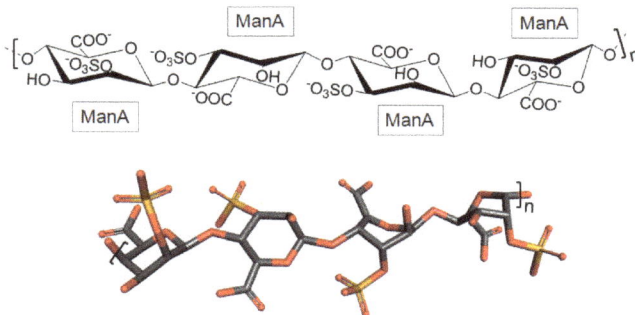

Figure 5. Structural representation of the brown algal sulfated polymannuronate (SPM). It is composed of 4-linked β-D-mannuronate (ManA) units in polymers with mean MW of 10 kDa. Sulfation can occur at either C-2 or C-3.

SPM has shown anti-HIV property [74]. SPM entered into the Phase II clinical trial in China, becoming the first marine sulfated polysaccharide with the potential to become a real anti-AIDS drug [75]. Several authors have focused on the elucidation of the molecular mechanism involved in the anti-HIV activity of SPM and their beneficial effects on the human cells of the immune system [75]. The particular study of Miao et al. has reported that CD4 is one of the possible targets for the specific binding of SPM on lymphocytes [75]. SPM-derived oligosaccharides have shown the capacity to interact, in multiple ways, with gp120, and therefore, present an anti-HIV outcome [74]. SPM can also inhibit the adhesion of the HIV Trans-activator of transcription (Tat) on SLK cells by direct binding to the KKR site (high-affinity heparin binding region) of Tat [73]. This structural information facilitates the elucidation of the structure-activity relationship of sulfated polysaccharides in the fight against HIV-1 infection.

3.2.4. Glycosaminoglycans

Glycosaminoglycans (GAGs) are linear and heterogeneous sulfated glycans. Although structurally complex, the skeletons of these polysaccharides are simply constituted by repeated building blocks of disaccharides composed of alternating uronic acid (UroA) or Gal and hexosamine. The hexosamine may be glucosamine (GlcN) or *N*-acetylgalactosamine (GalNAc) and its differently substituted (mostly sulfated) derivatives. UroA can be either glucuronic acid (GlcA) or iduronic acid (IdoA) [76].

Heparin, heparan sulfate (HS), chondroitin sulfate (CS), dermatan sulfate (DS), keratan sulfate (KS) and hyaluronan (HA) are the major classes of GAGs found in animals. Although GAGs are all composed of repeating disaccharide units, the patterns of sulfation and the alternating monosaccharides that make up these units within the polymers vary significantly. The GAG classification is conventionally based on these structural variations. Interestingly, GAGs of marine organisms can present distinct structures from those from terrestrial animals, even considering the same class of GAGs [77]. Structural variations and heterogeneities of GAG chains (from either marine or terrestrial sources) especially in terms of sequence domains and the common occurrence in the extracellular matrix or on the surface of cells are all relevant contributing factors to the diversity of their biological and medicinal functions.

Heparin

Heparin is mostly composed of alternating *N*,6-di-*O*-sulfated α-D-GlcN (GlcNS6S) and 2-sulfated α-L-IdoA units (IodA2S), both 4-linked (Figure 6). Among its occurrence in marine invertebrates, heparin is found in several phyla such as mollusks, crustaceans, annelids, echinoderms, tunicates and other urochordates [78]. In some of these invertebrates the heparin-like structures have presented structural peculiarities which are unique and not commonly found in the commonest and well-known mammalian-derived heparins. These unique properties may comprise low-levels of *N*- and 6-sulfation content and high-levels of *N*-acetylation on the GlcN units together with consistent amounts of GlcA units [79]. Naturally occurring low MW heparins are also found in marine invertebrates [80]. Works have also suggested that marine heparin structures are related to the species of occurrence and the chemical differences lie mostly on the relative abundance of the various composing disaccharide units or different chains [81]. In addition to these structural variations, the marine invertebrate heparin-like compounds also show variable biological functions [78].

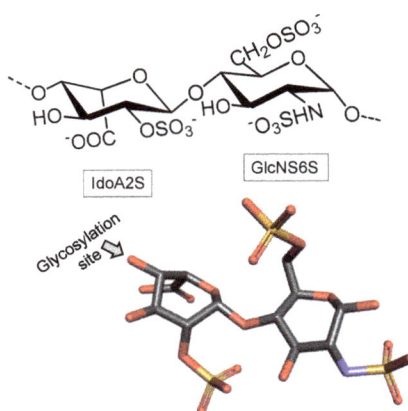

Figure 6. The heparin structure is mostly composed of alternating *N*,6-di-*O*-sulfated α- D-glucosamine (GlcNS6S) and 2-sulfated α-L-iduronate (IdoA2S) units, both 4-linked.

Dietrich et al. reported the presence of a heparin in the crustacean *Penaeus brasiliensis* [80]. Of particular importance were the findings that this low MW heparin (LMWH) is enriched with non-sulfated UroA residues and exhibits potent antithrombotic activity. In vitro anticoagulant activity have shown that its effect is exerted on the inhibition of factor Xa and inhibition of thrombin (IIa) mediated mainly by cofactor heparin II (HCII) as opposed to mammalian heparins which exert their anticoagulant activity mainly through the inhibition of IIa and factor Xa mediated by antithrombin (AT). This shrimp-derived heparin has also presented potent in vivo antithrombotic activity as compared to the mammalian LMWH. Oppositely to the shrimp heparin, another heparin isolated from the crab *Goniopsis cruentata* has shown insignificant in vitro anticoagulant activity and low bleeding potency [78].

The heparin-like compound extracted from the shrimp *Litopenaeus vannamei* has shown capacity to reduce the influx of inflammatory cells in the lesion sites of a model of acute inflammation because this marine GAG is able to reduce the activity of the matrix metalloproteinases (MMPs) in the peritoneal lavage of inflamed animals [79]. This molecule has been reported to reduce almost 90% of the activity of MMP-9 secreted by activated human leukocytes besides presenting low hemorrhagic potential [79]. Another study has shown that this shrimp "heparinoid" is capable of suppressing the neovascularization process [82].

An analogue of heparin isolated from the ascidian *Styela plicata* was investigated in a model of colitis in rats [83]. The result observed was a decrease in the production of TNF-α, TGF-β and vascular endothelial growth factor (VEGF), as well as reduced activation of NF-β and mitogen-activated protein kinase (MAPK) kinase. At the cellular level, this tunicate heparin analogue can attenuate the recruitment of lymphocytes and macrophages and reduce apoptosis levels in epithelial cells. A drastic reduction in collagen-mediated fibrosis has also been observed [83].

Heparan Sulfate

Heparin and Heparan sulfate (HS) are structurally related GAGs since both are composed of GlcN units in their backbones, although with different concentrations [84]. HS is typically considered a less-modified heparin version. Among the sulfated GAGs, HS has the greatest structural variability. Depending on the tissue and species of origin, such a polysaccharide may be composed of several distinct disaccharide units, containing either GlcA or IdoA and GlcN with different extents of *N*- and/or 6-*O*-sulfation besides *N*-acetylation and 3-*O*-sulfation [84].

For example, the HS isolated from shrimp *Artemia franciscana* possesses a high degree of *N*-sulfation and a relatively low degree of 6-*O*-sulfation of the GlcN residues. This compound exhibits high anticoagulant activity mediated by heparin cofactor II (HCII) [85]. In a study by Gomes et al., a novel HS structure with unique characteristics was isolated from the bivalve mollusk *Nodipecten nodosus* (Figure 7). This HS was reported to be formed by GlcA and GlcN units and by rare types of sulfation which can occur on C-2 or C-3 of the GlcA units [86]. This mollusk HS can inhibit thrombus growth without inducing the provoking hemorrhage. The same group reported later the action of this HS in inhibiting P-selectin-mediated events such as metastasis and recruitment of inflammatory cells [87].

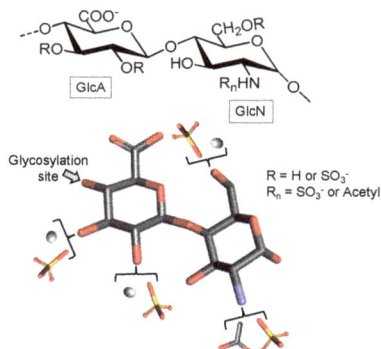

Figure 7. The heparan sulfate structure from the bivalve mollusk *Nodipecten nodosum* composed of alternating β-D-glucuronic acid (GlcA) and α-D-glucosamine (GlcN), both 4-linked. This molecule has a rare sulfation pattern on C-2 or C-3 of the GlcA units. The C-6 of GlcN can also be sulfated. The substituents of R_n can be either acetyl or sulfate.

Dermatan Sulfate

Dermatan sulfate (DS) is a linear variable-length polysaccharide composed of alternating disaccharide building blocks of 4-linked α-L-IdoA and 3-linked β-D-GalNAc units. These alternating disaccharide units can be variably sulfated at position C-2 of IdoA (IdoA2S) and/or C4 (GalNAc4S) and/or C6 (GalNAc6S) or both carbons (GalNAc4S6S) in the GalNAc unit, giving rise to different sulfated disaccharides [76].

In addition of being present in mammalian tissues, DS with high sulfation content was also found in different species of clam and tunicate [88–90]. The work of Pavão et al. [90] raised an interesting discussion about the structure-function relationship of DS, extracted from different species of ascidians (Figure 8). For example, DS isolated from *Ascidia nigra* is fully sulfated at C-6 of the GalNAc unit (100%) and at C-2 of IdoA (80%) (Figure 8). The DS from *S. plicata* however is less sulfated at C-2 (65%) and widely sulfated at the C-4 position of GalNAc (Figure 8). The DS, isolated from *Halocynthia pyriforms*, is similar to that of *S. plicata* (Figure 8).

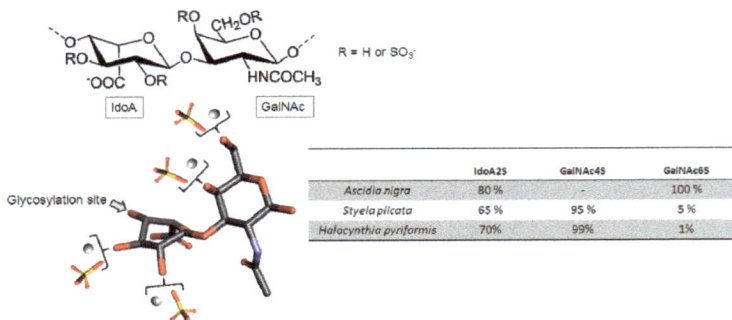

	IdoA2S	GalNAc4S	GalNAc6S
Ascidia nigra	80 %	-	100 %
Styela plicata	65 %	95 %	5 %
Halocynthia pyriformis	70%	99%	1%

Figure 8. Representative chemical structure of dermatan sulfate (DS) which is composed of a backbone of 4-linked α-L-Idorunate (IdoA) and 3-linked β-D-*N*-acetylgalactosamine (GalNAc) units. The different radicals represent different patterns of sulfate substitutions. Ascidian DS are highly sulfated at C-2 of IdoA, but differ in the sulfation pattern at GalNAc. The insert table displays the sulfation rates of the ascidian species *Ascidia nigra*, *Styela plicata* and *Halocynthia pyriformis*.

Sulfation patterns in ascidian DS play a decisive role in biological actions. For instance, in anticoagulation the DS molecules from *S. plicata*, *H. pyriformis*, which bear more GalNAc4S units, exhibited a significant HCII-mediated IIa inhibition as opposed to *A. nigra* DS which did not show considerable anticoagulant activity [90,91]. With the exception of *A. nigra*, the two ascidian DSs displayed 10- and 6-fold more activity for HCII-related inhibition than the mammalian-derived native and oversulfated DS, respectively [90].

DS from *S. plicata* was also investigated regarding its anti-inflammatory activity in a model of colitis in rats [83]. This GAG exhibited a superior anti-inflammatory effect to that of mammalian heparin. This DS can decrease recruitment of lymphocytes and macrophages and apoptosis of epithelial cells. It is important to note that no hemorrhagic propensity has been pointed out after treatment with the ascidian glycan [83].

Kozlowski et al. investigated the effect of two DSs, isolated from *S. plicata* and *Phallusia nigra*, in the events of thrombosis, inflammation and metastasis [92]. The study showed that both GAGs can reduce thrombus size in a model of arterial thrombosis induced by FeCl$_3$. In addition, they can also attenuate metastasis of MC-38 colon carcinoma, B16-BL6 melanoma cells and the infiltration of inflammatory cells in a mouse model of thioglycollate-induced peritonitis. The authors suggested that the observed effects are related to the inhibition of P-selectin [92].

Fucosylated Chondroitin Sulfate

Fucosylated chondroitin sulfate (fCS) is a distinct marine GAG found exclusively in sea cucumber (Echinodermata, Holothuroidea). This GAG is composed of the regular CS backbone with branches of α-L-Fuc units attached to C-3 of the GlcA residues (Figure 9). The lateral units of Fuc can show different patterns of sulfation according to the holothurian species [77,93].

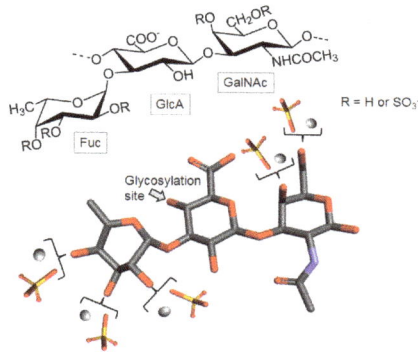

Figure 9. Structural representation of the holothurian fucosylated chondroitin sulfate (fCS). The structure is composed of α-L-fucose (Fuc), β-D-glucuronic acid (GlcA) and *N*-acetyl β-D-galactosamine (GalNAc).

With regard to the fCS' therapeutic properties, this glycan exhibits a wide range of applications: anticoagulant [94], anti-metastasis [95] anti-inflammatory [96] and antiviral activities [97]. For this reason several papers have focused on the study of fCS. One of the works investigated samples of fCS extracted from three species of sea cucumbers: *Apostichopus japonicus*, *Stichopus chloronotus* and *Acaudina molpadioidea* in order to carry out a structural comparison among the three molecules and their antioxidant and anti-inflammatory properties. Analysis of ^{1}H and ^{13}C NMR of the polysaccharide identified three patterns of sulfation of the fucose branches: 4-*O*-, 2,4-di-*O*- and 3,4-di-*O*-sulfation. In addition, their activities were affected by the sulfation patterns of the Fuc branches, revealing that sulfation in O-4 is particularly important [98].

In the work of Ustyzhanina et al., the fCS isolated from the sea cucumber *Cucumaria japonica* inhibited platelet aggregation in vitro, and demonstrated significant anticoagulant activity. The latter activity was associated with the ability of fCS to increase the inhibition of IIa and factor Xa by AT as well to influence von Willebrand factor activity. The platelet aggregation inhibition process significantly distinguishes fCS from the LMWH [99]. fCS isolated from sea cucumber *Holothuria mexicana* exhibited high affinity with fibroblast growth factors 1 and 2. These factors are important in the neovascularization event. In addition, it displays the intrinsic anticoagulant activity and inhibited the activation of IIa and factor Xa by AT [100]. Still regarding anticoagulant property, a new fCS, isolated from the sea cucumber *Holothuria scabra*, was tested in comparison to heparin, and was shown to prolong activated partial thromboplastin time [101].

As mentioned above, the fucosylated sulfated polysaccharide also presents some antiviral properties, including against HIV. The anti-HIV action of holothurian fCS has generated a patent filed in the European patent bank [102]. Recent studies have reported the anti-HIV activity of the fCS obtained from the sea cucumber *Thelenota ananas*, which inhibited several strains of HIV-1 replication with different potencies. This study also reported that *T. ananas* fCS can bind potently to the recombinant HIV-1 gp120 protein, but did not inhibit recombinant HIV-1 reverse transcriptase [97].

3.2.5. Propylene Glycol Alginate Sodium Sulfate

Propylene glycol alginate sodium sulfate (PSS) is a sulfated polysaccharide, prepared by the chemical sulfation of the low MW alginate [103]. The backbone of this carbohydrate is composed of 4-linked β-D-ManA and 4-linked α-L-GulA, with degrees of sulfation substitution of 0.8 to 1.5 in the hydroxyls C-2 and C-3. It can also bear partially C-6-linked propylene glycol group at the hexuronic residues [104,105]. As a similar molecule to alginate, the blocks of these units constituting the PSS molecule may be composed of consecutive GulA residues [GulA-GulA-GulA-GulA]$_n$, consecutive

ManA units [ManA-ManA-ManA-ManA]$_m$ residues or alternative residues of ManA and GulA [GulA-ManA-GulA-ManA]$_n$ (Figure 10) [105].

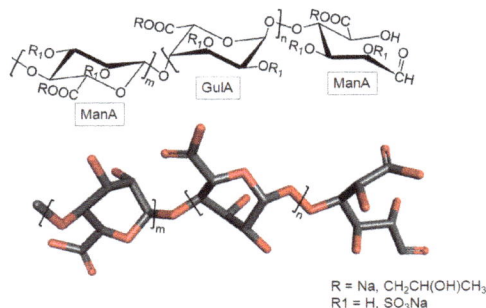

R = Na, CH$_2$CH(OH)CH$_3$
R1 = H, SO$_3$Na

Figure 10. Structural representation of the propylene glycol alginate sodium sulfate (PSS).

With respect to biological activity, PSS has been used as a heparinoid drug to prevent and treat hyperlipidemia and ischemic cardio-cerebrovascular diseases for almost 30 years [103,106]. Because it has many important bioactivities, PSS has been the subject of many studies. This is proven by recent literature, where the various applications of this compound have been reported.

In the work of Xin et al. the anticoagulant and antithrombotic activities of low MW PSS were shown [104]. The low-MW PSS were prepared by oxidative-reductive depolymerization, and the activity tests were performed in vitro and in vivo. For the tests, four PPS fragments (FPs) with different MWs were used. The bioactivity evaluation showed a positive correlation between the MW and the anticoagulant and antithrombotic activities of the FPs. It was observed that FPs prolonged coagulation time and significantly reduced platelet aggregation. FPs also exerted an effect on factor IIa in the presence of AT and HCII, in addition to decreasing the weight and size of the thrombus in vivo [104].

Besides the anticoagulant activity, other PSS potentials have been explored. For example, Zhang et al. studied the anti-inflammatory potential of PSS through models of acute pancreatitis induced by Cerulein in mice. The results obtained by the authors indicated that PSS attenuates pancreas lesion by inhibiting autophagy and apoptosis through a mechanism involving the ratio between the MAPK/extracellular signal-regulated kinase (ERK). Inhibition of inflammatory factors, such as TNF-α, IL-6 and IL-1β, was also observed during the PSS-suppressed pancreatitis [103].

Also regarding the anti-inflammatory activity, Xu et al. investigated the protective function and mechanism of PSS in a hepatic ischemic reperfusion injury (RI) model in mice [106]. Pretreatment was performed at doses of 25 or 50 mg/kg, which were injected intraperitoneally into the animals 1 h 45 min prior to the induction of injury. The results indicated that pretreatment of PSS at both doses reduced the serum levels of the enzymes aspartate transaminase (AST) and alanine transaminase (ALT) compared to those observed in animals that did not receive pretreatment. PSS doses were also able to decrease the extent of hepatic necrosis, congestion and edema produced by IR injury. The authors suggested that pretreatment with PSS protected against hepatic IR injury [106].

More recent studies have sought a way to improve the bioavailability and efficacy of PSS in the body, since the absorption of this compound can sometimes be impaired because of its high MW. Faced with this challenge, Li et al. tested a new formulation of PSS in the form of enteric-coated nanoparticle (enteric PSS-NP) [107]. The study showed that the PSS nanoparticle had targeted intestinal absorption and improved pharmacodynamics. When compared to the PSS solution, enteric PSS-NP had an improved effectiveness in controlling body weight. These data indicate that enteric PSS-NP could be promising in terms of product development in the future [107].

3.3. N-acetylated Sugars

Chitin and Chitosan

Chitin is an important constituent of the exoskeleton of many organisms such as crustaceans and insects. In the marine environment chitin is certainly the most abundant biopolymer, being structurally composed of GlcNAc and GlcN units bound by β-1,4 glycosidic bonds (Figure 11). In chitin, the GlcNAc content is higher than 70% of the total monosaccharide, making this polysaccharide highly N-acetylated. This, in turn, significantly decreases its water solubility property [24,108].

Chitosan is a cationic polysaccharide composed of the same units and the glycosidic linkage of chitin (Figure 11). However, low amounts of GlcNAc are found in chitosan, usually less than 50%. Physicochemical characteristics such as hydrophobicity and inter-chain interactions depend on the amount and distribution of the acetyl groups [24,108].

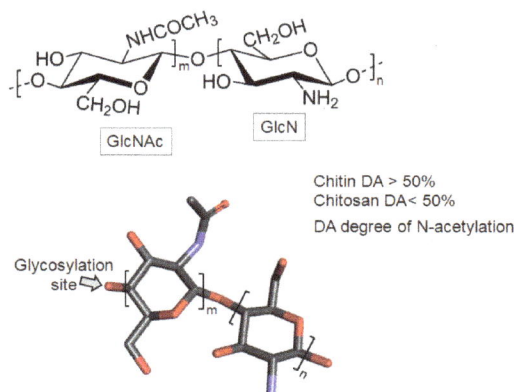

Figure 11. The chemical structures of chitin and chitosan. Chitin is consisting mainly of 2-acetamido-2-deoxy-D-β-glucose (N-acetylglucosamine, GlcNAc) units and partially of 2-amino-2-deoxy-β-D-glucose (glucosamine, GlcN) units, both 4-linked. When the degree of N-acetylation (DA) is less than 50% (GlcNAc content), the polymer is then named chitosan, otherwise, it is named chitin. DA is defined as the average number of N-acetylation per 100 monomers expressed as a percentage.

The chitosan molecule is non-toxic and has many biomedical applications, including bone tissue regeneration [109] and effects against a wide variety of pathogenic microorganisms [110–112]. Its proper use depends on many physicochemical factors and these factors can be managed accordingly to the levels of activity aimed for the chitosan. Examples of these factors are MW, degree of deacetylation, degree of substitution, length and position of a substituent in the GlcN units and pH [108].

The antineoplastic activity of chitin/chitosan and low MW chitin was evaluated using a human monocyte leukemia cell line, THP-1. Chitin and chitosan suppressed 100% growth of THP-1 tumor cells at concentrations equal to or greater than 1.5 mg/mL. The low MW chitin exhibited the same EC_{50} of 250 μg/mL [113].

Antioxidant property of chitosan was also investigated. Trung and Bao studied chitosan extracted from *L. vannamei* [114]. Their study suggested that the antioxidant effect observed was based on the free radical scavenging activity and the reduction potency. Another study related to the antioxidant effect of this marine glycan was carried out by Sarbon et al. [115]. In their work, the chitosan was extracted from the ladle shells species *Scylla olivacea*. The chitosan of *S. olivacea* exhibited a dose-dependent effect, where at the concentration of 10 mg/mL, the natural chitosan showed a greater reduction effect than the commercial chitosan.

Given the versatile applicability of this acetylated glycan, Divya et al. tested the antifungal and antioxidant activities of chitosan nanoparticles (ChNP) [116]. ChNP was tested in comparison to Amphotericin B, and showed good antifungal activity against all selected pathogens. The ChNP also exhibited significant antioxidant activity [116]. Previous work by the same group showed that chitosan nanoparticles inhibited the growth of clinically important microorganisms such as *Staphylococcus aureus*, *Pseudomona aeruginosa*, *Escherichia coli* and *Klebsiella pneumoniae* besides exhibiting antibiofilm activity with an inhibition rate of up to 98% [112].

A recent study was conducted with chitin/chitosan obtained from the shrimp shell *Penaeus monodon* [117]. These polysaccharides showed inhibitory effects on the proliferation of the human ovarian cancer cell line, PA-1. Chitin and chitosan can suppress 100% growth of PA-1 tumor cells at the respective concentrations of 50 µg/mL and 10 µg/mL, respectively [117].

3.4. Triterpene Glycosides

The glycosides consist of amphiphilic compounds which contain a sugar bound to another functional group through a glycosidic bond (Figure 12). While the sugar can be a simple unit (monosaccharide) or various units (oligosaccharide) and the aglycone (functional group) may be a terpene, a flavonoid, or any other naturally occurring molecules [2,118].

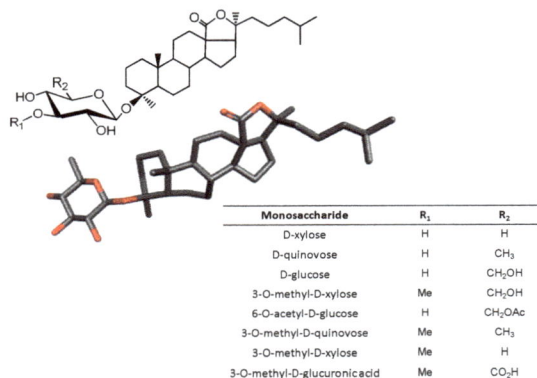

Monosaccharide	R_1	R_2
D-xylose	H	H
D-quinovose	H	CH_3
D-glucose	H	CH_2OH
3-O-methyl-D-xylose	Me	CH_2OH
6-O-acetyl-D-glucose	H	CH_2OAc
3-O-methyl-D-quinovose	Me	CH_3
3-O-methyl-D-xylose	Me	H
3-O-methyl-D-glucuronic acid	Me	CO_2H

Figure 12. Chemical structures of glycosides with a triterpene backbone of holostane type bound to a sugar unit (glucose, Glc, in the case) and the possible substituents shown at the insert table.

Glycosides of marine organisms can be isolated from sea cucumber [119], starfish [120], sponge [121], alga [122] and coral [123]. Due to the great diversity of marine glycosides, many studies have focused on the investigation of their therapeutic properties. For example, glycosides isolated from the edible red seaweed *Laurencia undulata*, called floridoside or D-isofloridoside, have their antioxidant property investigated by Li et al. The two compounds showed significant antioxidant activity and are potential inhibitors of MMP-2 and MMP-9 [124].

Aurantoside K (a tetramic acid glycoside isolated from a sponge belonging to the genus *Melophlus*) exhibited a broad spectrum of antifungal activity against strains of *Candida albicans*, with the minimum inhibitory concentration (MIC) of 31.25 µg/mL for a strain resistant to Amphotericin B, and 1.95 µg/mL for a wild-type strain. It also showed a zone of inhibition of 14 mm of diameter in the concentration of 100 µg/disc for yeast *Cryptococcus neoformans*, 28 mm for *Aspergillus niger*, 31 mm *Penicillium* sp., 21 mm *Rhizopus sporangia* and 29 mm *Sordaria* sp. [125]. Another study carried out with a class of triterpene glycosides, called variegatusides, isolated from the sea cucumber *Stichopus variegatus* (Holothuriidae), and showed that these compounds have potent in vitro antifungal activity [126].

Wang et al. verified the cytotoxic effects of 13 purified triterpenic glycosides of *Holothuria scabra* and *Cucumaria frondosa* (Holothuriidae) against four human cell lines in order to advance the structure-activity relationship of these compounds [127]. The results showed that the number of glycosyl residues in the sugar chains and the aglycone side chain may affect their cytotoxicity to tumor cells and selective cytotoxicity in neoplastic versus normal cells. Works like this arouse interests in the use of these glycosides for the development of new antitumor drugs [115].

Given a vast number of actions that these compounds can have, it is worth understanding the underlying mechanisms by which these molecules act. A good option to uncover their molecular mechanisms of action of the marine glycosides is by identifying the relationships between their structures and activities. In a review of Park et al. the relationship between their effects and their structures were attempted on several molecular types. For example, stichoposide C and D, both isolated from the holothurian *Stichopus chloronotus*, exert anticancer activity [128]. However, the activity of the compounds occurs by distinct mechanisms due to differences in the sugar content. Stichoposide C has quinovose, and induces apoptosis through the generation of ceramide by the activation of acidic sphingomyelinase (SMase) and neutral SMase. Stichoposide D, which possesses Glc as the second monosaccharide unit, induces apoptosis by the activation of ceramide 6 synthase leading to the increase of cellular levels of ceramide.

Following the same reasoning, a recent study compared the effects of three frondosides (A, B and C) extracted from *C. frondosa* and its aglycone against pancreatic cancer cells. What can be observed was that frondoside A potentially inhibited the growth of pancreatic cancer cells with an EC_{50} of ~1 μM. Frondoside B was less potent with an EC_{50} of ~2.5 μM. Frondoside C and aglycone had no effect [129]. Frondoside A has potent antiproliferative, anti-invasive and antiangiogenic effects on a variety of cancers [130–132].

Cyclic steroid glycosides isolated from the starfish *Echinaster luzonicus*, namely as luzonicoside A (LuzA) and D (LuzD), were tested for their potential inhibitory capacity against RPMI-7951 and SK-Mel-28 melanoma cell lines. LuzA inhibited proliferation, colony formation and migration of SK-Mel-28 cells more significantly than LuzD. The authors suggested that their mechanisms of action are related to the regulation of the activity of cleaved caspase-3 and poly (ADP-ribose) polymerase (PARP), together with the levels of Survivin, Bcl-2, p21 and cyclin D1 [120].

3.5. Glycoproteins

Glycoproteins are glycoconjugates in which various monosaccharides are covalently attached to the protein backbone. Two major types of sugar chains (*N*- and *O*-linked) are found in glycoproteins. *N*-linked sugar chains contain a GlcNAc residue at its reducing end which is attached to the amide group of an asparagine (Asn) residue of the polypeptide backbone. The *O*-linked sugar chains contain a residue of GalNAc at its reducing terminus which is attached to the hydroxyl group of either a serine (Ser) or threonine (Thr) residue of a polypeptide backbone (Figure 13) [133].

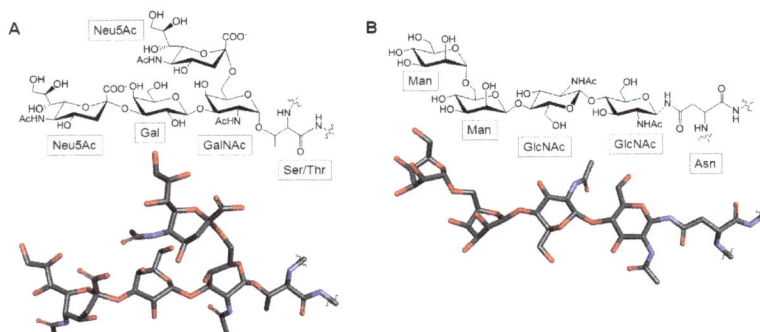

Figure 13. Chemical representatives of glycoproteins. While (**A**) *O*-linked glycans bind to the peptide chain by the hydroxyl group of a serine (Ser) or a threonine (Thr) residue, (**B**) *N*-linked glycans bind to the peptide chain by the amide group of an asparagine (Asn) residue.

Glycoproteins represent a large class of biomolecules. Many of the proteins that are components of cell membranes are glycosylated. Glycoproteins may have essential functions as receptors that capture various ligands into the cell such as transport proteins that are involved in the ingestion of various compounds, or as structures that mediate molecular recognition, signaling and interactions between cells [134]. For instance, lectins are excellent examples of biologically relevant glycoproteins found in marine organisms. Lectins are recognition proteins (glycosylated or not) of non-immune origin and endowed with the capacity to bind to the carbohydrate moieties of other glycoconjugates. Lectins play many varied biological functions including regulation of cell adhesion, recognition of molecules in cell-cell and cell-molecule interactions, and are also known to have vital immune functions [135]. Lectins are isolated from a variety of marine organisms including algae [136,137], sponges [138], mollusks [139] and echinoderms [140].

Many studies have reported the therapeutic effects of glycoproteins, especially lectins. For example, a study by Silva et al. aimed at the potential anti-inflammatory action of the lectin extracted from the red alga *Pterocladiella capillacea* [141]. The authors have observed a reasonable anti-inflammatory effect through both the paw edema model and the neutrophil migration model, based on the injection of carrageenan as an inflammation stimulus [141]. In a different work, the antinociceptive and anti-inflammatory effects of the lectin extracted from the red alga *Solieria filiformis* were evaluated [142]. In this work, the animals were pretreated with lectin by 30 min before receiving the nociceptive or inflammatory stimuli. The *S. filiformis* lectin significantly reduced the number of abdominal writhes and reduced the paw licking time in the formalin test. The lectin of *S. filiformis* also reduced neutrophil migration in a peritonitis model, in addition to reducing paw edema induced by carrageenan, dextran and serotonin [142]. In a recent work, Fontenelle et al. investigated the lectin extracted from the red seaweed *Bryothamnion triquetrum*, and reported its anti-inflammatory effect in mice [143].

Reports of anticancer activity of lectins have also been found in the literature. In one of the collected works, besides investigating the biological activity the authors also dealt with structural aspects of a lectin of the sea mollusk *Crenomytilus grayanus*. Cell viability assays have shown that *C. grayanus* lectin recognizes Gb3 globotriose on the surface of breast cancer cells, leading to cell death [144]. Also regarding anticancer activity, Liu et al. investigated the in vivo antitumor activity of hemocyanin (multifunctional glycoprotein) of the shrimp *L. vannamei* in Sarcoma-180 (S180) model of tumor-bearing mice [145]. After 8 days of treatment, the dose of 4 mg/kg significantly inhibited the growth of S180 to 49% compared to untreated animals [145].

In terms of antimicrobial activity, a new lectin was isolated from the green alga *Halimeda renschii*. The mannose-specificity lectin showed a potent activity against influenza virus in NCI-H292 cells at half maximal effective dose (ED$_{50}$) of 2.45 nM. Antiviral action occurred through high affinity binding to hemagglutinin from the viral envelope [137].

3.6. Glycolipids

Glycolipids comprise a large and diverse group of lipids that serve numerous cellular functions [146]. They are amphipathic lipids, containing a hydrophilic portion composed of units of carbohydrates, from which gives its name (the prefix "glyco"). The lipid moiety is referred to as the hydrophobic tail, generally constituted of aliphatic fatty acid chains [147].

Among the classes of glycolipids are glycosphingolipids that are constituents of cell membranes in a wide variety of organisms (either from terrestrial or marine habitat) [148]. These compounds have biotechnological potential and play an important physiological role due to variations in their sugar chains. They are classified into cerebrosides, ceramide oligohexosides, globosides and gangliosides based on the constituent sugars (Table 1). In recent years, some glycosphingolipids have been isolated from marine invertebrates such as echinoderms, porifera and mollusks [149].

Table 1. Classification of sphingolipids according to their sugar content.

Sugar Moiety	Glycosphingolipid
monosaccharide	cerebrosideo
disaccharide	ceramide dihexoside
oligosaccharide	ceramide oligohexoside
oligosaccharide + amino sugar	globoside
oligosaccharide + sulfate	sulfatide
oligosaccharide + sialic acid	ganglioside

Marine algae synthesize three major types of glycolipids, i.e., monogalactosil digliceride (MGDG), digalactosil diglyceride (DGDG) and sulfonoquinovosyl dipalmitoyl glyceride (SQDG) (Figure 14). These glycoglycerolipids are present in the chloroplasts of eukaryotic algae. MGDG and DGDG are the most abundant glycolipids of the thylakoid membrane and appear to play a crucial role in photosynthesis [150].

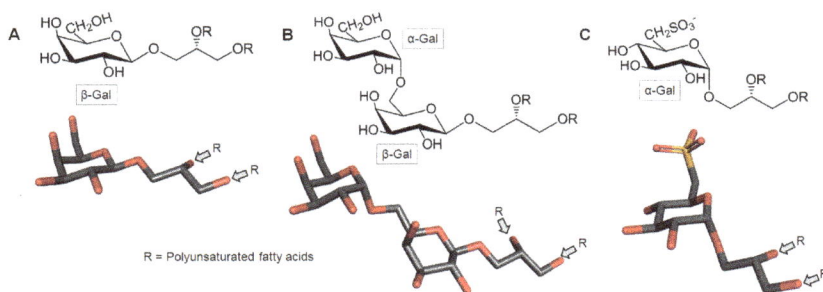

Figure 14. Representation of the general structure of the three main types of seaweed glycolipids. (**A**) Monogalactosil diglicerol (MGDG), (**B**) digalactosil diglicerol (DGDG) and (**C**) sulfonoquinovosyl dipalmitoyl glyceride (SQDG). R represents the acyl substituent chain.

Many researchers have sought biologically active glycolipids from marine organisms to elucidate the structure-function relationships of glycolipids and to develop new medicinal resources. A good example of this was the study where eight new cerebrosides named Renierosides were isolated from an extract of the marine sponge *Haliclona* (*Reniera*) sp. The isolated compounds exhibited cytotoxicity of five human tumor cell lines, including human lung cancer (A549), human ovarian cancer (SK-OV-3), human skin cancer (SK-MEL-2), cancer cell line of the human central nervous system (XF498) and human colon cancer (HCT15) [151].

Plouguerné et al. identified SGDGs in fractions obtained after the purification of the organic extract of the *Sargassum vulgare* brown alga [152]. These metabolites exhibited antiviral activity against the herpes simplex virus type 1 (HSV1) and 2 (HSV2) viruses. The main SQDG responsible for anti-HSV1 and anti-HSV2 activities was characterized as 1,2-di-*O*-palmitoyl-3-*O*-(6-sulfo-α-D-quinovopyranosyl) glycerol [152]. Two SQDGs isolated from the red alga *Palmaria palmata* showed potent anti-inflammatory activity. Bioactive compounds were identified as (2S) -1-*O*-eicosapentaenoyl-2-*O*-myristoyl-3-*O*-(6-sulfo-α-D-quinazopyranosyl)-glycerol and (2S) -1-*O*-eicosapentaenoyl-2-*O*-palmitoyl-3-*O*-(6-sulfo-α-D-quinovopyranosyl-glycerol and showed nitric oxide inhibitory activity with IC_{50} values of 36.5 and 11.0 µM, respectively [153].

In the paper by Reyes et al. the first characterization of the MGDGs, DGDGs and glycosylceramides from *Isochrysis galbana* (Haptophyte) was described together with a study of their anti-inflammatory property as inhibitors of tumor necrosis factor α (TNF-α), a protein of cell signaling involved in the inflammatory response of the acute systemic phase [154]. In a recent paper, Che et al. have described that sea cucumber cerebrosides have improved learning and memory deficits, protecting against oxidative stress in vivo, and increasing the survival rate of PC12 cells, a rat pheochromocytoma cell line [148].

Overall, the bioactivities of the glycoglycerides are directly related to the sugar moiety. The position of the glycerol binding to the sugar, the length and the location of the acyl chain and the anomeric sugar configuration are all key structural contributors [155].

3.7. Iminosugar

Naturally occurring imino- or azasugars are monosaccharides whose oxygen heteroatom in the ring structure is replaced by nitrogen. In 1960 the first member of this class of compounds was isolated and characterized, a 5-amino-5-deoxyglucose antibiotic called nojirimycin. Subsequently, more than 25 additional nojirimycin analogs were described from plant and microbial sources [156,157].

Iminosugars are commonly obtained from terrestrial sources or through chemical synthesis [158]. However, the work of Segraves and Crews described for the first time iminosugars from the marine environment [157]. In this work, three compounds were extracted from the sea sponge *Batzella sp.* and were presented as iminosugar nucleus with a long chain of alkyl substituent. They were identified as Batzellasides A, B and C (Figure 15). The identification of these compounds was made through comparison with the properties of known iminosugars derived from both natural and synthetic sources.

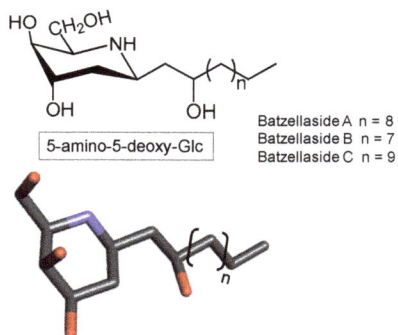

Figure 15. Representation of a nucleus of alkylated iminosugar. Batzellasides differ according to the length of the alkyl chain.

Iminosugars have potential therapeutic importance. These molecules can serve as antiviral [158], insecticidal [159], and nematicidal activities [160]. These potentials are associated with the ability of these molecules to selectively inhibit enzymes that degrade carbohydrates (glycosidases). The antiviral activity of iminosugars relies on its capacity to interfere with the glycoprotein processing [161].

Concerning the potential biomedical actions of iminosugars, the study of Segraves and Crews evaluated the antimicrobial action of the three iminosugars studied therein (batzellasides A, B and C) against the bacteria *Staphylococcus epidermidis* [157]. The three structures were able to inhibit the growth of this microorganism with MICs of 6.3 μg/mL [157].

The work of Sayce et al. has shown that the 1-deoxynojirimycin iminosugar bearing Glc and capable of inhibiting the production of infectious virus in vitro including dengue (DENV), hepatitis B, hepatitis C, HIV and influenza A viruses. Inhibition of endoplasmic reticulum α-glycosidases prevents virus release and is the main antiviral mechanism of action of iminosugars against DENV [161].

4. Concluding Remarks

The marine environment comprises a very rich source of biomedically potential compounds. Among these compounds, carbohydrate-based molecules and glycoconjugates are calling special attention, especially in light of the current development of the glycomics (sub) projects such as the marine medicinal glycomics [24]. Throughout this work we have seen a miscellany of investigations into the effects of marine glycans/glycoconjugate on human health. We have seen that in most of the time the beneficial effects of these molecules are related to their structural properties such as (a) length of the sugar chains, (b) monosaccharide composition, and above all, (c) the presence, (d) the type, and (e) the degree of substituents such as sulfation and/or acetylation. The chemical features of these molecules play a decisive role in their pharmacological properties. However, it is still necessary to understand the molecular mechanisms underlying these activities in order to understand the structural aspects of these molecules and what this diversity of structures may represent in the final effect. Despite advances in study techniques that have allowed a reasonable understanding of the structure-activity relationship and some underlying mechanisms of action of these compounds, clinical trials using marine glycans are still very scarce. At this point of the glycomics it is necessary to further evaluate the safety and efficacy of the carbohydrate-based molecules of marine origin, especially in the context of their large applications in potential formulation of new drugs and/or for the delivery of an end product to a specific site that a therapeutic intervention is required.

Author Contributions: Writing-Original Draft Preparation, A.A.V. & V.H.P.; Writing-Review & Editing, V.H.P.; Supervision & Initial Paper Outline, V.H.P.

Acknowledgments: The authors are grateful to the guest editor of the Special Issue "Marine Glycosides" Prof. Francisco Sarabia for the kind invitation to collaborate a paper from our authorship to this Special Issue.

Conflicts of Interest: The authors declare no conflict of interest.

References

1. Snelgrove, P.V.R. An ocean of discovery: Biodiversity beyond the census of marine life. *Planta Med.* **2016**, *82*, 790–799. [CrossRef] [PubMed]
2. Kang, H.K.; Seo, C.H.; Park, Y. The effects of marine carbohydrates and glycosylated compounds on human health. *Int. J. Mol. Sci.* **2015**, *16*, 6018–6056. [CrossRef] [PubMed]
3. Malve, H. Exploring the ocean for new drug developments: Marine pharmacology. *J. Pharm. Bioallied Sci.* **2016**, *8*, 83–91. [CrossRef] [PubMed]
4. Molinski, T.F.; Dalisay, D.S.; Lievens, S.L.; Saludes, J.P. Drug development from marine natural products. *Nat. Rev. Drug Discov.* **2009**, *8*, 69–85. [CrossRef] [PubMed]
5. Schumacher, M.; Kelkel, M.; Dicato, M.; Diederich, M. Gold from the sea: Marine compounds as inhibitors of the hallmarks of cancer. *Biotechnol. Adv.* **2011**, *29*, 531–547. [CrossRef] [PubMed]
6. Vo, T.S.; Ngo, D.H.; Ta, Q.V.; Kim, S.K. Marine organisms as a therapeutic source against herpes simplex virus infection. *Eur. J. Pharm. Sci.* **2011**, *44*, 11–20. [CrossRef] [PubMed]

7.   Pomin, V.H. Antimicrobial sulfated glycans: Structure and function. *Curr. Top. Med. Chem.* **2017**, *17*, 319–330. [CrossRef] [PubMed]

8.   Pomin, V.H.; Bezerra, F.F.; Soares, P.A.G. Sulfated glycans in HIV infection and therapy. *Curr. Pharm. Des.* **2017**, *23*, 3405–3414. [CrossRef] [PubMed]

9.   Vacquier, V.D. Evolution of gamete recognition proteins. *Science* **1998**, *281*, 1995–1998. [CrossRef] [PubMed]

10.   Vilela-Silva, A.C.E.S.; Alves, A.P.; Valente, A.P.; Vacquier, V.D.; Mourão, P.A.S. Structure of the sulfated α-L-fucan from the egg jelly coat of the sea urchin *Strongylocentrotus franciscanus*: Patterns of preferential 2-O and 4-O-sulfation determine sperm cell recognition. *Glycobiology* **1999**, *9*, 927–933. [CrossRef] [PubMed]

11.   Pomin, V.H. Sulfated glycans in sea urchin fertilization. *Glycoconj. J.* **2015**, *32*, 9–15. [CrossRef] [PubMed]

12.   Alpuchea, J.; Pereyrab, A.; Agundis, C.; Rosasa, C.; Pascuala, C.; Slomiannyc, M.C.; Vázquez, L.; Zentenob, E. Purification and characterization of a lectin from the white shrimp *Litopenaeus setiferus* (*Crustacea decapoda*) hemolymph. *Biochim. Biophys. Acta* **2005**, *1724*, 86–93. [CrossRef] [PubMed]

13.   Chiu, P.C.N.; Tsang, H.Y.; Koistinen, H.; Seppala, M.; Lee, K.F.; Yeung, W.S.B. The contribution of D-mannose, L-fucose, N-acetylglucosamine, and selectin residues on the binding of glycodenlin isoforms to human spermatozoa. *Biol. Reprod.* **2004**, *70*, 1710–1719. [CrossRef] [PubMed]

14.   Glavey, S.V.; Huynh, D.; Reagana, M.R.; Manier, S.; Moschetta, M.; Kawano, Y.; Roccaro, A.M.; Ghobrial, I.M.; Joshi, L.; O'Dwyer, M.E. The cancer glycome: Carbohydrates as mediators of metastasis. *Blood Rev.* **2015**, *29*, 269–279. [CrossRef] [PubMed]

15.   Kang, Y.; Wang, Z.J.; Xie, D.; Sun, X.; Yang, W.; Zhao, X.; Xu, N. Characterization and potential antitumor activity of polysaccharide from *Gracilariopsis lemaneiformis*. *Mar. Drugs* **2017**, *15*. [CrossRef] [PubMed]

16.   Zhou, G.; Sheng, W.; Yao, W.; Wang, C. Effect of low molecular λ-carrageenan from *Chondrus ocellatus* on antitumor H-22 activity of 5-Fu. *Pharmacol. Res.* **2006**, *53*, 129–134. [CrossRef] [PubMed]

17.   Hidari, K.I.P.J.; Takahashi, N.; Arihara, M.; Nagaoka, M.; Morita, K.; Suzuki, T. Structure and anti-dengue virus activity of sulfated polysaccharide from a marine alga. *Biochem. Biophys. Res. Commun.* **2008**, *376*, 91–95. [CrossRef] [PubMed]

18.   Talarico, L.B.; Damonte, E.B. Interference in dengue virus adsorption and uncoating by carrageenans. *Virology* **2007**, *363*, 473–485. [CrossRef] [PubMed]

19.   Pomin, V.H. Structure-function relationship of anticoagulant and antithrombotic well-defined sulfated polysaccharides from marine invertebrates. *Adv. Food. Nutr. Res.* **2012**, *65*, 195–209. [PubMed]

20.   Vinsová, J.; Vavríková, E. Chitosan derivatives with antimicrobial, antitumour and antioxidant activities—A review. *Curr. Pharm. Des.* **2011**, *17*, 3596–3607. [CrossRef]

21.   Lee, S.H.; Ko, C.I.; Ahn, G.; You, S.; Kim, J.S.; Heu, M.S.; Kim, J.; Jee, Y.; Jeon, Y.J. Molecular characteristics and anti-inflammatory activity of the fucoidan extracted from *Ecklonia cava*. *Carbohydr. Polym.* **2012**, *20*, 599–606. [CrossRef] [PubMed]

22.   Pomin, V.H. Sulfated glycans in inflammation. *Eur. J. Med. Chem.* **2015**, *6*, 353–369. [CrossRef] [PubMed]

23.   Ernst, B.; Magnani, J.L. From carbohydrate leads to glycomimetic drugs. *Nat. Rev. Drug Discov.* **2009**, *8*, 661–677. [CrossRef] [PubMed]

24.   Pomin, V.H. Marine medicinal glycomics. *Front. Cell. Infect. Microbiol.* **2014**, *4*, 1–13. [CrossRef] [PubMed]

25.   Sanjeewa, K.K.A.; Lee, J.S.; Kim, W.S.; Jeon, Y.J. The potential of brown-algae polysaccharides for the development of anticancer agents: An update on anticancer effects reported for fucoidan and laminaran. *Carbohydr. Polym.* **2017**, *177*, 451–459. [CrossRef] [PubMed]

26.   Rioux, L.E.; Turgeon, S.L.; Beaulieu, M. Structural characterization of laminaran and galactofucan extracted from the brown seaweed *Saccharina longicruris*. *Phytochemistry* **2010**, *71*, 1586–1595. [CrossRef] [PubMed]

27.   Rioux, L.E.; Turgeon, S.L.; Beaulieu, M. Effect of season on the composition of bioactive polysaccharides from the brown seaweed *Saccharina longicruris*. *Phytochemistry* **2009**, *70*, 1069–1075. [CrossRef] [PubMed]

28.   Kadam, S.U.; Tiwari, B.K.; O'Donnell, C.P. Extraction, structure and biofunctional activities of laminarin from brown algae. *Int. J. Food Sci. Technol.* **2015**, *50*, 24–31. [CrossRef]

29.   Usoltseva, P.V.; Shevchenko, N.M.; Malyarenko, O.S.; Ishina, I.A.; Ivannikova, S.I.; Ermakova, S.P. Structure and anticancer activity of native and modified polysaccharides from brown alga *Dictyota dichotoma*. *Carbohydr. Polym.* **2018**, *180*, 21–28. [CrossRef] [PubMed]

30.   Malyarenko, O.S.; Roza, V.; Usoltseva, R.V.; Shevchenko, N.M.; Isakov, V.V.; Zvyagintseva, T.N.; Ermakova, S.P. In vitro anticancer activity of the laminarans from Far Eastern brown seaweeds and their sulfated derivatives. *J. Appl. Phycol.* **2017**, *29*, 543–553. [CrossRef]

31. Lee, J.Y.; Kim, Y.J.; Kim, H.J.; Kim, Y.S.; Park, W. Immunostimulatory effect of laminarin on RAW 264.7 mouse macrophages. *Molecules* **2012**, *17*, 5404–5411. [CrossRef] [PubMed]
32. Kuda, T.; Kosaka, M.; Hirano, S.; Kawahara, M.; Sato, M.; Kaneshima, T.; Nishizawa, M.; Takahashi, H.; Kimura, B. Effect of sodium-alginate and laminaran on *Salmonella Typhimurium* infection in human enterocyte-like HT-29-Luc cells and BALB/c mice. *Carbohydr. Polym.* **2015**, *125*, 113–119. [CrossRef] [PubMed]
33. Ahmadi, A.; Zorofchian, S.; Moghadamtousi, S.Z.; Abubakar, S.; Zandi, K. Antiviral potential of algae polysaccharides isolated from marine sources: A review. *Biomed. Res. Int.* **2015**, *2015*, 1–10. [CrossRef] [PubMed]
34. Lee, K.Y.; Mooney, D.J. Alginate: Properties and biomedical applications. *Prog. Polym. Sci.* **2012**, *37*, 106–126. [CrossRef] [PubMed]
35. Draget, K.I.; Moe, S.T.; Skjak-Braek, G.; Smidsrod, O. Alginates. In *Food Polysaccharides and Their Applications*, 2nd ed.; Stephen, A.M., Phillips, G.O., Williams, P.A., Eds.; Taylor and Francis Group Press: Boca Raton, FL, USA, 2006.
36. So, M.J.; Kim, B.K.; Choi, M.J.; Park, K.Y.; Rhee, S.H.; Cho, E.J. Protective activity of fucoidan and alginic acid against free radical-induced oxidative stress under in vitro and cellular system. *J. Food Sci. Nutr.* **2007**, *12*, 191–196. [CrossRef]
37. Sarithakumari, C.H.; Renju, G.L.; Kurup, G.M. Anti-inflammatory and antioxidant potential of alginic acid isolated from the marine algae, *Sargassum wightii* on adjuvant-induced arthritic rats. *Inflammopharmacology* **2013**, *21*, 261–268. [CrossRef] [PubMed]
38. Endo, Y.; Aota, T.; Tsukui, T. Antioxidant activity of alginic acid in minced pork meat. *Food Sci. Technol. Res.* **2015**, *21*, 875–878. [CrossRef]
39. Neetoo, H.; Ye, M.; Chen, H. Bioactive alginate coatings to control *Listeria monocytogenes* on cold-smoked salmon slices and fillets. *Int. J. Food Microbiol.* **2010**, *136*, 326–331. [CrossRef] [PubMed]
40. Karunanithi, P.; Murali, M.R.; Samuel, S.; Raghavendran, H.R.B.; Abbas, A.A.; Kamarul, T. Three dimensional alginate-fucoidan composite hydrogel augments the chondrogenic differentiation of mesenchymal stromal cells. *Carbohydr. Polym.* **2016**, *147*, 294–303. [CrossRef] [PubMed]
41. Alea, M.T.; Meyer, A.S. Fucoidans from brown seaweeds: An update on structures, extraction techniques and use of enzymes as tools for structural elucidation. *RSC Adv.* **2013**, *3*, 8131–8141. [CrossRef]
42. Percival, E.G.V.; Ross, A.G. Fucoidin. Part 1. The isolation and purification of fucoidin from brown seaweeds. *J. Chem. Soc.* **1950**, *145*, 717–720. [CrossRef]
43. Patankar, M.S.; Oehninger, S.; Barnett, T.; Williams, R.L.; Clark, G.F. A revised structure for fucoidan may explain some of its biological activities. *J. Biol. Chem.* **1993**, *268*, 21770–21776. [PubMed]
44. Holtkamp, A.D.; Kelly, S.; Ulber, R.; Lang, S. Fucoidans and fucoidanases—Focus on techniques for molecular structure elucidation and modification of marine polysaccharides. *Appl. Microbiol. Biotechnol.* **2009**, *82*, 1–11. [CrossRef] [PubMed]
45. Bilan, M.I.; Grachev, A.A.; Ustuzhanina, N.E.; Shashkov, A.S.; Nifantiev, N.E.; Usov, A.I. Structure of a fucoidan from the brown seaweed *Fucus evanescens* C.Ag. *Carbohydr. Res.* **2002**, *337*, 719–730. [CrossRef]
46. Pomin, V.H.; Mourão, P.A. Structure, biology, evolution, and medical importance of sulfated fucans and galactans. *Glycobiology* **2008**, *18*, 1016–1027. [CrossRef] [PubMed]
47. Fitton, J.H.; Stringer, D.N.; Karpiniec, S.S. Therapies from fucoidan: An update. *Mar. Drugs* **2015**, *13*, 5920–5946. [CrossRef] [PubMed]
48. Fitton, J.H. Therapies from fucoidan; Multifunctional marine polymers. *Mar. Drugs* **2011**, *9*, 1731–1760. [CrossRef] [PubMed]
49. Cumashi, A.; Ushakova, N.A.; Preobrazhenskaya, M.E.; D'Incecco, A.; Piccoli, A.; Totani, L.; Tinari, N.; Morozevich, G.E.; Berman, A.E.; Bilan, M.I.; et al. Consorzio interuniversitario nazionale per la bio-oncologia, Italy. A comparative study of the anti-inflammatory, anticoagulant, antiangiogenic, and antiadhesive activities of nine different fucoidans from brown seaweeds. *Glycobiology* **2007**, *17*, 541–552. [CrossRef] [PubMed]
50. Ushakova, N.A.; Morozevich, G.E.; Ustyuzhanina, N.E.; Bilan, M.I.; Usov, A.I.; Nifantiev, N.E.; Preobrazhenskaya, M.E. Anticoagulant activity of fucoidans from brown algae. *Biochem. Suppl. Ser. B* **2009**, *3*, 77–83. [CrossRef]

51. Irhimeh, M.R.; Fitton, J.H.; Lowenthala, R.M. Pilot clinical study to evaluate the anticoagulant activity of fucoidan. *Blood Coagul. Fibrinolysis* **2009**, *20*, 607–610. [CrossRef] [PubMed]

52. Yang, Q.; Yang, R.; Li, M.; Zhou, Q.; Liang, X.; Elmada, Z.C. Effects of dietary fucoidan on the blood constituents, anti-oxidation and innate immunity of juvenile yellow catfish (*Pelteobagrus fulvidraco*). *Fish Shellfish. Immunol.* **2014**, *41*, 264–270. [CrossRef] [PubMed]

53. Ermakova, S.; Sokolova, R.; Kim, S.M.; Um, B.H.; Isakov, V.; Zvyagintseva, T. Fucoidans from brown seaweeds *Sargassum hornery*, *Ecklonia cava*, *Costaria costata*: Structural characteristics and anticancer activity. *Appl. Biochem. Biotechnol.* **2011**, *164*, 841–850. [CrossRef] [PubMed]

54. Vishchuk, O.S.; Ermakova, S.P.; Zvyagintseva, T.N. Sulfated polysaccharides from brown seaweeds *Saccharina japonica* and *Undaria pinnatifida*: Isolation, structural characteristics, and antitumor activity. *Carbohydr. Res.* **2011**, *346*, 2769–2776. [CrossRef] [PubMed]

55. Usoltsevaa, R.V.; Anastyuka, S.D.; Ishinaa, I.A.; Isakova, V.V.; Zvyagintsevaa, T.N.; Thinhb, P.D.; Zadorozhnyc, P.A.; Dmitrenok, P.S.; Ermakovaa, S.P. Structural characteristics and anticancer activity in vitro of fucoidan from brown algae *Padina boryana*. *Carbohydr. Polym.* **2018**, *184*, 260–268. [CrossRef] [PubMed]

56. Thuy, T.T.; Ly, B.M.; Van, T.T.; Quang, N.V.; Tu, H.C.; Zheng, Y.; Seguin-Devaux, C.; Mi, B.; Ai, U. Anti-HIV activity of fucoidans from three brown seaweed species. *Carbohydr. Polym.* **2015**, *115*, 122–128. [CrossRef] [PubMed]

57. Rajeshkumar, S. Phytochemical constituents of fucoidan (*Padina tetrastromatica*) and its assisted AgNPs for enhanced antibacterial activity. *IET Nanobiotechnol.* **2017**, *3*, 292–299. [CrossRef] [PubMed]

58. Pomin, V.H. Structural and functional insights into sulfated galactans: A systematic review. *Glycoconj. J.* **2010**, *1*, 1–12. [CrossRef] [PubMed]

59. Van de Velde, F.; Pereira, L.; Rollema, H.S. The revised NMR chemical shift data of carrageenans. *Carbohydr. Res.* **2004**, *339*, 2309–2313. [CrossRef] [PubMed]

60. Campo, V.L.; Kawano, D.F.; Silva, D.B., Jr.; Carvalho, I. Carrageenans: Biological properties, chemical modifications and structural analysis—A review. *Carbohydr. Polym.* **2009**, *77*, 167–180. [CrossRef]

61. Cash, M.J. New iota carrageenan allows gelatin replacement, simplified manufacturing, and new textures for confectionary applications. In Proceedings of the Abstract of IFT Annual Meeting, Dallas, TX, USA, 10–14 June 2000.

62. Sun, Y.; Yang, B.; Wu, Y.; Liu, Y.; Gu, X.; Zhang, H.; Wang, C.; Cao, H.; Huang, L.; Wang, Z. Structural characterization and antioxidant activities of κ-carrageenan oligosaccharides degraded by different methods. *Food Chem.* **2015**, *178*, 311–318. [CrossRef] [PubMed]

63. Lucille Abad, V.; Relleve, L.S.; Racadio, C.D.T.; Aranilla, C.T.; De la Rosa, A.M. Antioxidant activity potential of gamma irradiated carrageenan. *Appl. Radiat. Isot.* **2013**, *79*, 73–79. [CrossRef] [PubMed]

64. Diogo, J.V.; Novo, S.G.; González, M.J.; Ciancia, M.; Bratanich, A.C. Antiviral activity of lambda-carrageenan prepared from red seaweed (*Gigartina skottsbergii*) against BoHV-1 and SuHV-1. *Res. Vet. Sci.* **2015**, *98*, 142–144. [CrossRef] [PubMed]

65. Leibbrandt, A.; Meier, C.; König-Schuster, M.; Weinmüllner, R.; Kalthoff, D.; Pflugfelder, B.; Graf, P.; Frank-Gehrke, B.; Beer, M.; Fazekas, T.; et al. Iota-carrageenan is a potent inhibitor of influenza a virus infection. *PLoS ONE* **2010**, *5*. [CrossRef] [PubMed]

66. Luo, Z.; Tian, D.; Zhou, M.; Xiao, W.; Zhang, Y.; Li, M.; Sui, B.; Wang, W.; Guan, H.; Chen, H.; et al. λ-carrageenan P32 is a potent inhibitor of rabies virus infection. *PLoS ONE* **2015**, *10*. [CrossRef] [PubMed]

67. Prasedya, E.S.; Miyake, M.; Kobayashi, D.; Hazama, A. Carrageenan delays cell cycle progression in human cancer cells in vitro demonstrated by FUCCI imaging. *BMC Complement. Altern. Med.* **2016**, *16*, 2–9. [CrossRef] [PubMed]

68. Kalitnik, A.A.; Karetin, Y.A.; Kravchenko, A.O.; Khasina, E.I.; Yermak, I.M. Influence of carrageenan on cytokine production and cellular activity of mouse peritoneal macrophages and its effect on experimental endotoxemia. *J. Biomed. Mater. Res. A* **2017**, *105*, 1549–1557. [CrossRef] [PubMed]

69. Murad, H.; Ghannam, A.; Al-Ktaifani, M.; Abbas, A.; Hawat, M. Algal sulfated carrageenan inhibits proliferation of MDA-MB-231 cells via apoptosis regulatory genes. *Mol. Med. Rep.* **2014**, *11*, 2153–2158. [CrossRef] [PubMed]

70. Luo, M.; Shao, B.; Nie, W.; Wei, X.W.; Li, Y.L.; Wang, B.L.; He, Z.Y.; Liang, X.; Ye, T.H.; Wei, Y.Q. Antitumor and adjuvant activity of λ-carrageenan by stimulating immune response in cancer immunotherapy. *Sci. Rep.* **2015**, *5*. [CrossRef] [PubMed]

71. McKim, J.M., Jr.; Baas, H.; Rice, G.P.; Willoughby, J.A., Sr.; Weiner, M.L.; Blakemore, W. Effects of carrageenan on cell permeability, cytotoxicity, and cytokine gene expression in human intestinal and hepatic cell lines. *Food Chem. Toxicol.* **2016**, *96*, 1–10. [CrossRef] [PubMed]
72. Souza, R.B.; Frota, A.F.; Sousa, R.S.; Cezario, N.A.; Santos, T.B.; Souza, L.M.; Coura, C.O.; Monteiro, V.S.; Cristino Filho, G.; Vasconcelos, S.M.; et al. Neuroprotective effects of sulphated agaran from marine alga *Gracilaria cornea* in Rat 6-hydroxydopamine Parkinson's disease model: Behavioural, neurochemical and transcriptional alterations. *Basic Clin. Pharmacol. Toxicol.* **2017**, *120*, 159–170. [CrossRef] [PubMed]
73. Lu, C.X.; Li, J.; Sun, Y.X.; Qi, X.; Wanga, Q.J.; Xin, X.L.; Geng, M.Y. Sulfated polymannuroguluronate, a novel anti-AIDS drug candidate, inhibits HIV-1 Tat-induced angiogenesis in Kaposi's sarcoma cells. *Biochem. Pharmacol.* **2007**, *74*, 1330–1339. [CrossRef] [PubMed]
74. Liu, H.; Geng, M.; Xin, X.; Li, F.; Zhang, Z.; Li, J.; Ding, J. Multiple and multivalent interactions of novel anti-AIDS drug candidates, sulfated polymannuronate (SPMG)-derived oligosaccharides, with gp120 and their anti-HIV activities. *Glycobiology* **2005**, *15*, 501–510. [CrossRef] [PubMed]
75. Miao, B.; Geng, M.; Li, J.; Li, F.; Chen, H.; Guan, H.; Ding, J. Sulfated polymannuroguluronate, a novel anti-acquired immune deficiency syndrome (AIDS) drug candidate, targeting CD4 in lymphocytes. *Biochem. Pharmacol.* **2004**, *68*, 641–649. [CrossRef] [PubMed]
76. Pomin, V.H.; Mulloy, B. Glycosaminoglycans and proteoglycans. *Pharmaceuticals* **2018**, *11*, 27. [CrossRef] [PubMed]
77. Vasconcelos, A.A.; Pomin, V.H. The sea as a rich source of structurally unique glycosaminoglycans and mimetics. *Microorganisms* **2017**, *5*, 51. [CrossRef] [PubMed]
78. Andrade, G.P.V.; Lima, M.A.; Souza, A.A., Jr.; Fareed, J.; Hoppensteadt, D.A.; Santos, E.A.; Chavante, S.F.; Oliveira, F.W.; Rocha, H.A.O.; Nader, H.B. A heparin-like compound isolated from a marine crab rich in glucuronic acid 2-O-sulfate presents low anticoagulant activity. *Carbohydr. Polym.* **2013**, *94*, 647–654. [CrossRef] [PubMed]
79. Brito, A.S.; Arimatéia, D.S.; Souza, L.R.; Lima, M.A.; Santos, V.O.; Medeiros, V.P.; Ferreira, P.A.; Silva, R.A.; Ferreira, C.V.; Justo, G.Z.; et al. Anti-inflammatory properties of a heparin-like glycosaminoglycan with reduced anti-coagulant activity isolated from a marine shrimp. *Bioorg. Med. Chem.* **2008**, *16*, 9588–9595. [CrossRef] [PubMed]
80. Dietrich, C.P.; Paiva, J.F.; Castro, R.A.; Chavante, S.F.; Jeske, W.; Fareed, J.; Gorin, P.A.; Mendes, A.; Nader, H.B. Structural features and anticoagulant activities of a novel natural low molecular weight heparin from the shrimp *Penaeus brasiliensis*. *Biochim. Biophys. Acta* **1999**, *1428*, 273–283. [CrossRef]
81. Nader, H.B.; Lopes, C.C.; Rocha, H.A.; Santos, E.A.; Dietrich, C.P. Heparins and heparinoids: Occurrence, structure and mechanism of antithrombotic and hemorrhagic activities. *Curr. Pharm. Des.* **2004**, *10*, 951–966. [CrossRef] [PubMed]
82. Dreyfuss, J.L.; Regatieri, C.V.; Lima, M.A.; Paredes-Gamero, E.J.; Brito, A.S.; Chavante, S.F.; Belfort, R., Jr.; Farah, M.E.; Nader, H.B. A heparin mimetic isolated from a marine shrimp suppresses neovascularization. *J. Thromb. Haemost.* **2010**, *8*, 1828–1837. [CrossRef] [PubMed]
83. Belmiro, C.L.; Castelo-Branco, M.T.; Melim, L.M.; Schanaider, A.; Elia, C.; Madi, K.; Pavão, M.S.; de Souza, H.S. Unfractionated heparin and new heparin analogues from ascidians (chordate-tunicate) ameliorate colitis in rats. *J. Biol. Chem.* **2009**, *284*, 11267–11278. [CrossRef] [PubMed]
84. Pomin, V.H. ¹H and (15)N NMR analyses on heparin, heparan sulfates and related monosaccharides concerning the chemical exchange regime of the N-Sulfo-glucosamine sulfamate proton. *Pharmaceuticals* **2016**, *9*, 58. [CrossRef] [PubMed]
85. Chavante, S.F.; Santos, E.A.; Oliveira, F.W.; Guerrini, M.; Torri, G.; Casu, B.; Dietrich, C.P.; Nader, H.B. A novel heparan sulphate with high degree of N-sulphation and high heparin cofactor-II activity from the brine shrimp *Artemia franciscana*. *Int. J. Biol. Macromol.* **2000**, *27*, 49–57. [CrossRef]
86. Gomes, A.M.; Kozlowski, E.O.; Pomin, V.H.; de Barros, C.M.; Zaganeli, J.L.; Pavão, M.S. Unique extracellular matrix heparan sulfate from the bivalve *Nodipecten nodosus* (Linnaeus, 1758) safely inhibits arterial thrombosis after photochemically induced endothelial lesion. *J. Biol. Chem.* **2010**, *285*, 7312–7323. [CrossRef] [PubMed]
87. Gomes, A.M.; Kozlowski, E.O.; Borsig, L.; Teixeira, F.C.; Vlodavsky, I.; Pavão, M.S. Antitumor properties of a new non-anticoagulant heparin analog from the mollusk *Nodipecten nodosus*: Effect on P-selectin, heparanase, metastasis and cellular recruitment. *Glycobiology* **2015**, *25*, 386–393. [CrossRef] [PubMed]

88. Volpi, N.; Maccari, F. Structural characterization and antithrombin activity of dermatan sulfate purified from marine clam *Scapharca inaequivalvis*. *Glycobiology* **2009**, *4*, 356–367. [CrossRef] [PubMed]

89. Gandra, M.; Cavalcante, M.C.M.; Pavão, M.S.G. Anticoagulant sulfated glycosaminoglycans in the tissues of the primitive chordate *Styela plicata* (Tunicata). *Glycobiology* **2000**, *10*, 1333–1340. [CrossRef] [PubMed]

90. Pavão, M.S.G.; Mourão, P.A.S.; Mulloy, B.; Tollefsen, D.M. A unique dermatan sulfate-like glycosaminoglycan from ascidian. Its structure and the effect of its unusual sulfation pattern on anticoagulant activity. *J. Biol. Chem.* **1995**, *270*, 31027–31036. [CrossRef] [PubMed]

91. Pavão, M.S.; Aiello, K.R.; Werneck, C.C.; Silva, L.C.; Valente, A.P.; Mulloy, B.; Colwell, N.S.; Tollefsen, D.M.; Mourão, P.A. Highly sulfated dermatan sulfates from Ascidians. Structure versus anticoagulant activity of these glycosaminoglycans. *J. Biol. Chem.* **1998**, *273*, 27848–27857. [CrossRef] [PubMed]

92. Kozlowski, E.O.; Pavão, M.S.; Borsig, L. Ascidian dermatan sulfates attenuate metastasis, inflammation and thrombosis by inhibition of P-selectin. *J. Thromb. Haemost.* **2011**, *9*, 1807–1815. [CrossRef] [PubMed]

93. Pomin, V.H. Holothurian fucosylated chondroitin sulfate. *Mar. Drugs* **2014**, *1*, 232–254. [CrossRef] [PubMed]

94. Zhang, X.; Yao, W.; Xu, X.; Sun, H.; Zhao, J.; Meng, X.; Wu, M.; Li, Z. synthesis of fucosylated chondroitin sulfate glycoclusters: A robust route to new anticoagulant agents. *Chemistry* **2018**, *24*, 1694–1700. [CrossRef] [PubMed]

95. Liu, X.; Liu, Y.; Hao, J.; Zhao, X.; Lang, Y.; Fan, F.; Cai, C.; Li, G.; Zhang, L.; Yu, G. In vivo anti-cancer mechanism of low-molecular-weight fucosylated chondroitin sulfate (LFCS) from sea cucumber *Cucumaria frondosa*. *Molecules* **2016**, *21*, 625. [CrossRef] [PubMed]

96. Panagos, C.G.; Thomson, D.S.; Moss, C.; Hughes, A.D.; Kelly, M.S.; Liu, Y.; Chai, W.; Venkatasamy, R.; Spina, D.; Page, C.P.; et al. Fucosylated chondroitin sulfates from the body wall of the sea cucumber *Holothuria forskali*: Conformation, selectin binding, and biological activity. *J. Biol. Chem.* **2014**, *289*, 28284–28298. [CrossRef] [PubMed]

97. Huang, N.; Wu, M.Y.; Zheng, C.B.; Zhu, L.; Zhao, J.H.; Zheng, Y.T. The depolymerized fucosylated chondroitin sulfate from sea cucumber potently inhibits HIV replication via interfering with virus entry. *Carbohydr. Res.* **2013**, *380*, 64–69. [CrossRef] [PubMed]

98. Mou, J.; Li, Q.; Qi, X.; Yang, J. Structural comparison, antioxidant and anti-inflammatory properties of fucosylated chondroitin sulfate of three edible sea cucumbers. *Carbohydr. Polym.* **2018**, *185*, 41–47. [CrossRef] [PubMed]

99. Ustyuzhanina, N.E.; Bilan, M.I.; Dmitrenok, A.S.; Shashkov, A.S.; Kusaykin, M.I.; Stonik, V.A.; Nifantiev, N.E.; Usov, A.I. Structure and biological activity of a fucosylated chondroitin sulfate from the sea cucumber *Cucumaria japonica*. *Glycobiology* **2016**, *5*, 449–459. [CrossRef] [PubMed]

100. Li, Q.; Cai, C.; Chang, Y.; Zhang, F.; Linhardt, R.J.; Xue, C.; Li, G.; Yu, G. A novel structural fucosylated chondroitin sulfate from *Holothuria Mexicana* and its effects on growth factors binding and anticoagulation. *Carbohydr. Polym.* **2018**, *181*, 1160–1168. [CrossRef] [PubMed]

101. Yang, L.; Wang, Y.; Yang, S.; Lv, Z. Separation, purification, structures and anticoagulant activities of fucosylated chondroitin sulfates from *Holothuria scabra*. *Int. J. Biol. Macromol.* **2018**, *108*, 710–718. [CrossRef] [PubMed]

102. Hoshino, H.; Heiwamachi, M. Anti-HIV Drug. European Patent EP 0410002A1, 1991.

103. Zhang, H.; Li, Y.; Li, L.; Liu, H.; Hu, L.; Dai, Y.; Chen, J.; Xu, S.; Chen, W.; Xu, X.; et al. Propylene glycol alginate sodium sulfate alleviates cerulein-induced acute pancreatitis by modulating the MEK/ERK pathway in mice. *Mar. Drugs* **2017**, *15*, 45. [CrossRef] [PubMed]

104. Xin, M.; Ren, L.; Sun, Y.; Li, H.H.; Guan, H.S.; He, X.X.; Li, C.X. Anticoagulant and antithrombotic activities of low-molecular-weight propylene glycol alginate sodium sulfate (PSS). *Eur. J. Med. Chem.* **2016**, *114*, 33–40. [CrossRef] [PubMed]

105. Xue, Y.T.; Li, S.; Liu, W.J.; Xin, M.; Li, H.H.; Yu, G.L.; Guan, H.S.; He, X.X.; Li, C.X. The mechanisms of sulfated polysaccharide drug of propylene glycol alginate sodium sulfate (PSS) on bleeding side effect. *Carbohydr. Polym.* **2018**, *194*, 365–374. [CrossRef] [PubMed]

106. Xu, S.; Niu, P.; Chen, K.; Xia, Y.; Yu, Q.; Liu, N.; Li, J.; Li, S.; Wu, L.; Feng, J.; et al. The liver protection of propylene glycol alginate sodium sulfate preconditioning against ischemia reperfusion injury: Focusing MAPK pathway activity. *Sci. Rep.* **2017**, *7*. [CrossRef] [PubMed]

107. Li, P.; Hao, J.; Li, H.; Guan, H.; Li, C. Development of an enteric nanoparticle of marine sulfated polysaccharide propylene glycol alginate sodium sulfate for oral administration: Formulation design, pharmacokinetics and efficacy. *J. Pharm. Pharmacol.* **2018**. [CrossRef] [PubMed]

108. Kumirska, J.; Czerwicka, M.; Kaczyński, Z.; Bychowska, A.; Brzozowski, K.; Thöming, J.; Stepnowski, P. Application of spectroscopic methods for structural analysis of chitin and chitosan. *Mar. Drugs* **2010**, *8*, 1567–1636. [CrossRef] [PubMed]

109. Venkatesan, J.; Vinodhini, P.A.; Sudha, P.N.; Kim, S.K. Chitin and chitosan composites for bone tissue regeneration. *Adv. Food Nutr. Res.* **2014**, *73*, 59–81. [PubMed]

110. Liu, H.; Tian, W.; Li, B.; Wu, G.; Ibrahim, M.; Tao, Z.; Wang, Y.; Xie, G.; Li, H.; Sun, G. Antifungal effect and mechanism of chitosan against the rice sheath blight pathogen, *Rhizoctonia solani*. *Biotechnol. Lett.* **2012**, *34*, 2291–2298. [CrossRef] [PubMed]

111. Berger, L.R.R.; Stamford, N.P.; Willadino, L.G.; Laranjeira, D.; de Lima, M.A.B.; Malheiros, S.M.M.; de Oliveira, W.J.; Stamford, T.C.M. Cowpea resistance induced against *Fusarium oxysporum* f. sp. tracheiphilum by crustaceous chitosan and by biomass and chitosan obtained from Cunninghamella elegans. *Biol. Control* **2016**, *92*, 45–54. [CrossRef]

112. Divya, K.; Vijayan, S.; George, T.K.; Jisha, M. Antimicrobial properties of chitosan nanoparticles: Mode of action and factors affecting activity. *Fibers Polym.* **2017**, *18*, 221–230. [CrossRef]

113. Salah, R.; Michaud, P.; Mati, F.; Harrat, Z.; Lounici, H.; Abdi, N.; Drouiche, N.; Mameri, N. Anticancer activity of chemically prepared shrimp low molecular weight chitin evaluation with the human monocyte leukaemia cell line, THP-1. *Int. J. Biol. Macromol.* **2013**, *52*, 333–339. [CrossRef] [PubMed]

114. Trung, T.S.; Bao, H.N.D. Physicochemical properties and antioxidant activity of chitin and chitosan prepared from pacific white shrimp waste. *Int. J. Carbohydr. Chem.* **2015**, *2015*. [CrossRef]

115. Sarbon, N.M.; Sandanamsamy, S.; Kamaruzaman, S.F.; Ahmad, F. Chitosan extracted from mud crab (*Scylla olivicea*) shells: Physicochemical and antioxidant properties. *J. Food Sci. Technol.* **2015**, *7*, 4266–4275. [CrossRef] [PubMed]

116. Divya, K.; Smitha, V.; Jisha, M.S. Antifungal, antioxidant and cytotoxic activities of chitosan nanoparticles and its use as an edible coating on vegetables. *Int. J. Biol. Macromol.* **2018**, *114*, 572–577. [CrossRef] [PubMed]

117. Srinivasan, H.; Kanayairam, V.; Ravichandran, R. Chitin and chitosan preparation from shrimp shells *Penaeus monodon* and its human ovarian cancer cell line, PA-1. *Int. J. Biol. Macromol.* **2018**, *107*, 662–667. [CrossRef] [PubMed]

118. Mondol, M.A.M.; Shin, H.J.; Rahman, M.A.; Islam, M.T. Sea cucumber glycosides: Chemical structures, producing species and important biological properties. *Mar. Drugs* **2017**, *15*, 317–352. [CrossRef] [PubMed]

119. Aminin, D.L.; Menchinskaya, E.S.; Pisliagin, E.A.; Silchenko, A.S.; Avilov, S.A.; Kalinin, V.I. Anticancer activity of sea cucumber triterpene glycosides. *Mar. Drugs* **2015**, *13*, 1202–1223. [CrossRef] [PubMed]

120. Malyarenko, O.S.; Dyshlovoy, S.A.; Kicha, A.A.; Ivanchina, N.V.; Malyarenko, T.V.; Carsten, B.; Gunhild, V.A.; Stonik, V.A.; Ermakova, S.P. The inhibitory activity of luzonicosides from the starfish *Echinaster luzonicus* against human melanoma cells. *Mar. Drugs* **2017**, *15*, 227. [CrossRef] [PubMed]

121. Kalinin, V.I.; Ivanchina, N.V.; Krasokhin, V.B.; Makarieva, T.N.; Stonik, V.A. Glycosides from marine sponges (porifera, demospongiae): Structures, taxonomical distribution, biological activities and biological roles. *Mar. Drugs* **2012**, *10*, 1671–1710. [CrossRef] [PubMed]

122. Garcia, M.M.; van der Maarel, M.J.E.C. Floridoside production by the red microalga *Galdieria sulphuraria* under different conditions of growth and osmotic stress. *AMB Express* **2016**, *6*. [CrossRef]

123. Liu, C.Y.; Hwang, T.L.; Lin, M.-R.; Chen, Y.H.; Chang, Y.C.; Fang, L.S.; Wang, W.H.; Wu, Y.C.; Sung, P.J.; Carijoside, A. A bioactive sterol glycoside from an octocoral *Carijoa* sp. (Clavulariidae). *Mar. Drugs* **2010**, *8*, 2014–2020. [CrossRef] [PubMed]

124. Li, Y.X.; Li, Y.; Lee, S.H.; Qian, Z.J.; Kim, S.K. Inhibitors of oxidation and matrix metalloproteinases, floridoside, and D-isofloridoside from marine red alga *Laurencia undulata*. *J. Agric. Food Chem.* **2010**, *58*, 578–586. [CrossRef] [PubMed]

125. Kumar, R.; Subramani, R.; Feussner, K.D.; Aalbersberg, W.; Aurantoside, K. A new antifungal tetramic acid glycoside from a Fijian marine sponge of the genus *Melophlus*. *Mar. Drugs* **2012**, *10*, 200–208. [CrossRef] [PubMed]

126. Wang, X.H.; Zou, Z.R.; Yi, Y.H.; Han, H.; Li, L.; Pan, M.X. Variegatusides: New non-sulphated triterpene glycosides from the sea cucumber *Stichopus variegates* semper. *Mar. Drugs* **2014**, *4*, 2004–2018. [CrossRef] [PubMed]

127. Wang, J.; Han, H.; Chen, X.; Yi, Y.; Sun, H. Cytotoxic and apoptosis-inducing activity of triterpene glycosides from *Holothuria scabra* and *Cucumaria frondosa* against HepG2 cells. *Mar. Drugs* **2014**, *12*, 4274–4290. [CrossRef] [PubMed]

128. Park, J.I.; Bae, H.R.; Kim, C.G.; Stonik, V.A.; Kwak, J.Y. Relationships between chemical structures and functions of triterpene glycosides isolated from sea cucumbers. *Front. Chem.* **2014**, *2*. [CrossRef] [PubMed]

129. Al Shemaili, J.; Parekh, K.A.; Newman, R.A.; Hellman, B.; Woodward, C.; Adem, A.; Collin, P.; Adrian, T.E. Pharmacokinetics in mouse and comparative effects of frondosides in pancreatic cancer. *Mar. Drugs* **2016**, *14*, 115. [CrossRef] [PubMed]

130. Al Marzouqi, N.; Iratni, R.; Nemmar, A.; Arafat, K.; Al Sultan, A.M.; Yasin, J.; Collin, P.; Mester, J.; Adrian, T.E.; Attoub, S. Frondoside a inhibits human breast cancer cell survival, migration, invasion and the growth of breast tumor xenografts. *Eur. J. Pharmacol.* **2011**, *668*, 25–34. [CrossRef] [PubMed]

131. Attoub, S.; Arafat, K.; Gélaude, A.; Al Sultan, M.A.; Bracke, M.; Collin, P.L.; Takahashi, T.; Adrian, T.E.; De Wever, O. Frondoside a suppressive effects on lung cancer survival, tumor growth, angiogenesis, invasion, and metastasis. *PLoS ONE* **2013**, *8*. [CrossRef] [PubMed]

132. Ma, X.; Kundu, N.; Collin, P.D.; Goloubeva, O.; Fulton, A.M. Frondoside a inhibits breast cancer metastasis and antagonizes prostaglandin E receptors EP4 and EP2. *Breast Cancer Res. Treat.* **2011**, *132*, 1001–1008. [CrossRef] [PubMed]

133. Murray, R.K. Glycoproteins. In *Harper's Illustrated Biochemistry*, 26th ed.; Murray, R.K., Granner, D.K., Mayes, P.A., Rodwell, V.W., Eds.; McGraw-Hill Companies: New York, NY, USA, 2003.

134. Zanetta, J.P.; Kuchler, S.; Lehmann, S.; Badache, A.; Maschke, S.; Thomas, D.; Dufourcq, P.; Vincendon, G. Glycoproteins and lectins in cell adhesion and cell recognition processes. *Histochem. J.* **1992**, *24*, 791–804. [CrossRef] [PubMed]

135. Sharon, N.; Lis, H. History of lectins: From hemagglutinins to biological recognition molecules. *Glycobiology* **2004**, *14*, 53R–62R. [CrossRef] [PubMed]

136. Benevides, N.M.B.; Holanda, M.L.; Melo, F.R.; Freitas, A.L.P.; Sampaio, A.H. Purification and partial characterisation of the lectin from the marine red alga ***Enantiocladia duperreyi*** (C. Agardh) falkenberg. *Bot. Mar.* **1998**, *41*, 521–526. [CrossRef]

137. Mu, J.; Hirayama, M.; Sato, Y.; Morimoto, K.; Hori, K. A novel high-mannose specific lectin from the green alga *Halimeda renschii* exhibits a potent anti-influenza virus activity through high-affinity binding to the viral hemagglutinin. *Mar. Drugs* **2017**, *15*, 255. [CrossRef] [PubMed]

138. Gundacker, D.; Leys, S.P.; Schröder, H.C.; Müller, I.M.; Müller, W.E. Isolation and cloning of a C-type lectin from the hexactinellid sponge *Aphrocallistes vastus*: A putative aggregation factor. *Glycobiology* **2001**, *11*, 21–29. [CrossRef] [PubMed]

139. Bulgakov, A.A.; Park, K.I.; Choi, K.S.; Lim, H.K.; Cho, M. Purification and characterisation of a lectin isolated from the *Manila clam Ruditapes philippinarum* in Korea. *Fish Shellfish. Immunol.* **2004**, *4*, 487–499. [CrossRef] [PubMed]

140. Hatakeyama, T.; Kohzaki, H.; Nagatomo, H.; Yamasaki, N. Purification and characterization of four Ca^{2+}-dependent lectins from the marine invertebrate, *Cucumaria echinata*. *J. Biochem.* **1994**, *116*, 209–214. [CrossRef] [PubMed]

141. Silva, L.M.; Lima, V.; Holanda, M.L.; Pinheiro, P.G.; Rodrigues, J.A.; Lima, M.E.; Benevides, N.M. Antinociceptive and anti-inflammatory activities of lectin from marine red alga *Pterocladiella capillacea*. *Biol. Pharm. Bull.* **2010**, *33*, 830–835. [CrossRef] [PubMed]

142. Abreu, T.M.; Ribeiro, N.A.; Chaves, H.V.; Jorge, R.J.; Bezerra, M.M.; Monteiro, H.S.; Vasconcelos, I.M.; Mota, É.F.; Benevides, N.M. Antinociceptive and anti-inflammatory activities of the lectin from marine red alga *Solieria filiformis*. *Planta Med.* **2016**, *7*, 596–605. [CrossRef] [PubMed]

143. Fontenelle, T.P.C.; Lima, G.C.; Mesquita, J.X.; Lopes, J.L.S.; de Brito, T.V.; Vieira, F.D.C., Jr.; Sales, A.B.; Aragão, K.S.; Souza, M.H.L.P.; Barbosa, A.L.D.R.; et al. Lectin obtained from the red seaweed *Bryothamnion triquetrum*: Secondary structure and anti-inflammatory activity in mice. *Int. J. Biol. Macromol.* **2018**, *112*, 1122–1130. [CrossRef] [PubMed]

144. Liao, J.H.; Chien, C.T.; Wu, H.Y.; Huang, K.F.; Wang, I.; Ho, M.R.; Tu, I.F.; Lee, I.M.; Li, W.; Shih, Y.L.; et al. A multivalent marine lectin from *Crenomytilus grayanus* possesses anti-cancer activity through recognizing globotriose Gb3. *J. Am. Chem. Soc.* **2016**, *138*, 4787–4795. [CrossRef] [PubMed]

145. Liu, S.; Zheng, L.; Aweya, J.J.; Zheng, Z.; Zhong, M.; Chen, J.; Wang, F.; Zhang, Y. *Litopenaeus vannamei* hemocyanin exhibits antitumor activity in S180 mouse model in vivo. *PLoS ONE* **2017**, *12*. [CrossRef] [PubMed]

146. Róg, T.; Vattulainen, I. Cholesterol, sphingolipids, and glycolipids: What do we know about their role in raft-like membranes? *Chem. Phys. Lipids* **2014**, *184*, 82–104. [CrossRef] [PubMed]

147. Ratnayake, W.M.N.; Galli, C. Fat and fatty acid terminology, methods of analysis and fat digestion and metabolism: A background review paper. *Ann. Nutr. Metab.* **2009**, *55*, 8–43. [CrossRef] [PubMed]

148. Che, H.; Du, L.; Cong, P.; Tao, S.; Ding, N.; Wu, F.; Xue, C.; Xu, J.; Wang, Y. Cerebrosides from sea cucumber protect against oxidative stress in SAMP8 mice and PC12 cells. *J. Med. Food* **2017**, *20*, 392–402. [CrossRef] [PubMed]

149. Yamada, K. Chemo-pharmaceutical studies on the glycosphingolipid constituents from echinoderm, sea cucumbers, as the medicinal materials. *Yakugaku Zasshi* **2002**, *122*, 1133–1143. [CrossRef] [PubMed]

150. Hölzl, G.; Dörmann, P. Structure and function of glycoglycerolipids in plants and bacteria. *Prog. Lipid Res.* **2007**, *46*, 225–243. [CrossRef] [PubMed]

151. Mansoor, T.A.; Shinde, P.B.; Luo, X.; Hong, J.; Lee, C.O.; Sim, C.J.; Son, B.W.; Jung, J.H. Renierosides, cerebrosides from a marine sponge *Haliclona* (Reniera) sp. *J. Nat. Prod.* **2007**, *70*, 1481–1486. [CrossRef] [PubMed]

152. Plouguerné, E.; da Gama, B.A.P.; Pereira, R.C.; Barreto-Bergter, E. Glycolipids from seaweeds and their potential biotechnological applications. *Front. Cell. Infect. Microbiol.* **2014**, *4*. [CrossRef] [PubMed]

153. Banskota, A.H.; Stefanova, R.; Sperker, S.; Lall, S.P.; Craigie, J.S.; Hafting, J.T.; Critchley, A.T. Polar lipids from the marine macroalga *Palmaria palmata* inhibit lipopolysaccharide-induced nitric oxide production in RAW264.7 macrophage cells. *Phytochemistry* **2014**, *101*, 101–108. [CrossRef] [PubMed]

154. Reyes, C.; Ortega, M.J.; Rodríguez-Luna, A.; Talero, E.; Motilva, V.; Zubía, E. Molecular characterization and anti-inflammatory activity of galactosylglycerides and galactosylceramides from the microalga *Isochrysis galbana*. *J. Agric. Food Chem.* **2016**, *64*, 8783–8794. [CrossRef] [PubMed]

155. Zhang, J.; Li, C.; Yu, G.; Guan, H. Total synthesis and structure-activity relationship of glycoglycerolipids from marine organisms. *Mar. Drugs* **2014**, *12*, 3634–3659. [CrossRef] [PubMed]

156. Simmonds, M.S.J.; Klte, G.C.; Porter, E.A. Taxonomic distribution of iminosugars in plants and their biological activities. In *Iminosugars As Glycosidase Inhibitors: Nojirimycin and Beyond*; Stiitz, A.E., Ed.; Wiley-VCH Verlag GmbH: Weinheim, Germany, 1999.

157. Segraves, N.L.; Crews, P. A Madagascar Sponge *Batzella* sp. as a Source of Alkylated Iminosugars. *J. Nat. Prod.* **2005**, *68*, 118–121. [CrossRef] [PubMed]

158. Chang, J.; Wang, L.; Ma, D.; Qu, X.; Guo, H.; Xu, X.; Mason, P.M.; Bourne, N.; Moriarty, R.; Gu, B.; et al. Novel imino sugar derivatives demonstrate potent antiviral activity against flaviviruses. *Antimicrob. Agents Chemother.* **2009**, *53*, 1501–1508. [CrossRef] [PubMed]

159. Jüttner, F.; Wessel, H.P. Isolation of di(hydroxymethyl)dihydroxypyrrolidine from the cyanobacterial genus *Cylindrospermum* that effectively inhibits digestive glucosidases of aquatic insects and crustacean grazers. *J. Phycol.* **2003**, *39*, 26–32. [CrossRef]

160. Birch, A.N.E.; Robertson, W.M.; Geoghegan, I.E.; McGavin, W.J.; Alphey, T.J.W.; Phillips, M.S.; Fellows, L.E.; Watson, A.A.; Simmonds, M.S.J.; Porter, E.A. Dmdp—A plant-derived sugar analogue with systemic activity against plant parasitic nematodes. *Nematologica* **1993**, *39*, 521–535. [CrossRef]

161. Sayce, A.C.; Alonzi, D.S.; Killingbeck, S.S.; Tyrrell, B.E.; Hill, M.L.; Caputo, A.T.; Iwaki, R.; Kinami, K.; Ide, D.; Kiappes, J.L.; et al. Iminosugars inhibit dengue virus production via inhibition of ER alpha-glucosidases-not glycolipid processing enzymes. *PLoS Negl. Trop. Dis.* **2016**, *10*. [CrossRef] [PubMed]

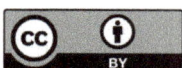

© 2018 by the authors. Licensee MDPI, Basel, Switzerland. This article is an open access article distributed under the terms and conditions of the Creative Commons Attribution (CC BY) license (http://creativecommons.org/licenses/by/4.0/).

marine drugs

MDPI

Review

Chemistry and Biology of Bioactive Glycolipids of Marine Origin

Iván Cheng-Sánchez * and Francisco Sarabia *

Department of Organic Chemistry, Faculty of Sciences, University of Málaga, Campus de Teatinos s/n, 29071 Málaga, Spain
* Correspondence: cheng@uma.es (I.C.-S.); frsarabia@uma.es (F.S.);
  Tel.: +34-952-131-939 (I.C.-S.); +34-952-134-258 (F.S.)

Received: 6 July 2018; Accepted: 15 August 2018; Published: 22 August 2018

check for
updates

Abstract: Glycolipids represent a broad class of natural products structurally featured by a glycosidic fragment linked to a lipidic molecule. Despite the large structural variety of these glycoconjugates, they can be classified into three main groups, i.e., glycosphingolipids, glycoglycerolipids, and atypical glycolipids. In the particular case of glycolipids derived from marine sources, an impressive variety in their structural features and biological properties is observed, thus making them prime targets for chemical synthesis. In the present review, we explore the chemistry and biology of this class of compounds.

Keywords: glycolipids; glycosphingolipids; glycoglycerolipids; natural products; total synthesis

1. Introduction

Glycolipids represent a broad class of biologically active natural products with a wide variety of molecular structures and biological functions, many of which are essential for life [1,2]. Despite their extensive structural diversity, glycolipids can be classified by the nature of the lipidic fragment. According to this classification, these glycoconjugates are divided into three main groups, i.e., glycoglycerolipids, glycosphingolipids, and those comprising the rest of the glycolipids possessing atypical lipidic moieties. Whereas glycoglycerolipids are mainly distributed in the realm of micro-organisms and plants, glycosphingolipids are extensively found in all living beings. In fact, these molecules are found on the surface of cell membranes and, together with glycoproteins and glycosaminoglycans, which are known as glycocalyx, play critical roles for cell growth, cellular recognition, adhesion, neuronal repair, and signal transduction, which are essential for health and involved in a number of diseases such as cancer and inflammatory processes and infections [3–5]. Given their molecular complexity and diversity, glycosphingolipids are classified into the following subgroups: (a) neutral, which can be subdivided into the cerebrosides that contain only one uncharged sugar, the diosylceramides with two sugar units, and the neutral glycosphingolipids with more than two (up to 30) uncharged sugars; and (b) acidic, which can be subdivided into the gangliosides, characterized by the presence of one or more neuraminic acid residues, and, finally the sulfatides, which contain at least one sugar residue with a sulfate group. In any case, all of the glycosphingolipids share a common ceramide lipid unit, consisting of a long-chain amino-alcohol fragment, which can be a sphingosine or a phytosphingosine unit (sphingoid base) linked to a fatty acid via an amide bond. In the case of the glycoglycerolipids, their core structure is comprised of a 1,2-diacyl glycerol attached to a mono- or an oligosaccharide molecule, although some variations with respect to this general structure can be found, as will be described later. In contrast to the glycosphingolipids, the glycoglycerolipids are present in nature in much lower abundance, which, combined with the difficulty of their isolation from natural sources, have significantly hampered extensive and detailed biological studies. The third group consists of the atypical glycolipids that include any glycoconjugate that contains a lipidic chain not present in the previous groups (Figure 1). The stunning and limitless wealth of secondary metabolites that marine organisms provide is extensive for this class of compounds, with a myriad of glycolipid-type natural products with impressive molecular diversity and a variety of biological activities, including antitumor, antiviral, and anti-inflammatory properties. Given the biological relevance and structural complexity of these classes of compounds, a large number of reviews [6–12], books, and book chapters [13–15] have been devoted to all aspects related to their chemistry and biology. More specifically, in the field of glycolipids of marine origin, several excellent reviews have been published, especially by Barnathan et al. [16], which represents an excellent description of all the glycolipids found in marine invertebrates, as well as by Li et al. [17], which focused on the chemistry and biology of glycoglycerolipids from marine organisms. In addition, numerous reviews have been reported on very specific compounds, such as KRN7000 [18] and related glycosphingolipids [19] due to their outstanding biological activities and their potential pharmacological activity. In light of this publication landscape, this review intends to give a chemical and biological perspective of these fascinating natural products with a particular emphasis on recent contributions that were not covered in the aforementioned reviews and highlighting the importance of their synthesis given the particularly intricate requirements to obtain sufficient amounts from their natural sources. This review also provides an updated state of the art of this field that can attract the interest of chemists and biologists, revealing the potential and prospects that these compounds may provide in biology, chemistry, and biomedicine for the future.

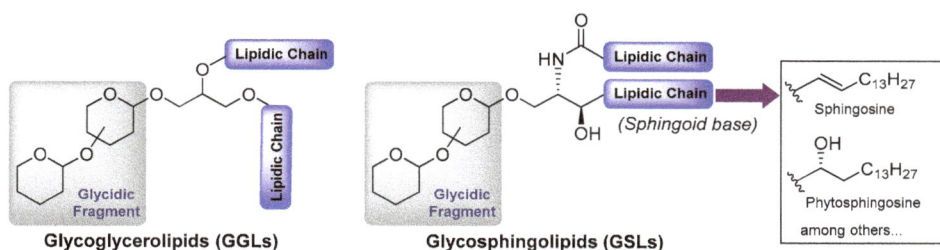

Figure 1. General structural feature of glycolipids.

2. Chemistry and Biology of Glycosphingolipids

2.1. Neutral Glycosphingolipids

2.1.1. Cerebrosides

Acanthacerebrosides, Astrocerebrosides, and Asteriacerebrosides

Among the wide and important family of marine glycosphingolipids containing a phytosphingosine unit, which confers the glycolipids outstanding immunostimulant properties, as will be described later, the acanthacerebrosides and astrocerebrosides represent interesting members isolated from different starfish species. It was in 1988 when Komori et al. [20] discovered the first members of the acanthacerebrosides (A–F, **1–6**) from the starfish *Acanthaster planci*. These compounds were isolated as a mixture, which hindered a complete structural elucidation and biological evaluations. However, subsequent purification efforts by the same group led to the isolation of one of their members, acanthacerebroside B (**2**), which could be isolated as a pure compound from the starfish *Asterina pectinifera* and allowed full structural characterization by a complete NMR spectroscopic analysis. In the same year, these authors described the first total synthesis of acanthacerebroside A (**1**), establishing unambiguously the structure and absolute configuration of this new family of cerebrosides [21]. In addition, the investigations of Komori et al. [22] with the starfish *Astropecten latespinosus* led to the discovery of three new related cerebrosides, which were named astrocerebrosides A (**7**), B (**8**), and C (**9**). Later, in 1991, the study of the starfish *Asterias amurensis versicolor* allowed Komori´s group to isolate new cerebrosides: asteriacerebrosides A–F (**10–15**) [23]. Ten years later, Ishii et al. [24] discovered a new member of this class, asteriacerebroside G (**16**), from the starfish *Asterias amurensis* (Figure 2).

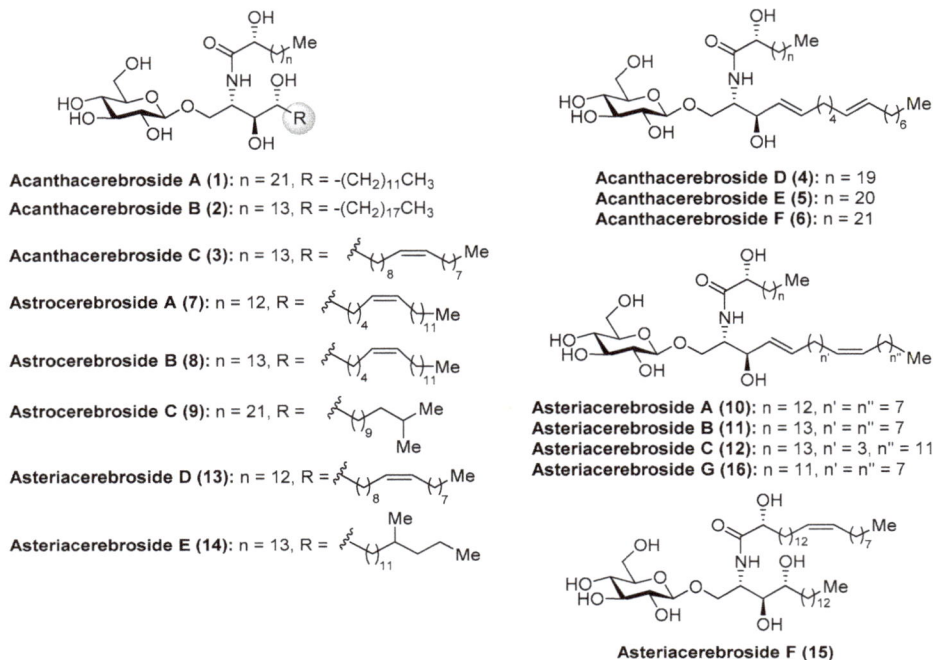

Acanthacerebroside A (**1**): n = 21, R = -(CH$_2$)$_{11}$CH$_3$
Acanthacerebroside B (**2**): n = 13, R = -(CH$_2$)$_{17}$CH$_3$

Acanthacerebroside C (**3**): n = 13, R =

Astrocerebroside A (**7**): n = 12, R =

Astrocerebroside B (**8**): n = 13, R =

Astrocerebroside C (**9**): n = 21, R =

Asteriacerebroside D (**13**): n = 12, R =

Asteriacerebroside E (**14**): n = 13, R =

Acanthacerebroside D (**4**): n = 19
Acanthacerebroside E (**5**): n = 20
Acanthacerebroside F (**6**): n = 21

Asteriacerebroside A (**10**): n = 12, n' = n" = 7
Asteriacerebroside B (**11**): n = 13, n' = n" = 7
Asteriacerebroside C (**12**): n = 13, n' = 3, n" = 11
Asteriacerebroside G (**16**): n = 11, n' = n" = 7

Asteriacerebroside F (**15**)

Figure 2. Structures of the acanthacerebrosides (**1–6**), astrocerebrosides (**7–9**), and asteriacerebrosides (**10–16**).

More recently, from the same starfish (*A. amurensis*), Kim et al. identified new members of related asteriacerebrosides, whose structures were established by mass spectrometric techniques [25]. After the synthesis of acanthacerebroside A (**1**) by Komori in 1998, the Chida group [26] reported a new synthesis for acanthacerebroside A (**1**) and astrocerebroside A (**7**), in which the preparation of the phytosphingosine moiety was achieved using the commercially available L-quebrachitol (**17**) (Scheme 1). Accordingly, L-quebrachitol (**17**) was transformed into the azide **18** in seven steps, which was directed towards the phytosphingosine fragment **20**, contained in acanthacerebroside A (**1**). The coupling of **20** with the donor trichloroacetimidate **21** via a glycosylation reaction mediated by BF$_3$·OEt$_2$ provided the corresponding acanthacerebroside A derivative, which was derivatized to the peracetylated **22** to facilitate purification. After removing the acetate protecting groups, natural acanthacerebroside A (**1**) was obtained. In a similar manner, astrocerebroside A (**7**) was efficiently prepared from the phytosphingosine **23**, synthesized from the common epoxide **19**, and the same glycosyl donor (**21**). From a biological standpoint, surprisingly only the asteriacerebrosides were evaluated, showing that asteriacerebrosides A (**10**), B (**11**), and G (**16**) displayed growth-promoting activity against the plant *Brassica campestris*. This was the first report of a promotive plant-growth activity of this class of compounds.

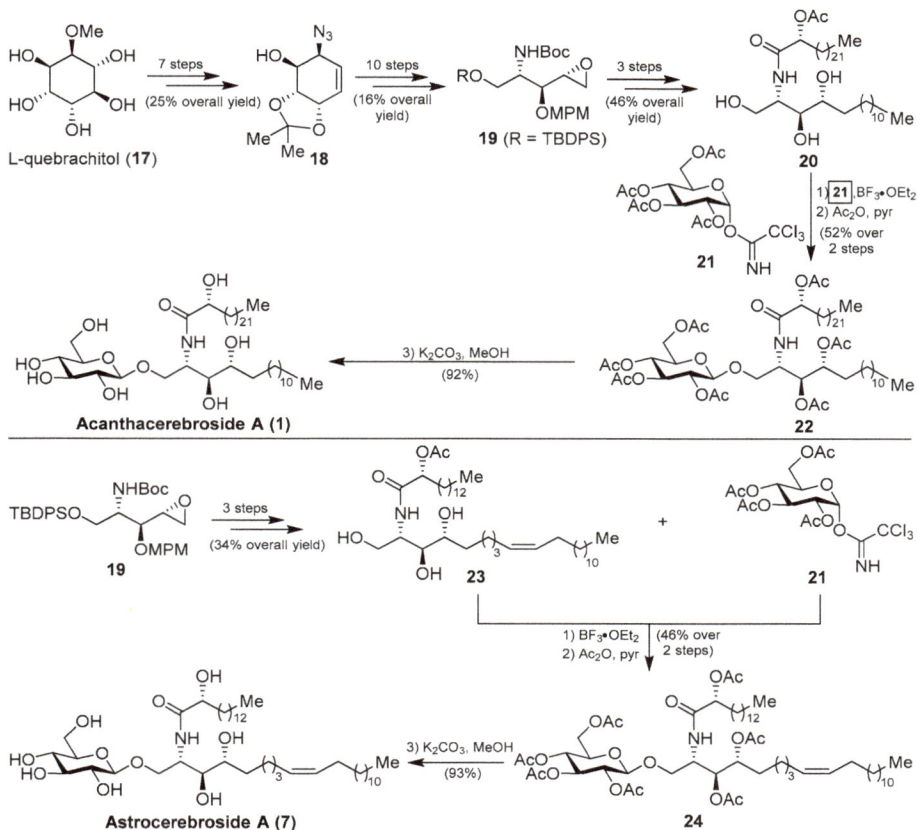

Scheme 1. Total syntheses of acanthacerebroside A (**1**) and astrocerebroside A (**7**).

Agelasphins

Within the family of phytosphingosine-containing cerebrosides of marine origin, the agelasphins (**25–31**) (Figure 3) occupy a privileged position by virtue of their striking and promising biological properties. The presence of a galactosyl fragment instead of a glucosyl moiety confers upon them unexpected and intriguing biological properties. After the isolation of the first members of this family by Natori et al. in 1993 [27] from the marine sponge *Agelas mauritianus*, the agelasphins were rapidly recognized as antitumor compounds with weak toxicity, which elicited a great interest in chemical and biological circles. Despite these antitumoral properties, the agelasphins did not exhibit cytotoxicity against B16 melanoma cells at 20 µg/mL, which led Natori, Koezuka, et al. [28] to undertake further biological studies for a rational explanation of these intriguing properties. These studies revealed that these compounds, for example agelasphin-11 (**28**), were capable of stimulating the immune system via activation of NK cells, which explained not only their potent antitumor activity but also their immunostimulatory property. These outstanding biological findings encouraged the Koezuka's group to achieve an extensive structure–activity relationship (SAR) study by preparation of a library of their analogues and subsequent antitumor activity evaluation from which the well-known analogue KRN7000 (**32**) was discovered [29]. At a molecular level, the activation of the immune system exerted by the agelasphins occurs because these compounds are potent ligands of the MHC class I-like CD1d protein, present on the surface of the antigen presenting cells (APCs), and, as a consequence of this potent interaction, an overwhelming response by the immune system is triggered. Thus, the invariant natural killer T cells (*i*NKT cells) are initially activated by producing high levels of cytokines, which, in turn, activate other antitumor effector cells, resulting in a strong immunological response by the organism against tumor cells. These important findings rapidly propelled KRN7000 (**32**) as a novel and promising anticancer agent, which recently entered into phase I clinical trials against various types of cancers [30]. As a consequence of its intriguing biological properties, KRN7000 has elicited widespread interest and excitement in both the biological and chemical fields. Indeed, an indication of this great interest is a flurry of activity directed toward the synthesis of a plethora of analogues for SAR studies [31,32]. Related to the agelasphins, Mangoni's group [33] has recently identified a disaccharide derivative, named damicoside (**33**), from the marine sponge *Axinella damicornis*. This glycolipid represents the first disaccharide, structurally related to that of agelasphins, and with an immunostimulatory activity similar to the agelasphins, allowing the completion of the structure–activity relationship study of this fascinating class of compounds.

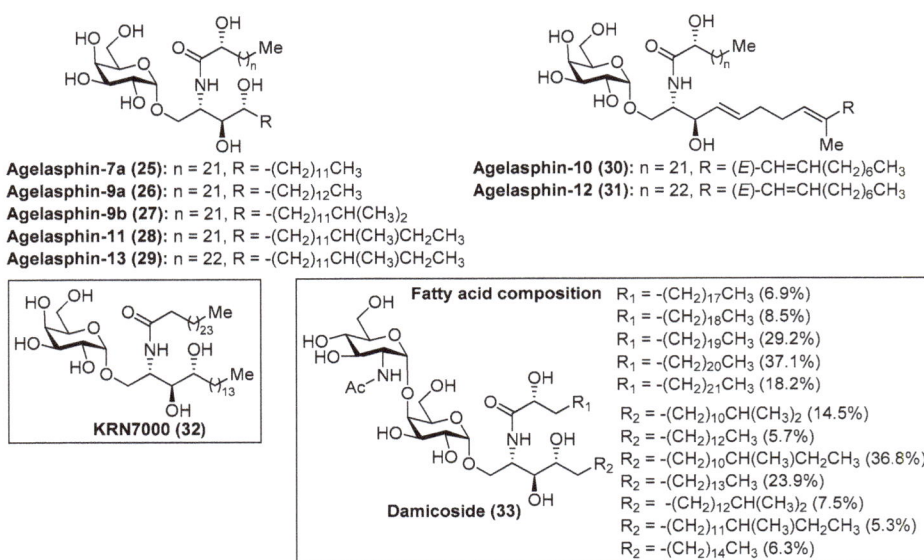

Agelasphin-7a (25): n = 21, R = -(CH$_2$)$_{11}$CH$_3$
Agelasphin-9a (26): n = 21, R = -(CH$_2$)$_{12}$CH$_3$
Agelasphin-9b (27): n = 21, R = -(CH$_2$)$_{11}$CH(CH$_3$)$_2$
Agelasphin-11 (28): n = 21, R = -(CH$_2$)$_{11}$CH(CH$_3$)CH$_2$CH$_3$
Agelasphin-13 (29): n = 22, R = -(CH$_2$)$_{11}$CH(CH$_3$)CH$_2$CH$_3$

Agelasphin-10 (30): n = 21, R = (*E*)-CH=CH(CH$_2$)$_6$CH$_3$
Agelasphin-12 (31): n = 22, R = (*E*)-CH=CH(CH$_2$)$_6$CH$_3$

KRN7000 (32)

Damicoside (33)

Fatty acid composition
R$_1$ = -(CH$_2$)$_{17}$CH$_3$ (6.9%)
R$_1$ = -(CH$_2$)$_{18}$CH$_3$ (8.5%)
R$_1$ = -(CH$_2$)$_{19}$CH$_3$ (29.2%)
R$_1$ = -(CH$_2$)$_{20}$CH$_3$ (37.1%)
R$_1$ = -(CH$_2$)$_{21}$CH$_3$ (18.2%)

R$_2$ = -(CH$_2$)$_{10}$CH(CH$_3$)$_2$ (14.5%)
R$_2$ = -(CH$_2$)$_{12}$CH$_3$ (5.7%)
R$_2$ = -(CH$_2$)$_{10}$CH(CH$_3$)CH$_2$CH$_3$ (36.8%)
R$_2$ = -(CH$_2$)$_{13}$CH$_3$ (23.9%)
R$_2$ = -(CH$_2$)$_{12}$CH(CH$_3$)$_2$ (7.5%)
R$_2$ = -(CH$_2$)$_{11}$CH(CH$_3$)CH$_2$CH$_3$ (5.3%)
R$_2$ = -(CH$_2$)$_{14}$CH$_3$ (6.3%)

Figure 3. Structures of the agelasphins (**25–31**), KRN7000 (**32**), and damicoside (**33**).

In order to confirm the structures of the agelasphins, Natori, together with Akimoto et al. [34], achieved the first total synthesis of an agelasphin member, agelasphin-9b (**27**). Accordingly, the construction of the phytosphingosine fragment commenced with the Wittig reaction of aldehyde **34** with phosphonium salt **35** to give a mixture of isomeric alcohols **36** in 68% yield. The alcohol **36** was then converted into the azide **37** in six steps in 45% overall yield. Subsequent reduction of the azide and acetylation of the corresponding amine with *p*-nitrophenyl ester **38** afforded a protected ceramide **39** in 40% overall yield. Reaction of **39** with galactosyl fluoride **40**, under Mukaiyama's glycosylation conditions, gave the corresponding α-galactoside in 36% yield, which was finally transformed into agelasphin-9b (**27**) after a deprotection of the protecting groups (Scheme 2). This synthesis was important not only because the authors were able to confirm the structures of these natural products, but also because the strategy for the future construction of these molecules was established and extended to the synthesis of other agelasphins and their analogues, such as KRN7000 (**32**) [18,19].

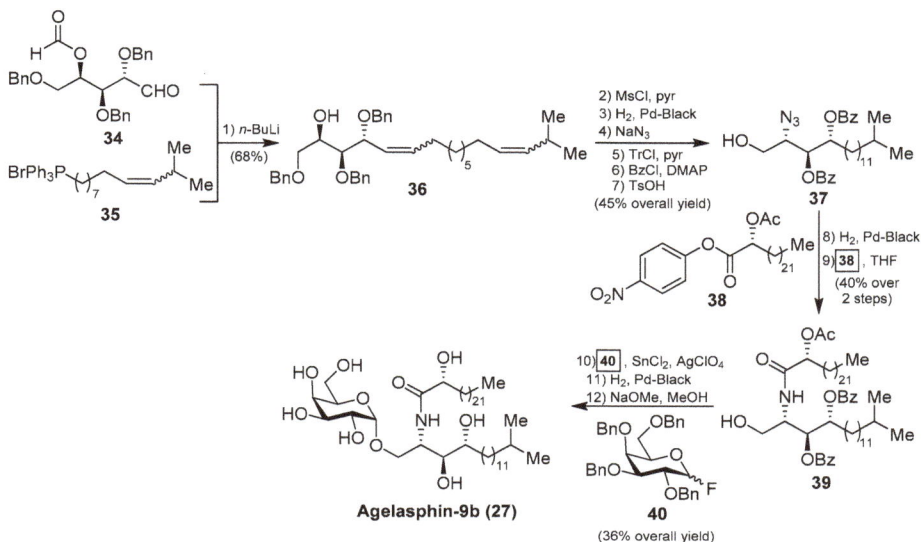

Scheme 2. Total synthesis of agelasphin-9b (**27**).

Axidjiferosides

Barnathan et al. [35] described the isolation of axidjiferosides A–C (**41–43**) (Figure 4) from the marine sponge *Axinyssa djiferi*, collected from mangrove tree roots in Senegal. Interestingly, the structure of these compounds contained the unusual Δ^6-phytosphingosine and also the unusual β-configuration of the galactopyranosyl unit. These compounds showed significant antimalarial activity, with an IC_{50} of 0.53 ± 0.2 μM against a chloroquine-resistant strain of *Plasmodium falciparum*. In addition, the axidjiferosides also showed antiplasmodial activity, with low cytotoxicity against various human cancer cell lines, and no significant antitrypanosomal and antileishmanial activities. In contrast to the α-galactosylceramide derivatives, such as the agelasphins, which displayed immunostimulating properties, the antimalarial activity exhibited by the axidjiferosides was ascribed by the authors to the β anomeric configuration present in these natural products.

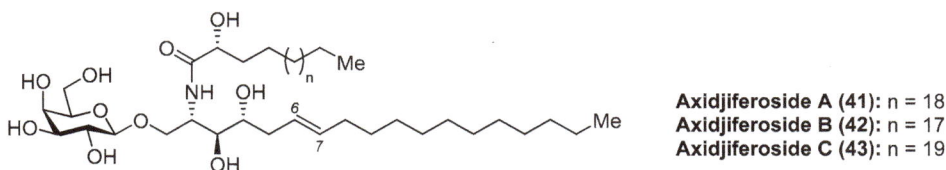

Axidjiferoside A (41): n = 18
Axidjiferoside B (42): n = 17
Axidjiferoside C (43): n = 19

Figure 4. Structures of the axidjiferosides (**41–43**).

Cerebrosides CE

Cerebrosides CE (**44–48**) (Figure 5) were isolated, together with ganglioside CG-1 (See Section Ganglioside CG-1), from the sea cucumber *Cucumaria echinata* [36]. These cerebrosides showed toxicity in a brine shrimp lethality assay with the rates of 11–27%. However, no further chemical and biological studies about these cerebrosides have been carried out so far.

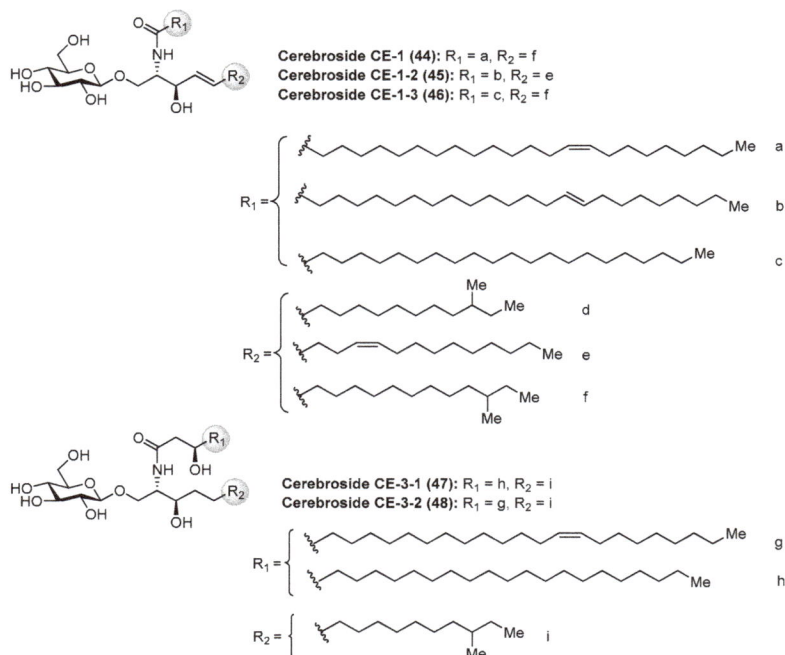

Figure 5. Structures of the cerebrosides CE (**44**–**48**).

Halicylindrosides

Within the family of cerebrosides of marine origin, the halicylindrosides (**49**–**58**) (Figure 6) were isolated and characterized by Fusetani´s group in 1995 from the marine sponge *Halichondria cylindrata* [37]. These structural studies revealed that the halicylindrosides were a new family of phytosphingosine-containing cerebrosides, which promoted a great deal of expectation by virtue of their antifungal activity against *Mortierella remanniana* at 250 µg/disk and citotoxity against P388 murine leukemia cells at 6.8 µg/mL, respectively.

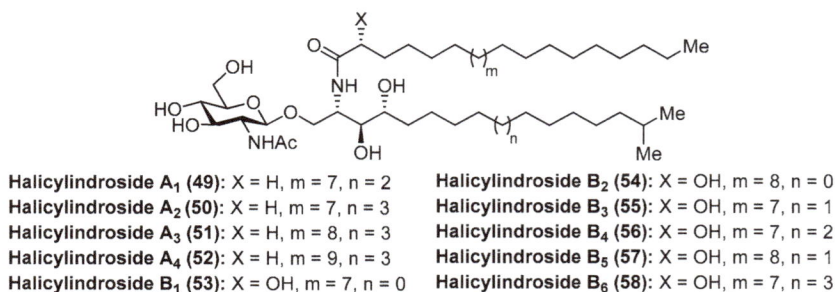

Halicylindroside A$_1$ (**49**): X = H, m = 7, n = 2   Halicylindroside B$_2$ (**54**): X = OH, m = 8, n = 0
Halicylindroside A$_2$ (**50**): X = H, m = 7, n = 3   Halicylindroside B$_3$ (**55**): X = OH, m = 7, n = 1
Halicylindroside A$_3$ (**51**): X = H, m = 8, n = 3   Halicylindroside B$_4$ (**56**): X = OH, m = 7, n = 2
Halicylindroside A$_4$ (**52**): X = H, m = 9, n = 3   Halicylindroside B$_5$ (**57**): X = OH, m = 8, n = 1
Halicylindroside B$_1$ (**53**): X = OH, m = 7, n = 0   Halicylindroside B$_6$ (**58**): X = OH, m = 7, n = 3

Figure 6. Structures of the halicylindrosides (**49**–**58**).

The synthesis of the halicylindroside A homologue **59** was carried out by Murakami et al. [38], paving the way for the synthesis of the natural congeners. Thus, **61**, which was prepared from *N*-benzoyl-D-glucosamine **60** in 87% over two steps, was transformed into the oxazoline derivative **63** in seven steps in 41% overall yield, involving regioselective *O*-methanesulfonation and diastereoselective

Grignard addition as key steps. The coupling between **63** and *N*-chloroacetyl glucosyl chloride **64**, which was chosen as a more efficient donor for the glycosylation reaction, was achieved by using silver trifluoromethanesulfonate as the promoter at 70 °C to obtain **65** in 75% yield. Reduction of the chloroacetyl **65** with *n*-Bu$_3$SnH afforded acetamide **66** in 90% yield. Subsequent acid-catalyzed ring opening of the oxazoline **66**, followed by reaction with palmitoyl chloride of the resulting amino alcohol provided **67**, which was finally transformed into halicylindroside A homologue (**59**) after a basic treatment (Scheme 3). In a similar manner, a homologue of halicyndroside B (**53**) was obtained by using (2*R*)-acetoxypalmitoyl imide.

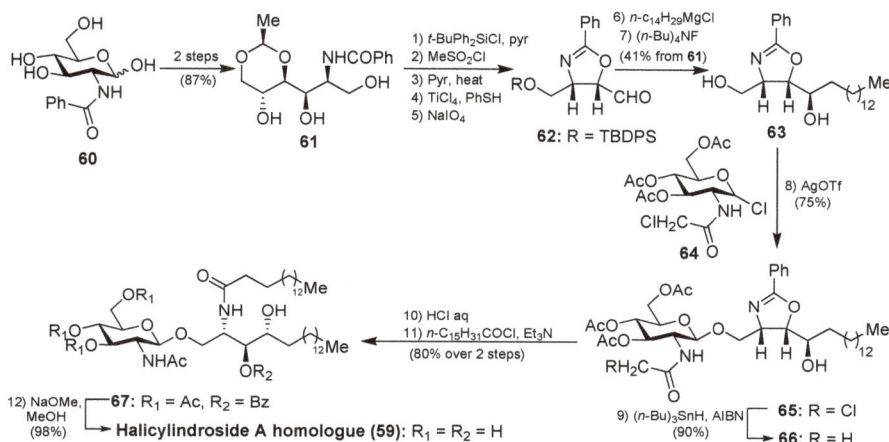

Scheme 3. Total synthesis of halicylindroside A homologue **59**.

Phallusides

Phallusides (**68–71**) (Figure 7) were isolated from the Mediterranean ascidian *Phallusia fumigata* and from the starfishes *Allostichaster inaequalis* and *Cosmasterias lurida* [39] and their structures were elucidated by a combination of spectroscopic and chemical degradation studies. These studies revealed the presence of an unusual sphingoid base, which corresponded to the 2-amino-9-methyl-D-*erythro*-(4*E*,8*E*,10*E*)-octadeca-4,8,10-triene-1,3-diol. Prior to these findings, Karlsson et al. [40] had described isolation and structure elucidation of a closely related glycosphingolipid from the sea anemone *Metridium senite*, which was assigned as Sch II (**72**). Interestingly, this compound was also isolated from the basidiomycete *Schizophyllum commune* some years later [41].

The biological activity evaluation of phallusides 1–3 (**68–70**) revealed that these compounds possessed significant activity as antifungal agents against several phytopathogenic fungi (*Fusarium oxysporum f.* sp. *Niveum, F. solani f.* sp. Cucurbitae, *Pythium ultimum*, and *Alternaria solani*) [42].

The first synthetic explorations of these compounds were attempted by Kocienski et al. [43] leading to the total syntheses of phalluside-1 (**68**) and Sch II (**72**) via a Cu (I)-mediated 1,2-metallate rearrangement of a lithiated glycal as a key step for the stereoselective synthesis of the sphingoid base. In this direction, the authors envisioned the synthesis of the azidosphingatrienine **79** from iodoalkene **73** through two sequentially 1,2-metallate rearrangements involving cyanocuprate intermediates, derived from lithium derivatives **74** and **77**, to obtain the triene triol **78**. Conversion of **78** into the azide **79** proceeded in eight steps in 17% overall yield. The key Schmidt glycosylation reaction of the alcohol **79** with the donor **80**, using BF$_3$·OEt$_2$ as a promoter, afforded the glycoside **81** in a modest 34% yield. To complete the synthesis, a Staudinger reaction of the azide **81**, followed by an *N*-acetylation of the resulting amine with the acid **82** generated protected phalluside **83** in 63% yield over two steps. Final debenzoylation under basic conditions gave phalluside **68** in a 72% yield. For the synthesis of

Sch II (**72**), the authors employed the same synthetic strategy using the same lithium derivatives **74** and **77** but starting from a different iodoalkene (Scheme 4).

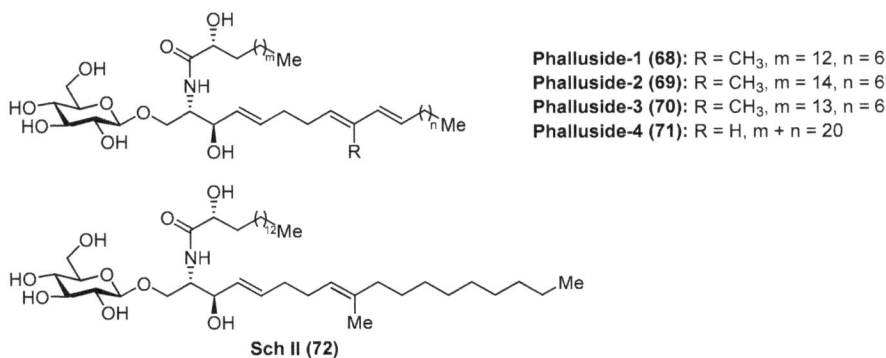

Phalluside-1 (68): R = CH$_3$, m = 12, n = 6
Phalluside-2 (69): R = CH$_3$, m = 14, n = 6
Phalluside-3 (70): R = CH$_3$, m = 13, n = 6
Phalluside-4 (71): R = H, m + n = 20

Sch II (72)

Figure 7. Structures of the phallusides (**68–71**) and Sch II (**72**).

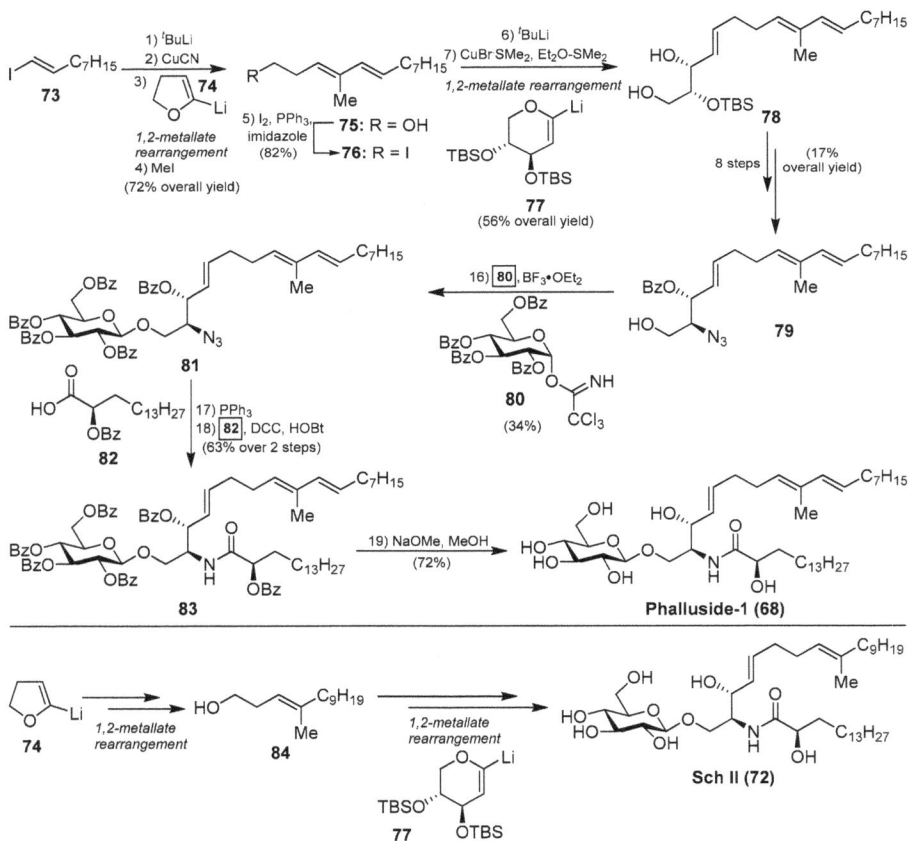

Scheme 4. Total synthesis of phalluside-1 (**68**) and Sch II (**72**).

2.1.2. Diosylceramides

Amphiceramides

Amphiceramides A (**85**) and B (**86**) were isolated from the Caribbean sponge *Amphimedon compressa* by Mangoni et al. [44] (Figure 8). The structures of both glycolipids contain an unusual Δ^6-phytosphingosine unit, which can be found in other secondary metabolites such as the aforementioned axidjiferosides A–C (**41–43**). In addition, amphiceramide A (**85**) contains an uncommon *N*-acetyl-β-glucosamine, which has never been found in any natural product. Amphiceramide B (**86**) was the first glycosphingolipid that possesses an allolactose [Gal(1 β→6)Glc] residue β-linked to the ceramide moiety.

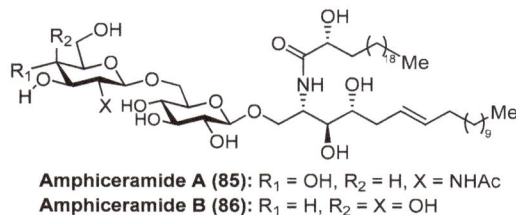

Amphiceramide A (85): R_1 = OH, R_2 = H, X = NHAc
Amphiceramide B (86): R_1 = H, R_2 = X = OH

Figure 8. Structures of the amphiceramides A (**85**) and B (**86**).

Plakosides

Fattorusso et al. [45] described the isolation of plakosides (**87–90**) (Figure 9) from the marine sponge *Plakortis simplex*, which featured the presence of a cyclopropane ring in the lipidic chain and a 2-*O*-prenylation of the carbohydrate moiety. Interestingly, in contrast to the immunostimulating property of related glycosphingolipids, such as agelasphins, the plakosides exhibited potent immunosuppressive activity, with plakosides A (**87**) and B (**88**) as inhibitors of the proliferative response of lymph-node cells when T cells were stimulated with concavaline A in all doses tested (0.01–10 µg/mL). In addition, these natural products did not display cytotoxic property. This intriguing immunosuppressive activity was ascribed to the presence of the susbstituent on C-2 of the inner monosaccharide. Some years later, the same authors isolated two new related glycosphingolipids, plakosides C (**89**) and D (**90**), from another marine-sponge species, *Ectyoplasia ferox* [46]. Further investigations led to the conclusion that the plakosides are in fact biosynthesized by sponge-associated bacterial symbionts and not from the sponge itself [46].

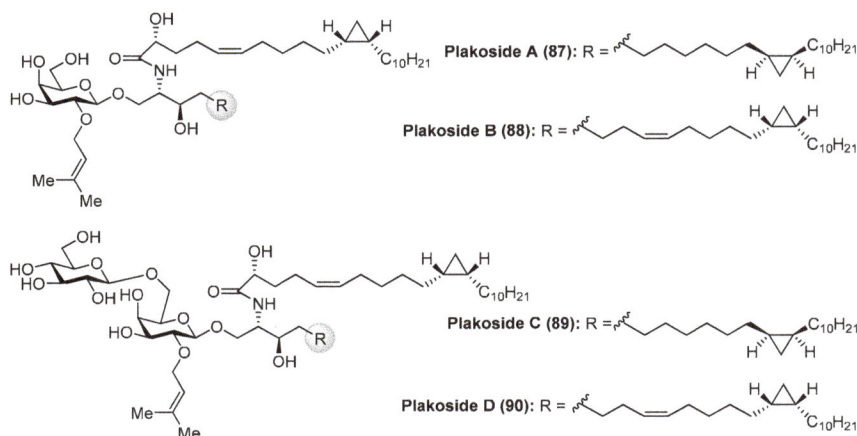

Plakoside A (87): R =
Plakoside B (88): R =
Plakoside C (89): R =
Plakoside D (90): R =

Figure 9. Structures of plakosides **87–90**.

The interesting molecular structures of the plakosides, combined with their intriguing immunosuppressive activity, have prompted their total synthesis to further investigate their biological properties. Thus, Nicolaou et al. [47] reported an efficient and stereoselective total synthesis of these glycosphingolipids, which provided not only sufficient amounts of the compounds for further biological studies, but also some analogues that allowed the determination of key structural factors for the immunosuppressive activity through a structure–activity-relationship study. Having prepared the cyclopropane-containing derivatives **91** and **92** in stereoselective manner, a first assembly of **91** with the corresponding galactosyl fluoride **93** was achieved in an excellent 93% yield in a stereoselective glycosylation reaction mediated by SnCl$_2$/AgOTf. The introduction of the prenyl group was then carried out in two steps to obtain the key intermediate **94**, which was prepared for the final steps (Scheme 5). These steps consisted of an amide coupling between **94** and the fatty acid **92**, followed by a global protecting group deprotection in two additional steps.

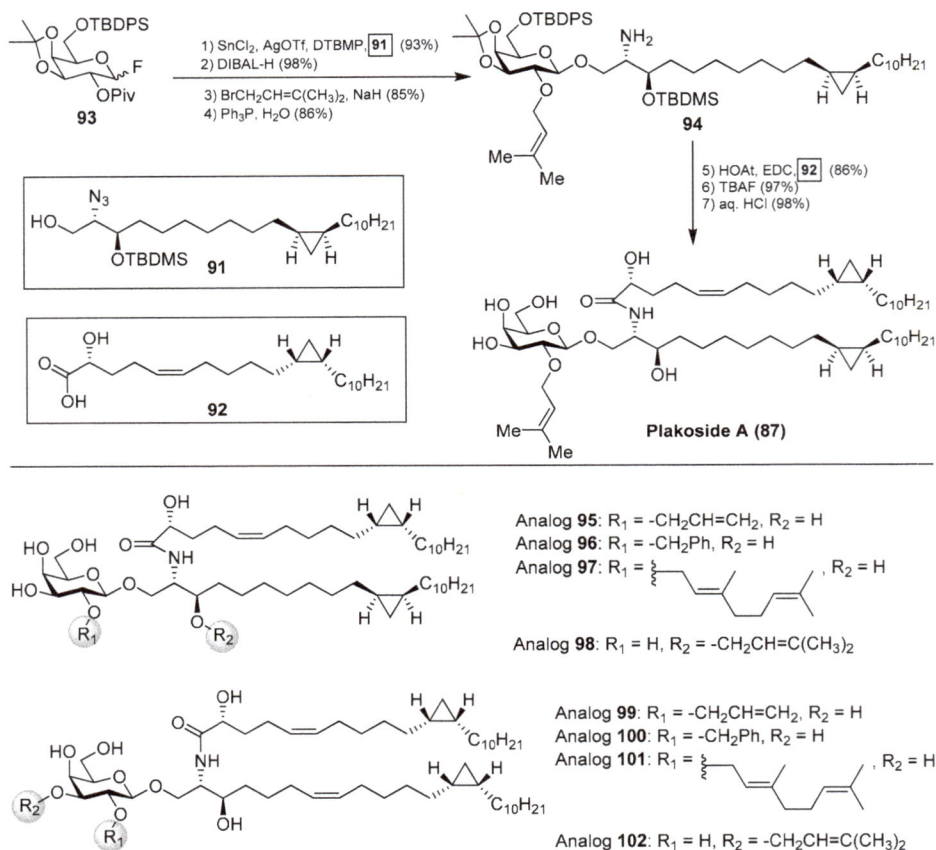

Scheme 5. Total syntheses of plakoside A (**87**) and its analogues **95–102**.

In a similar manner, the synthesis of plakoside B (**88**) was efficiently accomplished by using the suitable sphingosine derivative. This synthetic strategy was extended to the preparation of a small collection of plakoside analogues **95–102**, in which the effect of the prenyl group upon the biological activities was analysed by modification of this group. In fact, with all these plakosides in hand, their biological activities were evaluated in three in vitro assays (the mixed-lymphocyte-reaction proliferation (MLR) assay, the concanavalin A response assay, and the murine bone marrow cell proliferation assay). Surprisingly, the authors found that all these compounds (**95–102**), and the synthetic plakosides A (**87**) and B (**88**), displayed modest immunosuppressive activity compared to the reported activities for the natural compounds. Among them, analogue **95** was the most active in the series, albeit in a modest range, with an IC$_{50}$ value of 7.1 µM in the MLR proliferation assay. The discrepancy between the immunosuppressive activities of the synthetic plakosides and of the natural products reported in the literature could be explained by the work of Mori et al., who corrected the absolute configuration initially assigned for the plakosides [48,49]. These authors demonstrated, through their total synthesis described in Scheme 6, that the absolute configurations of the stereogenic carbons of the cyclopropane rings present in both lipidic chains, through compounds **103** and **104**, were opposite to those initially proposed by the Fattorusso's group [50,51]. The incorrect configurations assigned for plakoside A (**108**) could explain the poor immunosuppressive activity exhibited by the synthetic plakosides A and B prepared by Nicolaou et al. which corresponded to the stereoisomers of the naturally ocurring counterparts. It is interesting to point out that the structures of the synthetic plakosides obtained by Nicolaou's group possessed the same spectroscopic data and optical rotations as those from naturally occurring plakosides. This fact led them to conclude that the synthetic plakosides were the same as the naturally occurring counterparts.

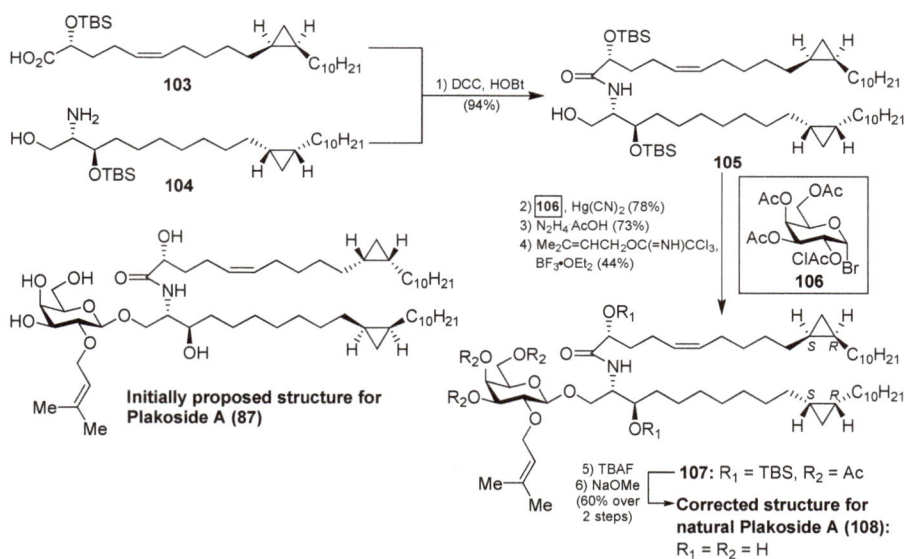

Scheme 6. Total synthesis of the corrected structure of plakoside A (**108**).

Terpiosides

Terpioside A (**109**) and B (**110**) (Figure 10) were isolated from the marine sponge *Terpios* sp. by Costantino et al. [52] and represent the first glycosphingolipids reported from sponges of the genus *Terpios*. Later, Cutignano et al. [53] reported the isolation of the terpiosides from the Antarctic sponge *Lyssodendoryx flabellata*. The structure of terpioside A (**109**) was secured by a combination of extensive spectroscopic analysis, as well as chemical degradation studies, revealing the presence of a unique sugar moiety, comprised of an α-fucofuranoside, linked to the 3-position of a β-glucopyranoside, which is the sugar residue linked to the ceramide. Thus, terpioside A (**109**) represents the first natural glycosphingolipid that contains an L-fucose in a furanose form. On the other hand, terpioside B (**110**) contains a pentasaccharide chain, which possesses two terminal α-L-fucofuranose units. The biological activity evaluation of terpioside B (**110**) led to the discovery that this compound was capable of inhibiting LPS-induced NO release, displaying higher activity than simpler glycosphingolipids, such as terpioside A (**109**) and monoglucosylceramide [54].

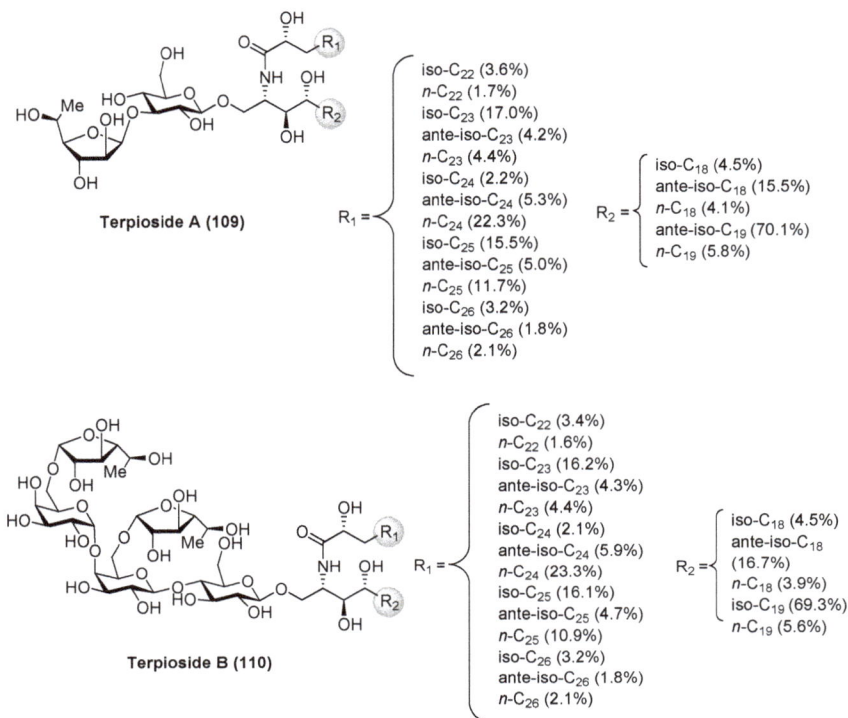

Figure 10. Structures of terpiosides A (**109**) and B (**110**).

2.1.3. Neutral Glycosphingolipids with Oligosaccharide Chains

Agelagalastatin

Agelagalastatin (**111**) was isolated from the Western-Pacific marine sponge *Agelas* sp. as a mixture of two isomers (**111a** and **111b**) through a human cancer cell line bioassay carried out by Pettit et al. [55]. Agelagalastatin showed significant in vitro antitumoral activity against various human cancer cell lines, including lung NCI-H460, brain SF-295, renal A498, colon KM20L2, melanoma SK-MEL-5, and the ovarian OVCAR-3, with a range of GI$_{50}$ values from 0.77 µg/mL to 2.8 µg/mL. Structurally, this natural product contains an unprecedented digalactofuranosyl unit, which has not been found before in a natural product.

This intriguing structure, in conjuction with its antitumor activity, drew the attention of many synthetic chemists and, as a consequence, a total synthesis of agelagalastatin (**111**) was reported by Kim et al. [56] based on an α-selective glycosylation of the ceramide **115a** or **115b** with the trisaccharide fluoride **114**, prepared from monosaccharide derivatives **112** and **113** after several steps. This key glycosylation reaction, performed in the presence of SnCl$_2$, AgClO$_4$, and DTBMP, furnished **116a** and **116b** in 72 and 73% yields, respectively. Completion of the synthesis involved the final deprotection of the benzyl, O-acetyl, and O-benzoyl groups in 70 and 74% overall yields to obtain agelagalastatins **111a** and **111b**, respectively (Scheme 7).

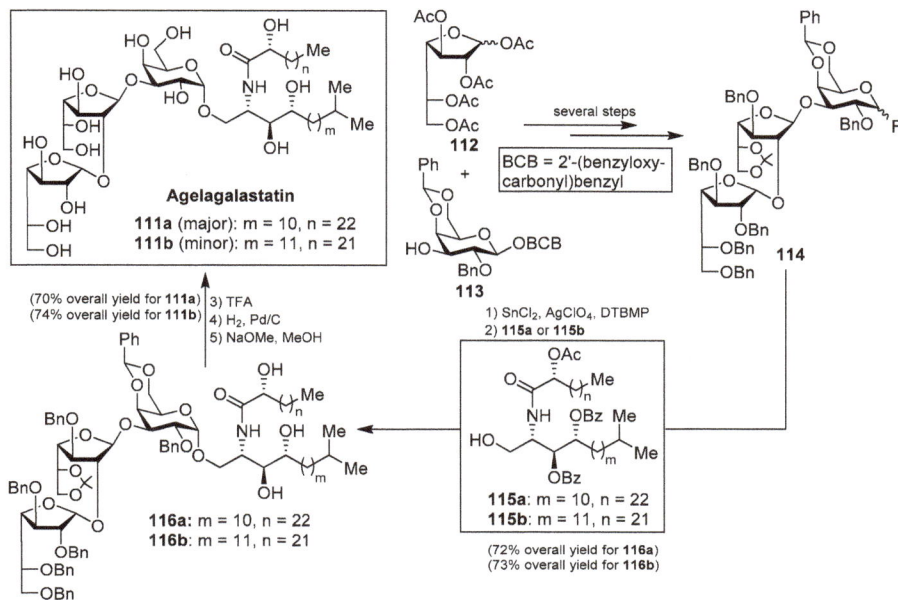

Scheme 7. Structures of agelagalastatins (**111a** and **111b**) and their total synthesis.

Clarhammosides

The clarhamnosides **117a$_x$b$_y$** (Figure 11) were isolated as an inseparable mixture of different members from the marine sponge *Agelas clathrodes* by Costantino et al. [57]. The combination of 2D NMR and CD spectroscopic techniques allowed the structural determination of this complex glycosphingolipid mixture. Clarhamnosides are the first α-galactoglycosphingolipids with a L-rhamnose unit in the sugar head. In addition, the sequential two 1,2-*cis*-α-D-galactopyranosidic linkages are also rare in nature.

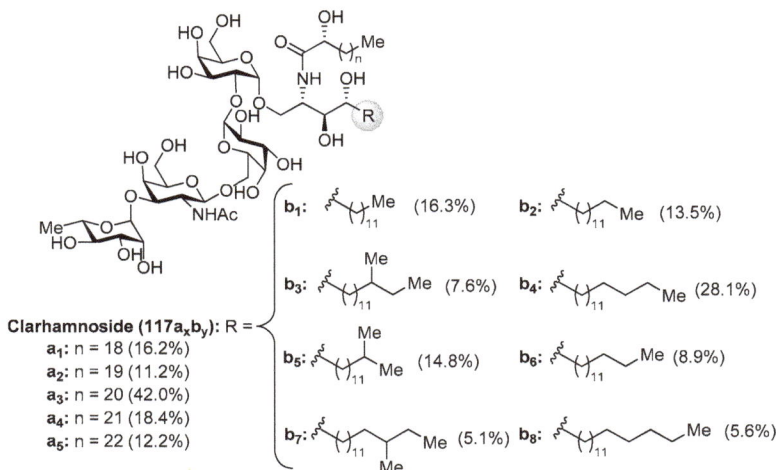

Figure 11. Structures of the clarhamnosides (**117a$_x$b$_y$**).

The first total synthesis of a clarhamnoside member (**117a₂b₆**) was carried out by Li et al. [58]. According to this work, the glycosylation reaction between **118** and **119**, promoted by the NIS/AgOTf system, afforded a 3:1 α:β separable mixture of the disaccharide **120** in 76% yield. Removal of the benzoyl group in **120** gave the disaccharide **121** in 86% yield, which was used as an acceptor for the next glycosylation reaction. In this reaction, **121** was reacted with donor trifluoroacetimidate **122** employing TMSOTf and 4 Å MS at −20 °C to provide the β-glycoside **123** in 76% yield. Conversion of the *N*-phthalimido group into an acetamido group by sequential treatment with ethylenediamine and Ac₂O afforded **124** in 72% yield in two steps. The reduction of **124**, employing H₂S in pyridine/water, was prior to the corresponding coupling of the resulting amine with α-hydroxy acid **125** to provide **126** in 66% yield in two steps. Final hydrogenolysis afforded the corresponding tetrasaccharide intermediate, which was acetylated to obtain clarhamnoside peracetate **127**. Removal of the acetyl groups furnished clarhamnoside **117a₂b₆** in a moderately good yield (Scheme 8).

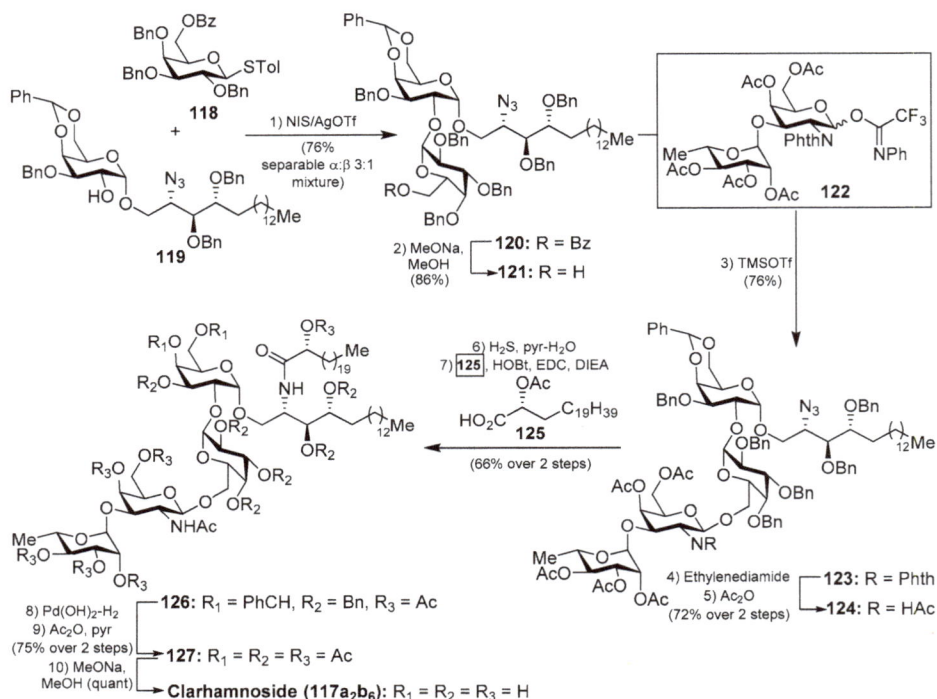

Scheme 8. Total synthesis of clarhamnoside **117a₂b₆**.

Vespariosides

After the isolation of vesparioside A (**128**) by Mangoni et al. [59] from *Spheciospongia vesparia* in 2005, the same authors in 2008 reported the isolation and structural elucidation of a unique furanose-rich glycosphingolipid that was named vesparioside B (**129**) (Figure 12) [60]. Through an exhaustive spectroscopic analysis, supported by theoretical and degradation studies, the authors were able to establish the absolute configuration of this stunning molecule, which was unambiguously confirmed through the total synthesis carried out by Yang et al. in 2016 [61]. In this total synthesis, after an extensive exploration of various strategies, the authors decided to construct initially the glycosphingolipid derivative **133**, via a glycosylation reaction of the donor trichloroacetimidate **131**, prepared from the disaccharide **130**, and the phytosphingosine acceptor **132**.

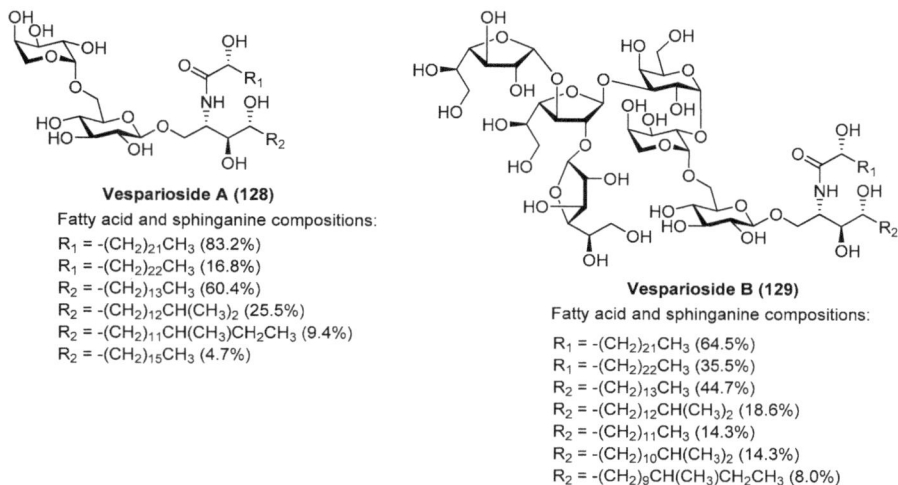

Figure 12. Structures of vespariosides A (**128**) and B (**129**).

The resulting glycosphingolipid **133** was then prepared for assembly with the tetrasaccharide fragment in the form of thioglycoside **135**. To this end, the removal of the PMB group of **133** by treatment with DDQ provided the alcohol **134**, which was reacted with the donor **135** under the action of the promoter NIS/TfOH. The resulting complex glycosphingolipid **136**, obtained in excellent yield and stereoselectively, was then transformed into natural vesparioside B (**129**) after removal of all the protecting groups in a 60% overall yield in three steps (Scheme 9).

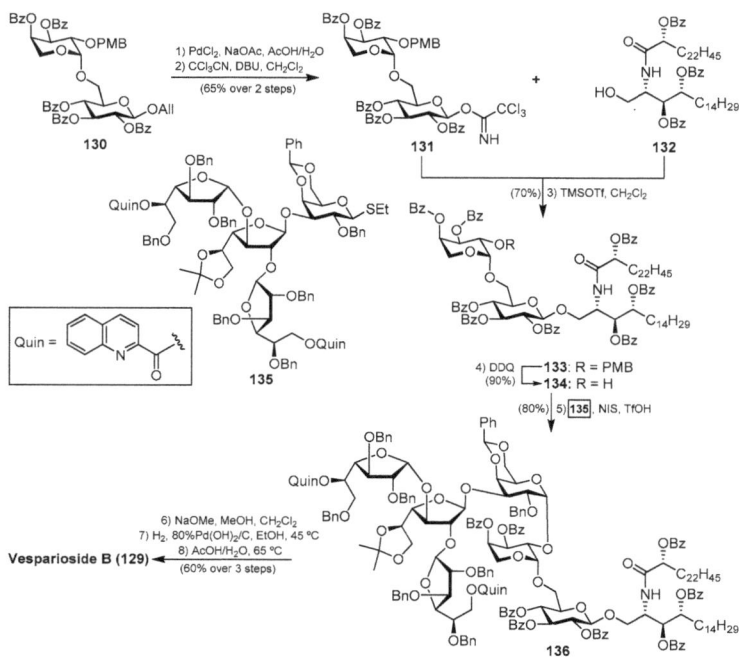

Scheme 9. Total synthesis of vesparioside B (**129**).

Interestingly, the preparation of the tetrasaccharide **135** required the stereoselective synthesis of 1,2-*cis*-α-galactofuranoside units, for which some methods have been recently developed. In this case, Yang's group has developed an elegant methodology based on a hydrogen-bond-mediated aglycone delivery (HAD) strategy for which they employed a 2-quinolinecarbonyl (Quin) functionality. This group, acting as an H-bond acceptor and incorporated in the α-face of the galactofuranoside ring, displays a strong α-stereocontrol effect in glycosylation reactions when furanosyl thioglycoside donors are employed in reactions with various acceptors. The application of this strategy in the synthesis of tetrasaccharide **135** commenced with the glycosylation reaction of the readily available galactofuranosyl acceptor **137** and the donor **138**, which was armed with the Quin group at the 5-position. This reaction delivered exclusively the α-disaccharide **139** in an excellent 95% yield, proving the reliability and validity of this strategy. The assembly of the third galactofuranosyl derivative proved more challenging, as the use of the 5-*O*-Quin derivative **138** as a donor did not work, resulting in recovered starting materials. Fortunately, when the 6-*O*-Quin derivative **141** was used instead, the reaction afforded the expected trisaccharide **142** as a 6:1 α/β separable mixture in an 85% combined yield. Finally, the fourth glycoside was incorporated through a glycosylation reaction with the trichloroacetamidate derivative of **142** and the thioglycoside acceptor **143** to deliver tetrasaccharide **135** in a 55% yield as a single β-anomer (Scheme 10). This total synthesis not only confirmed the molecular structure of this fascinating glycosphingolipid, but also, more importantly, provided the opportunity for further biological exploration of this class of compounds, which was not achievable due to the scarcity of material from natural sources. These biological studies with synthetic vespariosides are currently in progress.

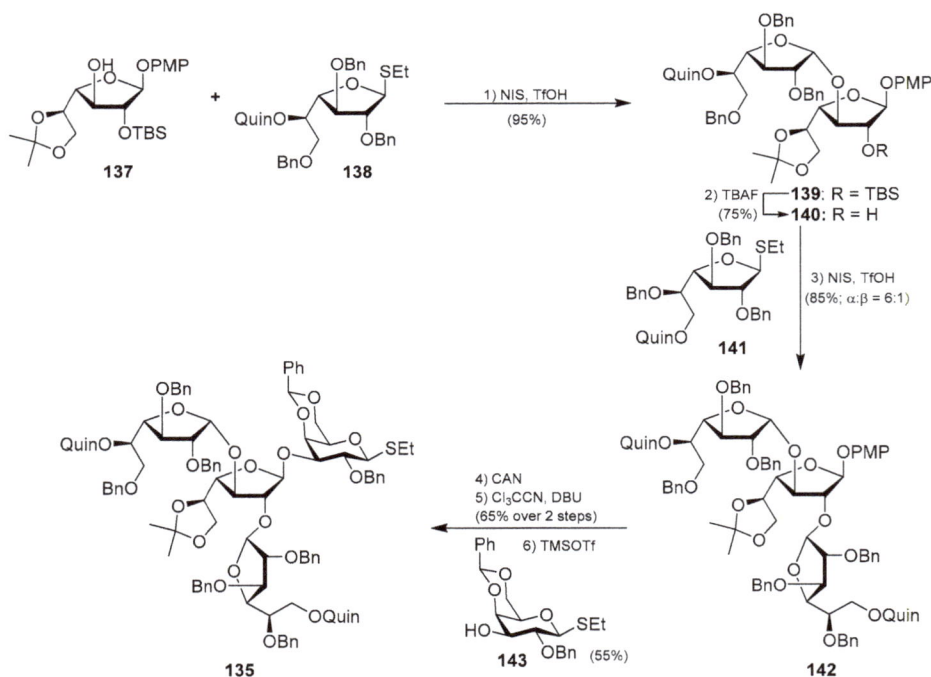

Scheme 10. Synthesis of the tetrasaccharide unit **135** of vespariosides.

2.2. Acidic Glycosphingolipids

2.2.1. Gangliosides

Structurally characterized by the presence of one or more sialic acid units, the gangliosides of a marine origin are almost exclusively found in echinoderms, mainly from urchins. In other marine invertebrates, it has been demonstrated that the sialic acid unit is replaced by a glucuronic acid residue. Despite the limited distribution of this class of glycosphingolipids in the marine realm, a huge number of natural products belonging to this category has been discovered. As a consequence, we have selected for this section the most biologically relevant gangliosides.

Ganglioside Hp-s1

Ganglioside Hp-s1 (**144**) was isolated from the ovary of the sea urchin *Diadema setosum* or from the sperm of the sea urchin *Hemicentrotus pulcherrimus* [62]. This compound showed an interesting neuritogenic activity towards the rat pheochromocytoma PC-12 cell line in the presence of nerve growth factor (NGF) and, when compared to ganglioside GM-1 (25.4%), its effect was better (34.0%). Together with ganglioside Hp-s1, ganglioside DSG-A (**145**) (Figure 13), isolated also from *D. setosum*, displayed similar neuritogenic activity, which can be useful for the treatment of neurodegenerative diseases [63].

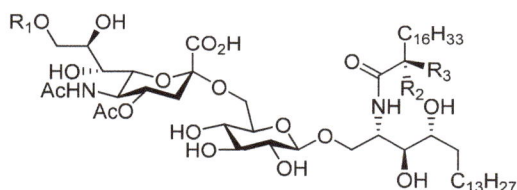

Ganglioside Hp-s1 (144): $R_1 = R_2 = R_3 = H$
Ganglioside DSG-A (145): $R_1 = Me$, $R_2 = H$, $R_3 = OH$

Figure 13. Structures of ganglioside Hp-s1 (**144**) and DSG-A (**145**).

Several syntheses of these natural products have been reported [64]. Initial synthetic efforts were carried out by Tsai et al. [65], who prepared the ganglioside Hp-s1 analogue **151**. The synthesis was accomplished by a sequence of chemoselective glycosylation reactions as key steps. Thus, the disaccharide **148** was obtained by the sialylation of the acceptor **147** with the sialyl donor **146a**, mediated by NIS/TfOH as a promoter at −30 °C in the presence of 4 Å molecular sieves, in 63% yield as an inseparable α:β 3.2:1 mixture. The next glycosylation reaction involved the resulting disaccharide **148** with the azidosphingosine derivative **149** in the presence of AgOTf and 3 Å molecular sieves at room temperature to obtain the resulting disaccharide derivative as a separable mixture of αβ and ββ anomers in 62% combined yield. From the corresponding αβ anomer, a Staudinger reaction was followed by an amidation process to obtain **150** in 54% yield in two steps. Final debenzylation and deacetylation reactions afforded the ganglioside Hp-s1 analogue **151** in 78% overall yield (Scheme 11). This analogue exhibited neurogenetic activity towards the human neuroblastoma cell line SH-SY5Y without the presence of NGF.

A different synthetic strategy was used in the first total synthesis of ganglioside Hp-s1 (**144**), achieved by Luo et al. [64], based on two key glycosylation reactions. According to this synthetic strategy, after an extensive optimization of the glycosylation reactions, the authors found that the first reaction of phytosphingosine **152** with benzyl protected imidate **153**, using TMSOTf as a promoter at −30 °C to room temperature, followed by a deacetylation step, afforded **154** in 82% (β:α 3.2:1) yield. The second glycosylation reaction involved the glycosyl acceptor **154** and the sialyl donor **146b**, mediated by NIS/TfOH as a promoter, to obtain **155** in 84% yield (αβ:ββ 3.9:1). From **155**, the conversion of the azide group into the corresponding amine, through a Staudinger reaction, followed by amide formation, and final deprotection of acetyl, benzyl, and acetonide groups delivered ganglioside Hp-s1 (**144**) in 43% overall yield from **155** (Scheme 12).

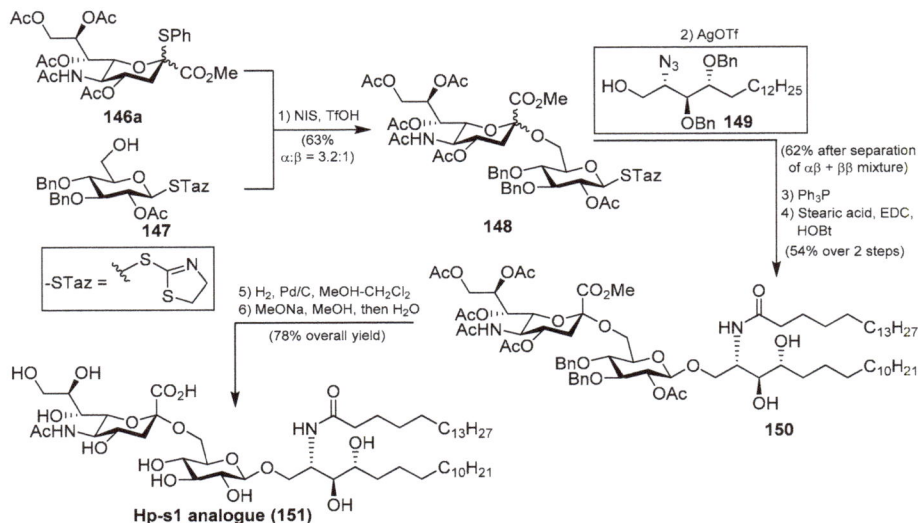

Scheme 11. Total synthesis of Hp-s1 analogue **151**.

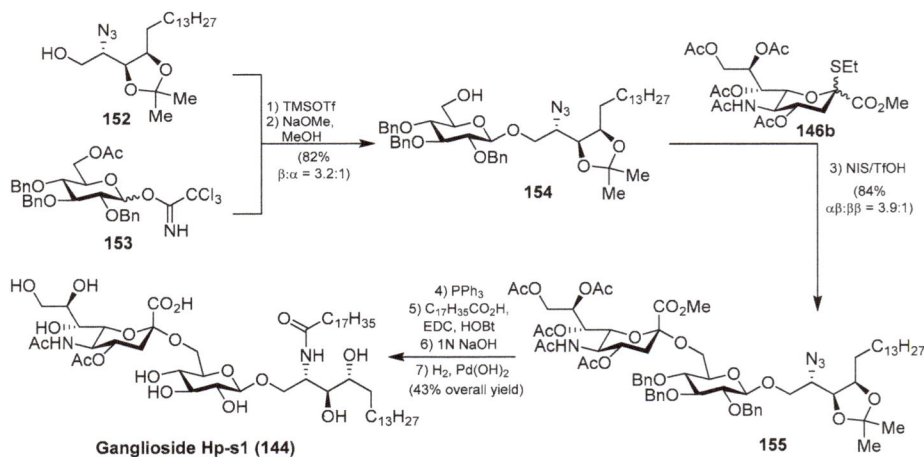

Scheme 12. Total synthesis of ganglioside Hp-s1 (**144**).

The same authors carried out an SAR study involving the synthesis of six Hp-s1 analogues (**156**–**161**) by replacing the glucosyl unit of Hp-s1 with α-glucose (**157**), α- and β-galactose (**158** and **159**), and α- and β-mannose (**160** and **161**), including the simple cerebroside **156** [66]. After the biological evaluation, the authors found that the C-2 hydroxyl group of the glucosyl unit played a crucial role in the stimulation of neurite outgrowth of SH-SY5Y cells. In addition, it was found that analogue **158** activated NKT cells, although it was inactive on neurite outgrowth of SH-SY5Y cells (Figure 14).

Based on these synthetic studies, the same authors developed an efficient method for α-selective sialylation based on a pre-activated 5-*N*,4-*O*-carbamate thiosialoside donor using *p*-TolSCl/AgOTf as promoters which was extended to the synthesis of gangliosides Hp-s1 and DSG-A [67]. Tsai et al. also achieved the total synthesis of ganglioside DSG-A (**145**) through a chemoselective glycosylation reaction in a [1 +1 + 2] synthetic strategy for the assembly of the four fragments of this molecule [68].

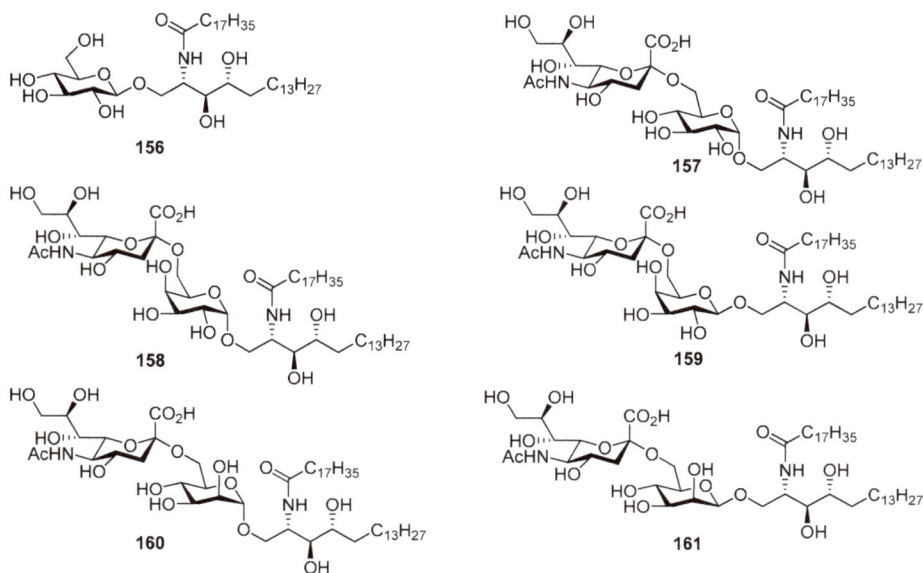

Figure 14. Gangliosides Hp-s1 analogues **156**–**161**.

Gangliosides HLG

Gangliosides HLG-1 (**162**), HLG-2 (**163**) and HLG-3 (**164**) (Figure 15) were isolated from the sea cucumber *Holothuria leucospilota* by Higuchi et al. [69]. These compounds showed similar neuritogenic activity toward the rat pheochromocytoma cell line, PC-12 cell, in the presence of NGF as other marine-derived gangliosides. Structurally, these gangliosides contain a unique α(2,4) linkage between sialic acids, which captured the attention of many synthetic chemists.

The first total synthesis of ganglioside HLG-2 (**163**) was carried out by Kiso et al. [70]. To construct the glycan unit, sialylation at C-4 hydroxyl group of the sialic acid residue was achieved using the 1,5-lactam-sialyl unit **166** as a novel glycosyl acceptor and readily prepared from **165** by a basic treatment (refluxing NaOMe in MeOH) in 95% yield. The glycosylation reaction of **166** with Troc-sialyl donor **167** in the presence of NIS/TfOH took place exclusively at C-4 hydroxyl group in a stereoselective manner to give the trisaccharide **168** in 69% yield (α:β 60:9). To complete the synthesis, the next glycosylation reaction involved the donor **169**, obtained in eight steps from the trisaccharide **168**, and the ceramide acceptor **170** in the presence of TMSOTf as a promoter, to obtain the corresponding ganglioside in 49% yield, which was finally transformed into ganglioside HLG-2 (**163**) in a quantitative yield after a basic treatment (Scheme 13).

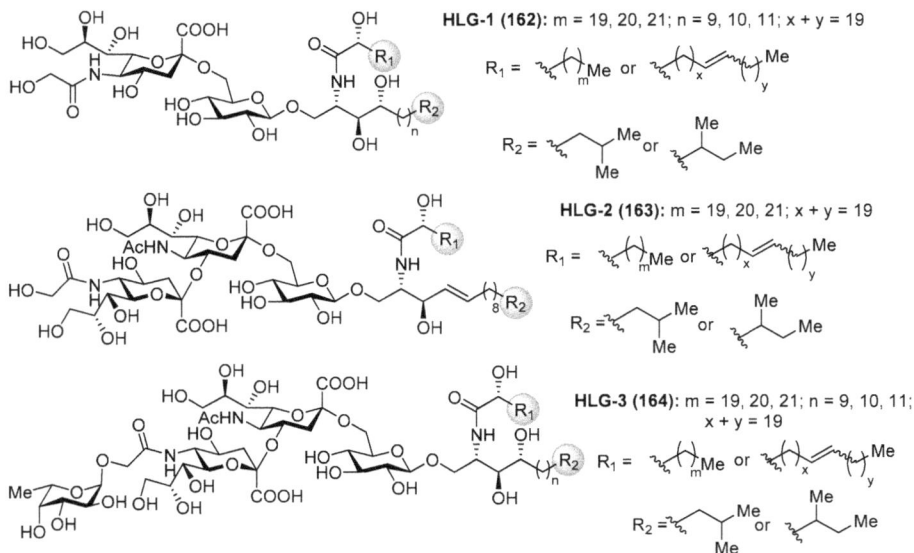

Figure 15. Structures of gangliosides HLG-1, -2, and -3 (**162–164**).

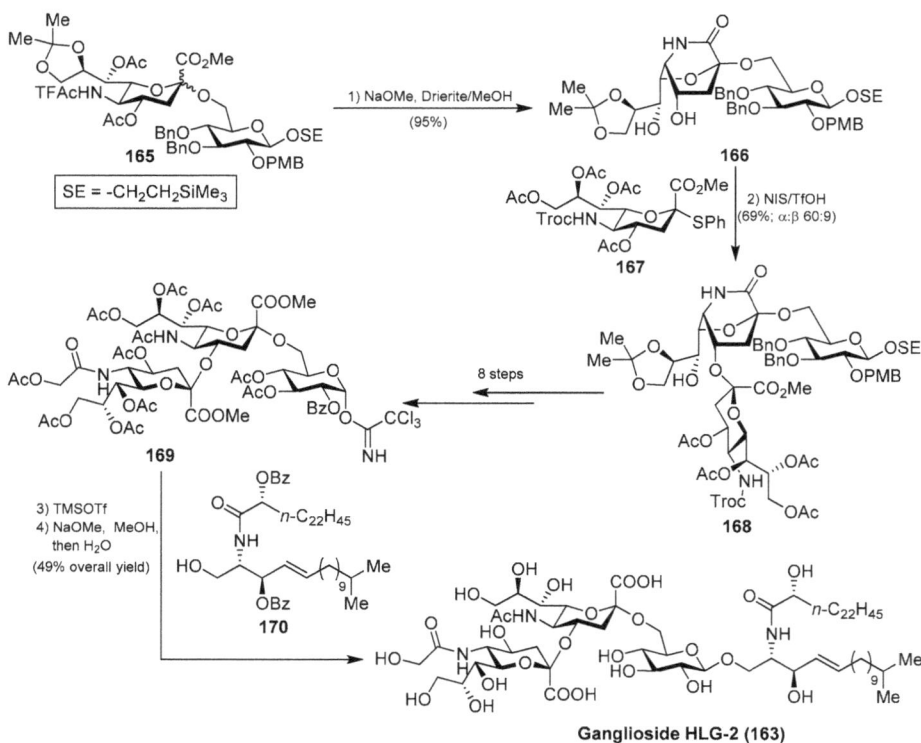

Scheme 13. Total synthesis of ganglioside HLG-2 (**163**).

Interesting was the synthetic approach by Ye et al., who achieved the synthesis of the glycan portion of ganglioside HLG-2 in a highly efficient and stereoselective manner, involving two key glycosylation reactions: first, for the construction of the disaccharide **173** using the phosphate donor **172**, in the presence of TMSOTf, in 95% yield; and, second, for the generation of the trisaccharide **176** by the use of NIS/TfOH in 96% yield, both with excellent α-stereoselectivity. From **176**, final conversion of functional groups and deprotection reactions afforded the trisaccharide core of ganglioside HLG-2 (**177**) [71] (Scheme 14).

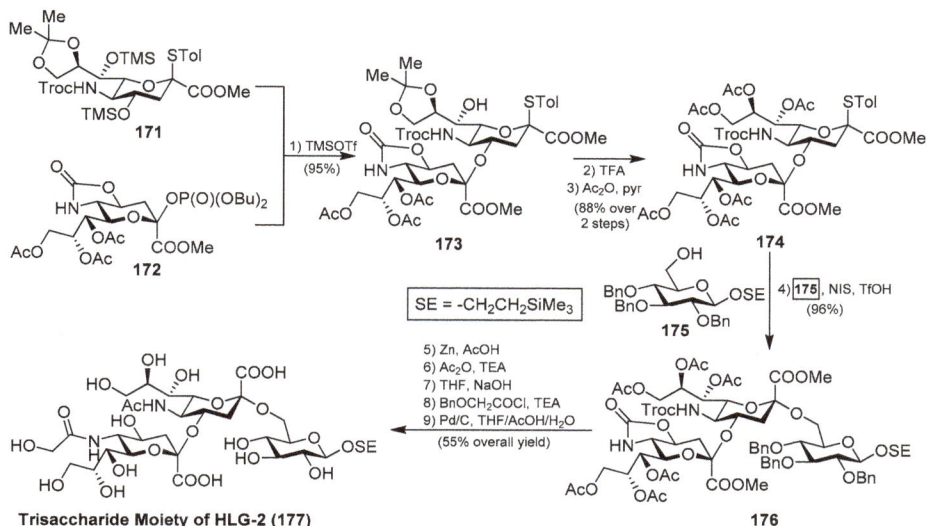

Scheme 14. Total synthesis of the trisaccharide core **177** of ganglioside HLG-2 (**163**).

Ganglioside GP-3

Ganglioside GP-3 (**178**) was isolated from the starfish *Asterina pectinifera* by Higuchi et al. [72]. As previous gangliosides, GP-3 also exhibited neuritogenic activity toward the rat pheochromocytoma PC-12 cells, in the presence of the NGF, displaying, in this case, a lower effect when compared with ganglioside GM-1. Structurally, the glycan part contains nine monosaccharide units in a unique saccharide sequence with two internal sialic acid residues and three furanose residues.

The total synthesis of ganglioside GP-3 (**178**) was achieved by Kiso et al. [73]. Briefly, the final glycosylation reaction of the octasaccharide donor **179** with the glucosphingolipic derivative **180** was promoted by TMSOTf to furnish the protected ganglioside GP-3 **181** in 77% yield. A final deprotection sequence, which included aqueous TFA and basic treatments, afforded ganglioside GP-3 (**178**) (Scheme 15).

Ganglioside CG-1

Ganglioside CG-1 (**183**), isolated from the sea cucumber *Cucumaria echinata* by Higuchi et al. [36], showed neuritogenic activity toward the rat pheochromocytoma PC-12 cells. The same authors carried out a partial synthesis of a related CG-1 ganglioside, which lacked the sulfate group in the natural product, by a coupling of 2-thioglycoside **185** with **184**, which was prepared from the natural acanthacerebroside (**1**), in the presence of NIS/TfOH, to obtain the corresponding α-sialoside in 31% yield. This advanced precursor of CG-1 was then subjected to stepwise deprotections to obtain the related CG-1 ganglioside **186** in 93% yield [74] (Scheme 16). This synthetic study can delineate the path towards the total synthesis of this natural product.

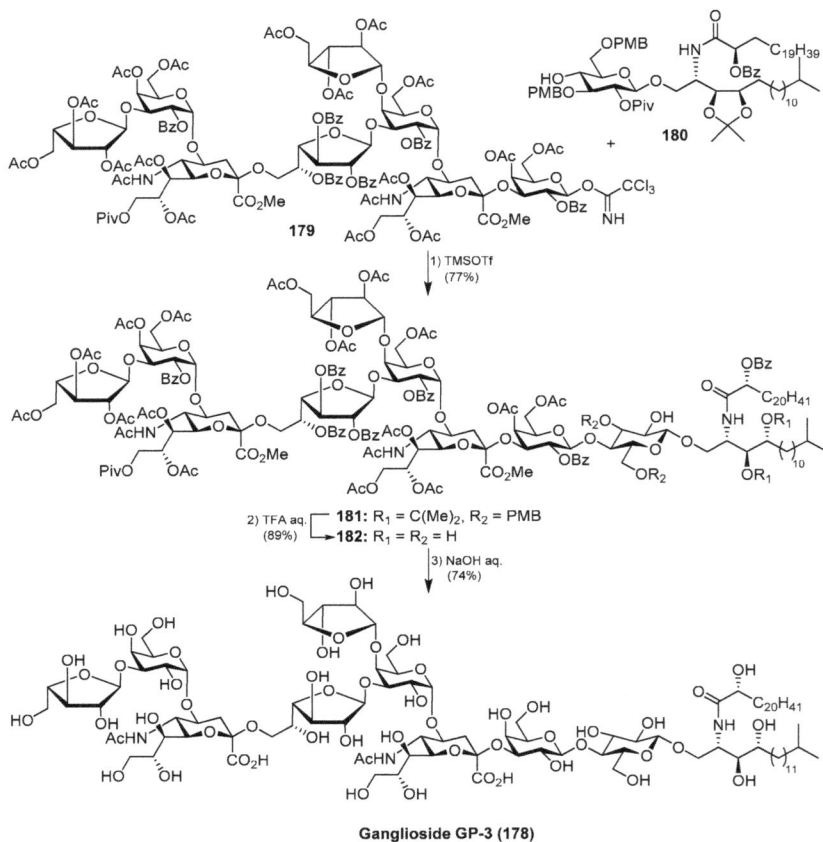

Scheme 15. Total synthesis of ganglioside GP-3 (**178**).

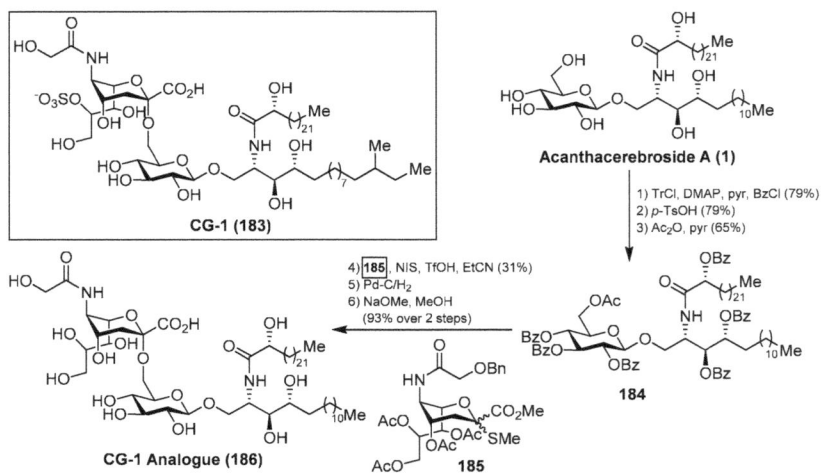

Scheme 16. Total synthesis of ganglioside CG-1 analogue **186**.

Gangliosides SJG

Gangliosides SJG-1 (**187**) and SJG-2 (**188**) were isolated from the sea cucumber *Stichopus japonicus* by Higuchi et al. [75,76] (Figure 16). As the gangliosides described in previous sections, the SJG gangliosides also showed neuritogenic activity toward the rat pheochromocytoma PC12 cells in the presence of NGF. The effect of SJG-2 was higher than that of mammalian ganglioside (proportion of neurite bearing cells SJG-2 64.8%, SJG-1 35.4%, and GM-1 47.0%).

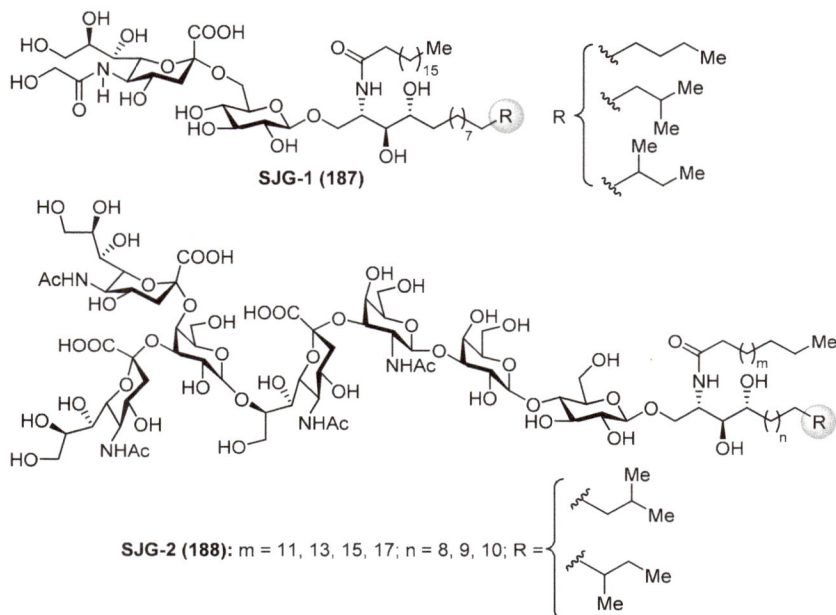

Figure 16. Structures of gangliosides SJG (**187** and **188**).

The same authors carried out an SAR study of a few gangliosides from Echinoderms involving trisialo-gangliosides (SJG-2 and LLG-5), disialo-gangliosides (LLG-3 [77], GAA-7 [78], HLG-2, LMG-4, HLG-3, and GP-3), and monosialo-gangliosides (AG-2, AG-3, HLG-1, SJG-1, LMG-2). Evaluation of the neuritogenic activity on a rat pheochromocytoma cell line (PC-12 cells) indicated that (a) the presence of sialic acid is essential; (b) the presence of two terminal sialic acids is key for strong activity; (c) gangliosides having an 8-O-Me sialic acid showed stronger activity; (d) gangliosides possessing sialic acid inside of the oligosaccharide unit showed better activity; (e) the different activity showed by HLG-1 and SJG-1 (44.7 and 35.4%, respectively), which have the same sugar unit, is due to the difference in the structure of their ceramide units; (f) SJG-2, LLG-5, LLG-3, and GAA-7 have better effect than mammalian ganglioside GM-1, which has positive effects in neuritogenical diseases; and (g) these gangliosides showed no activity without the presence of NGF [79].

Gangliosides CEG

Gangliosides CEG-3 (**189**), CEG-4 (**190**), CEG-5 (**191**), CEG-6 (**192**), CEG-8 (**193**), and CEG-9 (**194**) were isolated from the sea cucumber *Cucumaria echinata* by Higuchi et al. [80,81] (Figure 17). These compounds showed neuritogenic activity toward the rat pheochromocytoma cell line PC-12 in the presence of a nerve growth factor.

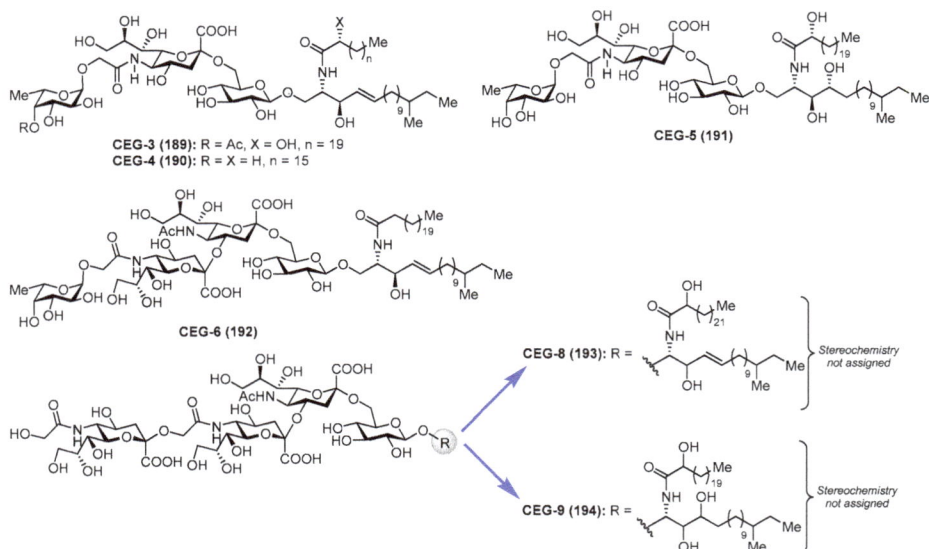

Figure 17. Structures of gangliosides CEG (**189–194**).

2.2.2. Sulfatides

Axinelloside A

Axinelloside A (**195**), a highly sulfated liposaccharide, was isolated from the lipophilic extract of the Japanease marine sponge *Axinella infundibula* by Fusetani et al. [82]. The structure of axinelloside A (**195**) was elucidated after an excellent spectroscopic work based on 2D NMR and MS techniques, determining the presence of twelve sugars including *scyllo*-inositol, D-arabinose, five D-galactoses, and five L-fucose units, to which one (*R*)-3-hydroxy-octadecanoic acid, three molecules of (*E*)-2-hexadecenoic acids and 19 sulfates groups were attached. This compound shows similar structure to sulfated polysaccharides from the marine sponge *Chondrilla nucula* and *Dysidea fragilis* (Figure 18).

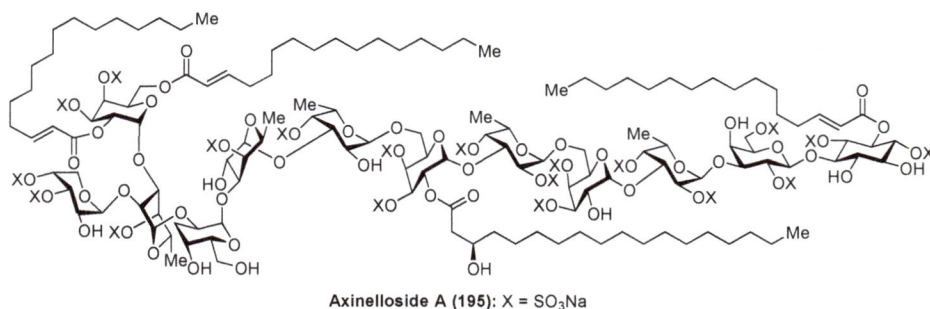

Axinelloside A (**195**): X = SO$_3$Na

Figure 18. Structure of axinelloside A (**195**).

From a biological standpoint, axinelloside A (**195**) strongly inhibited the activity of human telomerase with an IC$_{50}$ value of 0.4 µM (2 µg/mL). In this biological activity, it is possible that the sulfate groups play a key role, since it was proven that the dictyodendrins [83], a family of sulfated pyrrolocarbazoles isolated from the sponge *Dictyodendrilla verongiformis*, lost all telomerase inhibitory activity when their sulfate groups were removed. The mechanism of action of the telomerase inhibitory activity of axinelloside A (**195**) remains unknown.

Encouraged by the telomerase inhibitory activity of axinelloside A (**195**), Walczak et al. [84] achieved the synthesis of the *scyllo*-inositol fragment from D-glucose through a Ferrier rearrangement of a vinyl-acetate derivative and stereoslective reduction of the resulting ketone. The same authors established a synthetic sequence for the preparation of a series of simple sulfated D-galactosyl liposaccharides, inspired by axinelloside A (**195**), in order to evaluate their potential as new telomerase inhibitors [85]. However, the biological activities of these galactose derivatives have not been reported so far.

3. Chemistry and Biology of Glycoglycerolipids

3.1. Aminoglycoglycerolipids and Related Glycoglycerolipids

Within this class of glycoglycerolipids, it is noteworthy to mention avrainvilloside (**196**), isolated from the Dominican green alga *Avrainvillea nigricans* by Taglialatela-Scafati et al. [86]. Related to avrainvilloside (**196**), the aminoglycoglycerolipid 1,2-dipalmitoyl-3-(*N*-palmitoyl-6′-amino-6′-deoxy-α-D-glucosyl)-*sn*-glycerol (**197a**) was isolated from a marine alga, designated as UM2972M, by Kingston et al. This compound displayed potent inhibitory activity against the Myt1-kinase (IC_{50} = 0.12 mg/mL), an enzyme involved in the regulation of the cdc2/cyclin B kinase activity, which is essential for the growth of tumor cells [87]. Schmidt et al. [88] achieved the total synthesis of aminoglycoglycerolipid **197a** by glycosylation reaction of the imidate **198** and the alcohol **199**, promoted by TMSOTf, to obtain **200** in a 46% combined yield, as a separable α:β 78:22 mixture of anomers. Deprotection of the major α-anomer **200**, followed by an acylation step to introduce a palmitic-acid unit, afforded **201** in 55% yield in two steps. The final Staudinger reaction, followed by an amide coupling with the last palmitic acid unit and global deprotection, gave aminoglycoglycerolipid **197a** in 79% overall yield (Scheme 17).

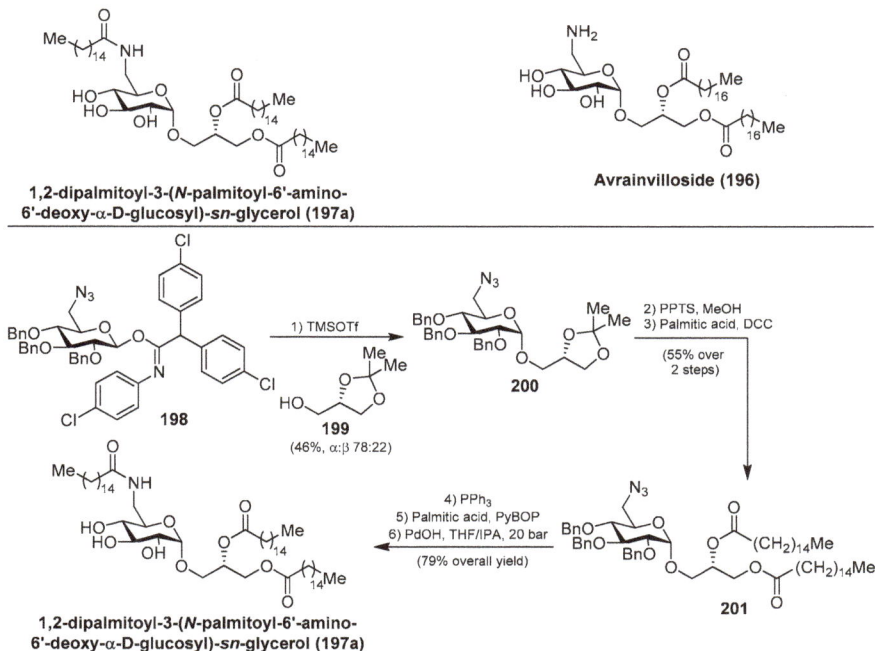

Scheme 17. Synthesis of 1,2-dipalmitoyl-3-(*N*-palmitoyl-6′-amino-6′-deoxy-α-D-glucosyl)-*sn*-glycerol **197a**.

Later, Li et al. [89] completed the synthesis of the aminoglycoglyceropilpid **197a** as well as its acyl analogues (**197b–h**) in an efficient method employing the trichloroacetimidate donor **202** to obtain **200**, by reaction with the glycerol derivative **199**, in 88% yield and high α-selectivity (α:β 33:1) as the key step. The same authors synthesized different mannosyl (**203a–h**) and galactosyl analogues related to **197** in a similar manner. Given the antiviral activity displayed by many glycoglycerolipids isolated from algae, the authors evaluated the inhibitory activity of these amino derivatives against the influenza A virus (IAV) by the cytophatic effects inhibition assay. These analogues displayed inhibition of the viral replication in MDCK cells and it was found that the type of the linkages and the length of the acids could influence the activity. Among them, **203g** showed the best activity with an IC_{50} of 69.9 μM [90,91]. Later, new analogues **204–207** (Figure 19) were prepared and tested for anti-IAV activity, and the authors concluded that acylamino and glycerol groups of the glycolipids were essential for the inhibitory activity on IAV multiplication [92]. From this new series, **204d** was the most potent, with an IC_{50} of 60.8 μM, and may provide a point of exploration of unique aminoglycoglycerolipids in drug discovery for pneumonia caused by viruses. In fact, this compound was selected for preliminary inhibitory studies on IAV infection *in vivo*. The results of this study showed that **204d** exhibited a significant reduction of viral titers in the lungs of IAV-infected mice at a dose of 5 mg/Kg/d, with a striking increase of the survival rate (90%) compared to the infected group treated with oseltamivir.

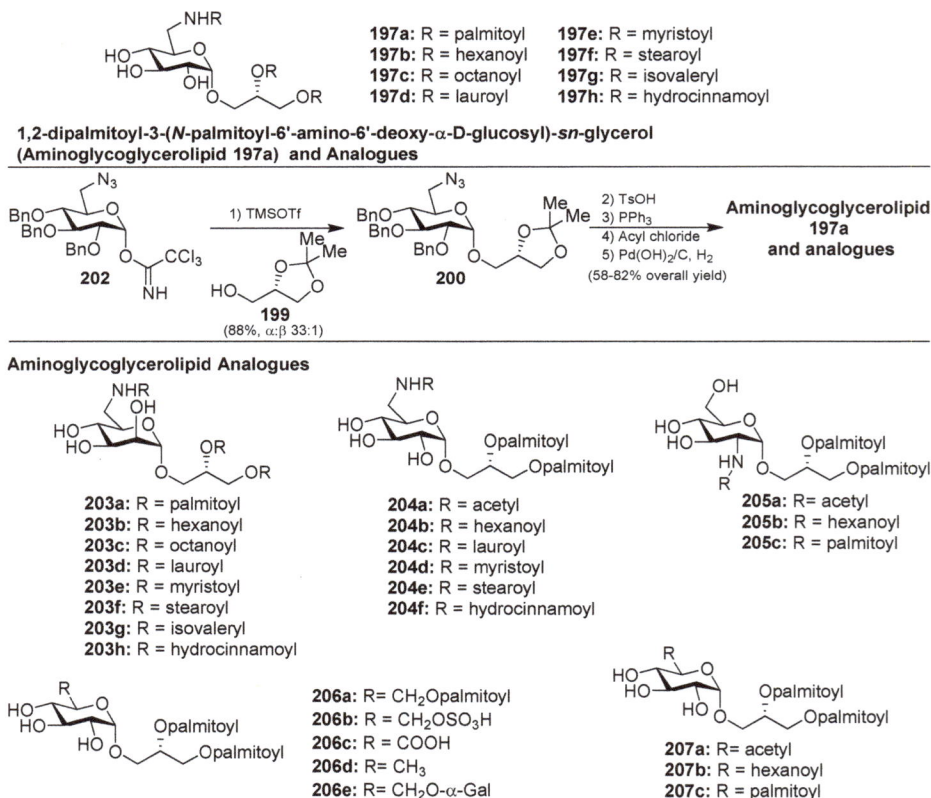

Figure 19. Structures of aminoglycoglycerolipids based on **197a**.

3.2. Crasserides and Isocrasserides

Crasserides (**208a–m**) (Figure 20), initially isolated by Fattorusso et al. [93] from the Caribbean sponge *Pseudoceratina crassa* (family Dysideidae), represent unique glycolipids that resemble common glycoglycerolipids by the replacement of an usual sugar by a five-membered cyclitol and the 1-*O*-acyl group present in the glycerol unit by an 1-*O*-alkyl group. Since their first isolation, the crasserides have been found in several families of sponges, including *Verongula gigantea* (family Dysideidae), *Aplysina fulva* (family Aplysinidae), *A. cauliformis* (family Aplysinidae), *Neofibularia nolitangere* (family Mycalidae), *Agelas clathrodes* (family Agelasidae), *A. dispar* (family Agelasidae), *A. conifera, A. longissima, Plakortis simplex* (family Plakinidae), *Ectyoplasia ferox* (family Raspailiidae), and *Siphonodictyon coralliphagum* (family Niphatidae) [94]. The structures of these interesting natural products were established and their stereochemistry was determined by exhaustive NMR spectroscopic analyses. Preliminary biological evaluations of these compounds revealed that the crasserides are potent feeding deterrents, with a concentration as low as 30 µg/cm^2 of food pellets according to the antifeedant assay on the fish *Carassius auratus*. Almost ten years later, the same authors discovered from the same sponges a new family of related compounds, which are termed isocrasserides (**209a–m**) [94], which accompanied the crasserides in minor amounts, demonstrating that these compounds are genuine natural metabolites and not artifacts, as initially suspected.

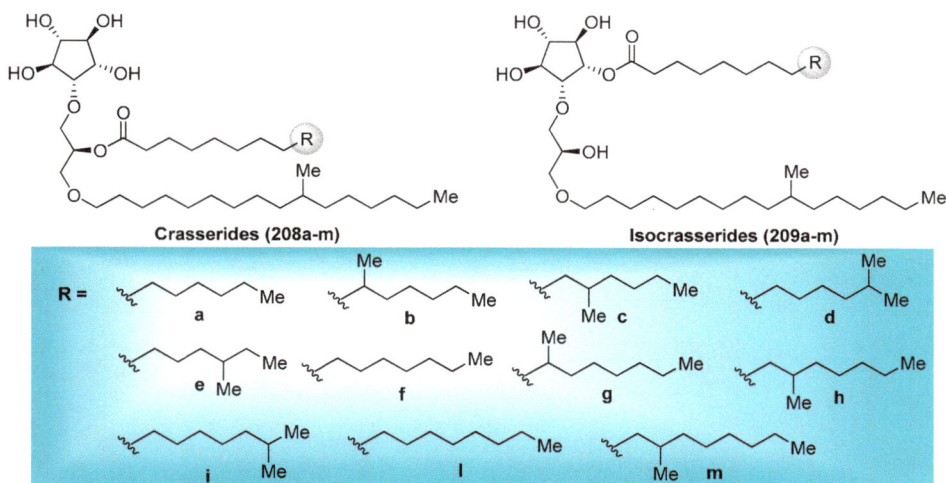

Figure 20. Structures of the crasserides (**208a–m**) and the isocrasserides (**209a–m**).

3.3. Myrmekiosides

The myrmekiosides (**210–212**) belong to the family of the glycoglycerolipids, isolated from the marine sponges *Myrmekioderma* sp. and *Trikentrion loeve* by Barnathan's group and displayed potent antitumor activity [95]. In fact, their preliminary biological evaluations revealed that myrmekiosides altered the tumor cell morphology of H-ras transformed NIH3T3 fibroblasts to normal at concentrations of 5 µg/mL. Later, Barnathan et al. isolated a new and related glycoglycerolipid from *M. dendyi*, which was named myrmekioside E (**213**), and found that its peracetylated derivative (**214**) exerted significant cytotocixity against NSCLC-N6 and lung tumor A549 cells with IC$_{50}$ values of 7.3 and 9.7 µM, respectively [96]. Like metabolites isolated from a marine origin, the scarcity of a bioactive material demanded its chemical synthesis as the only way to provide access in sufficient quantities for further biological evaluations. Prompted by this requirement, together with the unique mono-*O*-alkyl-diglycosylglycerol structure, Li's group published in 2015 in what represents the first and, so far, only total synthesis of myrmekioside A (**210**) [97]. Accordingly, careful inspection of this unprecedented molecular framework led the authors to prepare the xylosylglycerol **215** as the starting material to incorporate in subsequent steps other sugar units. Thus, the glycerol moiety was elaborated for the next glycosylation reaction with the trichloroacetimidate **216** to obtain, in very high yield, diglycosylglycerol **217**, after removal of the acetate group under basic conditions. Compound **217** was then reacted with thioglycoside **218**, using NIS/TfOH as a promoter, to give the corresponding glycoglycerol in an excellent 90% yield. At this point, the authors had to replace the acetyl protecting groups by benzyl ethers, and then the resulting derivative **219** was driven to the completion of the synthesis of myrmekioside A (**210**), for which the etherification reaction to introduce the pending lipidic chain was carried out by reaction of the alcohol resulting from the desilylation process of **219** with the mesylate **220** (Scheme 18). This synthesis demonstrated the proposed structure for this natural product and, in addition, that the modular character of the synthetic strategy could be useful for the preparation of other myrmekioside derivatives and analogues for further biological studies.

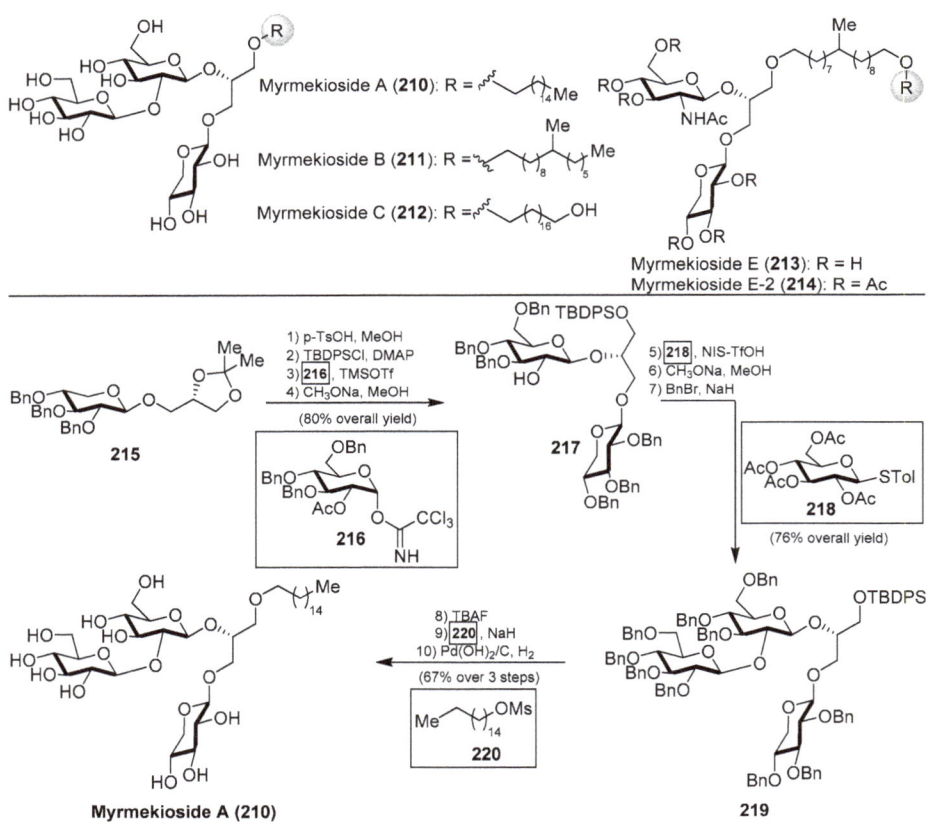

Scheme 18. Structures of the myrmekiosides (**210**–**214**) and total synthesis of myrmekioside A (**210**).

3.4. Nigricanosides

Isolated as methyl esters (**223** and **224**) from the green alga *Avrainvillea nigricans* in Dominica [98], the nigricanosides (**221** and **222**) represent a unique and unprecedented class of glycolipids with outstanding antitumoral activity in the low nM range with an IC_{50} value of 3 nM for **221** against human breast cancer MCF-7 and colon cancer HCT-116 cell lines (Figure 21). More intriguing was the recognition of the ability of the nigricanosides to promote a polimerization of tubulins as the mechanism of action of their antiproliferative property. However, the tremendous scarcity of these natural products from the natural sources (Only 800 µg and 400 µg of the methyl esters of nigricanosides A and B, **223** and **224**, respectively, were obtained from 28 Kg of wet material!) represents a significant hurdle to gain further insight into the biological properties and to establish the absolute configuration of the compounds. Consequently, the total synthesis represents the only means to determine unambiguously the stereochemistry of the chiral centers and to have enough material for further biological screenings.

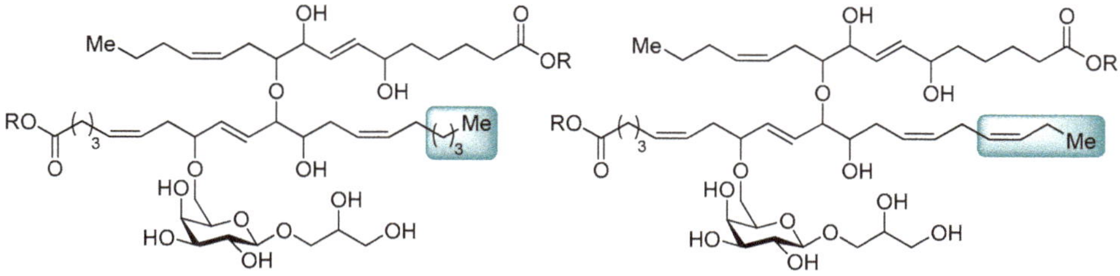

Nigricanoside A (**221**): R = H
Nigricanoside A dimethyl ester (**223**): R = Me

Nigricanoside B (**222**): R = H
Nigricanoside B dimethyl ester (**224**): R = Me

Figure 21. Structures of nigricanosides A (**221**), B (**222**), and their dimethyl esters, **223** and **224**.

Thus, several synthetic approaches have been initiated for the lipidic fragments [99–101], but many of them have not solved the stereochemical assignment problem. In fact, this stereochemical assignment represents a formidable synthetic challenge because of the presence of seven chiral centers in the lipidic unit, which could provide up to 128 possible stereoisomers, assuming that the configuration for the sugar unit and the geometry of the double bonds were correctly established (Scheme 19). This synthetic challenge was taken on by the McMillan [102] and Ready [103] groups, which used a flexible synthetic strategy capable of delivering all the possible stereoisomers. In addition, the knowledge of the stereochemistry of a related 20-C fatty acid, trioxilin A3 (**225**), isolated and identified as a hydrolysis product of the natural epoxide hepoxilin A3, led the authors to propose this stereochemistry for the 20-C unit of the nigricanosides. Thus, according to Scheme 19, they prepared the ester **226** in a convergent and efficient way from (*R*)-glycidol as the chiral source, which was prepared for the subsequent assembly of the 16-C fatty acid unit via an ether linkage. To this aim, the free alcohol of **226** was treated with 2-bromo acetic acid and, after the incorporation of the chiral auxiliary **227**, the alkylation with (*Z*)-1-iodo-2-hexene afforded, with a complete stereoselectivity, the corresponding alkylated product **228**. The use of the enantiomer *ent*-**227** provided the corresponding stereoisomer at this position. By continuation of the product **228**, the elongation of the second fatty acid was achieved in four additional steps, in which the chiral ester (*R*)-**229** was incorporated via a hydrozirconation reaction with the Schwartz reagent with a subsequent transmetalation with dimethylzinc. In a similar manner, the authors used the enantiomer (*S*)-**229** to generate all the possible stereochemical combinations of the lipidic fragment. The completion of the lipidic moiety was undertaken in five additional steps, in which the resulting product **230** was prepared for the introduction of the sugar moiety. In this event, the alcohol derived from the deprotection of the SEM group was treated with the galactosyl triflate **231** to obtain glycolipid **232**, which was finally directed towards the nigricanoside A methyl ester via a glycosylation reaction of the trichloroacetimidate derivative of **232** with the alcohol **199**. Unfortunately, the resulting synthetic nigricanoside **223a** did not match with the reported natural product and, furthermore, was inactive against HCT-116 and MCF7 tumoral cell lines. A detailed comparative analysis of the ^{1}H NMR spectra of synthetic diester **223a** and natural nigricanoside A dimethyl ester **223** revealed that the most important differences were located at the C7-C8 *trans* olefin region. These spectroscopic differences led the authors to propose a C6/C9 *syn* relationship for the natural product instead of the initially proposed *anti* relative configuration.

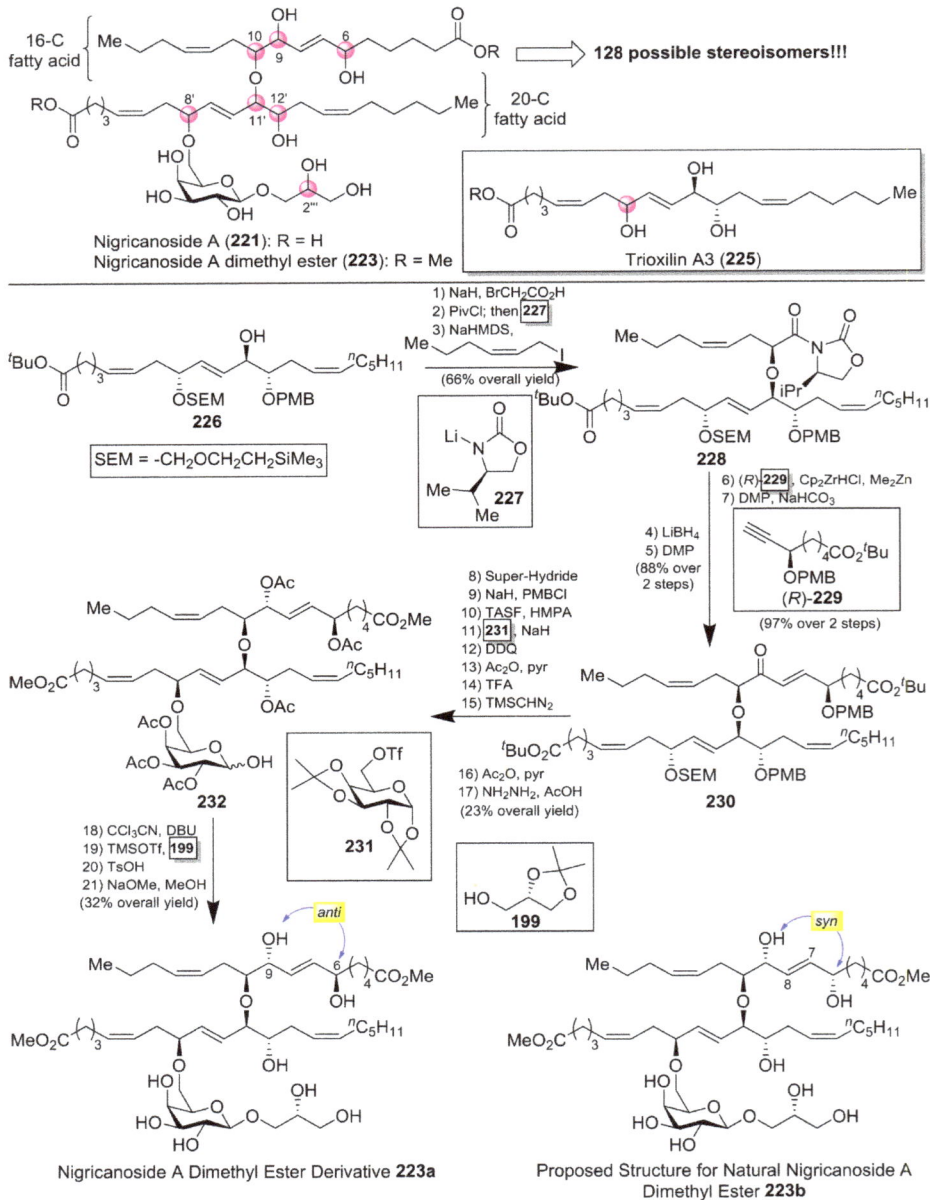

Scheme 19. Synthesis of proposed natural nigricanoside A dimethyl ester (**223a**).

Consequently, the nigricanoside derivative **223b** was prepared in the same way as for **223a**, and all its spectroscopic and physical properties matched with those reported for the natural product dimethyl ester. Despite this structural correspondence, it was surprising to find that neither **223b** nor its epimer at the glycerol subunit displayed cytotoxicity against HCT116 or MCF7 cells up to 10 μM. Due to the lack of cytotoxicity for the synthetic material compared to the reported activity for the natural product an explanation is warranted. One such explanation may be the presence of an unidentified product in the fractions corresponding to the natural nigrecanosides as the molecule responsible for the antitumoral activity exhibited by these natural products. The brilliant and outstanding synthetic work by McMillan and Ready's groups allowed the stereochemical assignment of these fascinating natural products. However, the biological properties of the synthetic nigricanosides have opened an important uncertainty about the identity of the compound responsible for the antitumoral activity detected for the isolated compounds, which must be resolved in future investigations.

4. Chemistry and Biology of Atypical Glycolipids

4.1. Agminosides

Agminosides A–E (**233**–**237**) were isolated from the New Zealand sponge *Raspailia agminata* by Northcote et al. [104] (Figure 22). Structurally, these compounds possess only one type of aglycone, and contain up to six partially acetylated glucose residues that differ only in the level of acetylation and the number of sugars. Their structural similarity made their separation challenging, which was achieved only after repetitive normal-phase chromatography, which was more difficult due to the lack of a chromophore. Mass spectrometry-guided isolation and extensive NMR analysis, together with chemical derivatization, were used for the identification of their structures.

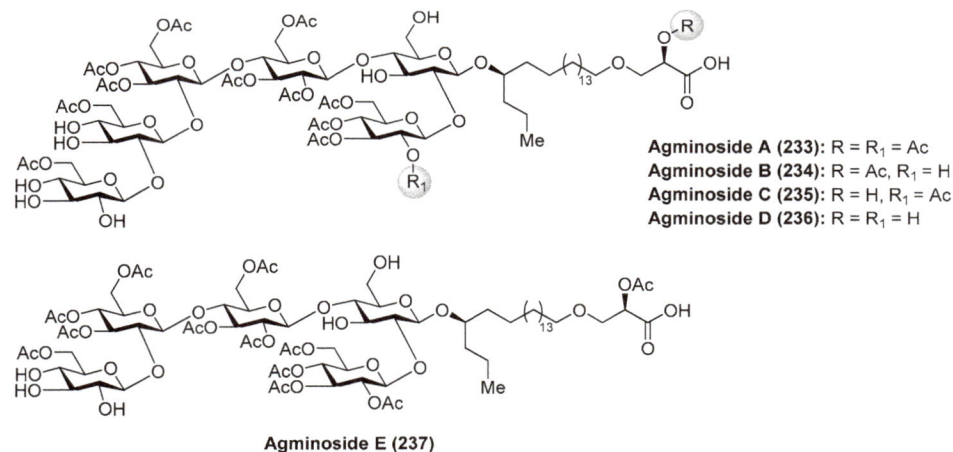

Agminoside A (233): R = R$_1$ = Ac
Agminoside B (234): R = Ac, R$_1$ = H
Agminoside C (235): R = H, R$_1$ = Ac
Agminoside D (236): R = R$_1$ = H

Agminoside E (237)

Figure 22. Structures of agminosides A–E (**233**–**237**).

4.2. Ancorinosides

Ancorinoside A (**238**) was isolated from the marine sponge *Ancorina* sp. by Ohta et al. [105] through bioassay-guided purification of the crude extract. This natural product is the first metabolite that possesses a tetramic acid ring derived from a D-amino acid, as well as a unique 21-methylene side chain. This compound was able to inhibit the blastulation of the starfish (*Asterina pectinifera*) embryo. Some years later, ancorinosides B–D (**239**–**241**) were isolated from the marine sponge *Penares sollasi* by Fusetani et al. [106] (Figure 23). Their structures were elucidated by spectroscopic and chemical methods, consisting of a tetramic acid glycoside related to ancorinoside A (**238**). In contrast to ancorinoside A (**238**), ancorinosides B–D (**239**–**241**) inhibited membrane type I matrix metalloproteinase (MT1-MMP) with IC$_{50}$ values in the range of 180–500 µg/mL. An SAR study carried out by the same authors, wherein the aglycone of ancorinoside B (**242a**), its methyl ester **242b**, and tenuazonic acid (**243**) were tested, showed that **243** exhibited the best results, while **242a** and **242b** were slightly more potent than ancorinoside B (**239**). These results indicated that the two carboxylic acid groups were irrelevant for the biological profile and pointed out the importance of the tetramic acid group for this biological activity. In the same year, Ikegami et al. [107] isolated the magnesium salt of ancorinoside A (**238**) from the marine sponge *Ancorina* sp., which exhibited an inhibitory activity of the blastulation of the starfish *Asterina pectinifera* embryo similar to ancorinoside A (**238**). This result indicated that the presence of Mg^{2+} ions, which act as transmembrane transport and influence the fluidity and permeability of the membrane, did not affect the inhibitory activity of ancorinoside A (**238**).

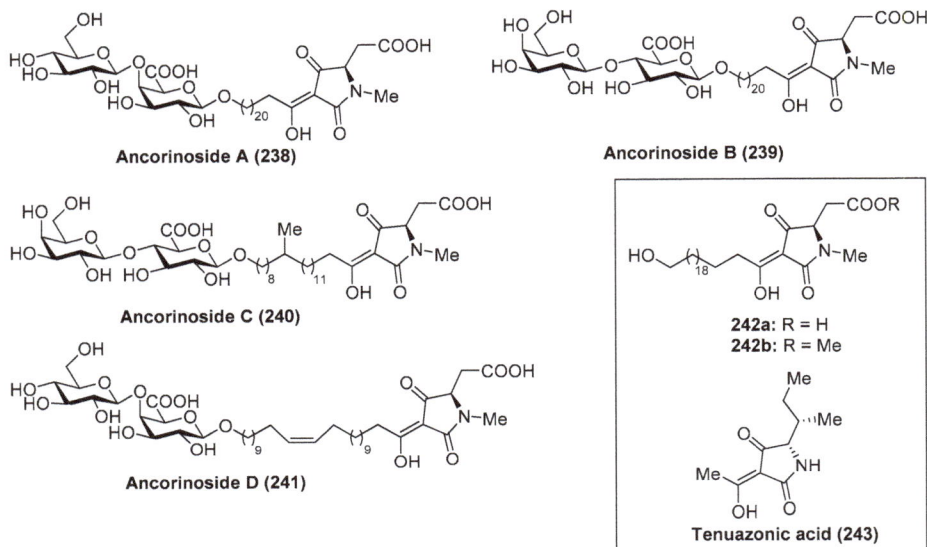

Figure 23. Structures of ancorinosides A–D (**238–241**).

A total synthesis of ancorinoside A (**238**) was achieved in 1.6% yield in 18 steps by Schobert et al. [108], as described in Scheme 20. The key steps were the Schmidt glycosylation for the introduction of the lipidic spacer, a TEMPO oxidation to the uronic acid, functionalisation of the spacer terminus, and final Dieckmann cyclisation for the construction of the tetramic residue. Thus, the authors started the synthesis from peracetylated β-D-galactose, which was rapidly transformed into the disaccharide **244** in six steps in 49% overall yield. Oxidative deprotection, employing CAN, followed by generation of the corresponding imidate, afforded a separable α/β mixture of **245** in 56% yield over two steps. From **245**, the glycosylation reaction with a spacer precursor **246** was achieved by the use of TMSOTf as an activator to obtain a mixture of the desired disaccharide **248** together with deacetyl **247**, which was reacetylated to generate **248** in a 73% yield in two steps. Subsequent debenzylation reaction, TEMPO oxidation of the alcohol to the corresponding uronic acid, esterification of the acid, removal of the silyl group, followed by Dess–Martin periodinane oxidation to the corresponding aldehyde, and a final *E*-olefination with Ley's β-ketophosphonate **249** afforded **250** in 29% overall yield. The coupling between **250** and **251** was achieved by the use of Ley's protocol mediated by a silver salt to obtain the β-ketoamide **252** in 63% yield. Debenzylation of **252**, followed by a final base-induced Dieckmann cyclisation with concomitant deacetylation, afforded ancorinoside A (**238**) (Scheme 20).

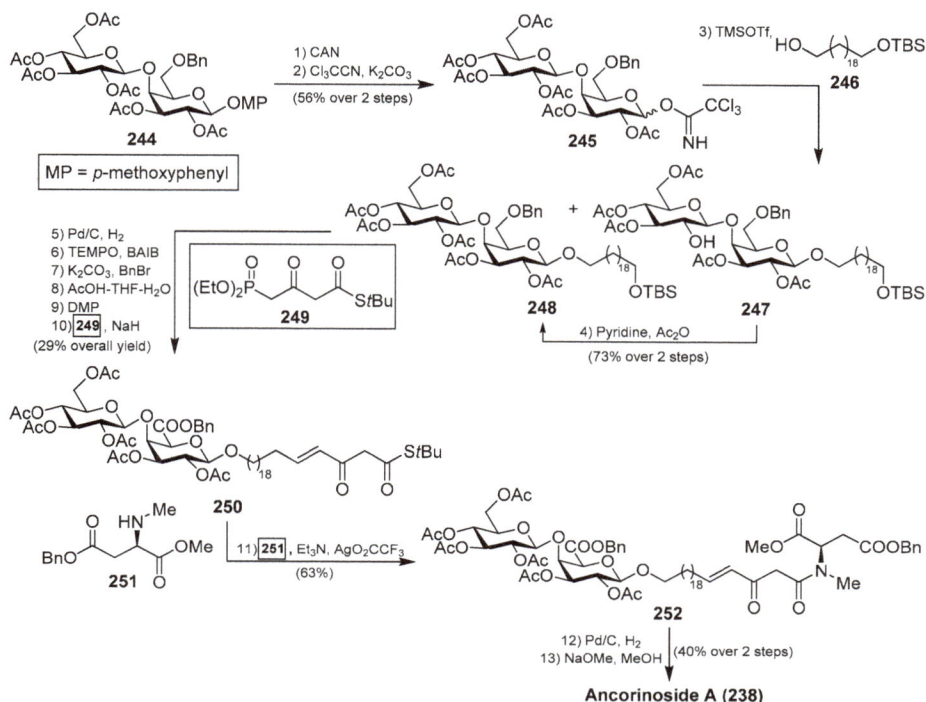

Scheme 20. Total synthesis of ancorinoside A (**238**).

4.3. Bartolosides

Bartoloside A (**253**) was isolated from the cyanobacterium *Nodosilinea* sp. LEGE 06102 [109] and bartolosides B–D (**254–256**) were isolated from the cyanobacterium *Synechocystis salina* LEGE 06155 through a bioassay-guided fractionation of the crude extract by Balskus et al. (Figure 24). A year later, Leao et al. [110] isolated bartolosides E–K (**257–263**) from the strain LEGE 06099 of *S. salina*.

Structurally, these glycolipids from marine cyanobacteria possess unique structures featured by the presence of a dialkyl-resorcinol core, decorated by one or two xylose units with chlorine groups in the aliphatic chains and a C-glycosyl moiety in the case of bartolosides B (**254**), C (**255**), and D (**256**). In the case of bartolosides E–K (**257–263**), these can be considered as analogues of bartoloside A (**253**) that differ in the alkyl chain lengths or halogenation patterns.

The chlorinated dialkylresorcinol core of the bartolosides conferred a challenge for their structural elucidation, which was finally established by combined biosynthetic and bioinformatic analysis. With regards to their biological features, the bartolosides are not known to possess strong biological activities, but their high abundance inside the cells suggests that they may have an important biological role that has to be investigated.

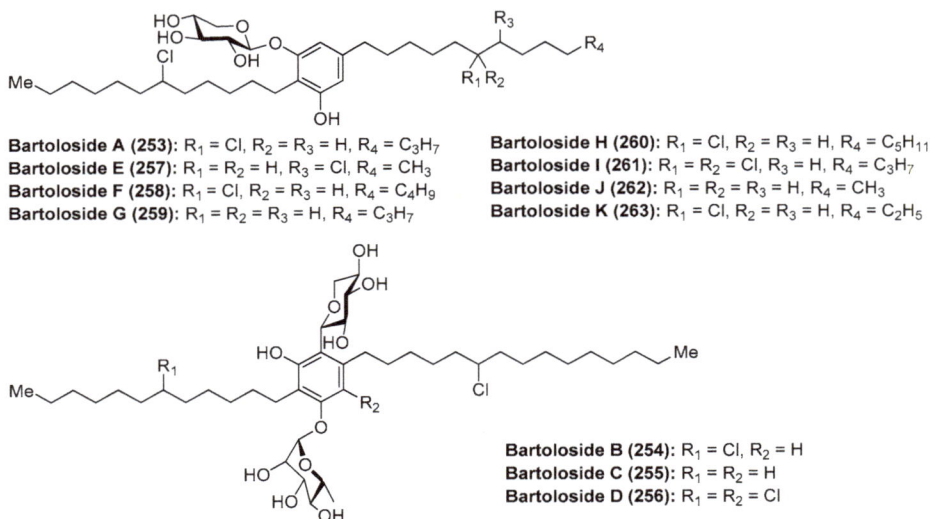

Bartoloside A (253): R_1 = Cl, R_2 = R_3 = H, R_4 = C_3H_7
Bartoloside E (257): R_1 = R_2 = H, R_3 = Cl, R_4 = CH_3
Bartoloside F (258): R_1 = Cl, R_2 = R_3 = H, R_4 = C_4H_9
Bartoloside G (259): R_1 = R_2 = R_3 = H, R_4 = C_3H_7

Bartoloside H (260): R_1 = Cl, R_2 = R_3 = H, R_4 = C_5H_{11}
Bartoloside I (261): R_1 = R_2 = Cl, R_3 = H, R_4 = C_3H_7
Bartoloside J (262): R_1 = R_2 = R_3 = H, R_4 = CH_3
Bartoloside K (263): R_1 = Cl, R_2 = R_3 = H, R_4 = C_2H_5

Bartoloside B (254): R_1 = Cl, R_2 = H
Bartoloside C (255): R_1 = R_2 = H
Bartoloside D (256): R_1 = R_2 = Cl

Figure 24. Structures of bartolosides A–K (**253–263**).

4.4. Caminosides

The caminosides (**264–270**) (Figure 25) are glycolipids with interesting antimicrobial activity isolated from the marine sponge *Caminus sphaeroconia* by Andersen et al. [111]. Firstly, caminoside A (**264**) was discovered after a biological screening of crude extracts of the marine sponge for its ability to inhibit the secretion of *Escherichia coli*-secreted proteins (Esps) by enteropathogenic *E. coli* (EPEC), a major cause of infantile diarrhea that actually represents the main cause of mortality of children in developing countries. Interestingly, pathogenic *E. coli*, and not nonpathogenic *E. coli*, employed the named type III secretory apparatus to deliver Esps. Thus, compounds capable of inhibiting the type III secretion system would affect the pathogenic *E. coli* and not the comensal *E. coli* flora. Actually, the inhibition of the type III secretion system produced the attenuation of the pathogenicity without killing the bacteria. Thus, caminoside A (**264**) displayed an IC_{50} of 20 μM, not inhibiting the growth of Gram-negative bacteria such as *E. coli* (MIC > 100 μg/mL). In addition, caminoside A (**264**) showed significant antibacterial activity against methicillin-resistant *Staphylococcus aureus* (MIC 12 μg/mL) and vancomycin-resistant *Enterococcus* (MIC 12 μg/mL). Some years later, the same authors isolated and identified new members of the caminosides (B–D, **265–267**) with similar biological activities [112]. In all the cases, the authors prepared the peracetylated derivatives **268–270** to facilitate their separation and structural determination. On the other hand, the unusual structure of these glycolipids is featured by the presence of a nonglycerol lipidic chain, whose stereochemistry at C-10 position was recently determined by circular dichroism [113].

The first synthesis of caminoside A (**264**) was reported by Yu et al. [114], wherein they succeeded in sorting out the different issues concerning the stereochemistry of the glycosidic bonds, particularly the 1,2-*cis*-β-mannopyranoside-type linkage of the 6-deoxy-talose unit. This issue was solved by the use of a 2-*O*-Lev (levulinyl) fucosyl derivative to obtain stereoselectively the β-glycosidic linkage with a glucopyranosyl derivative, and then an inversion of the C-2 configuration via oxidation/reduction of the alcohol. Having constructed the disaccharide **274**, its assembly with the glucosyl derivative **273**, prepared via glycosylation of the trichloroacetimidate **271** and alcohol **272**, was undertaken after removal of the acetate and Wacker oxidation of **273**. The resulting trisaccharide **275** was then prepared for the introduction of the 6-deoxy-L-glucosyl unit, for which **275** was benzylated at the 2-OH group of the deoxy-talose fragment, followed by the selective removal of the 2-(azidomethyl)benzoyl group (Azmb) that was possible in the presence of the acetate and butyrate groups by treatment with tributylphosphine. With the resulting acceptor **277** in hand, the reaction with the donor **278**, under the action of catalytic TMSOTf, provided the corresponding caminoside derivative in 53% yield, exclusively as the α-anomer, which was finally subjected to a global deprotection step and acetylation to obtain caminoside A peracetate (**268**) (Scheme 21). More recently, Li et al. have reported the total synthesis of caminoside B (**265**) in a closely related strategy, as summarized in Scheme 22, through key intermediates **282–285** and by efficient and stereoselective glycosylation reactions [115].

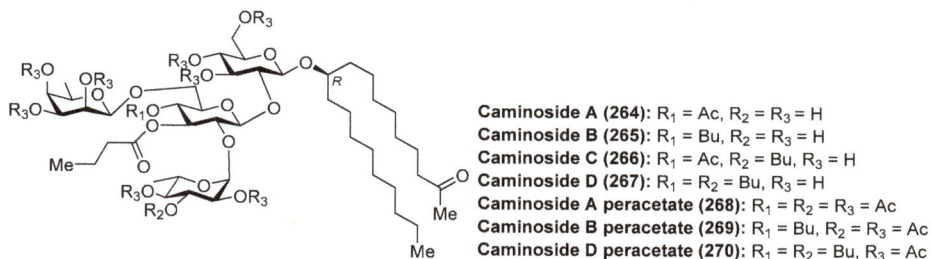

Figure 25. Structures of caminosides A–D (**264–267**) and their peracetylated derivatives (**268–270**).

Caminoside A (264): R_1 = Ac, R_2 = R_3 = H
Caminoside B (265): R_1 = Bu, R_2 = R_3 = H
Caminoside C (266): R_1 = Ac, R_2 = Bu, R_3 = H
Caminoside D (267): R_1 = R_2 = Bu, R_3 = H
Caminoside A peracetate (268): R_1 = R_2 = R_3 = Ac
Caminoside B peracetate (269): R_1 = Bu, R_2 = R_3 = Ac
Caminoside D peracetate (270): R_1 = R_2 = Bu, R_3 = Ac

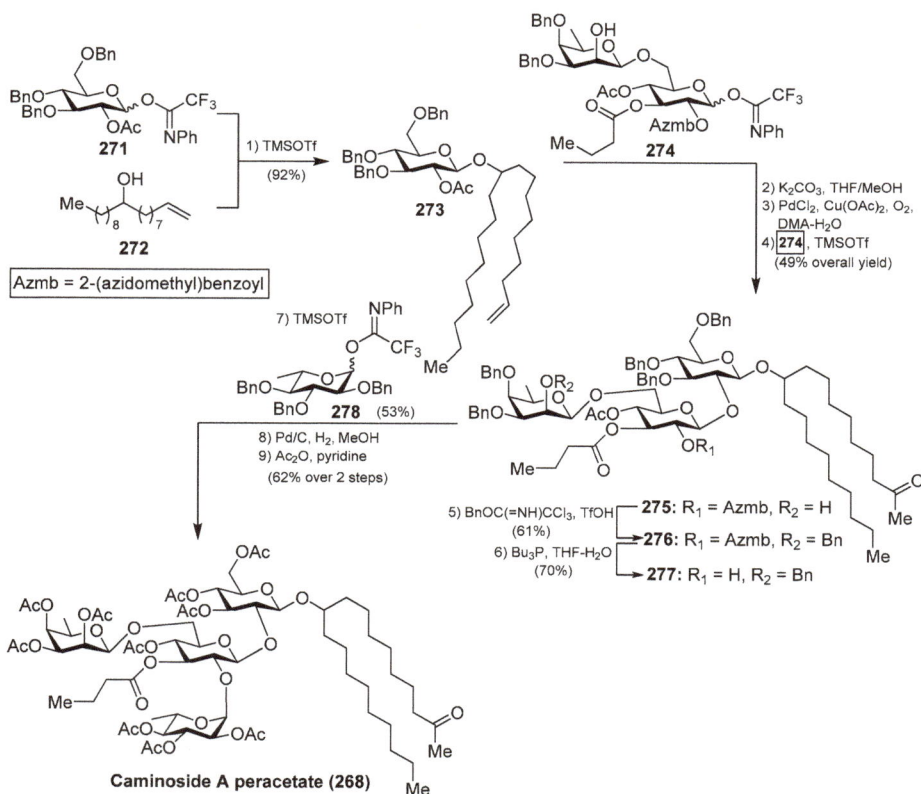

Scheme 21. Total synthesis of caminoside A peracetate (**268**).

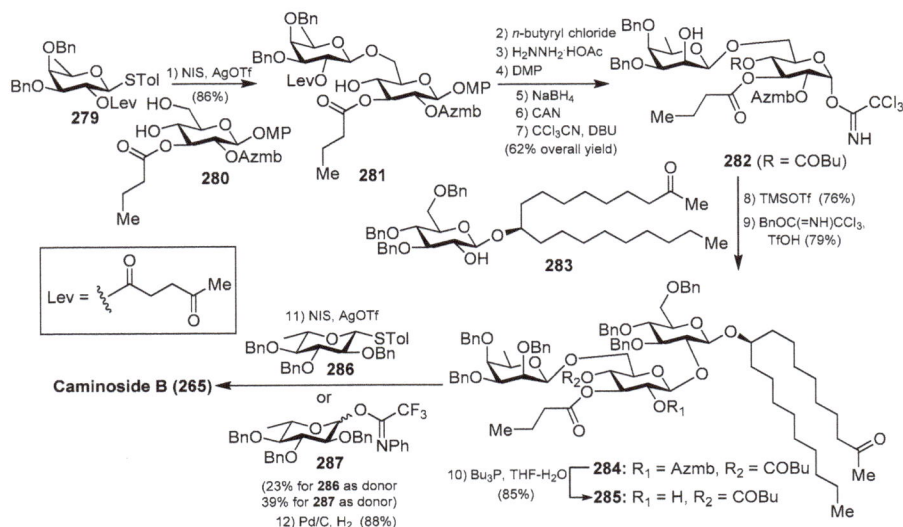

Scheme 22. Total synthesis of caminoside B (**265**).

4.5. Clathrosides and Isoclathrosides

Clathrosides A–C (**288**–**290**) and isoclathrosides A–C (**291**–**293**) (Figure 26), isolated from the Caribbean sponge *Agelas clathrodes* by Mangoni et al. [116], are glycosides containing a very long chain alcohol derived from fatty acids. The structural differences between the clathrosides and the isoclathrosides can be found in the configuration and in the branching of the alkyl chains. Stereostructures of the clathrosides were elucidated by NMR and CD spectroscopy, mass spectrometry, and chemical degradation studies. Clathroside A (**288**) and isoclathroside A (**291**) did not show significant activity on the immune system of mammals despite the structural similarity between clathrosides and the immunoactive simplexides, which will be described in the following section.

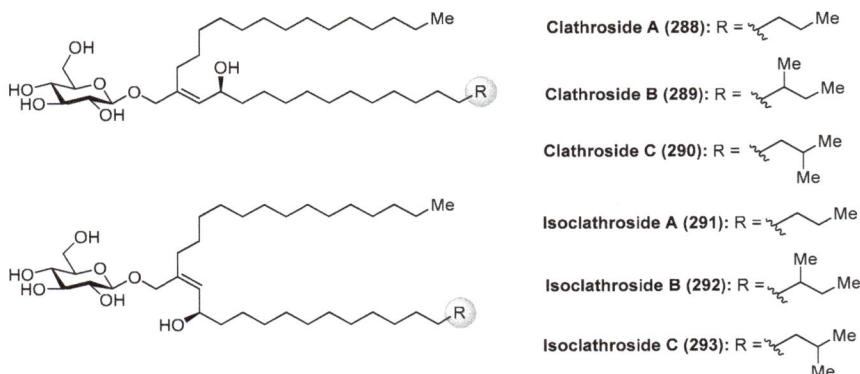

Figure 26. Structures of clathrosides A–C (**288**–**290**) and isoclathrosides A–C (**291**–**293**).

4.6. Discoside

Discoside (**294**) (Figure 27) was isolated as a mixture of homologues from the marine sponge *Discodermia dissoluta* by Fattorusso et al. [117]. The complete stereostructure of discoside was determined by mass spectrometric and NMR spectroscopic techniques, together with CD analysis of degradation products. Interestingly, discoside (**294**) represents the first reported glycolipid with a 4,6-O-diacylated α-linked to the 2-hydroxyl group of a *myo*-inositol unit [2-O-(4,6-di-O-acyl-α-D-mannopyranosyl)-*myo*-inositol]. The *myo*-inositol mannoside is a well-known building block of phosphatidylinositol mannosides and of their multiglycosylated form, lipomannans, which exhibit immunoregulatory effects. However, such types of compounds have never been reported from marine sponges, 1-O-pentadecanoyl-2-O-(6-O-heptadecanoyl-α-D-mannopyranosyl)-*myo*-inositol being the only closely discoside-type compound, which was isolated from various strains of *Propionibacterium*. This finding suggests that discoside is synthesized by symbiotic cyanobacteria associated with the marine sponge.

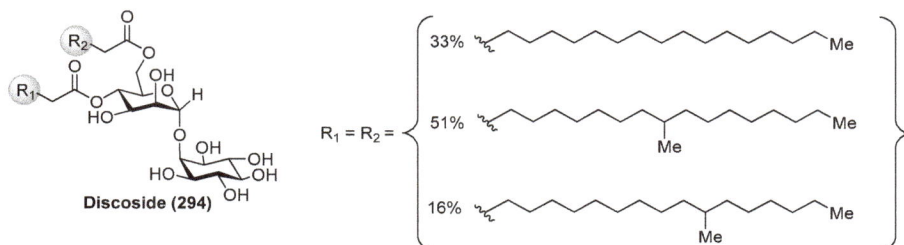

Figure 27. Structure of discoside (**294**).

The synthesis of 4,6-di-O-octadecanoyl discoside (**300**) was recently accomplished by Florence et al., starting with the preparation of the thiomannoside donor **296**. From α-D-phenylthiomannoside **295**, sequential protection of the 4- and 6-OH, benzylation of the remaining two hydroxyl groups, acidic methanolysis of the anisylidene acetal, followed by esterification under Steglich conditions, provided the donor **296** in 34% overall yield. The key glycosylation reaction between the donor **296** and the acceptor **297**, which was synthesized in six steps from a readily available orthoformate derivative of *myo*-inositol, was achieved with the activation of **296** using NIS and TESOTf, followed by the reaction with **297** to give a mixture of separable anomers **298** and **299** in 43% yield (α:β ratio 1:1.5). The total synthesis was completed by final debenzylation of the minor α isomer **299** to provide 4,6-di-O-octadecanoyl discoside (**300**) in a 98% yield (Scheme 23) [118].

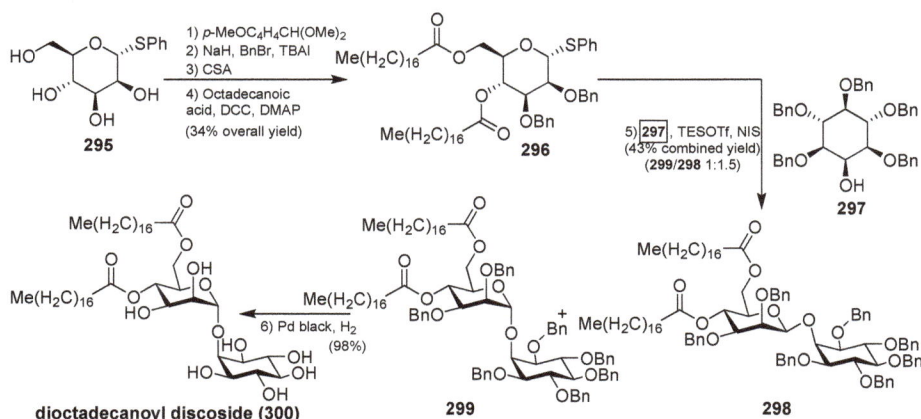

Scheme 23. Total synthesis of dioctadecanoyl discoside **300**.

4.7. Erylusamides

Erylusamides A–D (**301**–**304**) were isolated from the marine sponge *Erylus cf. deficiens* by Santos et al. through a bioassay-guided fractionation in order to find inhibitors of indoleamine 2,3-dioxygenase (IDO) [119]. The structures of erylusamides were established by NMR spectroscopy, HREIMS and chemical derivatization. These compounds possess a pentasaccharide moiety with unusual highly acetylated D-glucose, together with D-xylose and D-galactose units, and unprecedented aglycones, which are structurally featured by long chains of dihydroxyketo amides.

On the other hand, the related erylusamines A–E (**305**–**309**) were isolated from the marine sponge *Erylus placenta* by Fusetani et al. [120,121]. These compounds are interleukin-6 (IL-6) receptor antagonists. Erylusamine TA (**310**), erylusine (**311**), and erylusidine (**312**) (Figure 28) were isolated from *Erylus cf. lendenfeldi* by Kashman et al. [122]. These compounds were not tested for any biological activities due to the fact that they were not isolated as pure compounds but together with a small amount of other homologues.

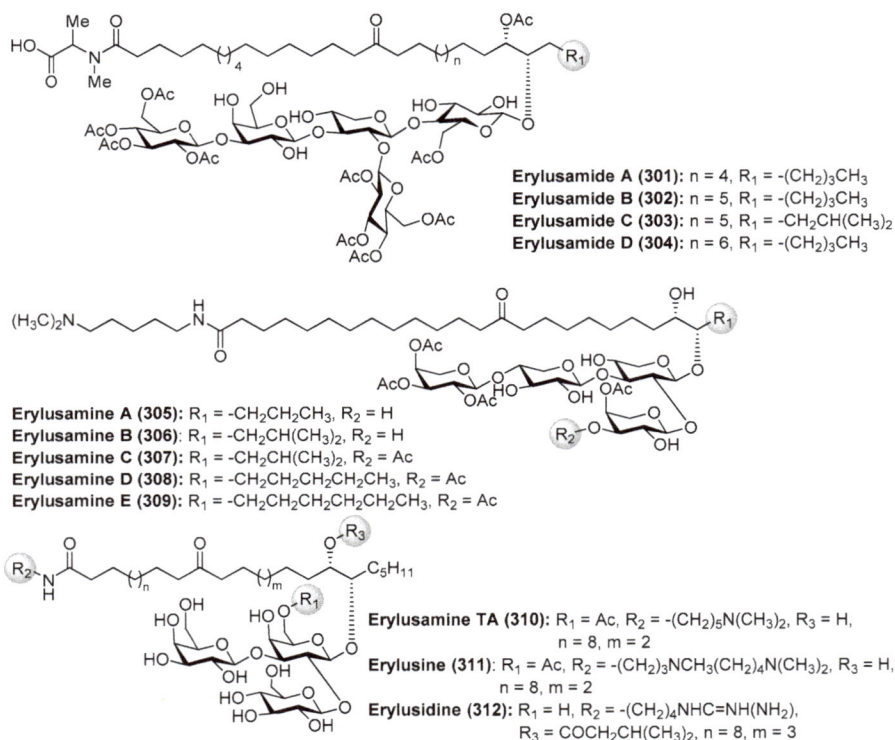

Figure 28. Structures of erylusamides A–D (**301**–**304**) and related glycolipids (**305**–**312**).

4.8. Ieodoglucomides and Ieodoglycolipid

Ieodoglucomides A (**313**) and B (**314**) (Figure 29) were isolated from a marine-derived bacterium, *Bacillus licheniformis*, in 2012 by Shin et al. [123] and their structures were elucidated by a combination of NMR spectroscopic analysis of the natural products with the spectroscopic and physical analyses of the products derived from their acid hydrolysis. Iedoglucomides are unique glycolipopeptides that contain an amino acid (L-ala for ieodoglucomide A and glycine for iedoglucomide B), an unprecedented fatty acid (14-hydroxy-15-methylhexadecanoic acid), succinic acid, and a sugar (β-D-glucose). Iedoglucomide B (**314**) showed moderate antimicrobial activity against Gram-positive and Gram-negative bacteria, antifungal as well as growth inhibition against lung cancer (NCI-H23) and stomach cancer (NUGC-3) cell lines with GI_{50} values of 25.18 and 17.78 μg/mL, respectively.

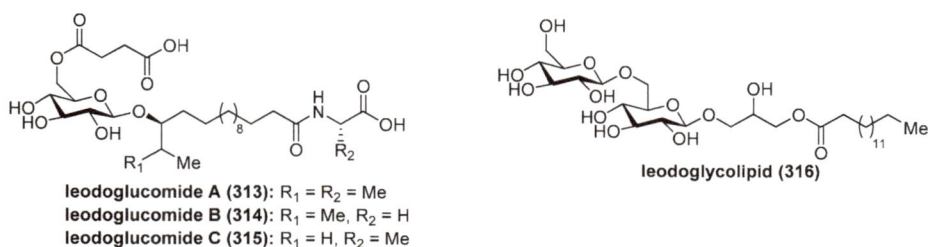

leodoglucomide A (**313**): $R_1 = R_2 = $ Me
leodoglucomide B (**314**): $R_1 = $ Me, $R_2 = $ H
leodoglucomide C (**315**): $R_1 = $ H, $R_2 = $ Me

leodoglycolipid (**316**)

Figure 29. Structures of ieodoglucomides A–C (**313–314**) and ieodoglycolipid (**316**).

Ieodoglucomide C (**315**) and ieodoglycolipid (**316**) were isolated from the fermentation broth of the marine-derived bacterium *Bacillus licheniformis* [124]. In contrast to ieodoglucomide B (**314**), these compounds showed good antibiotic properties against *Staphylococcus aureus*, *Bacillus subtilis*, *B. cereus*, *Salmonella typhi*, *Escherichia coli*, and *Pseudomonas aeruginosa* with MIC values in the 0.01–0.05 μM range. In addition, these compounds inhibit the mycelial growth of plant pathogenic fungi *Aspergillus niger*, *Rhizoctonia solani*, *Botrytis cinerea*, and *Colletotrichum acutatum* as well as the human pathogen *Candida albicans*, with MICs values of 0.03–0.05 μM. The antimicrobial profiles of ieodoglucomide C (**315**) and ieodoglycolipid (**316**) suggest that they could be potential bioprobes for the development of useful antibiotics and fungicides.

Total syntheses of ieodoglucomide A (**313**) and B (**314**) were carried out by Reddy et al. [125] starting from D-glucose and using β-glycosylation and olefin cross-methatesis reactions as the key steps. Thus, the synthesis started with the conversion of **317**, prepared from D-glucose in two steps, into the corresponding α-trichloroacetimidate, which was employed in the key glycosylation reaction, promoted by TMSOTf, with the alcohol **318** to obtain the β-glycoside **319** in 67% yield in two steps. The introduction of the succinyl group onto the sugar to generate **320** was accomplished in six steps in 41% overall yield from **319**. Next, the key olefin cross-metathesis between **320** and **321** or **322**, under the action of the Grubbs 2nd generation catalyst, gave the protected glycolipids **323** and **324** in excellent 86% and 85% yields, respectively. Final hydrogenation provided ieodoglucomides A (**313**) and B (**314**) in 92 and 90% yields, respectively (Scheme 24).

In order to identify analogs of ieodoglucomides with improved biological properties, the same authors prepared the α-isomers of ieodoglucomides A and B (**328** and **329**) and their C-14-epimers (**331** and **332**) (Scheme 25) [126]. As described in Scheme 25, the syntheses of these analogues were accomplished according to the same synthetic strategy employed for the synthesis of the natural products, starting from the α-anomer **325** for the synthesis of the analogues **328** and **329**, and from the epimer **330** for the syntheses of the analogues **331** and **332**. These stereochemical analogues, together with the natural ieodoglucomides, were tested for cytotoxicity against various cancer cell lines and found that ieodoglucomide A (**313**) and B (**314**), as well as their α-isomers (**328** and **329**), did not exhibit cytotoxicity in any cell lines tested. However, their α-C14 epimers (**331** and **332**) showed an inhibition of proliferation of DU145 and HeLa cells with IC_{50} values in the range of 15.2–35.5 μM. In addition, this biological study demonstrated that the activity of caspases-3 and -9 increased when these cell lines were treated with these compounds **331** and **332**, suggesting that the α-*epi* isomers of the ieodoglucomides led to the activation of pathway-initiating apoptosis in DU145 and HeLa cells.

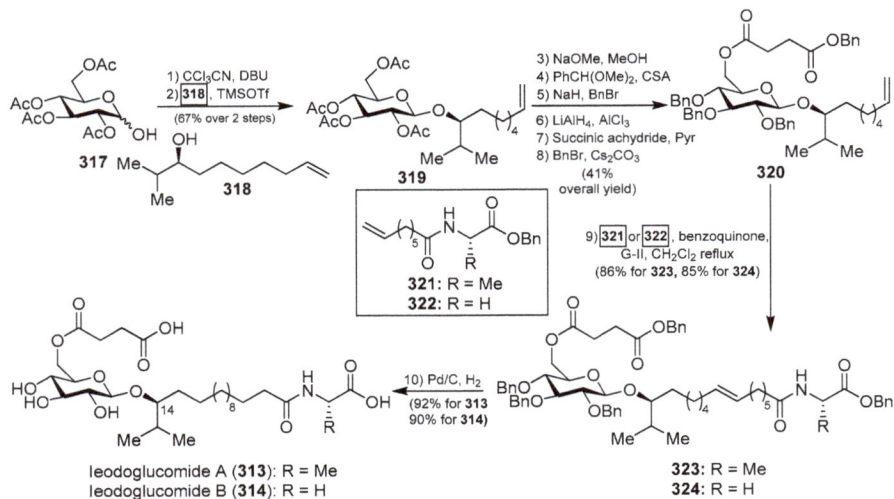

Scheme 24. Total synthesis of ieodoglucomides A (313) and B (314).

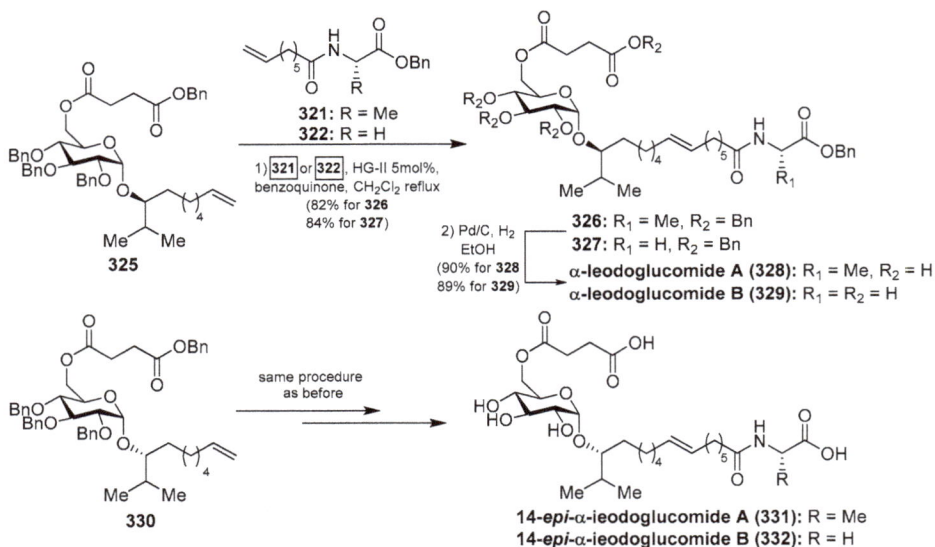

Scheme 25. Total synthesis of α-isomers of ieodoglucomide A (328) and B (329) and their α-14-*epi* analogues (331 and 332).

4.9. Pachymoside A

Pachymoside A (**333**) (Figure 30) was isolated from the North Sea marine sponge *Pachymatisma johnstonia* through a bioassay-guided fractionation in order to find inhibitors of the bacterial type III secretion system (TTSS), carried out by Andersen et al. [127]. Its structure was elucidated by NMR spectral analysis and chemical degradation. This structural study revealed that pachymoside A (**333**) possesses complete acetylation of the galactose residues (the eight galactose hydroxyls are acetylated) and only partial acetylation of the glucose residues (the C-6 hydroxyls of β-glucose and D-glucose are acetylated). Despite its promising activity as a TTSS inhibitor, pachymoside A (**333**) is not a true TTSS inhibitor. It seems that the biological activity exhibited is due to its ability to activate extracelular bacterial proteases that rapidly degrade the excreted Esps, resulting in a false indication of inhibition.

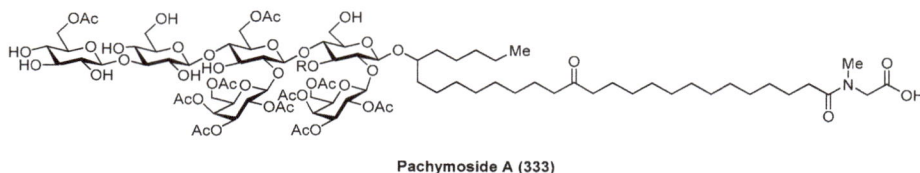

Pachymoside A (333)

Figure 30. Structure of pachymoside A (**333**).

4.10. Plaxyloside

Plaxyloside (**334**) (Figure 31) was isolated as its peracetate from the Caribbean sponge *Plakortis simplex* by Fattorusso et al. [128]. Its structure was established by NMR spectral analysis and chemical methods. Plaxyloside (**334**) is a glycolipid with a long linear polyisoprenoid alcohol aglycone and a linear carbohydrate chain of β-xylopyranose units and represents the first natural oligosaccharide that contains more than three (1→3) linked xylopyranosides. The biological activity of this compound was not evaluated.

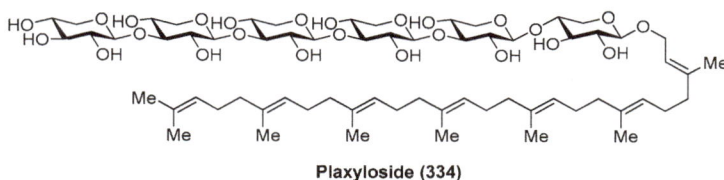

Plaxyloside (334)

Figure 31. Structure of plaxyloside (**334**).

4.11. Roselipins

Roselipins (**335–338**) (Figure 32) were isolated from the culture broth of fungus *Gliocladium roseum* KF-1040 by Omura et al. [129–131]. Later, a mixture of five new roselipins derivatives, separated in two fractions, named roselipins mixture 1–2 (**339a–b**) and mixture 3–5 (**340a–c**), were isolated from an extract of the fungus *Clonostachys candelabrum* by Singh et al. [132]. These compounds differ by the position of esterification of the arabinitol residue. Overall, the roselipins have a unique structure featured by a highly methylated C-20 fatty acid skeleton modified with D-mannose and D-arabinitol residues. Extensive biological evaluations of the roselipins revealed that these compounds displayed a broad range of biological activities. In particular, these compounds inhibit diacylglycerol acyltransferase (DGAT) with IC_{50} values ranging from 15 to 22 μM in an enzyme assay system using rat-liver microsomes, showing that are selective inhibitors of DGAT2 (IC_{50} = 30–50 μM) [133]. An SAR study carried out by Omura et al. [134] revealed that demannosyl roselipins 3A (**341**) and 3B (**342**), prepared from the natural products via enzymatic degradation, conserved DGAT inhibitory activity, in contrast to the dearabinitoyl derivatives (**343** and **344**), which completely lost their activity, suggesting that the arabinitoyl fatty acid core is essential for eliciting DGAT inhibitory activity. In addition, the roselipin derivatives 3A (**341**) and 3B (**342**) were more potent in the cell assay than the roselipins **335–338**, indicating that these derivatives are more membrane-permeable than natural roselipins. These compounds also exhibited antimicrobial activity against *Saccharomyces cervisiae* and *Aspergillus niger* and showed a cytotoxic effect on Raji cells at 39 μM. Furthermore, the mixture of roselipins

2A and 2B (**336** and **338**) inhibited HIV-1 integrase with IC$_{50}$ = 8.5 µM [135]. On the other hand, Ondeyka et al. [136] reported that roselipins 2A (**336**), 2B (**338**), and 1A (**335**) blocked the CXCR3 receptor interaction of IP-10 ligand with IC$_{50}$ = 14.6, 23.5, and 41 µM. The roselipins were also identified as anthelmintic compounds [133].

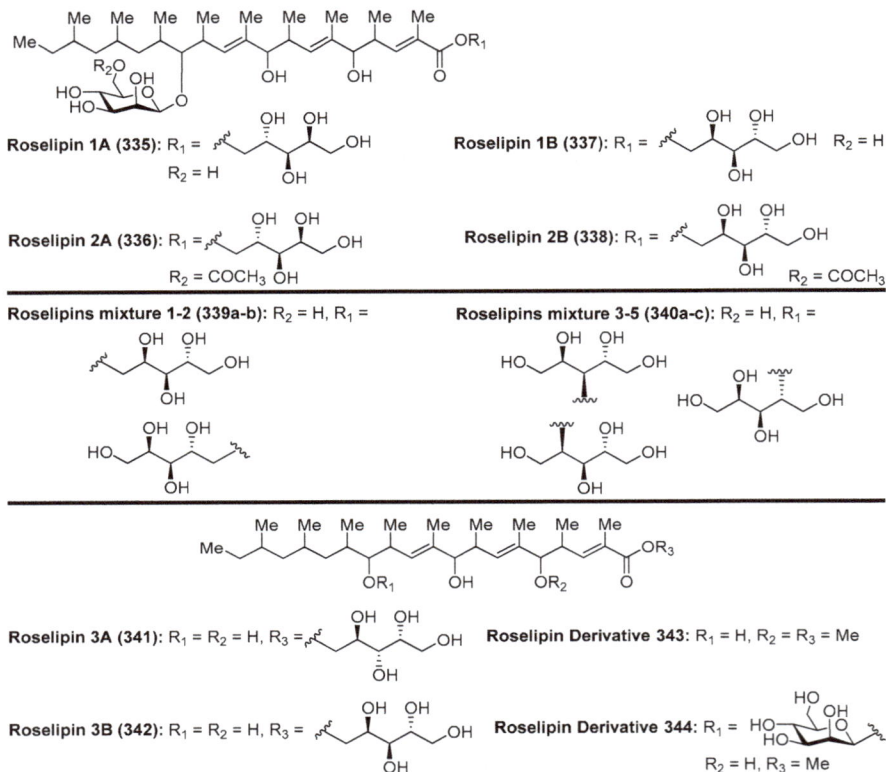

Figure 32. Structures of the roselipins (**335–340**) and derivatives **341–344**.

4.12. Simplexides

The same marine sponge that produces the plakosides and plaxyloside (Sections Plakosides and Plaxyloside), *Plakortis simplex*, has provided other types of glycolipids with immunosuppressive properties, the simplexides (**345a–e**), which were isolated as a mixture of related disaccharides [137]. Even though these compounds could not be separated by HPLC techniques, the authors were able to establish their structures via degradation and subsequent CG-MS analyses of the resulting methyl esters of the lipidic chains. Despite the remarkable structural differences with the plakosides, the simplexides share a very similar biological profile, showing potent inhibitory activity of the proliferarion of T cells in the murine immune system when stimulated with concanavalin A through a noncytotoxic mechanism. Further biological studies demonstrated that the immunosuppressive effects of the simplexides are due to the induction that they exert on the expression and release of cytokines and chemokines from human monocytes by direct interaction with the CD1d receptors, expressed in these cells [138]. In addition, the simplexides induce the expansion of *i*NKT (natural killer T cells with an invariant T cell receptor alpha chain). An interesting synthesis for the simplexides was recently developed by Yingxia et al. [139], in which thioglycosides were employed to construct the complete simplexide scaffold in a one-pot glycosylation method. Thus, the armed donor **346** reacted with the disarmed acceptor **347** by the action of the promoter system NIS/AgOTf to obtain, with a high α-selectivity, the disaccharide **348**. Without isolation of this product, the corresponding alcohol **349** was added to the crude mixture with additional promoters (NIS/AgOTf) to proceed with a second glycosylation reaction to provide **350a–c**, which were finally isolated in excellent yields and stereoselectivity. Final deprotection of **350a–c** gave simplexides **345a–c** (Scheme 26).

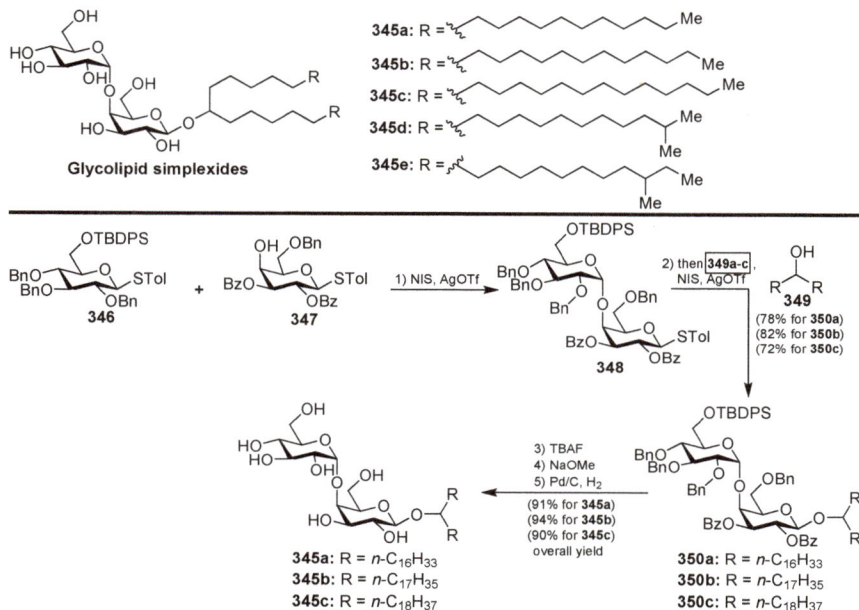

Scheme 26. Structures and synthesis of the simplexides (**345a–c**).

More recently, a synthesis of this class of glycolipids by Yu et al. [140] exploited the cross-metathesis reaction to build the lipidic chain from the allyl disaccharide **356**, efficiently prepared from glycosyl derivatives **351** and **352** via trichloroacetimidates. The crucial cross-metathesis reaction was achieved by the action of the Grubbs 2nd generation catalyst to obtain simplexides **357a–h** in very good yields, which were transformed into the final simplexides **345b** and **358a–g** in two additional steps (Scheme 27). This new efficient and concise synthesis of the simplexides and analogues will allow the determination of the structural factors that govern their interesting biological activities, a study that has yet to be completed by the authors.

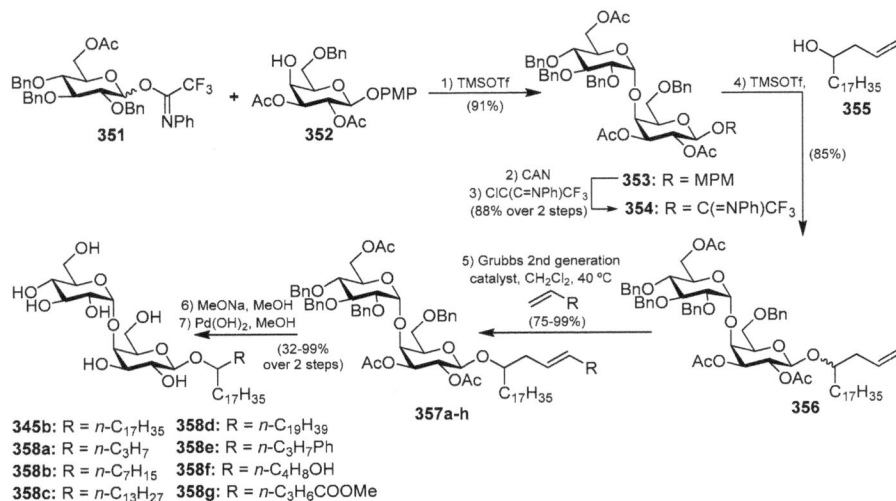

Scheme 27. Synthesis of the natural simplexide **345b** and analogues **358a–g**.

5. Conclusions

Carbohydrates are often found as primary metabolites in the form of monomers, oligomers, or polymers, and play essential functions for life. However, in the realm of natural products, carbohydrates can be found mainly as components of glycoconjugates. In this case, they play important roles in conferring certain physical, chemical, and biological properties to the carrier molecules, being essential in cellular-recognition processes. A relevant example of the glycoconjugates are glycolipids and, notably, the glycolipids from a marine origin, which represent an important class of natural products with wide structural diversity and a broad range of biological activities, including antitumoral, antibiotic, antiviral, antimalarial, immunostimulatory, and neuritogenic activities. However, their difficult accessibility from natural sources, coupled with their extreme scarcity, has made their chemical synthesis essential to provide their access for additional studies. In addition, further understanding of their mechanisms of biological action allows for the rational design and synthesis of new analogues. Through the present review, we have presented the molecular and biological diversity of the glycoclipids derived from marine sources, giving special emphasis on their syntheses as an important tool to confirm their molecular structures, gain insight into their biological activities, and the design of analogues for the development of new drugs. In conclusion, the readers have hopefully realized a greater interest in this class of natural products and the awesome power of chemical synthesis for the development of valuable bioactive compounds based on these natural products.

Funding: This research received no external funding.

Acknowledgments: This work was financially supported by the Ministerio de Economía y Competitividad (CTQ2014-60223-R). I.C.-S. thanks Ministerio de Educación, Cultura y Deporte for a fellowship (Programme FPU). We thank J. I. Trujillo from Pfizer (Groton, CT) for assistance in the preparation of this manuscript.

Conflicts of Interest: The authors declare no conflict of interest.

References

1.   Sasaki, D. *Glycolipids: New Research*; Nova Biomedical: New York, NY, USA, 2007; ISBN 978-1-60456-216-3.
2.   Sweely, C.C. *Biochemistry of Lipids, Lipoproteins and Membranes*; Benjamin/Elsevier: Amsterdam, The Netherlands, 1991.

3. Hakomori, S.-I. Structure and Function of Sphingolipids in Transmembrane Signalling and Cell-Cell Interactions. *Biochem. Soc. Trans.* **1993**, *21*, 583–595. [CrossRef] [PubMed]
4. Varki, A. Biological Roles of Oligosaccharides: All of the Theories are Correct. *Glycobiology* **1993**, *3*, 97–130. [CrossRef] [PubMed]
5. Kolter, T. A View on Sphingolipids and Disease. *Chem. Phys. Lipids* **2011**, *164*, 590–606. [CrossRef] [PubMed]
6. Wennekes, T.; van den Berg, R.J.B.H.N.; Boot, R.G.; van der Marel, G.A.; Overkleeft, H.S.; Aerts, J.M.F.G. Glycosphingolipids—Nature, Function, and Pharmacological Modulation. *Angew. Chem. Int. Ed.* **2009**, *48*, 8848–8869. [CrossRef] [PubMed]
7. Mori, K.; Tashiro, T. Sphingolipids and Glycosphingolipids—Their Synthesis and Bioactivities. *Heterocycles* **2011**, *83*, 951–1003. [CrossRef]
8. Vankar, Y.D.; Schmidt, R.R. Chemistry of Glycosphingolipids—Carbohydrate Molecules of Biological Significance. *Chem. Soc. Rev.* **2000**, *29*, 201–216. [CrossRef]
9. Farwanah, H.; Kolter, T. Lipidomics of Glycosphingolipids. *Metabolites* **2012**, *2*, 134–164. [CrossRef] [PubMed]
10. Tan, R.X.; Chen, J.H. The Cerebrosides. *Nat. Prod. Rep.* **2003**, *20*, 509–534. [CrossRef] [PubMed]
11. Barreto-Bergter, E.; Sassaki, G.L.; de Souza, L.M. Structural Analysis of Fungal Cerebrosides. *Front. Microbiol.* **2011**, *2*, 239. [CrossRef] [PubMed]
12. Kolter, T. Ganglioside Biochemistry. *ISRN Biochem.* **2012**, *2012*, 506160. [CrossRef] [PubMed]
13. Kates, M. *Glycolipids, Phosphoglycolipids and Sulfoglycolipis. Handbook of Lipid Research*; Springer: Boston, MA, USA, 1990; Volume 6.
14. Schnaar, R.L.; Suzuki, A.; Stanley, P. Glycosphingolipids. In *Essentials of Glycobiology*, 2nd ed.; Varki, A., Cummings, R.D., Esko, J.D., Freeze, H.H., Stanley, P., Bertozzi, C.R., Hart, G.W., Etzler, M.E., Eds.; Cold Spring Harbor Laboratory Press: Cold Spring Harbor, NY, USA, 2009; pp. 129–141.
15. Kulkarni, S.S. Synthesis of Glycosphingolipids. In *Glycochemical Synthesis: Strategies and Applications*; Hung, S.-C., Zulueta, M.M.L., Eds.; Wiley: Hoboken, NJ, USA, 2016; pp. 293–326.
16. Barnathan, G.; Couzinet-Mossion, A.; Wielgosz-Collin, G. Glycolipids from Marine Invertebrates. In *Outstanding Marine Molecules: Chemistry, Biology, Analysis*, 1st ed.; La Barre, S., Kornprobst, J.-M., Eds.; Wiley-VCH Verlag GmbH and Co., KGaA: Weinheim, Germany, 2014; pp. 99–162, ISBN 9783527681501.
17. Zhang, J.; Li, C.; Yu, G.; Guan, H. Total Synthesis and Structure–Activity Relationship of Glycoglycerolipids from Marine Organisms. *Mar. Drugs* **2014**, *12*, 3634–3659. [CrossRef] [PubMed]
18. Banchet-Cadeddu, A.; Hénon, E.; Dauchez, M.; Renault, J.-H.; Monneaux, F.; Haudrechy, A. The Stimulating Adventure of KRN7000. *Org. Biomol. Chem.* **2011**, *9*, 3080–3104. [CrossRef] [PubMed]
19. Anderson, B.L.; Teyton, L.; Bendelac, A.; Savage, P.B. Stimulation of Natural Killer T Cells by Glycolipids. *Molecules* **2013**, *18*, 15662–15688. [CrossRef] [PubMed]
20. Kawano, Y.; Higuchi, R.; Isobe, R.; Komori, T. Isolation and Structure of Six New Cerebrosides. *Liebigs Ann. Chem.* **1988**, *1988*, 19–24. [CrossRef]
21. Sugiyama, S.; Honda, M.; Komori, T. Synthesis of Acanthacerebroside A. *Liebigs Ann. Chem.* **1990**, *1990*, 1063–1068. [CrossRef]
22. Higuchi, R.; Kagoshima, M.; Komori, T. Structures of Three New Cerebrosides, Astrocerebroside A, B, and C and of Related Nearly Homogeneous Cerebrosides. *Liebigs Ann. Chem.* **1990**, *1990*, 659–663. [CrossRef]
23. Higuchi, R.; Jhou, J.X.; Inukai, K.; Komori, T. Isolation and Structure of Six New Cerebrosides, Asteriacerebrosides A–F, and Two Known Cerebrosides, Astrocerebroside A and Acanthacerebroside C. *Liebigs Ann. Chem.* **1991**, *1991*, 745–752. [CrossRef]
24. Ishii, T.; Okino, T.; Mino, Y. A Ceramide and Cerebroside from the Starfish *Asterias amurensis* Lütken and Their Plant-Growth Promotion Activities. *J. Nat. Prod.* **2006**, *69*, 1080–1082. [CrossRef] [PubMed]
25. Park, T.; Park, Y.S.; Rho, J.-R.; Kim, Y.H. Structural Determination of Cerebrosides Isolated from *Asterias amurensis* Starfish Eggs using High-Energy Collision-Induced Dissociation of Sodium-Adducted Molecules. *Rapid Commun. Mass Spectrom.* **2011**, *25*, 572–578. [CrossRef] [PubMed]
26. Chida, N.; Sakata, N.; Murai, K.; Tobe, T.; Nagase, T.; Ogawa, S. Total Synthesis of Acanthacerebroside A and Astrocerebroside A via a Chiral Epoxide Intermediate Derived from L-Quebrachitol. *Bull. Chem. Soc. Jpn.* **1998**, *71*, 259–272. [CrossRef]
27. Natori, T.; Koezuka, Y.; Higa, T. Agelasphins, Novel α-Galactosylceramides from the Marine Sponge *Agelas mauritianus*. *Tetrahedron Lett.* **1993**, *34*, 5591–5592. [CrossRef]

28. Natori, T.; Morita, M.; Akimoto, K.; Koezuka, Y. Agelasphins, Novel Antitumor and Immunostimulatory Cerebrosides from the Marine Sponge *Agelas mauritianus*. *Tetrahedron* **1994**, *50*, 2771–2784. [CrossRef]

29. Morita, M.; Motoki, K.; Akimoto, K.; Natori, T.; Sakai, T.; Sawa, E.; Yamaji, K.; Koezuka, Y.; Kobayashi, E.; Fukushima, H. Structure-Activity Relationship of α-Galactosylceramides against B16-Bearing Mice. *J. Med. Chem.* **1995**, *38*, 2176–2187. [CrossRef] [PubMed]

30. Giaccone, G.; Punt, C.J.A.; Ando, Y.; Ruijter, R.; Nishi, N.; Peters, M.; von Blomberg, B.M.E.; Scheper, R.J.; van der Vliet, H.J.J.; van den Eertwegh, A.J.M.; et al. A Phase I Study of the Natural Killer T-Cell Ligand α-Galactosylceramide (KRN7000) in Patients with Solid Tumors. *Clin. Cancer Res.* **2002**, *8*, 3702–3709. [PubMed]

31. Motoki, K.; Kobayashi, E.; Uchida, T.; Fukushima, H.; Koezuka, Y. Antitumor Activities of α-, β-Monogalactosylceramides and Four Diastereomers of an α-Galactosylceramide. *Bioorg. Med. Chem. Lett.* **1995**, *5*, 705–710. [CrossRef]

32. Reddy, B.G.; Silk, J.D.; Salio, M.; Balamurugan, R.; Shepherd, D.; Ritter, G.; Cerundolo, V.; Schmidt, R.R. Nonglycosidic Agonists of Invariant NKT Cells for Use as Vaccine Adjuvants. *ChemMedChem* **2009**, *4*, 171–175. [CrossRef] [PubMed]

33. Costantino, V.; D'Esposito, M.; Fattorusso, E.; Mangoni, A.; Basilico, N.; Parapini, S.; Taramelli, D. Damicoside from *Axinella damicornis*: The Influence of a Glycosylated Galactose 4-OH Group on the Immunostimulatory Activity of α-Galactoglycosphingolipids. *J. Med. Chem.* **2005**, *48*, 7411–7417. [CrossRef] [PubMed]

34. Akimoto, K.; Natori, T.; Morita, M. Synthesis and Stereochemistry of Agelasphin-9b. *Tetrahedron Lett.* **1993**, *34*, 5593–5596. [CrossRef]

35. Farokhi, F.; Grellier, P.; Clément, M.; Roussakis, C.; Loiseau, P.; Genin-Seward, E.; Kornprobst, J.-M.; Barnathan, G.; Wielgosz-Collin, G. Antimalarial Activity of Axidjiferosides, New β-Galactosylceramides from the African Sponge *Axinyssa djiferi*. *Mar. Drugs* **2013**, *11*, 1304–1315. [CrossRef] [PubMed]

36. Yamada, K.; Hara, E.; Miyamoto, T.; Higuchi, R.; Isobe, R.; Honda, S. Isolation and Structure of Biologically Active Glycosphingolipids from the Sea Cucumber *Cucumaria echinata*. *Eur. J. Org. Chem.* **1998**, *1998*, 371–378. [CrossRef]

37. Li, H.; Matsunaga, S.; Fusetani, N. Halicylindrosides, Antifungal and Cytotoxic Cerebrosides from the Marine Sponge *Halichondria cylindrata*. *Tetrahedron* **1995**, *51*, 2273–2280. [CrossRef]

38. Murakami, T.; Taguchi, K. Stereocontrolled Synthesis of Novel Phytosphingosine-type Glucosaminocerebrosides. *Tetrahedron* **1999**, *55*, 989–1004. [CrossRef]

39. Durin, R.; Zubia, E.; Ortega, M.J.; Naranjo, S.; Salv, J. Phallusides, New Glucosphingolipids from the Ascidian *Phallusia fumigata*. *Tetrahedron* **1998**, *54*, 14597–14602. [CrossRef]

40. Karlsson, K.-A.; Leffler, H.; Samuelsson, B.E. Characterization of Cerebroside (Monoglycosylceramide) from the Sea Anemone, *Metridium senile*. *Biochim. Biophys. Acta* **1979**, *574*, 79–93. [CrossRef]

41. Kawai, G.; Ikeda, Y. Fruiting-Inducing Activity of Cerebrosides Observed with *Schizophyllum commune*. *Biochim. Biophys. Acta* **1982**, *719*, 612–618. [CrossRef]

42. Hammami, S.; Bergaoui, A.; Boughalleb, N.; Romdhane, A.; Khoja, I.; Ben Halima Kamel, M.; Mighri, Z. Antifungal Effects of Secondary Metabolites Isolated from Marine Organisms Collected from the Tunisian Coast. *C. R. Chim.* **2010**, *13*, 1397–1400. [CrossRef]

43. Black, F.J.; Kocienski, P.J. Synthesis of Phalluside-1 and Sch II using 1,2-Metallate Rearrangements. *Org. Biomol. Chem.* **2010**, *8*, 1188–1193. [CrossRef] [PubMed]

44. Costantino, V.; Fattorusso, E.; Imperatore, C.; Mangoni, A.; Teta, R. Amphiceramide A and B, Novel Glycosphingolipids from the Marine Sponge *Amphimedon compressa*. *Eur. J. Org. Chem.* **2009**, *2009*, 2112–2119. [CrossRef]

45. Costantino, V.; Fattorusso, E.; Mangoni, A.; Di Rosa, M.; Ianaro, A. Glycolipids from Sponges. 6. Plakoside A and B, Two Unique Prenylated Glycosphingolipids with Immunosuppressive Activity from the Marine Sponge *Plakortis simplex*. *J. Am. Chem. Soc.* **1997**, *119*, 12465–12470. [CrossRef]

46. Costantino, V.; Fattorusso, E.; Mangoni, A. Glycolipids from Sponges. Part 9: Plakoside C and D, Two Further Prenylated Glycosphingolipids from the Marine Sponge *Ectyoplasia ferox*. *Tetrahedron* **2000**, *56*, 5953–5957. [CrossRef]

47. Nicolaou, K.C.; Li, J.; Zenke, G. Total Synthesis and Biological Evaluation of Glycolipids Plakosides A, B and Their Analogs. *Helv. Chim. Acta* **2000**, *83*, 1977–2006. [CrossRef]

48. Seki, M.; Kayo, A.; Mori, K. Synthesis of (2S,3R,11S,12R,2′′′R,11′′′S,12′′′R)-Plakoside A, a Prenylated and Immunosuppressive Marine Galactosphingolipid with Cyclopropane-Containing Alkyl Chains. *Tetrahedron Lett.* **2001**, *42*, 2357–2360. [CrossRef]

49. Seki, M.; Mori, K. Synthesis of a Prenylated and Immunosuppressive Marine Galactosphingolipid with Cyclopropane-Containing Alkyl Chains: (2S,3R,11S,12R,2′′′R, 5′′′Z,11′′′S,12′′′R)-Plakoside A and Its (2S,3R,11R,12S,2′′′R,5′′′Z,11′′′R,12′′′S) Isomer. *Eur. J. Org. Chem.* **2001**, *2001*, 3797–3809. [CrossRef]

50. Mori, K.; Tashiro, T.; Akasaka, K.; Ohrui, H.; Fattorusso, E. Determination of the Absolute Configuration at the Two Cyclopropane Moieties of Plakoside A, an Immunosuppressive Marine Galactosphingolipid. *Tetrahedron Lett.* **2002**, *43*, 3719–3722. [CrossRef]

51. Tashiro, T.; Akasaka, K.; Ohrui, H.; Fattorusso, E.; Mori, K. Determination of the Absolute Configuration at the Two Cyclopropane Moieties of Plakoside A, an Immunosuppressive Marine Galactosphingolipid. *Eur. J. Org. Chem.* **2002**, *2002*, 3659–3665. [CrossRef]

52. Costantino, V.; Fattorusso, E.; Imperatore, C.; Mangoni, A.; Teta, R. Terpioside from the Marine Sponge *Terpios* sp., the First Glycosphingolipid Having an L-Fucofuranose Unit. *Eur. J. Org. Chem.* **2008**, *2008*, 2130–2134. [CrossRef]

53. Cutignano, A.; De Palma, R.; Fontana, A. A Chemical Investigation of the Antarctic Sponge *Lyssodendoryx flabellata*. *Nat. Prod. Res.* **2012**, *26*, 1240–1248. [CrossRef] [PubMed]

54. Costantino, V.; Fattorusso, E.; Mangoni, A.; Teta, R.; Panza, E.; Ianaro, A. Terpioside B, a Difucosyl GSL from the Marine Sponge *Terpios* sp. is a Potent Inhibitor of NO Release. *Bioorg. Med. Chem.* **2010**, *18*, 5310–5315. [CrossRef] [PubMed]

55. Pettit, G.R.; Xu, J.; Gingrich, D.E.; Williams, M.D.; Doubek, D.L.; Chapuis, J.-C.; Schmidt, J.M. Antineoplastic agents. Part 395. Isolation and Structure of Agelagalastatin from the Papua New Guinea Marine Sponge *Agelas* sp. *Chem. Commun.* **1999**, 915–916. [CrossRef]

56. Lee, Y.J.; Lee, B.-Y.; Jeon, H.B.; Kim, K.S. Total Synthesis of Agelagalastatin. *Org. Lett.* **2006**, *8*, 3971–3974. [CrossRef] [PubMed]

57. Costantino, V.; Fatturusso, E.; Imperatore, C.; Mangoni, A. Glycolipids from Sponges. 13. Clarhamnoside, the First Rhamnosylated α-Galactosylceramide from *Agelas clathrodes*. Improving Spectral Strategies for Glycoconjugate Structure Determination. *J. Org. Chem.* **2004**, *69*, 1174–1179. [CrossRef] [PubMed]

58. Ding, N.; Li, C.; Liu, Y.; Zhang, Z.; Li, Y. Concise Synthesis of Clarhamnoside, a Novel Glycosphingolipid Isolated from the Marine Sponge *Agela clathrodes*. *Carbohydr. Res.* **2007**, *342*, 2003–2013. [CrossRef] [PubMed]

59. Costantino, V.; Fattorusso, E.; Imperatore, C.; Mangoni, A. Vesparioside from the Marine Sponge *Spheciospongia vesparia*, the First Diglycosylceramide with a Pentose Sugar Residue. *Eur. J. Org. Chem.* **2005**, *2005*, 368–373. [CrossRef]

60. Costantino, V.; Fattorusso, E.; Imperatore, C.; Mangoni, A. Glycolipids from Sponges. 20. J-Coupling Analysis for Stereochemical Assignments in Furanosides: Structure Elucidation of Vesparioside B, a Glycosphingolipid from the Marine Sponge *Spheciospongia vesparia*. *J. Org. Chem.* **2008**, *73*, 6158–6165. [CrossRef] [PubMed]

61. Gao, P.-C.; Zhu, S.-Y.; Cao, H.; Yang, J.-S. Total Synthesis of Marine Glycosphingolipid Vesparioside B. *J. Am. Chem. Soc.* **2016**, *138*, 1684–1688. [CrossRef] [PubMed]

62. Ijuin, T.; Kitajima, K.; Song, Y.; Kitazume, S.; Inoue, S.; Haslam, S.M.; Morris, H.R.; Dell, A.; Inoue, Y. Isolation and identification of novel sulfated and nonsulfated oligosialyl glycosphingolipids from sea urchin sperm. *Glycoconj. J.* **1996**, *13*, 401–413. [CrossRef] [PubMed]

63. Yamada, K.; Tanabe, K.; Miyamoto, T.; Kusumoto, T.; Inagaki, M.; Higuchi, R. Isolation and Structure of a Monomethylated Ganglioside Possessing Neuritogenic Activity from the Ovary of the Sea Urchin *Diadema setosum*. *Chem. Pharm. Bull.* **2008**, *56*, 734–737. [CrossRef] [PubMed]

64. Chen, W.-S.; Sawant, R.C.; Yang, S.-A.; Liao, Y.-J.; Liao, J.-W.; Badsara, S.S.; Luo, S.-Y. Synthesis of ganglioside Hp-s1. *RSC Adv.* **2014**, *4*, 47752–47761. [CrossRef]

65. Tsai, Y.-F.; Shih, C.-H.; Su, Y.-T.; Yao, C.-H.; Lian, J.-F.; Liao, C.-C.; Hsia, C.-W.; Shui, H.-A.; Rani, R. The Total Synthesis of a Ganglioside Hp-s1 Analogue Possessing Neuritogenic Activity by Chemoselective Activation Glycosylation. *Org. Biomol. Chem.* **2012**, *10*, 931–934. [CrossRef] [PubMed]

66. Hung, J.-T.; Yeh, C.-H.; Yang, S.-A.; Lin, C.-Y.; Tai, H.-J.; Shelke, G.B.; Reddy, D.M.; Yu, A.L.; Luo, S.-Y. Design, Synthesis, and Biological Evaluation of Ganglioside Hp-s1 Analogues Varying at Glucosyl Moiety. *ACS Chem. Neurosci.* **2016**, *7*, 1107–1111. [CrossRef] [PubMed]

67. Shelke, G.B.; Chen, B.-R.; Yang, S.-A.; Kuo, T.-M.; Syu, Y.-L.; Ko, Y.-C.; Luo, S.-Y. Mild and Highly α-Selective *O*-Sialylation Method Based on Pre-Activation: Access to Gangliosides Hp-s1, DSG-A, and Their Analogues. *Asian J. Org. Chem.* **2017**, *6*, 1556–1560. [CrossRef]

68. Wu, Y.-F.; Tsai, Y.-F.; Guo, J.-R.; Yu, C.-P.; Yu, H.-M.; Liao, C.-C. First Total Synthesis of Ganglioside DSG-A Possessing Neuritogenic Activity. *Org. Biomol. Chem.* **2014**, *12*, 9345–9349. [CrossRef] [PubMed]

69. Yamada, K.; Matsubara, R.; Kaneko, M.; Miyamoto, T.; Higuchi, R. Isolation and Structure of a Biologically Active Ganglioside Molecular Species from the Sea Cucumber *Holothuria leucospilota*. *Chem. Pharm. Bull.* **2001**, *49*, 447–452. [CrossRef] [PubMed]

70. Iwayama, Y.; Ando, H.; Ishida, H.; Kiso, M. A First Total Synthesis of Ganglioside HLG-2. *Chem. Eur. J.* **2009**, *15*, 4637–4648. [CrossRef] [PubMed]

71. Xu, F.-F.; Wang, Y.; Xiong, D.-C.; Ye, X.-S. Stereoselective Synthesis of the Trisaccharide Moiety of Ganglioside HLG-2. *J. Org. Chem.* **2014**, *79*, 797–802. [CrossRef] [PubMed]

72. Higuchi, R.; Inoue, S.; Inagaki, K.; Sakai, M.; Miyamoto, T.; Komori, T.; Inagaki, M.; Isobe, R. Isolation and Structure of a New Biologically Active Ganglioside Molecular Species from the Starfish *Asterina pectinifera*. *Chem. Pharm. Bull.* **2006**, *54*, 287–291. [CrossRef] [PubMed]

73. Goto, K.; Sawa, M.; Tamai, H.; Imamura, A.; Ando, H.; Ishida, H.; Kiso, M. The Total Synthesis of Starfish Ganglioside GP3 Bearing a Unique Sialyl Glycan Architecture. *Chem. Eur. J.* **2016**, *22*, 8323–8331. [CrossRef] [PubMed]

74. Higuchi, R.; Mori, T.; Sugata, T.; Yamada, K.; Miyamoto, T. Partial Synthesis of a Sea Cucumber Ganglioside Analogue from a Starfish Cerebroside. *Eur. J. Org. Chem.* **1999**, *1999*, 145–147. [CrossRef]

75. Kaneko, M.; Kisa, F.; Yamada, K.; Miyamoto, T.; Higuchi, R. Structure of Neuritogenic Active Ganglioside from the Sea Cucumber *Stichopus japonicus*. *Eur. J. Org. Chem.* **1999**, *1999*, 3171–3174. [CrossRef]

76. Kaneko, M.; Kisa, F.; Yamada, K.; Miyamoto, T.; Higuchi, R. Structure of a New Neuritogenic-Active Ganglioside from the Sea Cucumber *Stichopus japonicus*. *Eur. J. Org. Chem.* **2003**, *2003*, 1004–1008. [CrossRef]

77. Tamai, H.; Ando, H.; Tanaka, H.-N.; Hosoda-Yabe, R.; Yabe, T.; Ishida, H.; Kiso, M. The Total Synthesis of the Neurogenic Ganglioside LLG-3 Isolated from the Starfish *Linckia laevigata*. *Angew. Chem. Int. Ed.* **2011**, *50*, 2330–2333. [CrossRef] [PubMed]

78. Tamai, H.; Imamura, A.; Ogawa, J.; Ando, H.; Ishida, H.; Kiso, M. First Total Synthesis of Ganglioside GAA-7 from Starfish *Asterias amurensis versicolor*. *Eur. J. Org. Chem.* **2015**, *2015*, 5199–5211. [CrossRef]

79. Kaneko, M.; Yamada, K.; Miyamoto, T.; Inagaki, M.; Higuchi, R. Neuritogenic Activity of Gangliosides from Echinoderms and Their Structure-Activity Relationship. *Chem. Pharm. Bull.* **2007**, *55*, 462–463. [CrossRef] [PubMed]

80. Kisa, F.; Yamada, K.; Miyamoto, T.; Inagaki, M.; Higuchi, R. Isolation and Structure of Biologically Active Monosialo-Gangliosides from the Sea Cucumber *Cucumaria echinata*. *Chem. Pharm. Bull.* **2006**, *54*, 982–987. [CrossRef] [PubMed]

81. Kisa, F.; Yamada, K.; Miyamoto, T.; Inagaki, M.; Higuchi, R. Isolation and Structure of Biologically Active Disialo- and Trisialo-Gangliosides from the Sea Cucumber *Cucumaria echinata*. *Chem. Pharm. Bull.* **2006**, *54*, 1293–1298. [CrossRef] [PubMed]

82. Warabi, K.; Hamada, T.; Nakao, Y.; Matsunaga, S.; Hirota, H.; van Soest, R.W.M.; Fusetani, N. Axinelloside A, an Unprecedented Highly Sulfated Lipopolysaccharide Inhibiting Telomerase, from the Marine Sponge, *Axinella infundibula*. *J. Am. Chem. Soc.* **2005**, *127*, 13262–13270. [CrossRef] [PubMed]

83. Warabi, K.; Matsunaga, S.; van Soest, R.W.M.; Fusetani, N. Dictyodendrins A-E, the First Telomerase-Inhibitory Marine Natural Products from the Sponge *Dictyodendrilla verongiformis*. *J. Org. Chem.* **2003**, *68*, 2765–2770. [CrossRef] [PubMed]

84. Rodriguez, J.; Walczak, M.A. Synthesis of Asymmetrically Substituted *scyllo*-Inositol. *Tetrahedron Lett.* **2016**, *57*, 3281–3283. [CrossRef]

85. Guang, J.; Rumlow, Z.A.; Wiles, L.M.; O'Neill, S.; Walczak, M.A. Sulfated Liposaccharides Inspired by Telomerase Inhibitor Axinelloside A. *Tetrahedron Lett.* **2017**, *58*, 4867–4871. [CrossRef]

86. Andersen, R.J.; Taglialatela-Scafati, O. Avrainvilloside, a 6-Deoxy-6-aminoglucoglycerolipid from the Green Alga *Avrainvillea nigricans*. *J. Nat. Prod.* **2005**, *68*, 1428–1430. [CrossRef] [PubMed]

87. Zhou, B.-N.; Tang, S.; Johnson, R.K.; Mattern, M.P.; Lazo, J.S.; Sharlow, E.R.; Harich, K.; Kingston, D.G.I. New Glycolipid Inhibitors of Myt1 Kinase. *Tetrahedron* **2005**, *61*, 883–887. [CrossRef]

88.   Göllner, C.; Philipp, C.; Dobner, B.; Sippl, W.; Schmidt, M. First Total Synthesis of 1,2-dipalmitoyl-3-(N-palmitoyl-6′-amino-6′-deoxy-α-D-glucosyl)-sn-glycerol—A Glycoglycerolipid of a Marine Alga with a High Inhibitor Activity against Human Myt1-Kinase. *Carbohydr. Res.* **2009**, *344*, 1628–1631. [CrossRef] [PubMed]

89.   Sun, Y.; Zhang, J.; Li, C.; Guan, H.; Yu, G. Synthesis of Glycoglycerolipid of 1,2-dipalmitoyl-3-(N-palmitoyl-6′-amino-6′-deoxy-α-D-glucosyl)-sn-glycerol and its Analogues, Inhibitors of Human Myt1-Kinase. *Carbohydr. Res.* **2012**, *355*, 6–12. [CrossRef] [PubMed]

90.   Zhang, J.; Sun, Y.; Wang, W.; Zhang, X.; Li, C.; Guan, H. Synthesis and Antiviral Evaluation of 6′-acylamido-6′-deoxy-α-D-mannoglycerolipids. *Carbohydr. Res.* **2013**, *381*, 74–82. [CrossRef] [PubMed]

91.   Li, C.; Sun, Y.; Zhang, J.; Zhao, Z.; Yu, G.; Guan, H. Synthesis of 6′-acylamido-6′-deoxy-α-D-galactoglycerolipids. *Carbohydr. Res.* **2013**, *376*, 15–23. [CrossRef] [PubMed]

92.   Ren, L.; Zhang, J.; Ma, H.; Sun, L.; Zhang, X.; Yu, G.; Guan, H.; Wang, W.; Li, C. Synthesis and Anti-Influenza A Virus Activity of 6′-amino-6′-deoxy-glucoglycerolipids Analogs. *Mar. Drugs* **2016**, *14*, 116–130. [CrossRef] [PubMed]

93.   Costantino, V.; Fattorusso, E.; Mangoni, A. Isolation of Five-Membered Cyclitol Glycolipids, Crasserides: Unique Glycerides from the Sponge *Pseudoceratina crassa*. *J. Org. Chem.* **1993**, *58*, 186–191. [CrossRef]

94.   Costantino, V.; Fattorusso, E.; Imperatore, C.; Mangoni, A. Glycolipids from Sponge. 11. Isocrasserides, Novel Glycolipids with a Five-Membered Cyclitol Widely Distributed in Marine Sponges. *J. Nat. Prod.* **2002**, *65*, 883–886. [CrossRef] [PubMed]

95.   Aoki, S.; Higuchi, K.; Kato, A.; Murakami, N.; Kobayashi, M. Myrmekiosides A and B, Novel Mono-O-alkyl-diglycosylglycerols Reversing Tumor Cell Morphology of *ras*-Transformed Cells from a Marine Sponge of *Myrmekioderma* sp. *Tetrahedron* **1999**, *55*, 14865–14870. [CrossRef]

96.   Farokhi, F.; Wielgosz-Collin, G.; Robic, A.; Debitus, C.; Malleter, M.; Roussakis, C.; Kornprobst, J.-M.; Barnathan, G. Antiproliferative Activity against Human non-Small Cell Lung Cancer of Two O-alkyl-diglycosylglycerols from the Marine Sponges *Myrmekioderma dendyi* and *Trikentrion laeve*. *Eur. J. Med. Chem.* **2012**, *49*, 406–410. [CrossRef] [PubMed]

97.   Zhang, J.; Li, C.; Sun, L.; Yu, G.; Guan, H. Total Synthesis of Myrmekioside A, a Mono-O-alkyl-diglycosylglycerol from Marine Sponge *Myrmekioderma* sp.: Total Synthesis of Myrmekioside A. *Eur. J. Org. Chem.* **2015**, *2015*, 4246–4253. [CrossRef]

98.   Williams, D.E.; Sturgeon, C.M.; Roberge, M.; Andersen, R.J. Nigricanosides A and B, Antimitotic Glycolipids Isolated from the Green Alga *Avrainvillea nigricans* Collected in Dominica. *J. Am. Chem. Soc.* **2007**, *129*, 5822–5823. [CrossRef] [PubMed]

99.   Tsunoda, T.; Fujiwara, K.; Okamoto, S.; Kondo, Y.; Akiba, U.; Ishigaki, Y.; Katoono, R.; Suzuki, T. Double Bond Formation Based on Nitroaldol Reaction and Radical Elimination: A Prototype Segment Connection Method for the Total Synthesis of Nigricanoside A Dimethyl Ester. *Tetrahedron Lett.* **2018**, *59*, 1846–1850. [CrossRef]

100. Kinashi, N.; Fujiwara, K.; Tsunoda, T.; Katoono, R.; Kawai, H.; Suzuki, T. A stereoselective Method for the Construction of the C8′–O–C6″ Ether of Nigricanoside-A: Synthesis of Simple Models for the C20 Lipid Chain/Galactosyl Glycerol Segment. *Tetrahedron Lett.* **2013**, *54*, 4564–4567. [CrossRef]

101. Kurashina, Y.; Kuwahara, S. Stereoselective Synthesis of a Protected Form of (6R,7E,9S,10R,12Z)-6,9,10-trihydroxy-7,12-hexadecadienoic Acid. *Biosci. Biotechnol. Biochem.* **2012**, *76*, 605–607. [CrossRef] [PubMed]

102. Espindola, A.P.D.M.; Crouch, R.; DeBergh, J.R.; Ready, J.M.; MacMillan, J.B. Deconvolution of Complex NMR Spectra in Small Molecules by Multi Frequency Homonuclear Decoupling (MDEC). *J. Am. Chem. Soc.* **2009**, *131*, 15994–15995. [CrossRef] [PubMed]

103. Chen, J.; Koswatta, P.; DeBergh, J.R.; Fu, P.; Pan, E.; MacMillan, J.B.; Ready, J.M. Structure Elucidation of Nigricanoside A through Enantioselective Total Synthesis. *Chem. Sci.* **2015**, *6*, 2932–2937. [CrossRef] [PubMed]

104. Wojnar, J.M.; Northcote, P.T. The Agminosides: Naturally Acetylated Glycolipids from the New Zealand Marine Sponge *Raspailia agminata*. *J. Nat. Prod.* **2011**, *74*, 69–73. [CrossRef] [PubMed]

105. Ohta, S.; Ohta, E.; Ikegami, S. Ancorinoside A: A Novel Tetramic Acid Glycoside from the Marine Sponge, *Ancorina* sp. which Specifically Inhibits Blastulation of Starfish Embryos. *J. Org. Chem.* **1997**, *62*, 6452–6453. [CrossRef]

106. Fujita, M.; Nakao, Y.; Matsunaga, S.; Seiki, M.; Itoh, Y.; van Soest, R.W.M.; Fusetani, N. Ancorinosides B–D, Inhibitors of Membrane Type 1 Matrix Metalloproteinase (MT1-MMP), from the Marine Sponge *Penares sollasi* Thiele. *Tetrahedron* **2001**, *57*, 1229–1234. [CrossRef]

107. Ohta, E.; Ohta, S.; Ikegami, S. Ancorinoside A Mg Salt from the Marine Sponge, *Ancorina* sp., which Specifically Inhibits Blastulation of Starfish Embryos. *Tetrahedron* **2001**, *57*, 4699–4703. [CrossRef]

108. Petermichl, M.; Schobert, R. Total Synthesis of the Diglycosidic Tetramic Acid Ancorinoside A. *Chem. Eur. J.* **2017**, *23*, 14743–14746. [CrossRef] [PubMed]

109. Leão, P.N.; Nakamura, H.; Costa, M.; Pereira, A.R.; Martins, R.; Vasconcelos, V.; Gerwick, W.H.; Balskus, E.P. Biosynthesis-Assisted Structural Elucidation of the Bartolosides, Chlorinated Aromatic Glycolipids from Cyanobacteria. *Angew. Chem. Int. Ed.* **2015**, *54*, 11063–11067. [CrossRef] [PubMed]

110. Afonso, T.B.; Costa, M.S.; Rezende de Castro, R.; Freitas, S.; Silva, A.; Schneider, M.P.C.; Martins, R.; Leão, P.N. Bartolosides E–K from a Marine Coccoid Cyanobacterium. *J. Nat. Prod.* **2016**, *79*, 2504–2513. [CrossRef] [PubMed]

111. Linington, R.G.; Robertson, M.; Gauthier, A.; Finlay, B.B.; van Soest, R.; Andersen, R.J. Caminoside A, an Antimicrobial Glycolipid Isolated from the Marine Sponge *Caminus sphaeroconia*. *Org. Lett.* **2002**, *4*, 4089–4092. [CrossRef] [PubMed]

112. Linington, R.G.; Robertson, M.; Gauthier, A.; Finlay, B.B.; MacMillan, J.B.; Molinski, T.F.; van Soest, R.; Andersen, R.J. Caminosides B−D, Antimicrobial Glycolipids Isolated from the Marine Sponge *Caminus sphaeroconia*. *J. Nat. Prod.* **2006**, *69*, 173–177. [CrossRef] [PubMed]

113. MacMillan, J.B.; Linington, R.G.; Andersen, R.J.; Molinski, T.F. Stereochemical Assignment in Acyclic Lipids Across Long Distance by Circular Dichroism: Absolute Stereochemistry of the Aglycone of Caminoside A. *Angew. Chem. Int. Ed.* **2004**, *43*, 5946–5951. [CrossRef] [PubMed]

114. Sun, J.; Han, X.; Yu, B. First Total Synthesis of Caminoside A, an Antimicrobial Glycolipid from Sponge. *Synlett* **2005**, *3*, 437–440. [CrossRef]

115. Zhang, Z.; Zong, C.; Song, G.; Lv, G.; Chun, Y.; Wang, P.; Ding, N.; Li, Y. Total Synthesis of Caminoside B, a Novel Antimicrobial Glycolipid Isolated from the Marine Sponge *Caminus sphaeroconia*. *Carbohydr. Res.* **2010**, *345*, 750–760. [CrossRef] [PubMed]

116. Costantino, V.; Fattorusso, E.; Imperatore, C.; Mangoni, A. Glycolipids from Sponges. Part 17. Clathrosides and Isoclathrosides, Unique Glycolipids from the Caribbean Sponge *Agelas clathrodes*. *J. Nat. Prod.* **2006**, *69*, 73–78. [CrossRef] [PubMed]

117. Barbieri, L.; Costantino, V.; Fattorusso, E.; Mangoni, A. Glycolipids from Sponges. Part 16. Discoside, a Rare *myo*-Inositol-Containing Glycolipid from the Caribbean Sponge *Discodermia dissoluta*. *J. Nat. Prod.* **2005**, *68*, 1527–1530. [CrossRef] [PubMed]

118. Florence, G.J.; Aslam, T.; Miller, G.J.; Milne, G.D.S.; Conway, S.J. Synthesis of the Marine Glycolipid Dioctadecanoyl Discoside. *Synlett* **2009**, *19*, 3099–3102. [CrossRef]

119. Gaspar, H.; Cutignano, A.; Grauso, L.; Neng, N.; Cachatra, V.; Fontana, A.; Xavier, J.; Cerejo, M.; Vieira, H.; Santos, S. Erylusamides: Novel Atypical Glycolipids from *Erylus cf. deficiens*. *Mar. Drugs* **2016**, *14*, 179–192. [CrossRef] [PubMed]

120. Sata, N.; Asai, N.; Matsunaga, S.; Fusetani, N. Erylusamines, IL-6 Receptor Antagonists, from the Marine Sponge, *Erylus placenta*. *Tetrahedron* **1994**, *50*, 1105–1110. [CrossRef]

121. Fusetani, N.; Sata, N.; Matsunaga, S. Isolation and Structure Elucidation of Erylusamine B, a New Class of Marine Natural Products, which Blocked an IL-6 Receptor, from the Marine Sponge *Erylus placenta* Thiele. *Tetrahedron Lett.* **1993**, *34*, 4067–4070. [CrossRef]

122. Goobes, R.; Rudi, A.; Kashman, Y.; Ilan, M.; Loya, Y. Three New Glycolipids from a Red Sea Sponge of the Genus *Erylus*. *Tetrahedron* **1996**, *52*, 7921–7928. [CrossRef]

123. Tareq, F.S.; Kim, J.H.; Lee, M.A.; Lee, H.-S.; Lee, Y.-J.; Lee, J.S.; Shin, H.J. Ieodoglucomides A and B from a Marine-Derived Bacterium *Bacillus licheniformis*. *Org. Lett.* **2012**, *14*, 1464–1467. [CrossRef] [PubMed]

124. Tareq, F.S.; Lee, H.-S.; Lee, Y.-J.; Lee, J.S.; Shin, H.J. Ieodoglucomide C and Ieodoglycolipid, New Glycolipids from a Marine-Derived Bacterium *Bacillus licheniformis* 09IDYM23. *Lipids* **2015**, *50*, 513–519. [CrossRef] [PubMed]

125. Reddy, C.R.; Jithender, E.; Prasad, K.R. Total Syntheses of the Proposed Structure for Ieodoglucomides A and B. *J. Org. Chem.* **2013**, *78*, 4251–4260. [CrossRef] [PubMed]

126. Reddy, C.R.; Jithender, E.; Singh, A.; Ummanni, R. Stereoisomers of Ieodoglucomides A and B: Synthesis and Evaluation of Anticancer Activity. *Synthesis* **2014**, *46*, 822–827. [CrossRef]

127. Warabi, K.; Zimmerman, W.T.; Shen, J.; Gauthier, A.; Robertson, M.; Finlay, B.B.; van Soest, R.; Andersen, R.J. Pachymoside A—A Novel Glycolipid Isolated from the Marine Sponge *Pachymatisma johnstonia. Can. J. Chem.* **2004**, *82*, 102–112. [CrossRef]

128. Costantino, V.; Fattorusso, E.; Imperatore, C.; Mangoni, A. Plaxyloside from the Marine Sponge *Plakortis simplex*: An Improved Strategy for NMR Structural Studies of Carbohydrate Chains. *Eur. J. Org. Chem.* **2001**, *2001*, 4457–4462. [CrossRef]

129. Ōmura, S.; Tomoda, H.; Tabata, N.; Ohyama, Y.; Abe, T.; Namikoshi, M. Roselipins, Novel Fungal Metabolites Having a Highly Methylated Fatty Acid Modified with a Mannose and an Arabinitol. *J. Antibiot.* **1999**, *52*, 586–589. [CrossRef] [PubMed]

130. Tomoda, H.; Ohyama, Y.; Abe, T.; Tabata, N.; Namikoshi, M.; Yamaguchi, Y.; Masuma, R.; Ōmura, S. Roselipins, Inhibitors of Diacylglycerol Acyltransferase, Produced by *Gliocladium roseum* KF-1040. *J. Antibiot.* **1999**, *52*, 689–694. [CrossRef] [PubMed]

131. Tabata, N.; Ohyama, Y.; Tomoda, H.; Abe, T.; Namikoshi, M.; Ōmura, S. Structure Elucidation of Roselipins, Inhibitors of Diacylglycerol Acyltransferase Produced by *Gliocladium roseum* KF-1040. *J. Antibiot.* **1999**, *52*, 815–826. [CrossRef] [PubMed]

132. Ayers, S.; Zink, D.L.; Mohn, K.; Powell, J.S.; Brown, C.M.; Bills, G.; Grund, A.; Thompson, D.; Singh, S.B. Anthelmintic Constituents of *Clonostachys candelabrum. J. Antibiot.* **2010**, *63*, 119–122. [CrossRef] [PubMed]

133. Inokoshi, J.; Kawamoto, K.; Takagi, Y.; Matsuhama, M.; Ōmura, S.; Tomoda, H. Expression of Two Human Acyl-CoA: Diacylglycerol Acyltransferase Isozymes in Yeast and Selectivity of Microbial Inhibitors toward the Isozymes. *J. Antibiot.* **2009**, *62*, 51–54. [CrossRef] [PubMed]

134. Tomoda, H.; Tabata, N.; Ohyama, Y.; Ōmura, S. Core Structure in Roselipins Essential for Eliciting Inhibitory Activity against Diacylglycerol Acyltransferase. *J. Antibiot.* **2003**, *56*, 24–29. [CrossRef] [PubMed]

135. Guan, Z.; Collado, J.; Singh, S.B.; Jayasuriya, H.; Dewey, R.; Polishook, J.D.; Dombrowski, A.W.; Zink, D.L.; Platas, G.; Pelaez, F.; et al. Isolation, Structure, and HIV-1-Integrase Inhibitory Activity of Structurally Diverse Fungal Metabolites. *J. Ind. Microbiol. Biotechnol.* **2003**, *30*, 721–731. [CrossRef] [PubMed]

136. Ondeyka, J.G.; Herath, K.B.; Jayasuriya, H.; Polishook, J.D.; Bills, G.F.; Dombrowski, A.W.; Mojena, M.; Koch, G.; DiSalvo, J.; DeMartino, J.; et al. Discovery of Structurally Diverse Natural Product Antagonists of Chemokine Receptor CXCR3. *Mol. Divers.* **2005**, *9*, 123–129. [CrossRef]

137. Costantino, V.; Fattorusso, E.; Mangoni, A.; Di Rosa, M.; Ianaro, A. Glycolipids from Sponges. VII. Simplexides, Novel Immunosuppressive Glycolipids from the Caribbean Sponge *Plakortis simplex. Bioorg. Med. Chem. Lett.* **1999**, *9*, 271–276. [CrossRef]

138. Loffredo, S.; Staiano, R.I.; Granata, F.; Costantino, V.; Borriello, F.; Frattini, A.; Lepore, M.T.; Mangoni, A.; Marone, G.; Triggiani, M. Simplexide Induces CD1d-Dependent Cytokine and Chemokine Production from Human Monocytes. *PLoS ONE* **2014**, *9*, 111326. [CrossRef] [PubMed]

139. Lü, G.; Wang, P.; Liu, Q.; Zhang, Z.; Zhang, W.; Li, Y. Reactivity-based One-pot Synthesis of Immunosuppressive Glycolipids from the Caribbean Sponge *Plakortis simplex. Chin. J. Chem.* **2009**, *27*, 2217–2222.

140. Li, J.; Li, W.; Yu, B. A Divergent Approach to the Synthesis of Simplexides and Congeners via a Late-Stage Olefin Cross-Metathesis Reaction. *Org. Biomol. Chem.* **2013**, *11*, 4971–4974. [CrossRef] [PubMed]

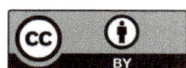

© 2018 by the authors. Licensee MDPI, Basel, Switzerland. This article is an open access article distributed under the terms and conditions of the Creative Commons Attribution (CC BY) license (http://creativecommons.org/licenses/by/4.0/).

marine drugs

Article

Distribution of Saponins in the Sea Cucumber *Holothuria lessoni*; the Body Wall Versus the Viscera, and Their Biological Activities

Yadollah Bahrami [1,2,3,4,*], **Wei Zhang** [1,4] and **Christopher M. M. Franco** [1,3,4,*]

1   Medical Biotechnology, School of Medicine, College of Medicine and Public Health, Flinders University, Adelaide, SA 5042, Australia; wei.zhang@flinders.edu.au
2   Pharmaceutical Sciences Research Center, Kermanshah University of Medical Sciences, Kermanshah 6714415185, Iran
3   Medical Biotechnology, Faculty of Medicine, Kermanshah University of Medical Sciences, Kermanshah 6714415185, Iran
4   Centre for Marine Bioproducts Development, College of Medicine and Public Health, Flinders University, Adelaide, SA 5042, Australia
*   Correspondence: ybahrami@mbrc.ac.ir or yadollah.bahrami@kums.ac.ir (Y.B.); chris.franco@flinders.edu.au (C.M.M.F.); Tel.: +61-872-218-563 (Y.B.); +61-872-218-554 (C.M.M.F.); Fax: +61-872-218-555 (Y.B. & C.M.M.F.)

Received: 6 October 2018; Accepted: 23 October 2018; Published: 1 November 2018

Abstract: Sea cucumbers are an important ingredient of traditional folk medicine in many Asian countries, which are well-known for their medicinal, nutraceutical, and food values due to producing an impressive range of distinctive natural bioactive compounds. Triterpene glycosides are the most abundant and prime secondary metabolites reported in this species. They possess numerous biological activities ranging from anti-tumour, wound healing, hypolipidemia, pain relieving, the improvement of nonalcoholic fatty livers, anti-hyperuricemia, the induction of bone marrow hematopoiesis, anti-hypertension, and cosmetics and anti-ageing properties. This study was designed to purify and elucidate the structure of saponin contents of the body wall of sea cucumber *Holothuria lessoni* and to compare the distribution of saponins of the body wall with that of the viscera. The body wall was extracted with 70% ethanol, and purified by a liquid-liquid partition chromatography, followed by isobutanol extraction. A high-performance centrifugal partition chromatography (HPCPC) was conducted on the saponin-enriched mixture to obtain saponins with a high purity. The resultant purified saponins were analyzed using MALDI-MS/MS and ESI-MS/MS. The integrated and hyphenated MS and HPCPC analyses revealed the presence of 89 saponin congeners, including 35 new and 54 known saponins, in the body wall in which the majority of glycosides are of the holostane type. As a result, and in conjunction with existing literature, the structure of four novel acetylated saponins, namely lessoniosides H, I, J, and K were characterized. The identified triterpene glycosides showed potent antifungal activities against tested fungi, but had no antibacterial effects on the bacterium *Staphylococcus aureus*. The presence of a wide range of saponins with potential applications is promising for cosmeceutical, medicinal, and pharmaceutical products to improve human health.

Keywords: triterpene glycosides; saponin; sea cucumber; mass spectrometry; MALDI; ESI; LC-MS; Holothuroidea; marine ginseng; structure elucidation; marine invertebrate; natural products; bioactive compounds; antifungal; antibacterial; antioxidant

1. Introduction

Sea cucumbers are known as slow-moving invertebrates, in which most species are nocturnal and benthic. They vary in size, shape, colour, and flavours. They have different pharmacological, nutraceutical, and medicinal activities due to the remarkable differences in the type and quantity of saponins, as well as the biodiversity of their species. These differences might also result from the localisation of saponins. Sea cucumbers are referred to as "marine ginseng" since they are a prolific source of bioactive compounds with many functions and are a potential source of biomedical and agrochemical products to treat or prevent many diseases.

Holothuria lessoni, commonly known as golden sandfish, belongs to the family Holothuriidae, class Holothuroidea, order Aspidochirotida, phylum Echinodermata. The colouration of this relatively new-identified holothurian is highly variable from dark greyish black to beige with black blotches and spots or beige without black spots [1,2]. Sea cucumbers are a delicacy in Chinese cuisine. This species is among the species with the highest demand for luxury seafood in Asia [3], which contains a high diversity of saponins in the viscera with a potential medicinal value. Purcell [3] also stated that *H. lessoni* and *H. scabra* are the most valuable tropical holothurians in dried (beche-de-mer) seafood markets in China. The processed (dried) *H. lessoni* is marketed in Hong Kong in retail markets with prices ranging from USD 242 to 787 per kg [1].

Holothurians, commonly known as sea cucumbers, generate a wide range of distinctive biologically and pharmacologically important compounds including triterpene glycosides, fatty acids, minerals, carotenoids, sphingosine, bioactive proteins (collagen, gelatine, peptides, amino acids), vitamins, mucopolysaccharides, glycosaminoglycan (chondroitin/fucan sulphates), fucoidan, phenolic, and flavonoids [4,5]. The presence and power of these active ingredients have led to a rapid growth and development in various biomedical and functional food industries, important to human health.

Sea cucumbers are a potential source of high-value-added substances with therapeutic applications in nutraceutical, cosmeceutical, medicinal and pharmaceutical products. Sea cucumber is consumed as traditional folk medicine in many Asian countries to cure diseases like rheumatoid arthritis, joint pain, tendonitis, osteoarthritis, cardiovascular, ankylosing spondylitis, arthralgia, tumours, fungal infection, gastric, impotence, frequent urination and kidney deficiency, high blood pressure and muscular disorders [6]. Thereby, the medicinal and beneficial influences of functional sea cucumbers on human health have been validated through scientific literature and have exhibited therapeutic value such as controlling excessive cholesterol levels, wound healing, neuroprotective, antimicrobial, anti-malaria, antithrombotic, anticoagulant, antioxidant, and anti-ageing (anti-melanogenic and anti-wrinkle) [4]. Many studies revealed that the health benefits and therapeutic properties of sea cucumbers are due to the presence of triterpene glycosides (saponins).

Saponins are water-soluble constituents. Among the marine organisms, triterpene glycosides (saponins) are predominantly identified in sea cucumber [7], starfish [8] and sponges. The chemical structures of saponins produced by sea cucumbers are unique and vary remarkably from those of terrestrial saponins. Triterpene glycosides, labelled as the most abundant glycosylated secondary metabolites in sea cucumbers, comprise of a carbohydrate moiety and an aglycone. The aglycone part of marine saponins is either triterpene (C30, sea cucumber) or steroid (C27, starfish). Triterpene molecules are assembled from six isoprene units containing 30 carbon atoms. Their aglycone possesses a molecular weight ranging from 400 to 1000 Da. Over 700 triterpene glycosides have been reported from various species of holothurians with a wide spectrum of chemical structures including sulfated, non-sulfated, and acetylated triterpene glycosides [7]. This diversity highlights their potential functions and commercial applications. Besides, the chemical diversity of saponins makes them more favourable as lead compounds for novel drug discovery.

Sea cucumber saponins are usually triterpene glycosides containing a holostane structure. The aglycone part of these glycosides are mainly derived from a tetracyclic triterpene lanosterol and possess a skeleton of a hypothetical lanostan-3-β-ol-(18-20)-lactone called as holostanol in that the D-ring contains a γ-18(20)-lactone. Besides a number of triterpene glycosides possessing aglycones with

18(16)-lactone or without a lactone ring are also reported [6,7]. Typically, their triterpene glycosides contain a polycyclic nucleus with 7(8)- or 9(11)-double bond, and oxygen-bearing substituents are prominently linked to C-12, C-17 or C-16. The lateral chain of aglycones may also contain different substituents namely hydroxy or acetate group, which can further enhance the diversity of saponins.

Their oligosaccharide moieties consist of up to six monosaccharide units, linked exclusively to the C-3 of the aglycone. The sugar residues mainly compose of D-xylose (Xyl, X), D-quinovose (Qui, Q), 3-*O*-methyl-D-glucose (MeGlc, MG), 3-*O*-methyl-D-xylose (MeXyl, MX) and D-glucose (Glc, G), and sometimes 3-*O*-methyl-D-quinovose (MeQui, MQ), 3-*O*-methyl-D-glucuronic acid (MeGlcA) and 6-*O*-acetyl-D-glucose (AcGlc). The molecular weight of prominent sugar residues are as hexose (162 Da), methylpentose or deoxyhexoses (146 Da), and pentose (132 Da) and methylhexose (176 Da). In the oligosaccharide chain, the first monosaccharide unit is always a Xyl, whereas the methylated monosaccharides, namely, MeGlc and/or MeXyl and/or MeQui are always the terminal sugars.

Saponins are widely distributed in sea cucumber species. In recent decades, these natural metabolites have gained great attention worldwide due to their unique features: rich sources, low toxicity, and high efficiency with few side effects [9]. Triterpene glycosides of sea cucumber are known to possess a broad range of medicinal and physiological activities [10,11]. The medical potency of sea cucumber saponins exhibits plentiful health benefits due to their cardiovascular, ant-diabetic, hypoglycaemia, anti-oxidant, anti-asthma, anti-eczema, anti-inflammatory, anti-arthritic, anti-diabetics, cholesterol-lowering effect, immunomodulator, cytotoxic, anti-parasitic, anti-viral, antifungal [7,12], anticancer [13,14], anti-angiogenesis, anti-proliferative [15], and anti-dementia activities [2]. According to the literature, saponins also possess neuroprotective effects on the diminution of central nervous system disorders, namely Alzheimer's disease, Huntington's disease, Parkinson's disease, and strokes [16]. Saponins are also able to stimulate apoptosis and prevent the growth of tumour cells [7]. Besides, sea cucumber saponins are also reported to have biological activities including lowering hyperlipidemia, regulating fat accumulation, restraining fatty liver, relieving hyperuricemia, controlling blood sugar, inhibiting gout and stimulating the hematopoietic function of bone marrow [9]. Various analytical techniques have been applied to study the structure of saponins.

Nuclear magnetic resonance (NMR) spectroscopy can provide extensive structural information for saponins, but high-quantities of high-purity samples are generally required. Saponins are often extracted as a complex mixture, needing a sequence of purification methods to fulfil the requirements for NMR analysis due to the relatively low concentration of saponins. Applying an NMR for analysing saponins in complex mixture generates signals for the most prominent metabolites, whereas signals of the low content metabolites remind either undetected or largely buried by dominant metabolites. In addition to the sample's complexity, the weak S/N ratio of NMR signals makes the structure elucidation of saponins very challenging. However, various mass spectrometry (MS) approaches have been documented to be rapid, reliable, sensitive and accurate for the direct analysis of saponins, both in terms of composition and relative proportion. Recently, Decroo et al. reported the successful application of ion mobility mass spectrometry for the analysis of saponins from different sources [17].

The combination of various MS-based approaches, such as matrix-assisted laser desorption/ionization mass spectrometry (MALDI-MS)/MS and electrospray ionization mass spectrometry (ESI-MS)/MS, affords a wealth of structural data on the saponin congeners, without applying sequential purifications. However, the structural determination of compounds is highly reliant on low kinetic energy collision-induced dissociation (CID) which cannot provide a comprehensive structure elucidation in terms of stereochemistry in some cases [18]. Accordingly, in this study, the integration of the counter-current chromatography and mass spectrometry techniques were utilised to purify and deduce the structure of saponins. We believe that it is a powerful and efficient technique for data interpretation of saponin congeners to tackle the structural complexity of saponin congeners. It can also differentiate the structure of isomeric compounds as they generate different MS/MS fingerprint patterns. It is notable that the mass transition of 132 Da, 146 Da, 162 Da, and 176 Da are due to the losses of Xyl (132), Qui (146), Glc (162 Da), and MeGlc (176), respectively. Usually, the simultaneous loss of two sugar units is also observed.

Previously, we thoroughly described the isolation and structure elucidation of a number of saponins in the viscera of *H. lessoni*. This study aims to purify and characterize the saponin congeners in the body wall of *H. lessoni*. This manuscript is the first to describe the distribution of saponins in the body wall of *H. lessoni*. In addition to their biological properties, it addresses the purification and structure elucidation of several holostane glycosides, including many new saponins along with multiple known compounds from the body wall of this species using the same methods as described previously [2,6,11], unless otherwise stated. Due to their structural diversity and amphiphilic nature, saponins provide a potent platform for pharmaceutical, medicinal, cosmeceutical, nutraceutical, and functional food applications.

2. Results

Despite the advanced developments in the extraction and purification methods, the isolation and identification of saponins in complex extracts remain challenging due to their similar physico-chemical and amphiphilic properties. We previously reported the isolation and purification of a number of saponins from the viscera of a sea cucumber species, *H. lessoni*, using standard chromatography and high-performance centrifugal partition chromatography (HPCPC) to overcome this issue [2,6,11]. The saponin constituents of the body wall of *H. lessoni* were also investigated using the same protocol to compare the saponin profiles and distribution of saponin congeners within these organs.

2.1. HPCPC Purification

One hundred and forty milligrams of the saponin-rich butanolic extract was fractionated by HPCPC in the ascending mode, and 130 fractions were collected and monitored by TLC as described previously [2,6,11]. The TLC profile of the saponin-enriched sample showed the presence of several bands Figure 1 (lane 1), whereas the TLC pattern of HPCPC fractions exhibited the existence of one band in the majority of fractions (Figure 1). Conducting HPCPC is critical for the separation of isomeric saponins. As a typical example, the TLC profile of HPCPC Fractions 89–102 is shown in Figure 1.

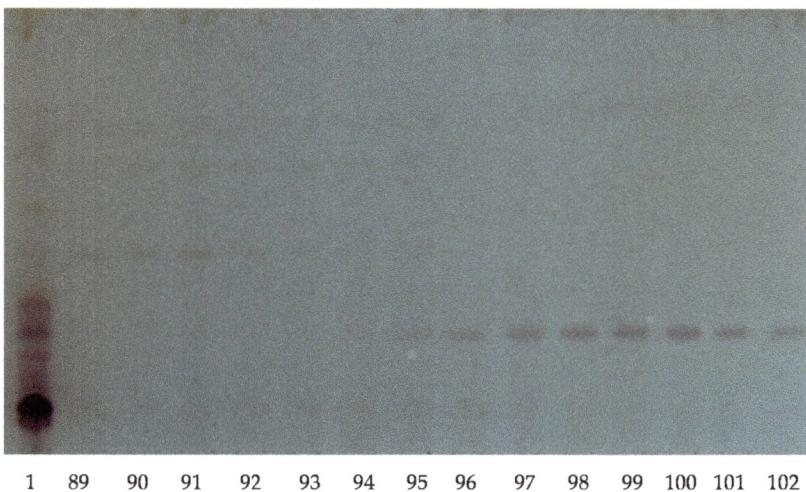

Figure 1. The thin-layer chromatography (TLC) pattern of the high-performance centrifugal partition chromatography (HPCPC) fractions from the purified extracts of the body wall of the *H. lessoni* sea cucumber using the lower phase of the $CHCl_3$–MeOH–H_2O (7:13:8) system. The numbers under each lane indicate the fraction number in the fraction collector. The Fractions 89 to 102 of one analysis (of 130 fractions) are shown. Lane 1 is the saponin enriched iso-butanol extract.

2.2. Mass Spectrometry Analysis of Saponins

The chemical profile of saponins was assigned by mass spectrometry using combinations of MALD-MS/(MS) and ESI-MS/(MS) in the positive and/or negative ion mode(s).

MALDI-MS and ESI-MS Analyses of Saponins from the Body Wall of *H. lessoni*

Saponin HPCPC fractions from the body wall of *H. lessoni* were analysed by MALDI-MS and ESI-MS, and MS/MS as described in detail previously [2,6,11]. The mass spectra were recorded within a *m/z* mass range of 400–2200 Da. The MALDI-MS and MS/MS were performed in the positive ion mode, while ESI-MS and MS/MS were conducted in both positive and negative ion modes. The observed ions clearly all correspond to ionized saponins. All detected ions in the positive ion mode were sodium-coordinated species such as $[M - H + 2Na]^+$ and $[M + Na]^+$ corresponding to sulphated and non-sulphated saponins, respectively. We have actually conducted a comprehensive literature review on the structure of saponins analysed by MS, and built an extensive MS library data to develop a stepwise protocol for the interpretation of MS spectra. The first step was performed to obtain the mass-to-charge ratio of all saponin ions and define the elemental composition of the corresponding saponin contents and their molecular weights. However, in the second step, MS/MS was applied to elucidate the structure of saponin ions by which ions of interest were mass-selected and subjected to CID, resulting in fragmented ions. The mass transition between the fragmented ion peaks is critical for reconstructing the structure of the parent ions.

MALDI and ESI-MS intensities were used to compare saponin compositions within each organ. Besides, they were used to estimate the relative proportion of saponin congeners in the extracts. More than 89 saponin congeners were found in the body wall of sea cucumber *H. lessoni*, which are summarised in Table 1. Around 80 saponins were common between the body wall and the viscera. Nine saponin congeners were found solely in the body wall as compared to the viscera (Table 1).

Twenty-three major saponin peaks were detected at *m/z* 905.4, 1069.5, 1071.5, 1087.5, 1107.5, 1109.5, 1123.5, 1125.5, 1141.5, 1199.5, 1211.5, 1227.5, 1229.5, 1243.5, 1287.6, 1289.6, 1303.6, 1305.6, 1361.7, 1461.7, 1463.7, 1475.7, and 1477.7 in the body wall of *H. lessoni* (Figure 2). These intense peaks could each correspond to at least one triterpene saponin congener. Compounds were assigned on the bases of the *m/z* values, isotope distributions, and fragmentation patterns.

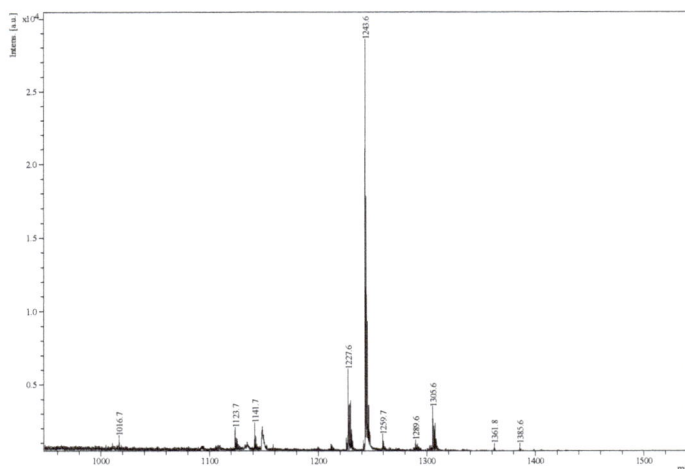

Figure 2. The matrix-assisted laser desorption/ionization mass spectrometry (MALDI-MS) fingerprint of saponin enriched iso-butanol extract over the mass range of 950–1550 *m/z* from the body wall of *H. lessoni*.

Table 1. The summary of saponins identified from the body wall of *H. lessoni* by MALDI- and ESI-MS^2. This table illustrates the 35 novel identified compounds (N) along with the 54 known compounds (P). This table also shows some identical saponins, which have been given different names by different researchers in which they might be isomeric congeners. Besides, it addresses the presence of specific saponins in the viscera or the body wall.

[M + Na]$^+$ m/z	MW	Formula	Compound Name	Body Wall	Viscera	Novel (N)/Published (P)	References
889.4	866	$C_{41}H_{63}NaO_{16}S$ $C_{42}H_{67}NaO_{15}S$	Holothurin B$_3$ Unidentified	Yes Yes	Yes Yes	P N	[19] –
905.4	882	$C_{41}H_{63}NaO_{17}S$	Holothurin B$_4$ Holothurin B Nobiliside B	Yes Yes Yes	Yes Yes Yes	P P P	[2,19] [20,21] [22]
907.4	884	$C_{41}H_{65}NaO_{17}S$	Holothurin B$_2$ Leucospilotaside B	No No	Yes Yes	P P	[19] [23]
911.6	888	$C_{45}H_{92}O_{16}$	Unidentified	Yes	Yes	N	–
917.4	994	$C_{44}H_{71}NaO_{15}S$	Unidentified	No	Yes	N	–
921.4	898	$C_{41}H_{63}NaO_{18}S$	Leucospilotaside A	No	Yes	P	[24]
1034.1	1011	a *	Unidentified	Yes	Yes	N	–
1065.5	1042	$C_{48}H_{82}O_{24}$	Unidentified	No	Yes	N	–
1069.5	1046	$C_{52}H_{86}O_{21}$	Unidentified	Yes	No	N	-
1071.5	1048	$C_{47}H_{93}NaO_{21}S$	Unidentified	Yes	Yes	N	[2,11]
1079.5	1056	$C_{53}H_{84}O_{21}$	Unidentified	Yes	Yes	N	-
1083.3	1060	$C_{58}H_{64}O_{25}$	Unidentified	No	Yes	N	[2,11]
1085.5	1062	$C_{53}H_{90}O_{21}$	Unidentified	No	Yes	N	-
1087.5	1064	$C_{52}H_{88}O_{22}$ $C_{47}H_{93}NaO_{22}S$	Unidentified	Yes	Yes	N	[2,11]
1101.6	1078	$C_{52}H_{86}O_{23}$	Unidentified	Yes	Yes	N	-
1103.5	1080	$C_{52}H_{88}O_{23}$	Unidentified	Yes	No	N	-
1107.7	1084	$C_{54}H_{84}O_{22}$	Unidentified	Yes	Yes	N	-
1109.5	1086	$C_{54}H_{86}O_{22}$	DS-pervicoside B	Yes	Yes	P	[25]
1111.5	1088	$C_{54}H_{88}O_{22}$	Bivitoside B	Yes	Yes	P	[26,27]
1121.5	1098	$C_{54}H_{82}O_{23}$	Unidentified	No	Yes	N	-
1123.5	1100	$C_{54}H_{84}O_{23}$	Unidentified	Yes	Yes	N	[2,11]
1125.5	1102	$C_{54}H_{86}O_{23}$	Holothurinosides C/C$_1$	Yes	Yes	P	[28,29]
1127.6	1104	$C_{53}H_{84}O_{24} C_{54}H_{88}O_{23}$	Holothurinosides X/Y/Z	Yes	Yes	P	[2,11]

Table 1. *Cont.*

[M + Na]$^+$ m/z	MW	Formula	Compound Name	Body Wall	Viscera	Novel (N)/Published (P)	References
1139.5	1116	$C_{54}H_{84}O_{24}$	Unidentified	No	Yes	N	-
1141.5	1118	$C_{54}H_{86}O_{24}$	Desholothurin A (Nobiliside 2a), Desholothurin A$_1$ (Arguside E)	Yes	Yes	P	[2,28–33]
1149.2	1126	a *	Holothurinoside T	No	Yes	P	–
1157.5	1134	$C_{54}H_{86}O_{25}$	Holothurinoside J$_1$ / Unidentified	Yes	Yes	P / N	[2,11,34]
1163.5	1140	$C_{54}H_{92}O_{25}$	Unidentified	Yes	Yes	N	-
1167.8	1144	$C_{56}H_{88}O_{24}$	Arguside A	No	Yes	P	[35]
1173.5	1150	$C_{57}H_{82}O_{24}$	Unidentified	Yes	Yes	N	-
1179.5	1156	$C_{57}H_{88}O_{24}$ $C_{54}H_{85}NaO_{23}S$	Unidentified	Yes	Yes	N	-
1181.4	1158	$C_{57}H_{90}O_{24}$	Unidentified	No	Yes	N	-
1189.5	1166	$C_{59}H_{97}O_{24}$	Unidentified	Yes	No	N	-
1193.5	1170	$C_{54}H_{83}NaO_{24}S$	Unidentified	Yes	Yes	N	[2,11]
1197.5	1174	$C_{54}H_{87}NaO_{24}S$	Unidentified	Yes	Yes	N	-
1199.5	1176	$C_{54}H_{64}O_{29}C_{56}H_{88}O_{26}$	Unidentified / Arguside D	Yes	Yes	N / P	[2,31]
1205.5	1182	$C_{57}H_{82}O_{26}$ $C_{55}H_{83}NaO_{24}S$	Unidentified	Yes	Yes	N	-
1207.5	1184	$C_{55}H_{83}NaO_{24}S$	Unidentified	Yes	Yes	N	-
1211.5	1188	$C_{54}H_{85}NaO_{25}S$	Unidentified	Yes	Yes	N	-
1221.5	1198	$C_{56}H_{79}O_{28}C_{55}H_{83}NaO_{25}S$	Unidentified / Intercedenside A	Yes	Yes	N / P	[2,36]
1223.5	1200	$C_{55}H_{85}NaO_{25}S$	Unidentified	No	Yes	N	-
1225.5	1202	$C_{54}H_{83}NaO_{26}S$	Unidentified	No	Yes	N	–
1227.5	1204	$C_{54}H_{85}NaO_{26}S$	Fuscocinerosides B/C, Scabraside A or 24-dehydroechinoside A, Unidentified	Yes	Yes	P	[1,28,37–42]
1229.5	1206	$C_{54}H_{87}NaO_{26}S$	Holothurin A$_2$, Echinoside A, Pervicoside B	Yes	Yes	P	[20,26,40,43–46]
1237.5	1214	$C_{56}H_{79}O_{29}C_{55}H_{83}NaO_{26}S$	Unidentified	Yes	Yes	N	-

Table 1. Cont.

[M + Na]+ m/z	MW	Formula	Compound Name	Body Wall	Viscera	Novel (N)/Published (P)	References
1243.5	1220	$C_{54}H_{85}NaO_{27}S$	Holothurin A Scabraside B 17-Hydroxy fuscocineroside B, 25-Hydroxy fuscocinerosiden B	Yes	Yes	P	[19,20,33,38,39,46–52]
1245.5	1222	$C_{54}H_{87}NaO_{27}S$	Holothurin A1 Holothurin A4 Scabraside D	No	Yes	P	[40,41,53]
1259.5	1236	$C_{54}H_{85}NaO_{28}S$	Holothurin A3 Holothurin D	Yes	Yes	P P	[2,11,53]
1261.5	1238	$C_{54}H_{87}NaO_{28}S$	Unidentified	No	Yes	N	–
1265.5	1242	$C_{56}H_{83}NaO_{27}S$	Unidentified	Yes	Yes	N	[2]
1269.5	1246	$C_{60}H_{94}O_{27}$	Cousteside G	No	Yes	P	[32]
1271.6	1248	$C_{60}H_{96}O_{27}$	Impatienside B Cousteside H	Yes	Yes	P	[32,54]
1273.6	1250	$C_{60}H_{98}O_{27}$	Cousteside J	Yes	Yes	P	[2,32]
1281.4	1258	$C_{54}H_{87}NaO_{29}S$	Unidentified	No	Yes	N	-
1283.4	1260	$C_{54}H_{89}NaO_{29}S$ $C_{61}H_{96}O_{27}$	Unidentified	No	Yes	N	-
1285.6	1262	$C_{56}H_{87}NaO_{28}S$	Fuscocineroside A	Yes	Yes	P	[37]
1287.6	1264	$C_{60}H_{96}O_{28}$	Holothurinoside E,	Yes	Yes	P	[30,55]
			Holothurinoside E1	Yes	Yes	P	[30,55]
			Holothurinoside O	Yes	Yes	P	[2,11]
			Holothurinoside P	Yes	Yes	P	[2,11]
			17-dehydroxy holothurinoside A	Yes	Yes	P	[32,56]
			Cousteside E	Yes	Yes	P	[32]
			Cousteside F	Yes	Yes	P	[32]
		$C_{56}H_{89}NaO_{28}S$	22-acetoxy-echinoside A	Yes	Yes	P	[57]

Table 1. *Cont.*

[M + Na]+ m/z	MW	Formula	Compound Name	Body Wall	Viscera	Novel (N)/Published (P)	References
1289.6	1266	C60H98O28	Griseaside A	Yes	Yes	P	[56]
			Cousteside I	Yes	Yes	P	[32]
1301.6	1278	C61H98O28-C60H94O29	Holothurinoside M	Yes	Yes	P	[11,58]
			Unidentified		Yes	N	–
			Holothurinoside A	Yes	Yes	P	[29,30]
			Holothurinoside A1	Yes	Yes	P	[29,30]
1303.6	1280	C60H96O29	Holothurinoside Q	Yes	Yes	P	[2,11]
			Holothurinoside S	Yes	Yes	P	[2,11]
			Holothurinoside R	Yes	Yes	P	[2,11]
			Holothurinoside R1	Yes	Yes	P	[2,11]
			Cousteside C	Yes	Yes	P	[32]
1305.6	1282	C60H98O29	Unidentified	Yes	Yes	N	[2]
1307.6	1284	C60H100O29	Unidentified	Yes	Yes	N	[2]
1317.6	1294	C61H98O29	Unidentified	Yes	Yes	N	[2,11,26]
			Holothurinoside L			P	
1319.5	1296	C60H96O30	Unidentified	Yes	Yes	N	–
1329.7	1306	C62H98O29	Arguside F	No	Yes	P	[54]
1335.3	1312	C60H96O31	Unidentified	Yes	Yes	N	[2]
1349.8	1326	C61H98O31	Unidentified	No	Yes	N	–
1356.4	1333	a *	Unidentified	No	Yes	N	–
1361.7	1338	C63H102O30	Unidentified	Yes	Yes	N	–
1377.3	1354	C63H102O31	Unidentified	No	Yes	N	–
1409.4	1386	C61H78O36	Unidentified	Yes	Yes	N	[2]
1411.7	1388	C62H116O33	Unidentified	No	Yes	N	–
1415.7	1392	C66H104O31	Unidentified	No	Yes	N	–
1417.7	1394	C66H106O31	Unidentified	Yes	Yes	N	–
1419.7	1396	C66H108O31	Unidentified	Yes	Yes	N	[2]
1431.4	1408	C66H104O32	Unidentified	No	Yes	N	–
1435.7	1412	C66H108O32	Unidentified	Yes	Yes	N	[2]

Table 1. Cont.

$[M + Na]^+$ m/z	MW	Formula	Compound Name	Body Wall	Viscera	Novel (N)/Published (P)	References
1447.7	1424	$C_{67}H_{108}O_{32}$	Unidentified Impatienside A Marmoratoside A	Yes	Yes	N P	- [59]
1449.7	1426	$C_{67}H_{110}O_{32}$	Bivittoside D	No	Yes	P	[27]
1453.6	1430	$C_{66}H_{94}O_{34}$	Unidentified	Yes	Yes	N	-
1459.7	1436	$C_{68}H_{108}O_{32}$	Unidentified	Yes	No	N	-
1461.7	1438	$C_{68}H_{110}O_{32}$	Unidentified	Yes	No	N	-
1463.7	1440	$C_{67}H_{108}O_{33}$	Holothurinosides H/H$_1$ Holothurin C Cousteside A 17α-hydroxy impatienside A Marmoratoside B	Yes	No	P	[26,55] [32] [59]
1465.7	1442	$C_{67}H_{110}O_{33}$	Argusides B/C	No	Yes	P	[60]
1475.7	1452	$C_{68}H_{108}O_{33}C_{65}H_{112}O_{35}$	Unidentified	Yes	Yes	N	[11]
1477.7	1454	$C_{68}H_{110}O_{33}C_{65}H_{114}O_{35}$	Lessoniosides A/B/C/D/E Unidentified	Yes	Yes	P	[6]
1479.7	1456	$C_{67}H_{108}O_{34}$	Holothurinosides I/I$_1$	No	Yes	P	[55]
1481.7	1458	$C_{66}H_{106}O_{35}C_{67}H_{110}O_{34}$	Unidentified	Yes	Yes	N	[2]
1489.7	1466	$C_{68}H_{106}O_{34}$	Unidentified	Yes	No	N	-
1491.5	1468	$C_{68}H_{108}O_{34}$	Unidentified	No	Yes	N	-
1493.7	1470	$C_{68}H_{110}O_{34}C_{65}H_{114}O_{36}$	Unidentified	No	Yes	N	-
1495.7	1472	$C_{67}H_{108}O_{35}$	Holothurinoside K$_1$ Unidentified	No	Yes	P N	[34]
1507.7	1484	$C_{69}H_{112}O_{34}$	25-acetoxy bivittoside D	Yes	Yes	P	[59]
1521.7	1498	$C_{69}H_{110}O_{35}$	Unidentified	Yes	Yes	N	-
1535.7	1412	$C_{69}H_{108}O_{36}$	Unidentified	Yes	No	N	-
1539.7	1416	$C_{69}H_{112}O_{36}$	Unidentified	Yes	No	N	-
1591.7	1568	$C_{66}H_{120}O_{41}$	Unidentified	No	Yes	N	-

a * The composition was not measured through the ESI analysis.

The most abundant saponin peaks were detected at *m/z* 1141.5, 1227.5, 1229.5, and 1243.5, which corresponded to Desholothurin A (Nobiliside 2a) (*m/z* 1141.5) [28,29], Fuscocinerosides B or C (*m/z* 1227.5)—which are isomers [2,28,37]—Holothurin A_2 (*m/z* 1229.5) [43], and Holothurin A (*m/z* 1243.5) [11,28,38,39,47,61], respectively. These abundant saponin congeners were sulphated triterpene glycosides (Table 1) except for the ions monitored at *m/z* 1141.7. Likewise, in the viscera, the most predominant peak at *m/z* 1243.5 corresponded to Holothurin A, which was followed by the ions at *m/z* 1227.5, 1229.5, 1305.6, and 1141.7. However, in the viscera, the ions at *m/z* 1243.5, 1141.5, 1305.6, 1259.5, and 1227.5 were from the five most intense saponins. In all the sulphated saponins ranging from *m/z* 900 to 1400, it was xylose that was sulphated.

The distribution of saponin in the cuvierian tubules and body wall of *H. forskali*, in the same family as *H. lessoni*, was investigated using both conventional MALDI and MALDI mass spectrometric imageing (MALDI-MSI) analyses [30,55]. This group reported eight major intense peaks at *m/z* 1125, 1141, 1287, 1303, 1433, 1449, 1463, and 1479. All of these glycosides were defined as non-sulphated saponins, while the major abundant saponins in the *H. lessoni* were sulphated congeners (except the ions at *m/z* 1141.5).

HPCPC fractions were also analysed. For instance, the positive ion mode MALDI-MS of Fraction 110 over a mass range of 950–1400 *m/z* is shown in Figure 3. This spectrum illustrates the presence of one major peak at *m/z* 1141.7 corresponding to Desholothurin A [29].

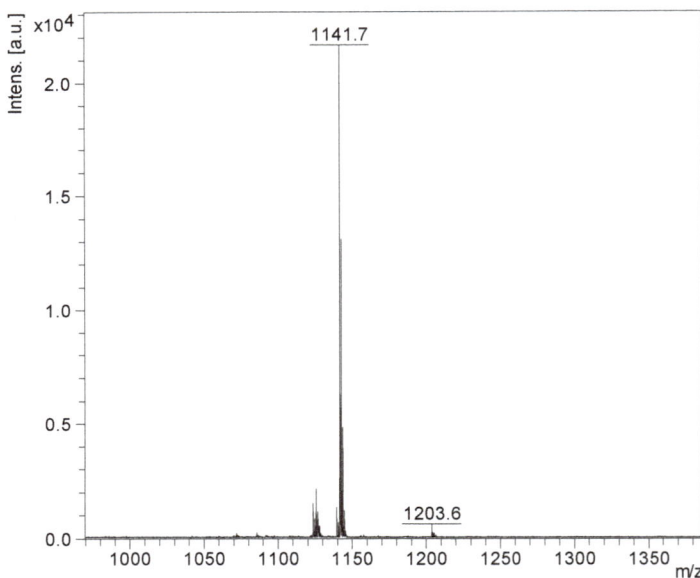

Figure 3. The MALDI-MS fingerprint of Fraction 110. The major peak at *m/z* 1141.7 corresponded to Desholothurin A.

Both positive and negative ion modes ESI-MS were also performed on the fractions. As an example, the positive ion mode ESI-MS spectrum of Fraction 110 is shown in Figure 4. This spectrum indicated the presence of the major ions at *m/z* 1141.5, corresponding to Desholothurin A. Therefore, the MALDI-MS data was corroborated by ESI-MS analysis.

A chemical analysis by MALDI- and ESI-MS/MS of the HPCPC fractions identified several novel along with multiple known saponins. The molecular structures of some of the identified compounds are illustrated in Figure 5. The isobutanol and HPCPC fractionated samples indicated 26 sulphated and 63 non-sulphated saponin ions.

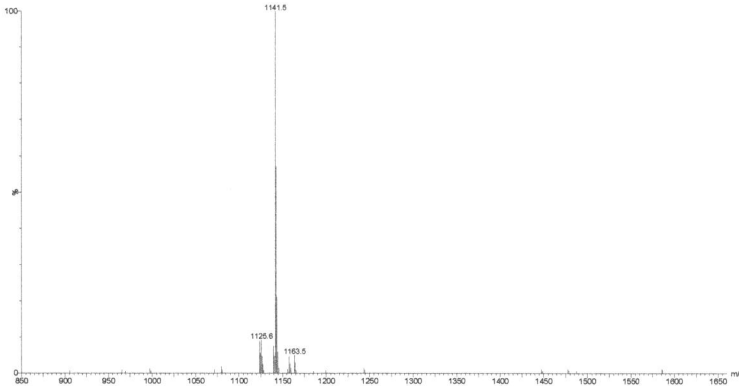

Figure 4. The electrospray ionization mass spectrometry (ESI-MS) spectrum of Fraction 110. The major peaks corresponded to Desholothurin A.

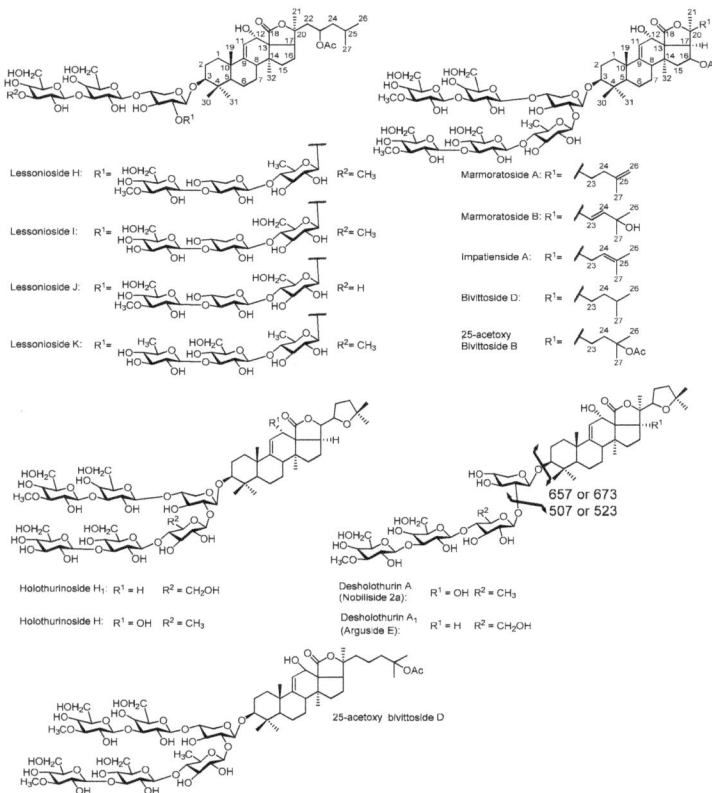

Figure 5. The structures of some of the newly identified saponins from the body wall of *H. lessoni*, as representative.

2.3. Saponin Profiles by Negative-Ion ESI-MS

The result of the positive ion mode was validated by the negative ion mode under conditions similar to those used for the positive ion mode. The analysis of saponins in the negative ion mode facilitated the calculation of the molecular formula of compounds as it showed the presence of the number of Na ions in the molecules, and also the presence or absence of sulphate groups. For instance, the ions detected in both the positive and negative ion modes ESI-MS of HPCPC Fraction 110 are displayed in Figure 6, which demonstrated ions detected in both positive $[M + Na]^+$ (Figure 6a,b) and negative $[M - H]^-$ (Figure 6c) ion modes between 1050 and 1275 Da. Three main peaks at m/z 1125, 1141, and 1163 in ESI-MS$^+$ generated peaks at m/z 1101, 1117, and 1139 in the negative ion mode $[M - H - Na]^-$ ESI-MS, respectively, indicating the presence of only one Na atom in their chemical formulae. The analysis of saponins in the negative ion mode involves the loss of a proton. As can be noted from the spectra, the mass discrepancy between the positive and negative ion modes for an individual ion was 24 u or Da, representing the loss of a sodium atom and a proton, and showing that there was no sulphur present. Therefore, the mass discrepancy between the sodiated saponins and the deprotonated saponins is 24 u. However, in the case of a sulphated saponin, the mass discrepancy between these two modes of ionisation was 46 u, showing the presence of two Na atoms which implies the presence of sulphur in the molecule.

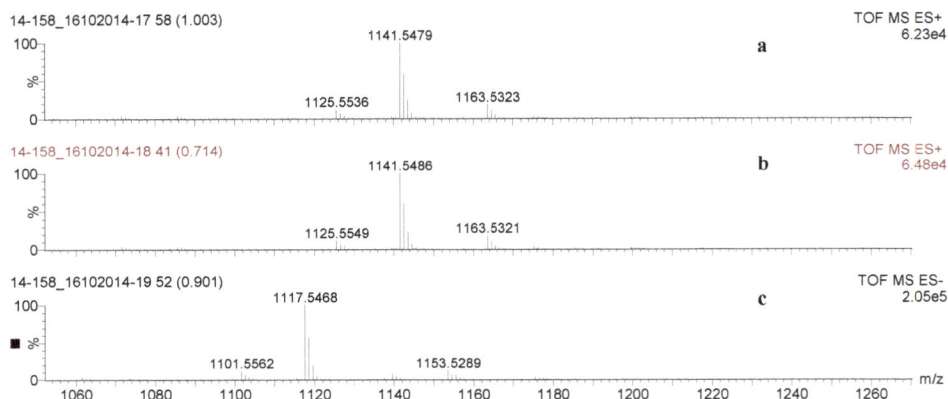

Figure 6. The saponin profile of Fraction 110 by ESI-MS in both the positive (**a**,**b**) and negative (**c**) ion modes. The 24 u or Da mass discrepancy between the positive and negative ion modes for an individual ion indicates the compound is non-sulphated saponin.

2.4. Structure Elucidation of Saponins by Tandem Mass Spectrometry Analysis

The appropriate HPCPC fractions were pooled on the basis of their similar Rf values on TLC and concentrated to dryness. The saponin content of each HPCPC fraction was then profiled by MALDI-MS, ESI-MS, and -MS^2. Tandem mass spectrometry analysis (MALDI and ESI) afforded crucial information about the chemical structure and elemental composition of individual saponins. Isomeric saponins were also differentiated following HPCPC purification [2,11,62]. However, in some cases, the definitive structure elucidation of saponins requires NMR analysis. It is notable that the low kinetic energy CID used here had no fragment in the core of the aglycone, whereas the side chain of the aglycone was cleaved in some cases, which was consistent with observations by Demeyer, et al. [63]. To describe the procedure, the tandem mass spectrometry analysis of a few saponin ions will be discussed.

Our previous MS^2 analyses of saponins revealed the key diagnostic ion peaks, namely the main fragmentation ions, generated by the cleavage of the glycosidic bonds, yielding oligosaccharide and monosaccharide fragments [2,6,11]. These characteristic peaks and unique fragmentation pattern provide vital structural information about the MW of the aglycones, the glycoside linkage, nature, number, sequence, and type of monosaccharaide units in the carbohydrate moiety, as well as the presence or absence of different groups such as acetoxy and/or sulphated moieties and their positions. Besides, other visible peaks originated from the cleavage of the lateral chain of aglycone and the loss of other neutral molecules, including H_2O and CO_2. In some cases, we observed the simultaneous loss of two sugar units.

Collisional induced-dissociation can also cleave the lateral chain of the aglycone and generate a wealth of information about the structure of the nucleus and side chain. For instance, the typical mass transitions of 60 and 104 u from the parent ions correspond to the losses of acetoxy group (acetic acid, $C_2H_4O_2$) and [$C_2H_4O_2$ + CO_2] in the aglycone of acetylated triterpene glycosides, respectively. The latter one is a characteristic feature of compounds having an acetoxy group and an 18(20)-lactone moiety. The presence of ion peaks at m/z 230.15 and 204.13 in the spectrum of triterpene glycosides corresponding to the losses of [$C_{12}H_{22}O_4$] and [$C_{10}H_{20}O_4$] are the common characteristic fragments of saponins with a saturated lateral chain. The side chain fragmentation with 23-oxo substitution led to losses of 100 Da, due to the low energy McLafferty rearrangement of 6-member transition states, which generates the neutral molecule $C_6H_{12}O$ (4-methylpent-1-en-2-ol). Having knowledge of these fragmentation ions enable us to elucidate the structure of novel aglycones.

2.5. Structural Determination of Saponins by MALDI MS/MS

To validate the structure of saponins, tandem mass spectrometry was conducted on the detected ions. As a typical example, the MALDI-MS/MS profile of the ions at m/z 1141 from Fraction 55 is shown in Figure 7. The chemical analysis of this ion revealed the structure of desholothurin A_1 [34]. This conclusion was established by fragment ion peaks at m/z 673, 523, 361, and 185 in the positive ion mode MALDI-MS^2, corresponding to the sequential losses of aglycone, Xyl, Glc, MeGlc, and Glc residues, respectively.

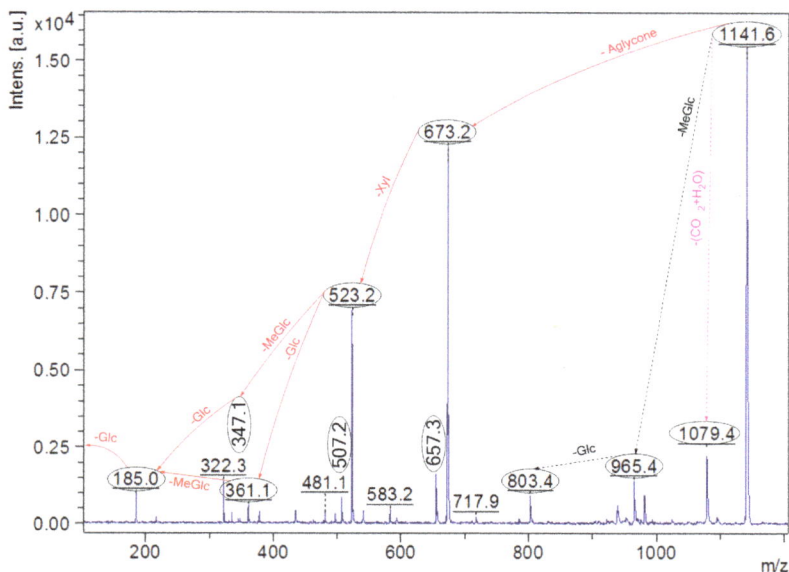

Figure 7. The MALDI-MS/MS profile of the ions at m/z 1141 from Fraction 55 corresponding to desholothurin A_1. The sequential losses of aglycone (Agl), Xyl, MeGlc, Glc, and Glc residues yielded the product ions at m/z 673, 523, 347, and 185, respectively. However, the ion peaks at m/z 507 and 657 corresponded to the sodiated key diagnostic peak [MeGlc-Glc-Qui + Na]$^+$, and the entire sodiated hydrated sugar residues [MeGlc-Glc-Qui-Xyl + H_2O + Na]$^+$ of desholothurin A, respectively.

2.5.1. Chemical Analysis of Saponins by ESI-MS/MS

The effective capability of HPCPC in purifying saponins and isomeric saponins was described previously [6,11]. The separation of ions detected at m/z 1141 is exemplified in Figure 8.

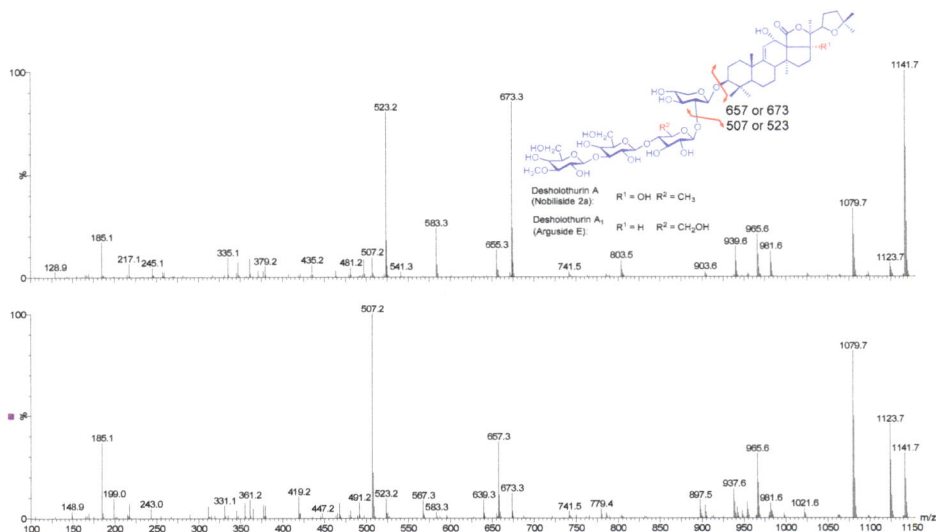

Figure 8. (+) The ESI-MS/MS spectra of the ions at m/z 1141.7 in Fractions 55 (top) and 110 (bottom). The figure indicates the presence of isomeric compounds. The key diagnostic peak at m/z 523 corresponding to [MeGlc-Glc-Glc + Na]$^+$ revealed the structure of desholothurin A$_1$, while the key diagnostic peak at m/z 507 corresponding to [MeGlc-Glc-Qui + Na]$^+$ indicted the structure of esholothurin A. The peak at m/z 481.2 corresponds to [Glc-Qui-Xyl + Na + H$_2$O].

The positive ion mode ESI-MS^2 spectra of the ions detected at m/z 1141 from the Fractions 55 (the top spectrum) and 110 (the bottom spectrum) are shown in Figure 8 as representative. These ions corresponded to desholothurin A$_1$ (arguside E) and desholothurin A (nobiliside 2a), respectively, which were different in both aglycone and sugar moieties from each other [2,31]. The presence of m/z 507 and/or 523 ions as the key fragment ions were observed in the MS^2 spectra of these compounds.

These isomeric compounds showed different MS/MS spectra. The major peak at m/z 523 (the top spectrum, Figure 8) corresponded to the sodiated key diagnostic peak [MeGlc-Glc-Glc + Na]$^+$, and the peak at m/z 673 generated by the loss of the Agl moiety corresponded to the entire sodiated hydrated sugar residue [MeGlc-Glc-Glc-Xyl + Na]$^+$. Therefore, this compound had an aglycone with a molecular weight of 468 Da. Our analysis inferred a tetraoside structure for these ions. This analysis revealed the structure of tetrasaccharide triterpene glycoside, corresponding to Desholothurin A$_1$.

The prominent peaks at m/z 507 and 657 (the bottom spectrum, Figure 8) corresponded to the sodiated key diagnostic peak [MeGlc-Glc-Qui + Na]$^+$, and the entire sodiated hydrated sugar residues [MeGlc-Glc-Qui-Xyl + Na]$^+$, respectively. The latter ion indicated that this compound had an aglycone with a molecular weight of 484 Da. The consecutive losses of the aglycone, Xyl, Qui, and Glc residues followed the MeGlc afford product ions at m/z 657.3, 507.2, 361.2, and 199.0. These findings revealed the structure of this compound as desholothurin A. Therefore, the analysis of data showed that HPCPC could separate the isomeric congeners in some cases. The integration of the counter-current chromatography and mass spectrometry techniques was an efficient and reliable approach for the purification and structure elucidation of saponins.

As an example, the positive ion mode ESI-MS/MS for the ions detected at m/z 1461 [M + Na]$^+$ from Fraction 95 is shown in Figure 9. These ions displayed an m/z value of 1437 [M − H]$^−$ in the negative ion mode ESI-MS, indicating that there was no sulphur group in the molecular structure.

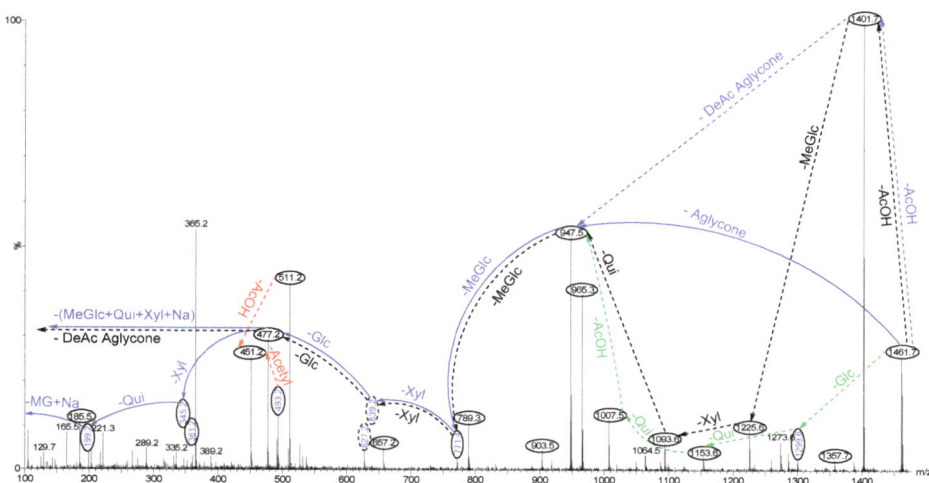

Figure 9. The positive ion mode ESI-MS/MS spectrum of ions detected at m/z 1461.7 from Fraction 95. The spectrum reveals the presence of different aglycones and sugar residues in the isomeric saponins. The full and dotted arrows demonstrate the three main feasible fragmentation pathways. The fragmentation pattern of ions at m/z 1461.7 reveals the structure of acetylated saponins lessoniosides H and K as a representative. The blue arrows show the decomposition of the isomeric congeners Lessonioside H, whereas the green arrows indicate the fragmentation patterns of lessonioside K. The loss of the acetoxy group from the ions at m/z 511.2 generates ions at m/z 451.2, which corresponds to hydrated three sugar units [Xyl-Xyl-MeXyl + H$_2$O + Na].

CID triggers three feasible independent fragmentation pathways of cationised parent ions shown in full and dotted arrows (for more details please refer to References [2,5–7,11]). The successive losses of the acetic acid (AcOH), deacetylated aglycone (DeAc Agl), 3-O-methyl-D-glucose (MeGlc), D-xylose (Xyl), D-glucose (Glc), Xyl, and D-quinovose (Qui) residues (blue arrows) were followed by MeGlc yielded ion fragments at m/z 1401.7, 947.5, 771.4, 639.2, 477.2, 345.2, and 199.2, respectively, in one of the new isomers for which we propose the name lessonioside H. Further, the sequential losses of MeGlc, Xyl, Qui, acetyl group, MeGlc, Xyl, Glc, and the deacetylated aglycone from the parent ions generated the fragment ions at m/z 1285.6, 1153.6, 1007.5, 965.3, 789.2, 657.2, and 477.2, respectively. This sequence of fragmentation confirms the structure of the new saponin, lessonioside H. As Figure 9 illustrates this triterpene glycoside contains the ion at m/z 493.2, corresponding to the key diagnostic sugar residue [MeGlc-Glc-Xyl + Na]$^+$. The black dotted arrows also corroborated the structure of lessonioside H. Alternatively, the consecutive losses of the deacetylated aglycone and acetic acid (AcOH) followed by sugar residues yielded ion fragments at m/z 1007.5 and 947.5, respectively. The latter ion corresponded to the sodiated sugar moiety generated by the loss of the Agl. This sequence of fragmentation confirmed the presence of an acetoxy group. The green dotted arrows indicate the decomposition patterns of lessonioside K, a new acetylated triterpene glycoside.

One of the new isomers was found to be identical with intercedenside A (C$_{55}$H$_{83}$NaO$_{25}$S), a sulfo-acetylated saponin was isolated from *Mensamaria intercedens* sea cucumber [36]. The MS^2 analyses of ions at m/z 1461.7 revealed a similar fingerprint profile with those reported for lessoniosides, which were isolated and characterised from the viscera of this species, in particular with Lessonioside A where the signals were coincident [6]. In addition, the sugar moiety of this novel isomeric compound was found to be identical to those of lessonioside A, confirming the constituents of the hexasaccharide chain. This novel triterpene glycoside had a holostane aglycone containing an 18(20)-lactone with a 9(11)-double bond and acetoxy group at C-23. We named these isomeric compounds lessoniosides H, I, J, and K.

Further, these isomers differed from holothurinoside H (marmoratoside B) in the sugar moieties. holothurinoside H generates a peak at m/z 507 corresponding to MeGlc-Glc-Qui under a positive ion mode mass spectrometry [30]. However, no peak was detected at m/z 507 corresponding to the key diagnostic ion [MeGlc-Glc-Qui + Na]$^+$ from the ions at m/z 1461.

Moreover, Sun, et al. [64] reported a lanostane-type triterpene glycoside, impatienside A, with a molecular weight [M + Na]$^+$ of 1447 ($C_{67}H_{108}O_{32}$), which had a peak at m/z 1423 [M − H]$^-$ in the negative ESI-MS, isolated from the sea cucumber *Holothuria impatiens*, and contained a double bond at the C24 position (ions 507 and 493), along with a structurally related known compound, bivittoside D [M + Na]$^+$ 1449 ($C_{67}H_{110}O_{32}$) and by negative ESI-MS m/z 1425 [M − H]$^-$, similar to impatienside A, without a double bond. However, Yuan, et al. [59] described a structure with a double bond at the position of C25 instead of C24 for this compound. This compound was detected in both the viscera and body wall of *H. lessoni*. However, it was found to be more intense in the body wall than the viscera.

Yuan et al. [59] isolated several saponins including marmoratoside A [M + Na]$^+$ 1447 ($C_{67}H_{108}O_{32}$), 17α-hydroxy impatienside A [M + Na]$^+$ 1463 ($C_{67}H_{108}O_{33}$), marmoratoside B [M + Na]$^+$ 1463 ($C_{67}H_{108}O_{33}$), 25-acetoxy bivittoside D [M + Na]$^+$ 1507 ($C_{69}H_{112}O_{34}$), together with known glycosides impatienside A and bivittoside D from the sea cucumber *B. marmorata*. These compounds were also identified in *H. lessoni*.

Our analysis revealed the presence of an ion peak at m/z 1435 [M + Na]$^+$ in the positive ion mode MS which showed a signal at m/z 1411 [M − H]$^-$ in the negative-ion mode ESI-MS. Tandem mass spectrometry revealed the isomeric structure of the ions at m/z 1435. The assignment of fragments revealed that these ions were isomeric compounds. These saponins were also common between the body wall and viscera. Wang, et al. [65] reported variegatuside D with a chemical formula $C_{59}H_{96}O_{27}$ at m/z 1259 [M + Na]$^+$, which might be produced by loss of MeGlc from the ions at m/z 1435.

Another novel isomeric saponin ion detected at m/z 1221.5 was common between the viscera and body wall. This novel saponin contained four sugar residues. Silchenko, et al. [66] also reported an acetylated-sulphated tetraosides triterpene glycoside, Typicosides A$_1$, isolated from the sea cucumber *Actinocucumis typica* (Family Cucumariidae, Order Dendrochirotida) with an identical m/z value (1221.5). However, the MS^2 spectrum of the ions at m/z 1221.5 had a different fragmentation pattern from that recorded for Typicosides A$_1$ even though they had the same m/z value which indicated the presence of a new saponin congener.

2.5.2. Negative Ion Mode ESI-MS/MS

Negative ion mode MS/MS analyses were also performed on compounds under experimental conditions similar to those used for the positive ion mode. It is clear that fragmentation patterns produced in the negative ion mode MS/MS were different from those in the positive mode.

As a typical example, the ESI-MS^2 fingerprints of the ions at m/z 1117.6 [M − H]$^-$ in the negative ion mode from fraction 110 is shown in Figure 10. These ions were observed at m/z 1141.5 [M + Na]$^+$ in positive mode, which corresponded to desholothurin A (nobiliside 2a). This peak detected at m/z 1117 in the negative ion mode ESI-MS with molecular formula $C_{54}H_{85}O_{24}$ [M − H]$^-$, indicates the presence of one Na atom (sodium adduct in the positive mode) which means no sulphate group exists in this compound.

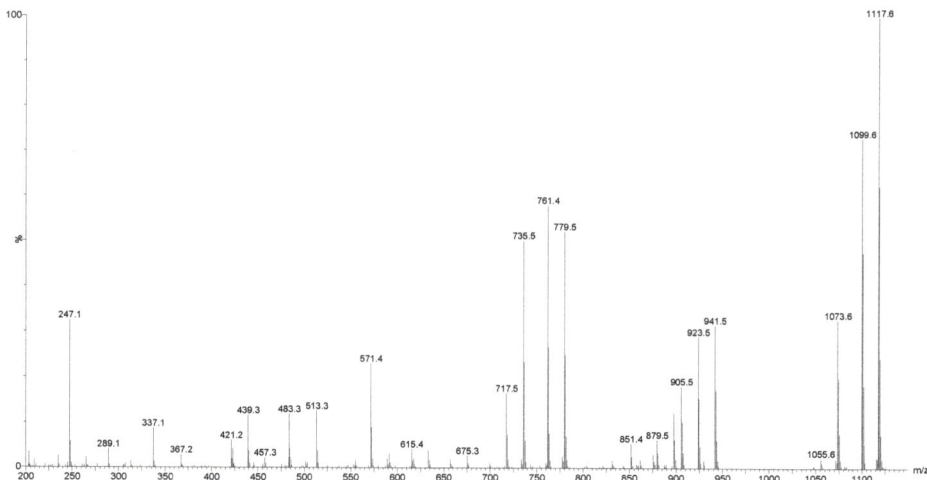

Figure 10. The ESI-MS/MS spectrum of desholothurin A in the negative ion mode.

The mass discrepancy among these peaks and associated peaks in the positive ion mode were 24 u. For instance, the ions at m/z 337 and 483 corresponded to the ions at m/z 361 and 507 in the positive mode ESI-MS/MS, respectively. This analysis determined that the sugar compartment of this saponin comprised of four sugar residues. This analysis further validated our results.

2.6. Common Saponins between the Viscera and Body Wall

Over 89 saponin congeners were found in the body wall, of which 54 saponin congeners have been reported previously. The comparison of saponins in the viscera and body wall of *H. lessoni*, showed that a large number (around 80 saponins) are shared between the body wall and the viscera as summarised in Table 1. Holothurin A was the major saponin in both body wall and viscera (Figure 11).

Even though the ions at m/z 1227.7 and 1229.5 were reported in both the body wall and viscera as major glycosides, our results revealed a higher abundance of these saponins in the body wall than in the viscera (Figure 11). The other compounds which gave a more intense signal in the body wall sample than the viscera sample were the ions at m/z 1291.5 and 1199.6, which corresponded to an unidentified saponin and arguside D, respectively. In contrast, the ions at m/z 1259.5 which corresponded to the sulphated isomeric compounds holothurins A_3 and D [2,11,53,67], were more intense in the viscera as compared to the body wall.

Some saponin congeners including the ions detected at m/z 1123.5, 1125.5, 1141.5 1301.6, 1303.5, 1305.6, and 1307.5 were apparently found with similar intensities in both the body wall and viscera. These findings suggested that saponins were generated in both the body wall and viscera in various concentrations, which proposes a diverse function of saponins with different mechanisms of action. These data were in good agreement with the findings of Van Dyck et al. [55] who reported that saponins originated from different cells for different purposes.

The presence of a high percentage of saponins in both the organs indicated the main acceptable role for saponins: namely, the defensive function against different predators. However, the relative quantities of saponins were much higher in the viscera than in the body wall, which is in a good agreement with the literature. They might be responsible for unknown biological functions. In addition, there was a correlation between the content of saponins and their biological activities.

The saponin congeners identified in this species contained different key diagnostic peaks at 493, 507, 511, 523, 639, 657, and 673. For instance, the ion at m/z 1305 was a novel pentasaccharide triterpene glycoside which contained the key diagnostic peaks at *m/z* 507.2 and 639.6 corresponded to [MeGlc-Glc-Qui + Na]$^+$ and [MeGlc-Glc-Qui-Xyl + Na]$^+$, respectively. Further, it had an aglycone with a molecular weight of 486 Da.

A large number of identified saponins have been also reported in other species (Table 1). For instance, Kitagawa et al. [28] were the first to report the presence of 24-dehydroechinoside A or scabraside A in the cuvierian tubules of the sea cucumber *Actinopyga agassizi* Selenka. Han et al. [41] also found this compound in *H. scabra*. The structure of scabraside A was also described in the sea cucumber *H. scabra* using NMR and ESI techniques by Han et al. [38]. Fuscocineurosides A/B/C and pervicoside C were reported in the sea cucumber *Holothuria fuscocinerea* in which they differed in the lateral chains of their aglycones [37]. Fuscocineroside A is defined as an acetylated-sulphated tetraosides triterpene glycoside. Fuscocineroside C was also reported in the *H. scabra* [41]. Bondoc et al. [67] investigated saponin congeners in three species of Holothuriidae (*H. scabra* Jaeger 1833, *H. fuscocinerea* Jaeger 1833, and *H. impatiens* Forskal 1775). This group assigned peaks at *m/z* 1227 for fuscocineurosides B/C, 24-dehydroechinoside A or scabraside A and another isomer.

Chanley et al. [48] were the first to report the sugar components of holothurin A in the sea cucumber *A. agassizi* Selenka. Later, Kitagawa et al. [39] described the structure of holothurin A extracted from the cuvierian tubules of *H. leucospilota* using spectroscopy methods.

Holothurin A$_3$, along with holothurin A$_4$, were isolated primarily from the methanol extract of the sea cucumber *H. scabra* by Dang et al. [53]. This group indicated both holothurins A$_3$ and A$_4$ as sulphated tetrasaccharide triterpene glycosides, contacting sulXyl, Qui, Glc, and MeGlc at a ratio of 1:1:1:1, which were different in the lateral chain of their aglycone moieties.

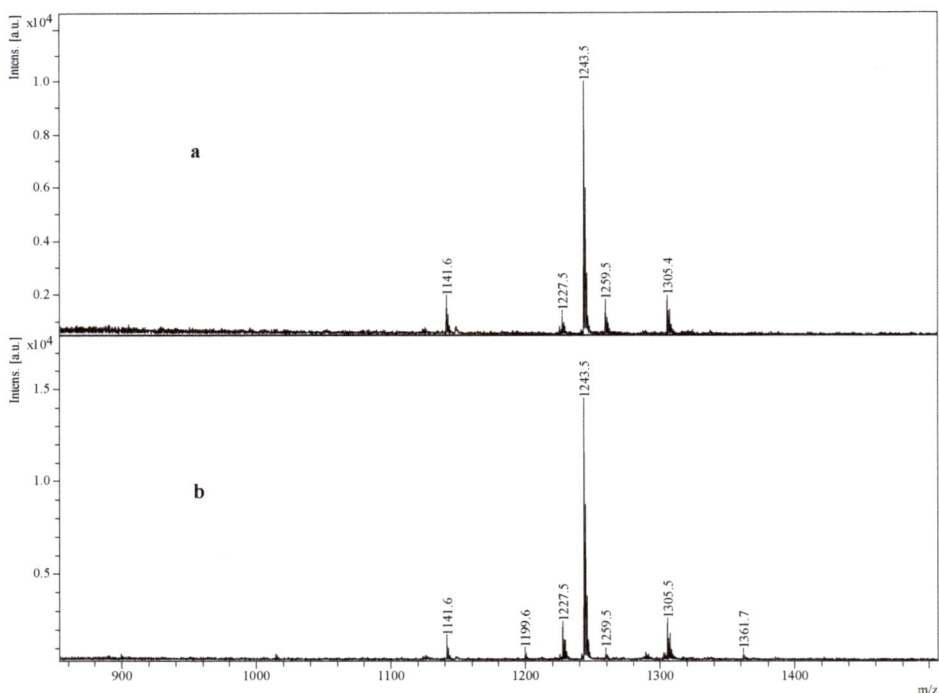

Figure 11. (+) MALDI spectra of butanolic saponin-enriched extract from viscera (**a**) and body wall (**b**) of *H. lessoni*.

2.6.1. Unique Saponins in the Body Wall

The integrated HPCPC-MS analysis indicated the presence of 35 new and 54 reported saponins in the body wall. Of these, nine ions m/z 1069, 1103, 1189, 1459, 1461, 1463, 1489, 1535, and 1539, were found exclusively in the body wall as compared to the viscera. Most of them had high molecular weights ranging from m/z 1400 to 1600. This result indicated epidermal or adjacent epidermal states for these saponins (the outer body wall epithelium directing sea water) as Caulier, et al. [26] reported the ions at m/z 1463 in the seawater surrounding *H. lessoni*. Over 30 saponin congeners were found exclusively in the viscera compared to the body wall. These saponins could be involved in the regulation of the reproductive systems, acting as natural emulsifiers, and assisting the absorption of food in digestive organs or having defence mechanism [68,69].

Mass spectrometry analysis revealed that a saponin observed at m/z 1463.7, corresponding to holothurinosides H/H_1, was localised exclusively in the body wall, probably in the epidermis. This observation was consistent with the findings proposed by Caulier, et al. [26] and Van Dyck, et al. [58] for the body wall of *H. lessoni* and *H. forskali*, respectively. Caulier et al. [26] reported the presence of this glycoside in the water surrounding the animal, which might have been released from the epidermis. Further, Van Dyck et al. [58] found this saponin congener localised in the epidermis of the body wall. Van Dyck, et al. [55] also indicated the presence of holothurinosides H/H_1 in the cuvierian tubules of *H. forskali*, while cuvierian tubules were absent in *H. lessoni*. However, these ions (1463.7) were not detected in the viscera, indicating a particular localisation of this saponin, which might be generated by the further glycosylation of other saponins. Mitu et al. also reported the presence of three saponins in the conditioned water of *H. scabra* and stated they were generated by the body wall [16].

2.6.2. Distribution of Saponin (Body Wall vs. Viscera)

Some of the identified saponins have been reported in several genera. For instance, the ion at m/z 1141 which corresponds to desholothurin A (synonymous with nobiliside 2a) or desholothurin A_1 (synonymous with arguside E) was also reported in different species of sea cucumbers independently [28–30,32,40,55]. Desholothurin A was first detected in the sea cucumber *Actinopyga agassizi* Selenka [28].

Van Dyck and associates [58] examined the secretion of saponins in the challenged and non-stressed holothuroids. Holothurinoside G (m/z 1449) was the only saponin detected in the seawater surrounding non-stressed holothuroids, originating from the epidermis, while holothurinosides C (m/z 1125) and F (m/z 1433), and desholothurin A (m/z 1141) were secreted when the animals were stressed [58]. Further, they noted the presence of two saponins at m/z 1301 and 1317 (holothurinosides M and L, respectively) in water surroundings stressed holothuroids, which stemmed from an internal organ such as the respiratory trees rather than the epidermis. They concluded that the ions at m/z 1125, 1141, 1301, 1317, and 1433 were stress-specific saponins, which could play more vital defensive roles. However, these glycosides were noted in both the viscera and body wall of *H. lessoni*.

Van Dyck, et al. [58] reported saponins detected at m/z 1125 (holothurinosides C/C_1), 1433 (holothurinosides F/F_1), and 1449 (holothurinosides G/G_1) present only in the epidermis, whereas saponins observed at m/z 1303 (Holothurinosides A/A_1) were localised exclusively in the mesothelium, and saponins at m/z 1141 and 1287 were present in both epithelia of body wall of relaxed holothuroids. A saponin observed at m/z 1463 was mainly located in the epidermis, whereas one with an m/z value of 1479 showed no particular localisation.

A MALDI-MSI analysis of saponins from the cuvierian tubules showed that the prolonged stress situation modified Holothurinosides C/C_1 (m/z 1125) to holothurinosides F/F_1 and H/H_1 (m/z 1433 and 1463, respectively), and desholothurins A/A_1 (m/z 1141) to holothurinosides G/G_1 and I/I_1 (m/z 1449 and 1479, respectively) [55,58]. This occurred by the addition of a disaccharide; either Qui-Glc or MeGlc-Glc. This modification, addition of a disaccharide, increased the saponins hydrophobicity and membranolysis (i.e., more toxic) [70].

Ions at m/z 1287 and 1303 were localised in the mesothelial or near mesothelial (the inner body wall epithelium toward the coelomic cavity), while saponins at m/z 11xx and 14xx had an epidermal or adjacent epidermal state (the outer body wall epithelium) [55,58].

Van Dyck, et al. [55] also studied the cuvierian tubules of *H. forskali* in both relaxed and stressed conditions by MALDI-MSI to determine the localisation of saponins. Likewise in the body wall, they found eight major peaks at m/z 1125, 1141, 1287, 1303, 1433, 1449, 1463, and 1479 [55], and categorised them into three different groups, corresponding to the isomeric saponins, which corresponded to different physiological states. Further, they found saponin ions at m/z 1125 and 1141 in low concentrations exclusively in non-stimulated tissues. The second group, the most abundant saponins, noticed at m/z 1287 and 1303, was more localised in the connective tissue of both the stimulated and non-stimulated individuals' tissues with the same concentration (expression level). They observed the third group of saponin ions at m/z 1433, 1449, 1463, and 1479 in the outer part of the connective tissue of the stressed specimen. They stated that the third group (m/z 14xx) were stress-specific and might originate from the first group (m/z 11xx) via glycosylation modifications. They also reported that different cell populations corresponded to generate different sets of saponins involving in a complex chemical defence mechanism [55]. For instances, holothurinosides A/A$_1$ (m/z 1303) and E/E$_1$ (m/z 1287) were produced by the vacuolar cells, while the other congeners generated by the neurosecretory-like cells. Recently, Popov and co-workers also investigated the distribution of saponin congeners in various organs of sea cucumber *Eupentacta fraudatrix* by LC-ESI QTOF-MS and stated the same metabolite profile for the whole body extract and the other individual analysed parts [71]. However, they reported the maximal content of the vast majority of detected compounds in the body wall as compared to other studied body components of sea cucumber. All the above findings support our data in which some saponin congeners were exclusively localised in the viscera or the body wall (present in only one type of organ), likely representing the specific and particular biological functions of these substances, while common congeners in the viscera and body wall might play the same role.

2.7. Bioactivity of Sea Cucumber Fractions and Saponins

2.7.1. Antifungal and Antibacterial Activities of Purified Saponins

Sea cucumbers have been used as a traditional remedy to cure infectious diseases. Previous studies have shown that some triterpene glycosides isolated from sea cucumber species possess antifungal activity [72]. The antifungal activity of isobutanol-enriched saponin and HPCPC fractions from *H. lessoni* viscera and body wall were assessed against *Fusarium. pseudograminearum, Pythium. irregulare*, and *Rhizoctonia. solani*. Our results revealed that several tested saponin congeners (fractions) have strong antifungal activities against *F. pseudograminearum* and *R. solani*. The antifungal activities were defined by the diameter of the zones of inhibition.

However, the examined triterpene glycosides had no effect on *P. irregulare*. Our data indicated that holothurian glycosides exhibit different activities against different fungal strains, which might be associated with the chemical composition and cellular structures of fungi.

Our result suggested that saponins having a linear sugar moiety, a sulphate group and/or an acetoxy group in their structures possess high antifungal activity. For instance, fractions that contained holothurin A and/or intercedenside A, which are sulphated compounds bearing a linear sugar residue, showed strong antifungal activity.

In contrast, the examined saponins had no inhibitory effect on the bacterial strain *S. aureus*, using the same concentration as used for the antifungal activity assay. This observation was consistent with the antibacterial findings of sea cucumber extracts reported by Mokhlesi et al. [73] and Kuznetsova et al. [74]. However, some studies reported antibacterial activity of sea cucumber saponins in crude extracts [75,76], which might be associated with other chemical classes rather than saponins.

2.7.2. Anti-Oxidant Activity of Sea Cucumber Extracts

The antioxidant activities of different extracts (70% EtOH, MeOH, H$_2$O, *i*-BuOH) of sea cucumber were evaluated by DPPH (2,2-Diphenyl-1-picrylhydrazyl) assay to determine their intrinsic antioxidant activity using α-tocopherol as the standard. Human immortalized keratinocytes (HaCat cells) were chosen as the target cells. Preliminary results indicated that sea cucumber extracts possess a high antioxidant activity in that the water extract and isobutanol fractions possess the highest antioxidant activity, which was consistent with the antioxidant findings reported by Husni et al. [77]. In summary, sea cucumber extracts tested in this experiment showed antioxidants activity comparable to other natural antioxidants.

3. Materials and Methods

3.1. Sea Cucumber Sample

Twenty sea cucumber samples of *Holothuria lessoni* were collected off Lizard Island (latitude 14°41′29.46″ S; longitude 145°26′23.33″ E), Queensland, Australia, in September 2010. The body wall was separated from the viscera (all internal organs) and kept separately in zip-lock plastic bags which were snap-frozen, then transferred to the laboratory and kept at −20 °C until use. The material and methods were the same as our previous publications [2,6,11], except for a small modification in the ESI-MS analysis as the samples were analysed in both the negative and positive ion modes.

3.2. Chemicals

All organic solvents were purchased from Merck (Darmstadt, Germany) except when the supplier was mentioned and was either of HPLC grade or the highest degree of purity. All aqueous solutions were prepared with ultrapure water generated by a Milli-Q system (18.2 MΩ, Millipore, Bedford, MA, USA).

3.3. Extraction and Purification Protocols

The saponins were extracted and purified as described previously [6,11], but by replacing the viscera with the body wall. The specimens were cut into small pieces, lyophilised and pulverised by a blonder and extracted with aqueous 70% EtOH (4 × 400 mL) on a shaker followed by filtration through Whatman filter paper (No.1, Whatman Ltd., Maidstone, UK) at room temperature overnight. The extract was concentrated under reduced pressure at 30 °C using a rotary evaporator (Büchi AG, Flawil, Switzerland) to remove the ethanol, and the residual sample was freeze dried. The dried extract (30 g) was re-dissolved in aq 90% MeOH (400 mL) and partitioned against 400 mL of n-hexane (v/v) twice. The water content of the hydromethanolic phase was then adjusted to 20% (v/v) and then to 40% (v/v) and the solutions partitioned against CH$_2$Cl$_2$ (450 mL) and CHCl$_3$ (350 mL), respectively. The hydromethanolic phase was concentrated to dryness using a rotary evaporator and freeze drier. The dried powder was solubilized in 10 mL of MilliQ water (the aqueous extract) in readiness to undergo chromatographic purification.

3.4. Purification of the Extract

The aqueous extract was then subjected to Amberlite® XAD-4 column chromatography (250 g XAD-4 resin 20–60 mesh; Sigma-Aldrich, MO, USA; 4 × 30 cm), washed extensively with water (1 L) to remove salts and impurities, and eluted sequentially with MeOH (450 mL), acetone (350 mL), and water (250 mL) [2,6,11]. The eluates were then concentrated, dried, and redissolved in 5 mL of MilliQ water. Finally, the aqueous extract was partitioned with 5 mL isobutanol (v/v). The isobutanolic saponin-enriched fraction was either stored for subsequent mass spectrometry analyses or concentrated to dryness and the components of the extract were further examined by HPCPC and RP-HPLC.

3.5. High-Performance Centrifugal Partition Chromatography (HPCPC or CPC)

The solvent system containing $CHCl_3$:MeOH:H_2O–0.1% HCO_2H (7:13:8) was mixed vigorously in a separating funnel and allowed to reach hydrostatic equilibration [6,11]. Following the separation of the two-immiscible phase solvent systems, both phases were degassed using a sonicator-degasser (Soniclean Pty Ltd., Adelaide, SA, Australia). Then the rotor column of the dual mode HPCPC™, CPC240 (Ever Seiko Corporation, Tokyo, Japan) was filled with the lower stationary phase in the ascending mode at a flow rate of 5 mL min^{-1} by a Dual Pump model 214 (Tokyo, Japan), with a revolution speed of 300 rpm. The aqueous upper mobile phase was pumped in the ascending mode at a flow rate of 1.2 mL min^{-1} with a rotation speed of 900 rpm within 2 h. One hundred and forty milligrams of an isobutanol-enriched saponin mixture was then injected into the machine in the ascending mode. The injected sample was carried by the mobile phase. The chromatogram was developed for 3 h at 1.2 mL min^{-1} and 900 rpm using the Variable Wavelength UV-VIS Detector S-3702 (Soma optics, Ltd., Tokyo, Japan) and chart recorder (Ross Recorders, Model 202, Topac Inc., Cohasset, MA, USA). The fractions were collected in 3.5 mL tubes using a Fraction collector. At Fraction 73, the elution mode was switched to a descending mode and the lower organic phase was pumped at the same flow rate for 3 h to recover saponins. The profile of fractions was also monitored by TLC. Monitoring of the fractions was necessary as most of the saponins could not be detected by UV due to the lack of a chromophore structure. Fractions were concentrated with nitrogen gas.

3.6. Thin Layer Chromatography (TLC)

Ten microliters of all fractions were applied on silica gel 60 F_{254} aluminium sheets (Merck # 1.05554.0001, Darmstadt, Germany) and developed with the lower phase of a $CHCl_3$:MeOH:H_2O (7:13:8 *v/v/v*) biphasic solvent system. The profile of separated compounds on the TLC plate was visualized by UV light, and by spraying with a 15% sulfuric acid in EtOH solution and heating for 10 min at 110 °C until maroon-dark purple spots developed.

3.7. Mass Spectrometry

The isobutanol saponin-enriched fractions and the resultant HPCPC purified polar samples were further analyzed by MALDI and ESI MS to elucidate and characterize the molecular structures of compounds. Mass spectrometry analyses combined with the existing literature led to the discovery of many known and new glycosides.

3.7.1. MALDI

MALDI mass spectra were acquired using a Bruker Autoflex III Smartbeam (Bruker Daltonik, Bremen, Germany). All MALDI MS equipment, software, and consumables were from Bruker Daltonics. The laser (355 nm) had a repetition rate of 200 Hz and operated in the positive reflectron ion mode for MS data over the mass range of 400 to 2200 Da under the control of the Flexcontrol and FlexAnalysis software (V3.3 build 108) (Bruker Daltonik, Bremen, Germany). External calibration was conducted using the sodium-attached ions from a Polyethylene Glycol (PEG) of average molecular weight 1000. MS spectra were processed in FlexAnalysis (V3.3, Bruker Daltonik, Bremen, Germany). MALDI MS^2 spectra were acquired in the LIFT mode of the Bruker Autoflex III with the aid of CID. The mass-selected ions were subjected to collision against argon in the collision cell to be fragmented, affording intense product ion signals. For MALDI, a laser was used to provide both good signal levels and mass resolution with the laser energy for MS^2 analysis being generally 25% higher than for MS analysis.

The samples were loaded onto a MALDI stainless steel MPT Anchorchip TM 600/384 target plate. Alpha-cyano-4-hydroxycinnamic acid (CHCA) in acetone/iso-propanol in a ratio of 2:1 (15 mg mL^{-1}) was used as a matrix to produce gas-phase ions. The matrix solution (1 µL) was spotted on the MALDI target plate and air-dried. Subsequently, 1 µL of sample was added to the matrix crystals and air-dried [2,6,11]. Finally, 1 µL of a NaI (Sigma-Aldrich # 383112, St Louis, MI, USA) solution (2 mg/mL in acetonitrile) was applied to the sample spots. The samples were mixed on the probe surface and dried prior to analysis. The dried samples were then introduced to MALDI for analysis.

Typically, the analysis of saponins by MALDI and ESI in the positive ion mode yields sodium adducts ions $[M + Na]^+$, however, protonated $[M + H]^+$ and potassium-cationized $[M + K]^+$ saponin ions are also observed.

3.7.2. ESI MS

The ESI mass spectra were attained with a Waters Synapt HDMS (Waters, Manchester, UK). Mass spectra were acquired in both the positive and negative ion modes with a capillary voltage of 3.0 kV and a sampling cone voltage of 60 V.

The other conditions were as follows: extraction cone voltage, 4.0 V; ion source temperature, 80 °C; desolvation temperature, 350 °C; desolvation gas flow rate, 500 L·h^{-1} [2,11]. Data acquisition was performed using a Waters MassLynx (V4.1, Waters Corporation, Milford, CT, USA). Positive ion mass spectra were obtained in the V resolution mode over a mass range of 600–1600 *m/z* using the continuum mode acquisition. Mass calibration was performed by infusing a sodium iodide solution (2 µg/µL, 1:1 (*v/v*) water:isopropanol). An accurate mass analysis was conducted in the positive ion mode, a lock mass signal from the sodium attached molecular ion of Raffinose (1 ng/µL in 50% aq acetonitrile, *m/z* 527.1588) was used through the LockSpray source of the Synapt instrument.

MS^2 spectra were acquired by mass selection of the ions of interest using the quadrupole fragmentation in the trap cell where argon was used as collision gas. The typical collision energy (Trap) was 50.0 eV. Samples were infused at a flow rate of 5 µL/min; if the dilution of the sample was required then acetonitrile was used.

3.8. Antifungal Activity Assay (Plug Type Diffusion Assay)

The antifungal activities of the isobutanol-saponin enriched and HPCPC fractions (pure saponins) were tested against three strains including *Fusarium pseudograminearum*, *Pythium irregulare*, and *Rhizoctonia solani* using a modified disc diffusion agar assay [78]. The test fungi were grown on an HPDA medium for 7 days, and a plug of the radial growth of each fungus was cut (0.5 × 0.5 cm cubes). The cubes were then placed onto the centre of a new HPDA plate and incubated at 27 °C for 24 h, or until the fungal growth surrounding the cube extended to a 1.5 cm diameter. At this stage, 40 µL of the samples (in methanol, in duplicate) were spotted onto standard paper discs and air-dried. The six discs were then placed onto the fungal growth plates about 1.5 cm from the edge and pressed into the agar using sterile tweezers. The plates were then re-incubated at 27 °C and checked for inhibition zones every 24 h for four days. The negative controls were methanol and plates of each fungus culture with tested samples, while Benomyl ® (Sigma-Aldrich, Castle Hill, Australia; 50 µg/mL) was used as a positive control.

3.9. Antibacterial Activity Assay

The antibacterial activity of saponin extracts was examined against Gram-positive bacterium *Staphylococcus aureus* using a typical agar diffusion assay. An antibiotic assay medium No.1 (AAM) was used for the antibacterial activity assay modified from Almuzara, et al. [79] and Wikler [80]. The test culture was grown in tryptone soy broth (TSB) and incubated at 37 °C for 18–22 h. The growth of the culture was evaluated by measuring the optical density (OD) using a Shimadzu UV-160A spectrophotometer at 600 nm (OD600 nm), and the OD was adjusted to 0.2. The AAM was seeded with the culture (1% *v/v*) and dispensed into 9-cm petri dish plates at 25 mL/plate, and cut using a cork borer to make 10 wells (6 mm). Each well was then filled with 40 µL of samples (in methanol) and the plates were incubated at 37 °C for 18–24 h. Vancomycin (0.25 µg/mL) was used as a positive control.

4. Conclusions

Sea cucumbers have been utilised as traditional folk remedies to treat various ailments by traditional practitioners. Sea cucumbers are a rich source of novel and bioactive metabolites. They are commercially important and contain various potent substances that can be used as a health care product in the markets. Among them, saponins are the most important and prime secondary metabolites reported in sea cucumbers. Likewise, the viscera, a highly diverse range of saponin congeners was identified in the body wall. This vast diversity could be associated with the different roles of saponins in sea cucumbers including kairomones; as chemical communicates to attract symbionts, chemical defence mechanism; the most acceptable biological functions for these bioactive compounds, or aposematic signal; threatening potential predators of the unpalatability food. Saponins are considered as a defence mechanism in which they are deleterious for most organisms, based on either adhesive defence or toxic mechanisms. The presence of a large number of the common saponins in both organs demonstrates their multifunctionality, representing the different internal and external biological roles of these metabolites.

Profiling of *H. lessoni* was conducted by MALDI and ESI-MS. The integration of HPCPC, MALDI-MS, ESI-MS, and tandem mass spectrometry proved to be a very efficient combination for structure elucidation of saponin congeners. The interpretation of fragmentation patterns of MS/MS spectra of triterpene glycosides allowed for the characterisation of the chemical structure of saponins. Accordingly, this analysis revealed the presence of 89 saponins. Knowledge of the chemical structure of saponins is critical for better understating of their structural/ activity relationships as well as the biosynthesis and biological roles of these compounds.

This study highlighted the diversity of saponin congeners in the viscera and body wall. This species produced a diverse range of saponin congeners, many of which were common between the body wall and the viscera. The results also revealed that some saponins are organ-specific. In other words, the different organs are characterised by different saponin congeners or specific saponin contents. Some of them were specific to either the viscera or the body wall. Further, the MS analyses also indicated that this species produced a mixture of common and unique saponin types. This specific localisation might be attributed to a particular function of these congeners, which will require further studies. The viscera had the highest number of specific congeners, which interestingly the majority belonged to non-sulphated triterpene glycosides. The role of viscera-specific triterpene glycosides may associate with regulating the reproduction of sea cucumbers, which is in a very good corroboration of the internal biological function of saponins. This indicated that the identity of saponins generated by sea cucumbers are different from species to species.

The most abundant ions observed under positive ion conditions were mainly sulphated compounds, which were common between the viscera and the body wall. This study suggested that saponins were synthesised in both the viscera and body wall, but further studies are warranted to investigate the biosynthesis of these secondary metabolites to discover which cells are in charge of producing saponins.

Saponin extracts are complex mixtures and, as such, the isolation and purification of these natural compounds are tedious, labour-consuming, and multistage due to their low content and a large number of saponin isomers. However, the identification of a large number of saponin congeners was not only due to the availability, development, and implementation of cutting-edge analytical equipment such as mass spectrometry and HPCPC based-procedures, but was also due to the presence of isomeric congeners in the experimental extract.

Many analytical methods have been used to purify, determine and elucidate the structure of saponin congeners in marine animals. As such a high diversity of saponin congeners were reported in this organism. In the current work, a large number of saponin congeners were detected for the first time using both the positive and negative modes of mass spectrometry. The structure of four novel acetylated saponins, namely lessoniosides H, I, J, and K were characterized.

In conclusion, our data revealed that there were differences in the distribution of saponins between the body wall and viscera, and showed a higher number of saponins for the viscera than the body wall, and highlighted some saponin congeners were found exclusively in the viscera.

However, some highly glycosylated saponins, such as ions at m/z 1461 and 1463, were found only in the body wall. In fact, having large sugar moieties increase the water solubility of these molecules. The examined saponins indicted a strong antifungal and antioxidant activities. This study revealed that sea cucumbers produce a wide spectrum of saponins with potential applications as valuable functional food or nutraceuticals as well as functional ingredients for cosmeceutical, medicinal, pharmaceutical products to improve human health.

Author Contributions: Y.B. and C.M.M.F. designed the experiments. Y.B. carried out the experiments with guidance of C.M.M.F., and W.Z., Y.B. set up the HCPCP analysis and worked on chemical structure elucidation. Y.B. prepared the original draft and all authors contributed in editing the manuscript.

Funding: This research was funded by the Australian SeaFood CRC and the Iranian Ministry of Health and Medical Education. This research received no external funding for (the APC) covering the costs to publish in open access.

Acknowledgments: We would like to express our sincerest thanks to the Australian SeaFood CRC for financially supporting this project and the Iranian Ministry of Health and Medical Education, and Kermanshah University of Medical Sciences for their scholarship to Y.B. The authors gratefully acknowledge the technical assistance provided by Daniel Jardine and Jason Young at Flinders Analytical Laboratory, Elham Kakaei and Associate Prof. Michael Perkins at Flinders. The authors also would like to thank Ben Leahy and Tasmanian SeaFoods for providing the sea cucumber samples.

Conflicts of Interest: The authors declare no conflict of interest.

References

1. Purcell, S.W.; Samyn, Y.; Conand, C. *Commercially Important Sea Cucumbers of the World*; FAO Species Catalogue for Fishery Purposes No. 6; FAO: Rome, Italy, 2012; p. 150.
2. Bahrami, Y.; Zhang, W.; Franco, C. Discovery of novel saponins from the viscera of the sea cucumber *Holothuria lessoni*. *Mar. Drugs* **2014**, *12*, 2633–2667. [CrossRef] [PubMed]
3. Purcell, S.W. Value, market preferences and trade of beche-de-mer from Pacific Island sea cucumbers. *PLoS ONE* **2014**, *9*, e95075. [CrossRef] [PubMed]
4. Pangestuti, R.; Arifin, Z. Medicinal and health benefit effects of functional sea cucumbers. *J. Tradit. Complement. Med.* **2018**, *8*, 341–351. [CrossRef] [PubMed]
5. Bahrami, Y. *Discovery of Novel Saponins as Potential Future Drugs from Sea Cucumber Viscera*; Flinders University: Adelaide, Australia, 2015.
6. Bahrami, Y.; Franco, M.M.C. Structure elucidation of new acetylated saponins, Lessoniosides A, B, C, D, and E, and non-acetylated saponins, Lessoniosides F and G, from the viscera of the sea cucumber *Holothuria lessoni*. *Mar. Drugs* **2015**, *13*, 597–617. [CrossRef] [PubMed]
7. Bahrami, Y.; Franco, C.M.M. Acetylated triterpene glycosides and their biological activity from holothuroidea reported in the past six decades. *Mar. Drugs* **2016**, *14*, 147. [CrossRef] [PubMed]
8. Demeyer, M.; Wisztorski, M.; Decroo, C.; De Winter, J.; Caulier, G.; Hennebert, E.; Eeckhaut, I.; Fournier, I.; Flammang, P.; Gerbaux, P. Inter- and intra-organ spatial distributions of sea star saponins by MALDI imaging. *Anal. Bioanal. Chem.* **2015**. [CrossRef] [PubMed]
9. Zhao, Y.-C.; Xue, C.-H.; Zhang, T.-T.; Wang, Y.-M. Saponins from sea cucumber and their biological activities. *J. Agric. Food Chem.* **2018**, *66*, 7222–7237. [CrossRef] [PubMed]
10. Silchenko, A.S.; Kalinovsky, A.I.; Avilov, S.A.; Kalinin, V.I.; Andrijaschenko, P.V.; Dmitrenok, P.S.; Chingizova, E.A.; Ermakova, S.P.; Malyarenko, O.S.; Dautova, T.N. Nine new triterpene glycosides, magnumosides A_1–A_4, B_1, B_2, C_1, C_2 and C_4, from the vietnamese sea cucumber *Neothyonidium (=Massinium) magnum*: Structures and activities against tumor cells independently and in synergy with radioactive irradiation. *Mar. Drugs* **2017**, *15*, 256. [CrossRef] [PubMed]
11. Bahrami, Y.; Zhang, W.; Chataway, T.; Franco, C. Structural elucidation of novel saponins in the sea cucumber *Holothuria lessoni*. *Mar. Drugs* **2014**, *12*, 4439–4473. [CrossRef] [PubMed]

12. Kalinin, V.I.; Aminin, D.L.; Avilov, S.A.; Silchenko, A.S.; Stonik, V.A. Triterpene glycosides from sea cucucmbers (Holothuroidea, Echinodermata). Biological activities and functions. *Stud. Nat. Prod. Chem.* **2008**, *35*, 135–196.

13. Yun, S.-H.; Sim, E.-H.; Han, S.-H.; Han, J.-Y.; Kim, S.-H.; Silchenko, A.S.; Stonik, V.A.; Park, J.-I. Holotoxin A$_1$ induces apoptosis by activating acid sphingomyelinase and neutral sphingomyelinase in K562 and human primary leukemia cells. *Mar. Drugs* **2018**, *16*, 123. [CrossRef] [PubMed]

14. Aminin, D.L.; Menchinskaya, E.S.; Pisliagin, E.A.; Silchenko, A.S.; Avilov, S.A.; Kalinin, V.I. Anticancer activity of sea cucumber triterpene glycosides. *Mar. Drugs* **2015**, *13*, 1202–1223. [CrossRef] [PubMed]

15. Zhang, J.-J.; Zhu, K.-Q. A novel antitumor compound nobiliside D isolated from sea cucumber (*Holothuria nobilis* Selenka). *Exp. Ther. Med.* **2017**, *14*, 1653–1658. [CrossRef] [PubMed]

16. Mitu, S.A.; Bose, U.; Suwansa-ard, S.; Turner, L.H.; Zhao, M.; Elizur, A.; Ogbourne, S.M.; Shaw, P.N.; Cummins, S.F. Evidence for a saponin biosynthesis pathway in the body wall of the commercially significant sea cucumber *Holothuria scabra*. *Mar. Drugs* **2017**, *15*, 349. [CrossRef] [PubMed]

17. Decroo, C.; Colson, E.; Lemaur, V.; Caulier, G.; De Winter, J.; Cabrera-Barjas, G.; Cornil, J.; Flammang, P.; Gerbaux, P. Ion mobility mass spectrometry of saponin ions. *Rapid Commun. Mass Spectrom.* **2018**. [CrossRef] [PubMed]

18. Decroo, C.; Colson, E.; Demeyer, M.; Lemaur, V.; Caulier, G.; Eeckhaut, I.; Cornil, J.; Flammang, P.; Gerbaux, P. Tackling saponin diversity in marine animals by mass spectrometry: Data acquisition and integration. *Anal. Bioanal. Chem.* **2017**, *409*, 3115–3126. [CrossRef] [PubMed]

19. Silchenko, A.S.; Stonik, V.A.; Avilov, S.A.; Kalinin, V.I.; Kalinovsky, A.I.; Zaharenko, A.M.; Smirnov, A.V.; Mollo, E.; Cimino, G. Holothurins B$_2$, B$_3$, and B$_4$, new triterpene glycosides from mediterranean sea cucumbers of the genus *holothuria*. *J. Nat. Prod.* **2005**, *68*, 564–567. [CrossRef] [PubMed]

20. Kobayashi, M.; Hori, M.; Kan, K.; Yasuzawa, T.; Matsui, M.; Suzuki, S.; Kitagawa, I. Marine natural products. XXVII: Distribution of lanostane-type triterpene oligoglycosides in ten kinds of Okinawan Sea cucumbers. *Chem. Pharm. Bull.* **1991**, *39*, 2282–2287. [CrossRef]

21. Kitagawa, I.; Nishino, T.; Matsuno, T.; Akutsu, H.; Kyogoku, Y. Structure of holothurin B a pharmacologically active triterpene-oligoglycoside from the sea cucumber *Holothuria leucospilota* Brandt. *Tetrahedron Lett.* **1978**, *19*, 985–988. [CrossRef]

22. Wu, J.; Yi, Y.H.; Tang, H.F.; Wu, H.M.; Zou, Z.R.; Lin, H.W. Nobilisides A–C, three new triterpene glycosides from the sea cucumber *Holothuria nobilis*. *Planta Med.* **2006**, *72*, 932–935. [CrossRef] [PubMed]

23. Han, H.; Zhang, W.; Yi, Y.H.; Liu, B.S.; Pan, M.X.; Wang, X.H. A novel sulfated holostane glycoside from sea cucumber *Holothuria leucospilota*. *Chem. Biodivers.* **2010**, *7*, 1764–1769. [CrossRef] [PubMed]

24. Han, H.; Yi, Y.H.; Li, L.; Wang, X.H.; Liu, B.S.; Sun, P.; Pan, M.X. A new triterpene glycoside from sea cucumber *Holothuria leucospilota*. *Chin. Chem. Lett.* **2007**, *18*, 161–164. [CrossRef]

25. Kitagawa, I.; Kobayashi, M.; Son, B.W.; Suzuki, S.; Kyogoku, Y. Marine natural products. XIX: Pervicosides A, B, and C, lanostane-type triterpene-oligoglycoside sulfates from the sea cucumber *Holothuria pervicax*. *Chem. Pharm. Bull.* **1989**, *37*, 1230–1234. [CrossRef]

26. Caulier, G.; Flammang, P.; Gerbaux, P.; Eeckhaut, I. When a repellent becomes an attractant: Harmful saponins are kairomones attracting the symbiotic *Harlequin* crab. *Sci. Rep.* **2013**, *3*, 1–5. [CrossRef] [PubMed]

27. Kitagawa, I.; Kobayashi, M.; Hori, M.; Kyogoku, Y. Marine natural products. XVIII. Four lanostane-type triterpene oligoglycosides, bivittosides A, B, C and D, from the Okinawan sea cucumber *Bohadschia bivittata* mitsukuri. *Chem. Pharm. Bull.* **1989**, *37*, 61–67. [CrossRef]

28. Kitagawa, I.; Kobayashi, M.; Kyogoku, Y. Marine natural products. IX. Structural elucidation of triterpenoidal oligoglycosides from the Bahamean sea cucumber *Actinopyga agassizi* Selenka. *Chem. Pharm. Bull.* **1982**, *30*, 2045–2050. [CrossRef]

29. Rodriguez, J.; Castro, R.; Riguera, R. Holothurinosides: New antitumour non sulphated triterpenoid glycosides from the sea cucumber *Holothuria forskalii*. *Tetrahedron* **1991**, *47*, 4753–4762. [CrossRef]

30. Van Dyck, S.; Gerbaux, P.; Flammang, P. Elucidation of molecular diversity and body distribution of saponins in the sea cucumber *Holothuria forskali* (Echinodermata) by mass spectrometry. *Comp. Biochem. Physiol. B Biochem. Mol. Biol.* **2009**, *152*, 124–134. [CrossRef] [PubMed]

31. Liu, B.S.; Yi, Y.H.; Li, L.; Sun, P.; Han, H.; Sun, G.Q.; Wang, X.H.; Wang, Z.L. Argusides D and E, two new cytotoxic triterpene glycosides from the sea cucumber *Bohadschia argus* Jaeger. *Chem. Biodivers.* **2008**, *5*, 1425–1433. [CrossRef] [PubMed]

32. Elbandy, M.; Rho, J.; Afifi, R. Analysis of saponins as bioactive zoochemicals from the marine functional food sea cucumber *Bohadschia cousteaui*. *Eur. Food Res. Technol.* **2014**, *238*, 937–955. [CrossRef]

33. Wu, J.; Yi, Y.; Zou, Z. Two new triterpene glycosides from sea cucumber *Holothuria nobilis*. *Chin. Tradit. Herb. Drugs* **2006**, *37*, 497.

34. Van Dyck, S.; Gerbaux, P.; Flammang, P. Qualitative and quantitative saponin contents in five sea cucumbers from the Indian ocean. *Mar. Drugs* **2010**, *8*, 173–189. [CrossRef] [PubMed]

35. Liu, B.S.; Yi, Y.H.; Li, L.; Zhang, S.L.; Han, H.; Weng, Y.Y.; Pan, M.X. Arguside A: A new cytotoxic triterpene glycoside from the sea cucumber *Bohadschia argus* Jaeger. *Chem. Biodivers.* **2007**, *4*, 2845–2851. [CrossRef] [PubMed]

36. Zou, Z.; Yi, Y.; Wu, H.; Wu, J.; Liaw, C.-C.; Lee, K.-H. Intercedensides A−C, three new cytotoxic triterpene glycosides from the sea cucumber *Mensamaria intercedens* Lampert. *J. Nat. Prod.* **2003**, *66*, 1055–1060. [CrossRef] [PubMed]

37. Zhang, S.-Y.; Yi, Y.-H.; Tang, H.-F. Bioactive triterpene glycosides from the sea cucumber *Holothuria fuscocinerea*. *J. Nat. Prod.* **2006**, *69*, 1492–1495. [CrossRef] [PubMed]

38. Han, H.; Yi, Y.; Xu, Q.; La, M.; Zhang, H. Two new cytotoxic triterpene glycosides from the sea cucumber *Holothuria scabra*. *Planta Med.* **2009**, *75*, 1608–1612. [CrossRef] [PubMed]

39. Kitagawa, I.; Nishino, T.; Kyogoku, Y. Structure of holothurin A a biologically active triterpene-oligoglycoside from the sea cucumber *Holothuria leucospilota* Brandt. *Tetrahedron Lett.* **1979**, *20*, 1419–1422. [CrossRef]

40. Han, H.; Yi, Y.H.; Li, L.; Liu, B.S.; La, M.P.; Zhang, H.W. Antifungal active triterpene glycosides from sea cucumber *Holothuria scabra*. *Acta Pharm. Sin.* **2009**, *44*, 620–624.

41. Han, H.; Li, L.; Yi, Y.; Wang, X.; Pan, M. Triterpene glycosides from sea cucumber *Holothuria scabra* with cytotoxic activity. *Chin. Herb. Med.* **2012**, *4*, 183–188.

42. Caulier, G.; Van Dyck, S.; Gerbaux, P.; Eeckhaut, I.; Flammang, P. Review of saponin diversity in sea cucumbers belonging to the family Holothuriidae. *SPC Beche-de-Mer. Inf. Bull.* **2011**, *31*, 48–54.

43. Kalinin, V.I.; Stonik, V.A. Glycosides of marine invertebrates. Structure of Holothurin A$_2$ from the holothurian *Holothuria edulis*. *Chem. Nat. Compd.* **1982**, *18*, 196–200. [CrossRef]

44. Dong, P.; Xue, C.; Du, Q. Separation of two main triterpene glycosides from sea cucumber *Pearsonothuria graeffei* by high-speed countercurrent chromatography. *Acta Chromatogr.* **2008**, *20*, 269–276. [CrossRef]

45. Kitagawa, I.; Kobayashi, M.; Inamoto, T.; Fuchida, M.; Kyogoku, Y. Marine natural products. XIV. Structures of echinosides A and B, antifungal lanostane-oligosides from the sea cucumber *Actinopyga echinites* (Jaeger). *Chem. Pharm. Bull.* **1985**, *33*, 5214–5224. [CrossRef] [PubMed]

46. Thanh, N.V.; Dang, N.H.; Kiem, P.V.; Cuong, N.X.; Huong, H.T.; Minh, C.V. A new triterpene glycoside from the sea cucumber *Holothuria scabra* collected in Vietnam. *Asean J. Sci. Technol. Dev.* **2006**, *23*, 253–259. [CrossRef]

47. Yuan, W.H.; Yi, Y.H.; Tang, H.F.; Xue, M.; Wang, Z.L.; Sun, G.Q.; Zhang, W.; Liu, B.S.; Li, L.; Sun, P. Two new holostan-type triterpene glycosides from the sea cucumber *Bohadschia marmorata* Jaeger. *Chem. Pharm. Bull.* **2008**, *56*, 1207–1211. [CrossRef] [PubMed]

48. Chanley, J.D.; Ledeen, R.; Wax, J.; Nigrelli, R.F.; Sobotka, H.; Holothurin, I. The isolation, properties and sugar components of holothurin A1. *J. Am. Chem. Soc.* **1959**, *81*, 5180–5183. [CrossRef]

49. Elyakov, G.B.; Stonik, V.A.; Levina, E.V.; Slanke, V.P.; Kuznetsova, T.A.; Levin, V.S. Glycosides of marine invertebrates—I. A comparative study of the glycoside fractions of pacific sea cucumbers. *Comp. Biochem. Physiol. B* **1973**, *44*, 325–336. [CrossRef]

50. Elyakov, G.B.; Kuznetsova, T.A.; Stonik, V.A.; Levin, V.S.; Albores, R. Glycosides of marine invertebrates. IV. A comparative study of the glycosides from Cuban sublittoral holothurians. *Comp. Biochem. Physiol. B* **1975**, *52*, 413–417. [CrossRef]

51. Yasumoto, T.; Nakamura, K.; Hashimoto, Y. A new saponin, holothurin B, isolated from sea-cucumber, *Holothuria vagabunda* and *Holothuria lubrica*. *Agric. Biol. Chem.* **1967**, *31*, 7–10. [CrossRef]

52. Matsuno, T.; Iba, J. Studies on the saponins of the sea cucumber. *Yakugaku Zasshi* **1966**, *86*, 637–638. [PubMed]

53. Dang, N.H.; Thanh, N.V.; Kiem, P.V.; Huong le, M.; Minh, C.V.; Kim, Y.H. Two new triterpene glycosides from the Vietnamese sea cucumber *Holothuria scabra*. *Arch. Pharm. Res.* **2007**, *30*, 1387–1391. [CrossRef] [PubMed]

54. Yuan, W.H.; Yi, Y.H.; Tan, R.X.; Wang, Z.L.; Sun, G.Q.; Xue, M.; Zhang, H.W.; Tang, H.F. Antifungal triterpene glycosides from the sea cucumber *Holothuria (Microthele) axiloga*. *Planta Med.* **2009**, *75*, 647–653. [CrossRef] [PubMed]

55. Van Dyck, S.; Flammang, P.; Meriaux, C.; Bonnel, D.; Salzet, M.; Fournier, I.; Wisztorski, M. Localization of secondary metabolites in marine invertebrates: Contribution of MALDI MSI for the study of saponins in Cuvierian tubules of *H. forskali*. *PLoS ONE* **2010**, *5*, e13923. [CrossRef] [PubMed]

56. Sun, G.Q.; Li, L.; Yi, Y.H.; Yuan, W.H.; Liu, B.S.; Weng, Y.Y.; Zhang, S.L.; Sun, P.; Wang, Z.L. Two new cytotoxic nonsulfated pentasaccharide holostane (=20-hydroxylanostan-18-oic acid γ-lactone) glycosides from the sea cucumber *Holothuria grisea*. *Helv. Chim. Acta* **2008**, *91*, 1453–1460. [CrossRef]

57. Bhatnagar, S.; Dudouet, B.; Ahond, A.; Poupat, C.; Thoison, O.; Clastres, A.; Laurent, D.; Potier, P. Marine-invertebrates. 4. Saponins and sapogenins from a seacucumber, *Actinopyga flammea*. *Bull. Soc. Chim. Fr.* **1985**, *1*, 124–129.

58. Van Dyck, S.; Caulier, G.; Todesco, M.; Gerbaux, P.; Fournier, I.; Wisztorski, M.; Flammang, P. The triterpene glycosides of *Holothuria forskali*: Usefulness and efficiency as a chemical defense mechanism against predatory fish. *J. Exp. Biol.* **2011**, *214 Pt 8*, 1347–1356. [CrossRef]

59. Yuan, W.H.; Yi, Y.H.; Tang, H.F.; Liu, B.S.; Wang, Z.L.; Sun, G.Q.; Zhang, W.; Li, L.; Sun, P. Antifungal triterpene glycosides from the sea cucumber *Bohadschia marmorata*. *Planta Med.* **2009**, *75*, 168–173. [CrossRef] [PubMed]

60. Liu, B.S.; Yi, Y.H.; Li, L.; Sun, P.; Yuan, W.H.; Sun, G.Q.; Han, H.; Xue, M. Argusides B and C, two new cytotoxic triterpene glycosides from the sea cucumber *Bohadschia argus* Jaeger. *Chem. Biodivers.* **2008**, *5*, 1288–1297. [CrossRef] [PubMed]

61. Stonik, V.A.; Chumak, A.D.; Isakov, V.V.; Belogortseva, N.I.; Chirva, V.Y.; Elyakov, G.B. Glycosides of marine invertebrates. VII. Structure of holothurin B from *Holothuria atra*. *Chem. Nat. Compd.* **1979**, *15*, 453–457. [CrossRef]

62. Liu, J.; Yang, X.; He, J.; Xia, M.; Xu, L.; Yang, S. Structure analysis of triterpene saponins in *Polygala tenuifolia* by electrospray ionization ion trap multiple-stage mass spectrometry. *J. Mass Spectrom.* **2007**, *42*, 861–873. [CrossRef] [PubMed]

63. Demeyer, M.; De Winter, J.; Caulier, G.; Eeckhaut, I.; Flammang, P.; Gerbaux, P. Molecular diversity and body distribution of saponins in the sea star *Asterias rubens* by mass spectrometry. *Comp. Biochem. Physiol. B Biochem. Mol. Biol.* **2014**, *168*, 1–11. [CrossRef] [PubMed]

64. Sun, P.; Liu, B.S.; Yi, Y.H.; Li, L.; Gui, M.; Tang, H.F.; Zhang, D.Z.; Zhang, S.L. A new cytotoxic lanostane-type triterpene glycoside from the sea cucumber *Holothuria impatiens*. *Chem. Biodivers.* **2007**, *4*, 450–457. [CrossRef] [PubMed]

65. Wang, X.-H.; Zou, Z.-R.; Yi, Y.-H.; Han, H.; Li, L.; Pan, M.-X. Variegatusides: New non-sulphated triterpene glycosides from the sea cucumber *Stichopus variegates* Semper. *Mar. Drugs* **2014**, *12*, 2004–2018. [CrossRef] [PubMed]

66. Silchenko, A.S.; Kalinovsky, A.I.; Avilov, S.A.; Andryjaschenko, P.V.; Dmitrenok, P.S.; Martyyas, E.A.; Kalinin, V.I.; Jayasandhya, P.; Rajan, G.C.; Padmakumar, K.P. Structures and biological activities of Typicosides A_1, A_2, B_1, C_1 and C_2, triterpene glycosides from the sea cucumber *Actinocucumis typica*. *Nat. Prod. Commun.* **2013**, *8*, 301–310. [PubMed]

67. Bondoc, K.G.V.; Lee, H.; Cruz, L.J.; Lebrilla, C.B.; Juinio-Meñez, M.A. Chemical fingerprinting and phylogenetic mapping of saponin congeners from three tropical holothurian sea cucumbers. *Comp. Biochem. Physiol. B Biochem. Mol. Biol.* **2013**, *166*, 182–193. [CrossRef] [PubMed]

68. Bakus, G.J. Defensive mechanisms and ecology of some tropical holothurians. *Mar. Biol.* **1968**, *2*, 23–32. [CrossRef]

69. Mercier, A.; Sims, D.W.; Hamel, J.F. *Advances in Marine Biology: Endogenous and Exogenous Control of Gametogenesis and Spawning in Echinoderms*; Academic Press: New York, NY, USA, 2009; Volume 55.

70. Kalinin, V.I. System-theoretical (Holistic) approach to the modelling of structural-functional relationships of biomolecules and their evolution: An example of triterpene glycosides from sea cucumbers (Echinodermata, Holothurioidea). *J. Theor. Biol.* **2000**, *206*, 151–168. [CrossRef] [PubMed]

71. Popov, R.S.; Ivanchina, N.V.; Silchenko, A.S.; Avilov, S.A.; Kalinin, V.I.; Dolmatov, I.Y.; Stonik, V.A.; Dmitrenok, P.S. Metabolite profiling of triterpene glycosides of the far eastern sea cucumber eupentacta fraudatrix and their distribution in various body components using LC-ESI QTOF-MS. *Mar. Drugs* **2017**, *15*, 302. [CrossRef] [PubMed]

72. Kitagawa, I.; Kobayashi, M.; Imamoto, T.; Yasuzawa, T.; Kyogoku, Y. The structures of six antifungal oligoglycosides, stichlorosides A_1, A_2, B_1, B_2, C_1 and C_2, from the sea cucumber *Stichopus chloronotus* Brandt. *Chem. Pharm. Bull.* **1981**, *29*, 2387–2391. [CrossRef]

73. Mokhlesi, A.; Saeidnia, S.; Gohari, A.R.; Shahverdi, A.R.; Nasrolahi, A.; Farahani, F.; Khoshnood, R.; Es'haghi, N. Biological activities of the sea cucumber *Holothuria leucospilota*. *Asian J. Anim. Vet. Adv.* **2012**, *7*, 243–249.

74. Kuznetsova, T.A.; Anisimov, M.M.; Popov, A.M.; Baranova, S.I.; Afiyatullov, S.; Kapustina, I.I.; Antonov, A.S.; Elyakov, G.B. A comparative study in vitro of physiological activity of triterpene glycosides of marine invertebrates of echinoderm type. *Comp. Biochem. Physiol. C* **1982**, *73*, 41–43. [CrossRef]

75. Abraham, T.J.; Nagarajan, J.; Shanmugam, S.A. Antimicrobial substances of potential biomedical importance from holothurian species. *Indian J. Mar. Sci.* **2002**, *31*, 161–164.

76. Park, S.Y.; Lim, H.K.; Lee, S.; Cho, S.K.; Park, S.; Cho, M. Biological effects of various solvent fractions derived from Jeju Island red sea cucumber (*Stichopus japonicus*). *J. Korean Soc. Appl. Biol. Chem.* **2011**, *54*, 718–724. [CrossRef]

77. Husni, A.; Shin, I.-S.; You, S.; Chung, D. Antioxidant properties of water and aqueous ethanol extracts and their crude saponin fractions from a far-eastern sea cucumber, *Stichopus japonicus*. *Food Sci. Biotechnol.* **2009**, *18*, 419–424.

78. Raza, W.; Yang, X.; Wu, H.; Wang, Y.; Xu, Y.; Shen, Q. Isolation and characterisation of fusaricidin-type compound-producing strain of *Paenibacillus polymyxa* SQR-21 active against *Fusarium oxysporum* f.sp. nevium. *Eur. J. Plant Pathol.* **2009**, *125*, 471–483. [CrossRef]

79. Almuzara, M.; Limansky, A.; Ballerini, V.; Galanternik, L.; Famiglietti, A.; Vay, C. In vitro susceptibility of *Achromobacter spp.* isolates: Comparison of disk diffusion, Etest and agar dilution methods. *Int. J. Antimicrob. Agents* **2010**, *35*, 68–71. [CrossRef] [PubMed]

80. Wikler, M.A. *Methods for Dilution Antimicrobial Susceptibility Tests for Bacteria that Grow Aerobically*, 9th ed.; CLSI Document M07-A9; Clinical and Laboratory Standards Institute: Wayne, PA, USA, 2012; Volume 32.

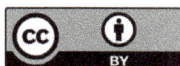

© 2018 by the authors. Licensee MDPI, Basel, Switzerland. This article is an open access article distributed under the terms and conditions of the Creative Commons Attribution (CC BY) license (http://creativecommons.org/licenses/by/4.0/).

![marine drugs logo] *marine drugs*

MDPI

Article

Angucycline Glycosides from an Intertidal Sediments Strain *Streptomyces* sp. and Their Cytotoxic Activity against Hepatoma Carcinoma Cells

Aihong Peng [1,2], Xinying Qu [1], Fangyuan Liu [1], Xia Li [1], Erwei Li [2,*] and Weidong Xie [1,*]

1   Department of Pharmacy, College of Marine Science, Shandong University, Weihai 264209, China;
    pengahsdu@163.com (A.P.); quxinying321@163.com (X.Q.); fangyuan617@outlook.com (F.L.);
    xiali@sdu.edu.cn (X.L.)
2   State Key Laboratory of Mycology, Institute of Microbiology, Chinese Academy of Sciences,
    Beijing 100101, China
*   Correspondence: liew@im.ac.cn (E.L.); wdxie@sdu.edu.cn
    (W.X.); Tel.: +86-10-6480-6141 (E.L.); +86-631-568-8303 (W.X.)

Received: 4 November 2018; Accepted: 25 November 2018; Published: 27 November 2018

check for
updates

Abstract: Four angucycline glycosides including three new compounds landomycin N (**1**), galtamycin C (**2**) and vineomycin D (**3**), and a known homologue saquayamycin B (**4**), along with two alkaloids 1-acetyl-β-carboline (**5**) and indole-3-acetic acid (**6**), were isolated from the fermentation broth of an intertidal sediments-derived *Streptomyces* sp. Their structures were established by IR, HR-ESI-MS, 1D and 2D NMR techniques. Among the isolated angucyclines, saquayamycin B (**4**) displayed potent cytotoxic activity against hepatoma carcinoma cells HepG-2, SMMC-7721 and plc-prf-5, with IC_{50} values 0.135, 0.033 and 0.244 µM respectively, superior to doxorubicin. Saquayamycin B (**4**) also induced apoptosis in SMMC-7721 cells as detected by its morphological characteristics in 4′,6-diamidino-2-phenylindole (DAPI) staining experiment.

Keywords: *Streptomyces*; angucycline glycosides; saquayamycin; cytotoxicity; apoptosis; SMMC-7721

1. Introduction

Angucycline is a group of aromatic polyketides containing a benz[a]anthraquinone framework of the aglycone which is mostly attached with C-glycosidic moiety [1]. Naturally occurring angucyclines are exclusively produced by terrestrial and marine actinomycetes, especially *Streptomycetes* species, in which a decaketide initially derived from acetyl-CoA is catalytically cyclized to four-ring core of angucycline by polyketide cyclase [2]. The structures of angucycline glycosides always vary in the oxidation degree of aglycones along with the number and position of diverse deoxy sugars [1–4]. In some cases, e.g., galtamycin B [5], grincamycin B [6], and vineomycin B_2 [7], the angular four-ring of typical angucycline is rearranged to linear tetracyclic or tricyclic system by enzymatic or non-enzymatic modification. Although firstly discovered half a century ago and possessing potent antibacterial, antiproliferative, and cytotoxic activities [6–11], so far, none of angucycline compounds has been successfully developed into clinical drug due to toxicity or solubility issues, which is unlike their biogenetic relatives tetracycline and anthracycline antibiotics [2]. Recent researches on angucyclines mainly concentrated on the understanding of their biosynthetic pathways in order to obtain modified analogues with medicinal potentiality through genetic manipulation [12–14].

Intertidal ecosystems are significantly different from those of seafloor. Regular tide immersion and emersion result in the dissolution of more organic carbon as well as oxygen and sulfate into intertidal sediment, which is beneficial to microbes' survival, particularly to aerobic actinomycetes. Both metagenomes and culture-dependent isolation have verified the abundance and diversity of

Actinobacteria in intertidal sediment [15]. Thus, we exploited the Actinobacteria resources from the intertidal sediment of Xiaoshi Island in Weihai, China, to screen for new antitumor agents. As a result, a *Streptomyces* sp., designated OC1610.4, was obtained, and its 16S rRNA nucleotide sequence (Accession no. MK045847) shared only 81.8% and 81.6% similarity, respectively, with those of *Streptomyces chromofuscus* (FJ486284) and *Streptomyces lannensis* (KM370050) in GenBank. The thin layer chromatography (TLC) analysis of its EtOAc extract of liquid culture medium displayed several yellow and brown spots, presumably due to aromatic polyketides. Subsequent large-scale fermentation and chromatographic isolation led to the identification of four angucycline glycosides including three new compounds, namely landomycin N (**1**), galtamycin C (**2**) and vineomycin D (**3**), and the previously reported saquayamycin B (**4**) (Figure 1), along with two alkaloids 1-acetyl-β-carboline (**5**) and indole-3-acetic acid (**6**) [16,17]. Saquayamycin B (**4**) displayed potent cytotoxic activity against hepatoma carcinoma HepG-2, SMMC-7721 and plc-prf-5 cell lines, and it caused apoptosis in SMMC-7721 cells.

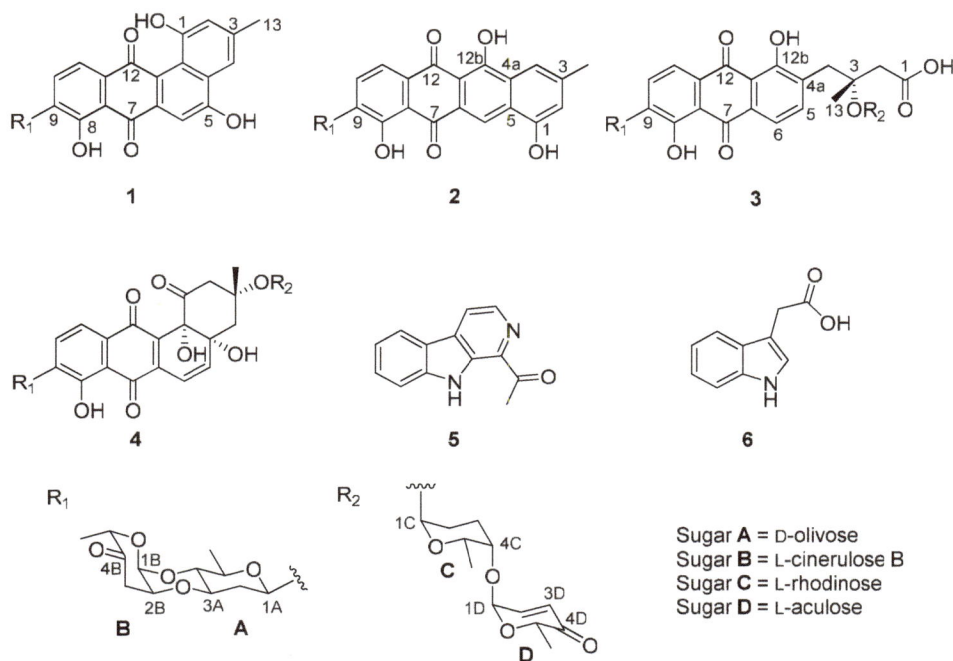

Figure 1. Structures of **1**–**6**.

2. Results and Discussion

From 30 L liquid fermentation broth of the strain *Streptomyces* sp. OC1610.4, cultured for 9 days, 4.6 g of EtOAc extract was obtained. After fractionation by column chromatography and preparative HPLC purification, six yellow or brown amorphous powdered-compounds were isolated from the crude EtOAc extract. The major constituent in the extract was firstly purified and whose molecular formula $C_{43}H_{48}O_{16}$ was established by the HR-ESI-MS m/z 838.3298 ([M + NH$_4$]$^+$, calcd for $C_{43}H_{52}NO_{16}$, 838.3286) and m/z 843.2842 ([M + Na]$^+$, calcd for $C_{43}H_{48}NaO_{16}$, 843.2840) (Figure S1). Its ^{1}H NMR spectrum displayed complex signals including three pairs of aromatic or olefinic protons from δ_H 6.06 to 7.91, more than a dozen methylene and methine protons from δ_H 1.40 to 5.39 and five methyl groups (Figure S2). The four oxygenated methine proton signals between δ_H 5.01 and 5.40 which, through HSQC spectrum, directly attached to the carbons signals at δ_C 96.0, 92.8, 92.1 and

72.0 (Figure S3), along with four doublets of methyl groups are the characteristic of four deoxy sugar molecules, one of which probably formed a C-glycoside since its anomeric carbon appeared at δ_C 72.0 [18,19]. These data, especially the signals of the deoxy sugar C-glycosidic moiety suggested the structure of angucycline glycoside [1]. Detailed comparison of its ^1H and ^{13}C NMR data with those previously reported in the literature and analysis of the 2D NMR sprectra (Figures S5–S8), led to the identification of this compound as saquayamycin B (**4**) [3,18].

Landomycin N (**1**) was a minor constituent of the crude extract. Its molecular formula $C_{31}H_{28}O_{10}$ was established by the m/z 561.1753 ([M + H]$^+$, calcd for $C_{31}H_{29}O_{10}$, 561.1761) from HR-ESI-MS. The IR spectrum showed the absorption band of hydroxyl (3203 cm^{-1}), carbonyl (1726, 1629 cm^{-1}) and aromatic (1607, 1578 cm^{-1}) groups. The ^1H and ^{13}C NMR, in combination with APT and HMQC spectra (Figures S11 and S12), revealed the presence of five aromatic protons, seven oxygenated methines, two methylenes and three methyl groups (Table 1). The five aromatic protons at δ_H 7.84 (d, J = 7.9 Hz), 7.72 (d, J = 7.9 Hz), 7.62 (brs), 7.46 (s) and 6.96 (brs), similar to those of urdamycin N4 [4], were assigned to the benz[a]anthraquinone nucleus of angucycline aglycone. The COSY spectrum exhibited the correlations from δ_H 7.84 (H-10) to δ_H 7.72 (H-11) and from δ_H 7.62 (H-2) to δ_H 6.96 (H-4) (Figure 2 and Figure S14). The HMBC correlations from δ_H 7.84 (H-10) to C-8 (δ_C 156.9) and C-11a (δ_C 134.7), δ_H 7.72 (H-11) to C-7a (δ_C 114.1), C-9 (δ_C 135.0) and C-12 (δ_C 182.6), and δ_H 7.46 (H-6) to C-4a (δ_C 130.6), C-7 (δ_C 188.9) and C-12a (δ_C 119.6) supported the presence of anthraquinone nucleus of angucycline aglycone. Although C-12 signal was not observed in the ^{13}C NMR spectrum, its chemical shift value was assigned as δ_C 182.6 through the correlation from H-11 to this signal in the HMBC spectrum. The presence of the hydroxyl substituent on C-8 on the anthraquinone nucleus was supported by the HMBC correlations from H-10 (δ_H 7.84) to C-8 (δ_C 156.9), and 8-OH (δ_H 12.53) to C-7a (δ_C 114.1), C-8 (δ_C 156.9) and C-9 (δ_C 135.0). The HMBC correlations from CH$_3$ (δ_H 2.40) to C-2 (δ_C 119.4), C-3 (δ_C 139.0), C-4 (δ_C 114.2), H-2 (δ_H 6.96) to C-1 (δ_C 155.4), C-4 (δ_C 114.2) and C-12b (δ_C 122.1), and H-4 (δ_H 7.62) to C-2 (δ_C 119.4), C-4a (δ_C 130.6) and C-12b (δ_C 122.1) confirmed the structure of the fourth ring conjugated to anthraquinone nucleus and the attachment of hydroxyl group at C-1 (δ_C 155.4) (Figure 2). The chemical shift of C-5 (δ_C 166.4) along with the HMBC correlation from H-4 (δ_H 7.26) to C-5 suggested the presence of the hydroxyl group at C-5.

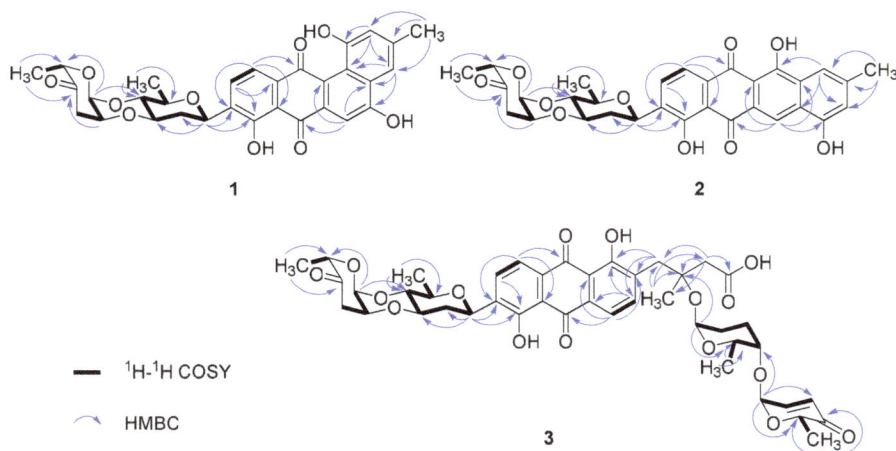

Figure 2. COSY and selected HMBC correlations for **1**–**3**.

Table 1. The ^{1}H and ^{13}C NMR data of **1–3** (500 MHz and 125 MHz) [a].

No.	1 [b] δC type	δH, mult (J in Hz)	2 [b] δC type	δH, mult (J in Hz)	3 [c] δC type	δH, mult (J in Hz)
1	155.4 C	-	155.9 C	-	172.1 C	-
2	119.4 CH	6.96, brs	116.2 CH	6.95, brs	44.6 CH$_2$	2.63, d (15.0) 2.72, d (15.0)
3	139.0 C	-	141.8 C	-	78.0 C	-
4	114.2 CH	7.26, brs	114.2 CH	7.52, brs	39.0 CH$_2$	3.19, d (13.4) 3.23, d (13.4)
4a	130.6 C	-	128.2 C	-	136.4 C	-
5	166.4 C	-	124.1 C	-	140.9 CH	7.84, d (7.8)
6	106.4 CH	7.46, s	116.7 CH	8.39, s	119.2 CH	7.75, d (7.8)
6a	137.3 C	-	125.1 C	-	132.5 C	-
7	188.9 C	-	187.3 C	-	189.1 C	-
7a	114.1 C	-	116.2 C	-	116.3 C	-
8	156.9 C	-	158.4 C	-	159.6 C	-
9	135.0 C	-	136.3 C	-	138.8 C	-
10	133.7 CH	7.84, d (7.9)	133.2 CH	7.87, d (7.8)	134.3 CH	7.94, d (7.8)
11	119.6 CH	7.72, d (7.9)	118.4 CH	7.73, d (7.8)	119.9 CH	7.80, d (7.8)
11a	134.7 C	-	132.4 C	-	133.0 C	-
12	182.6 C	-	186.3 C	-	189.2 C	-
12a	119.6 C	-	108.8 C	-	116.4 C	-
12b	122.1 C	-	162.1 C	-	162.4 C	-
13	20.9 CH$_3$	2.40, s	21.9 CH$_3$	2.40, s	23.5 CH$_3$	1.43, s
OH	-	12.53, brs	-	14.40, brs	-	13.14, brs
OH	-	12.08, brs	-	13.41, brs	-	13.10, brs
OH	-	-	-	10.92, brs	-	-
Sugar A, β-D-olivose						
1A	70.4 CH	4.97, brd (10.5)	70.5 CH	4.96, brd (10.8)	72.1 CH	5.01, brd (10.9)
2A	35.9 CH$_2$	1.63, ddd (11.6, 11.6, 10.5) 2.22, m	35.8 CH$_2$	1.61, ddd (11.7, 11.7, 10.8) 2.24, m	37.4 CH$_2$	1.60, ddd (11.6, 11.6, 10.9) 2.40, m
3A	75.7 CH	3.85, ddd (11.6, 9.0, 4.4)	75.7 CH	3.86, ddd (11.7, 9.0, 4.3)	77.4 CH	3.88, ddd (11.6, 8.9, 4.4)
4A	73.6 CH	3.51, dd (9.0, 9.0)	73.6 CH	3.51, dd (9.0, 9.0)	75.1 CH	3.58, dd (8.9, 8.9)
5A	73.5 CH	3.59, m	73.5 CH	3.60, m	75.1 CH	3.62, m
6A	17.4 CH$_3$	1.26, d (6.0)	17.4 CH$_3$	1.27, d (6.0)	17.9 CH$_3$	1.34, d (5.8)
Sugar B, α-L-cinerulose B						
1B	90.5 CH	5.22, d (2.6)	90.2 CH	5.23, d (2.4)	92.2 CH	5.26, d (2.8)
2B	70.8 CH	4.34, m	70.8 CH	4.35, m	72.3 CH	4.33, m
3B	39.6 CH$_2$	2.47, dd (17.4, 2.6) 2.90, dd (17.4, 2.6)	39.8 CH$_2$	2.47, dd (17.3, 3.4) 2.91, dd (17.4, 2.6)	40.6 CH$_2$	2.53, dd (17.3, 3.6) 2.84, dd (17.3, 2.7)
4B	208.7 C	-	208.7 C	-	208.5 C	-
5B	76.9 CH	4.72, q (6.6)	76.9 CH	4.72, q (6.6)	78.2 CH	4.76, q (6.8)
6B	16.0 CH$_3$	1.24, d (6.6)	16.0 CH$_3$	1.25, d (6.6)	16.5 CH$_3$	1.26, d (6.8)
Sugar C, α-L-rhodinose						
1C					92.0 CH	5.20, brs
2C					26.2 CH$_2$	1.40, m 1.95, m
3C					25.3 CH$_2$	1.90, m 2.10, m
4C					77.4	3.65, m
5C					67.0 CH	4.09, m
6C					17.5 CH$_3$	1.10, d (6.6)
Sugar D, α-L-aculose						
1D					96.0 CH	5.31, d (3.5)
2D					145.2 CH	7.03, dd (10.2, 3.5)
3D					127.2 CH	6.02, d (10.2)
4D					197.3 C	-
5D					71.0 CH	4.56, q (6.8)
6D					15.5 CH$_3$	1.27, d (6.8)

[a] Residual signals of solvent as reference. [b] Measured in DMSO-d_6. [c] Measured in acetone-d_6.

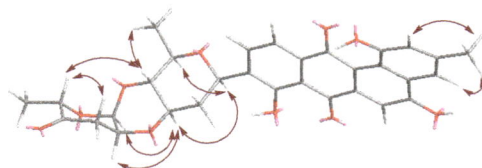

Figure 3. Key NOESY correlations for **1**.

The ^{1}H and ^{13}C NMR spectra of **1** showed that its aliphatic proton and carbon signals were very similar to those of marangucycline B which has a disaccharide composed of β-D-olivose and α-L-cinerulose B [20]. The observed COSY correlations from H-1A (δ_H 4.97) through H-6A (δ_H 1.26) confirmed the presence of an olivose (Figure 2). The COSY correlations from H-1B (δ_H 5.22) through H-3B (δ_H 2.47, 2.90), along with the HMBC correlations from CH$_3$-6B (δ_H 1.24) to C-4B (δ_C 208.7) and C-5B (δ_C 76.9), H-1B (δ_H 5.22) to C-5B (δ_C 76.9), and H-2B (δ_H 4.34) to C-4B (δ_C 208.7) confirmed the structure of cinerulose B. The linkage of two deoxy sugars was deduced by the HMBC correlations from H-1B to C-4A, and the NOESY correlation between H-2B to H-3A in the most stable conformation obtained by optimizing the molecule to minimized energy by MM2 in ChemBio3D Ultra 14.0 software (Figure 3). The relative configurations of both deoxy sugars were identified as β-D-olivose and α-L-cinerulose B, respectively, by NOESY correlations H-1A/H-5A,3A, H-3A/H-1B,2B, and H-4A/H-6A,5B (Figure 3). Based on the HMBC correlations from H-1A to C-8, H-1A to C-9 and H-1A to C-10, this disaccharide was linked to the aglycone at C-9 through C-1 of β-D-olivose moiety. Thus, the structure of **1** was established and named as landomycin N according to the structural classification code of angucycline initially proposed by Rohr et al. [1] (Figure 1).

Galtamycin C (**2**) is an isomer of **1**, due to its HRESIMS data *m/z* 561.1752 [M + H]$^+$ (calcd for C$_{31}$H$_{29}$O$_{10}$, 561.1761). The ^{1}H and ^{13}C NMR spectra showed that its aliphatic proton and carbon signals were similar to those of **1**, suggesting the presence of the disaccharide α-L-cinerulose B-(1→4, 2→3)-β-D-olivosyl moiety (Table 1). The ^{1}H NMR of **2** also showed five aromatic proton signals at δ_H 8.39 (s), 7.87 (d, *J* = 7.8 Hz), 7.73 (d, *J* = 7.8 Hz), 7.52 (brs) and 6.95 (brs), where the singlet at δ_H 8.39 (s) has higher frequency than the corresponding singlet of **1**. The ^{13}C NMR spectrum (Table 1) displayed sixteen aromatic carbons with chemical shifts ranging from δ_C 108.8 to 162.1 and two quinone carbonyl carbons at δ_C 187.3 and 186.3 were similar to those of rearranged linear angucycline glycosides, galtamycinone, grincamycin and grincamycin H [7,21]. Hence, **2** was suggested to possess a linear tetracyclic system. The structure of the compound and the relative configurations of the two deoxysugars were confirmed by COSY, HMBC and NOESY correlations (Figures 2 and 4). Therefore, **2** was named galtamycin C (Figure 1).

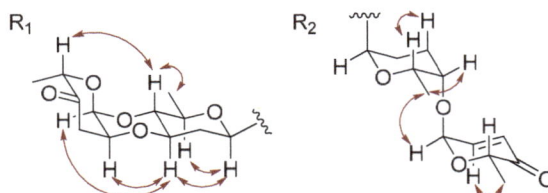

Figure 4. Key NOESY correlations in the sugar moiety of **2** and **3**.

Vineomycin D (**3**) was isolated as a yellow powder. Its HR-ESI-MS displayed the quasimolecular ion at *m/z* 838.3292 ([M + NH$_4$]$^+$, calcd for C$_{43}$H$_{52}$NO$_{16}$, 838.3286) and *m/z* 843.2838 ([M + Na]$^+$, calcd for C$_{43}$H$_{48}$NaO$_{16}$, 843.2840), indicating the same molecular formula (C$_{43}$H$_{48}$O$_{16}$) as saquayamycin B (**4**). Similar to that of saquayamycin B, the ^{1}H NMR of **3** also showed two pairs of coupling protons signals at δ_H 7.94 (d, *J* = 7.8 Hz, H-10) and 7.80 (d, *J* = 7.8 Hz, H-11), and δ_H 7.84 (d, *J* = 7.8 Hz, H-5) and 7.75 (d, *J* = 7.8 Hz, H-6), along with a pair of olefinic protons signals of α,β-conjugated carbonyl group at δ_H 7.03 (dd, *J* = 10.2, 3.5 Hz, H-2D) and 6.02 (d, *J* = 10.2 Hz, H-3D) (Table 1). The ^{1}H and ^{13}C NMR spectra also revealed the presence of three O-glycosidic anomeric proton and carbon signals at δ_H 5.31 (d, *J* = 3.5 Hz)/δ_C 96.0 (CH-1D), δ_H 5.26 (d, *J* = 2.8 Hz)/δ_C 92.2 (CH-1B), and δ_H 5.20 (brs)/δ_C 92.0 (CH-1C), and one C-glycosidic anomeric proton and carbon signals at δ_H 5.01 (brd, *J* = 10.9 Hz)/δ_C 72.1 (CH-1A). The most obvious difference in ^{13}C NMR spectra of **3** and **4** is the absence of a signal above δ_C 200 in **3**, and the presence of a signal at δ_C 172.2, characteristic of a carboxylic acid or ester group. Accordingly, **3** was suggested to have a tricyclic system with a side chain, probaly due to the opening of the cyclohexanone ring of saquayamycin B (**4**) [6,7,22].

The skeleton of anthraquinone and the positions of two hydroxyl groups at C-8 and C-12b were confirmed by the HMBC correlations associated with the two pairs of aromatic protons. In HMBC spectrum, the correlations from δ_H 7.94 (H-10) to C-8 (δ_C 159.6) and C-11a (δ_C 133.0), δ_H 7.80 (H-11) to C-7a (δ_C 116.3), C-9 (δ_C 138.8) and C-12 (δ_C 189.2), δ_H 7.84 (H-5) to C-6a (δ_C 132.5) and C-12b (δ_C 162.4), δ_H 7.75 (H-6) to C-4a (δ_C 136.4), C-7 (δ_C 189.1) and C-12a (δ_C 116.4) were observed (Figure 2). The correlations from the methyl protons at δ_H 1.43 (H-13) to C-2 (δ_C 44.6), C-3 (δ_C 78.0) and C-4 (δ_C 39.0), along with the correlations from the methylene protons appearing as a couple of AB system at δ_H 2.72 and 2.63 (H-2) to C-1 (δ_C 172.1), confirmed the side chain. The linkage between the anthraquinone and side chain was deduced to be at C-4a by the HMBC correlations from methylene protons at δ_H 3.23 and 3.19 (H-4) to C-4a (δ_C 136.4), C-5 (δ_C 140.9) and C-12b (δ_C 162.4). The presence of two disaccharides α-L-cinerulose B-(1→4, 2→3)-β-D-olivosyl and α-L-aculose-(1→4)-α-L-rhodinosyl groups were further deduced by COSY, HMBC and NOESY correlations (Figures 2 and 4). The HMBC correlations from H-1A (δ_H 5.01) to C-8 (δ_C 159.6), C-9 (δ_C 138.2) and C-10 (δ_C 134.3) suggested that the α-L-cinerulose B-(1→4, 2→3)-β-D-olivosyl group was linked to C-9 through C-1 of D-olivose moiety. The HMBC correlation from H-3A (δ_H 5.20) to C-3 (δ_C 78.0) indicated that α-L-aculose-(1→4)-α-L-rhodinosyl group was linked to C-3. In general, tricyclic angucyclines are derived from typical angucyclines with the same tetracyclic core structure under acidic conditions [1]. Accordingly, the absolute configuration of C-3 is proposed to be same as that of saquayamycin B (**4**) and other tricyclic angucyclines, e.g., grincamycin B, vineomycin B_2 and fridamycin D [6,7,22]. Thus, the structure of **3** was established and named vineomycin D (Figure 1).

A few anguclines, such as saquayamycin B, landomycin E, vineomycin A_1 etc., have been reported to exhibit remarkable antitumor activity against a series of tumor cell lines [3,7,10]. Though, the distinct in vivo toxicity restricted the further development of these compounds to be clinical drugs. Recently, an atypical angucycline, lomaiviticin A, was reported to be under preclinical evaluation for antitumor treatment due to its prominent cytotoxicity and effects of inducing double-strand breaks in DNA [14,23]. In present work, **1–4** were assayed for their cytotoxic activity against normal liver cell LO_2, hepatoma carcinoma HepG-2, SMMC-7721 and plc-prf-5 cell lines by 3-(4,5-dimethylthiazol-2-yl)-2,5-diphenyltetrazolium bromide (MTT) method (Table 2). At the concentrations of 40 μM, **1–3** displayed no cytotoxicity against any of the tested cell lines. Saquayamycin B (**4**) displayed potent cytotoxic activity against HepG-2, SMMC-7721 and plc-prf-5 cells, with IC_{50} values 0.135, 0.033 and 0.244 μM, respectively, which are less than the IC_{50} of doxorubicin. Treatment of SMMC-7721 cells with saquayamycin B at concentrations ranging from 0.025 to 0.100 μM for 24 h, SMMC-7721 cells resulted in chromatin dispersion and formation of apoptotic body in DAPI staining test (Figure 5a). The apoptotic ratio of SMMC-7721 cells was dependent on the concentrations of saquayamycin B (Figure 5b).

Table 2. Cytotoxicity of **1–4** against LO_2, HepG-2, SMMC-7721 and plc-prf-5 cells (IC_{50}, μM).

Compounds	Cell Lines			
	LO_2	HepG-2	SMMC-7721	plc-prf-5
1	>40	>40	>40	>40
2	>40	>40	>40	>40
3	>40	>40	>40	>40
4	0.343 ± 0.081	0.135 ± 0.056	0.033 ± 0.005	0.244 ± 0.001
Doxorubicin	2.26 ± 0.16	0.919 ± 0.599	0.706 ± 0.004	1.03 ± 0.99

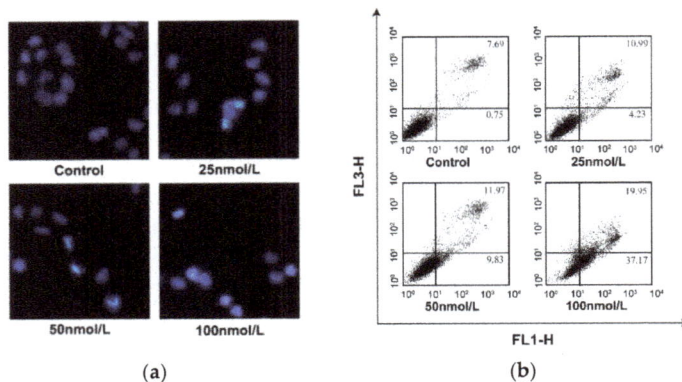

Figure 5. (**a**) Fluorescence micrographs of untreated and saquayamycin B-treated SMMC-7721 cells (24 h) stained with DAPI, Magnification: 100×; (**b**) Quantification of saquayamycin B-induced apoptosis in SMMC-7721 cell using flow cytometric analysis. ** $p < 0.01$ versus saquayamycin B 0 μM group.

3. Materials and Methods

3.1. General Experimental Procedures

Optical rotations were measured with an Anton Paar MCP 200 polarimeter with a sodium lamp (589 nm) (Anton Paar GmbH, Graz, Austria). UV spectra were obtained on Genesys 10S UV-Vis spectrometer (Thermo Fisher Scientific Ltd, Waltham, MA, USA); IR spectra were recorded with a Nicolet IS5 FT-IR spectrometer (Thermo Fisher Scientific Ltd, Waltham, MA, USA); NMR spectra were recorded on Bruker AVANCE III 500 spectrometer (Bruker Inc., Karlsruhe, Germany). HPLC-MS were acquired on Agilent 1200HPLC/6520QTOFMS (Agilent Technologies Inc., Santa Clara, CA, USA). Semi-preparative HPLC isolation was performed on Agilent 1260 Infinity II (Agilent Technologies Inc., Santa Clara, USA) with an ODS column (YMC-Triart C18, 10 mm × 250 mm, YMC Co. Ltd., Tokyo, Japan). Silica gel (200–300 and 300–400 mesh) used in column chromatography (CC) and silica gel GF$_{254}$ (10–40 μm) used in thin layer chromatography (TLC) were supplied by Qingdao Marine Chemical Factory in China.

3.2. Actinomycetes Strain

The intertidal sediment was collected after the tide has ebbed in Xiaoshi Island, Weihai, China in September 2016. The strain OC1610.4 was isolated from this sediment using Gause's synthetic medium (20 g/L amylogen, 1 g/L KNO$_3$, 0.5 g/L NaCl, 0.5 g/L K$_2$HPO$_4$·H$_2$O, 0.5 g/L MgSO$_4$·H$_2$O, 0.01 g/L FeSO$_4$·H$_2$O, and 3.0% sea salt) containing potassium dichromate (6 μg/mL) and nalidixic acid (20 μg/mL) as antifungal and antibacterial agents. The procedures of DNA extraction and PCR amplification of 16S rRNA were same as described in reference [24]. The nucleotide sequence of the OC1610.4 strain was sequenced at the Shanghai Sangon Biotech Co., China, and deposited at GenBank (Accession no. MK045847). Voucher strain (No. OC1610.4) was deposited at Laboratory of Natural Products Chemistry, Department of Pharmacy, Shandong University at Weihai.

3.3. Fermentation, Extraction and Isolation

The spore and mycelia suspension of strain OC1610.4 was inoculated in Erlenmeyer flasks (500 mL) each of which contains 100 mL S-medium (10 g/L glucose, 4 g/L yeast extract, 4 g/L K$_2$HPO$_4$, 2 g/L KH$_2$PO$_4$, 0.5 g/L MgSO$_4$·7H$_2$O, and 3.0% sea salt). Total 30 L medium was shaking-cultured at 140 rpm and 28 °C for 9 days. The fermentation broth including mycelia was extracted with equal volume of EtOAc five times to give 4.6 g crude extract. The extract was subjected to silica gel CC (60 g, 200–300 mesh) eluting with n-hexane-acetone (10:1, 5:1, 2:1 and acetone) to give four fractions

F_1–F_4. Part (72 mg) of fraction F_1 (n-hexane-acetone 10:1) was isolated by semi-preparative HPLC eluting with CH_3OH-H_2O (70:30, *v*/*v*) to give **5** (5.6 mg). Fraction F_2 (n-hexane-acetone 5:1, 267 mg) was further purified by silica gel CC (1 g, 300–400 mesh) eluting with n-hexane-acetone (10:1) to give sub-fractions F_{2a} and F_{2b}. Sub-fractions F_{2a} (67 mg) was purified by semi-preparative HPLC eluting with CH_3OH-H_2O (38:62, *v*/*v*) to give **6** (4.6 mg). The sub-fractions F_{2b} (26 mg) was a mixture presenting two brown spots on TLC, and was isolated by semi-preparative HPLC eluting with CH_3CN-H_2O (70:30, *v*/*v*) to give **1** (4.2 mg) and **2** (3.4 mg). Fraction F_3 (n-hexane-acetone 2:1, 670 mg) was subjected to a silica gel CC (10 g, 200–300 mesh) eluting with CH_3Cl-CH_3OH (20:1) to give two subfractions F_{3a} and F_{3b}. From F_{3a} (220 mg), compound **4** (18 mg) was purified using a low pressure silica gel CC (1 g, 300–400 mesh) eluting with n-hexane-acetone (4:1). Subfractions F_{3b} (67 mg) was isolated by semi-preparative HPLC eluting with CH_3CN-H_2O (65:35, *v*/*v*) to give **3** (5 mg).

Landomycin N (**1**): brown amorphous powder; $[\alpha]_D^{25}$ +92 (*c* 0.002, MeOH); UV (MeOH) λ_{max} (log ε) 225 (2.99), 327 (2.65) nm; IR (KBr) ν_{max} 3203, 2974, 2916, 1726, 1629, 1607, 1578, 1433, 1295, 1111, 1075, 852, 791 cm^{-1}; ^1H NMR (500 MHz, DMSO-d_6) and ^{13}C NMR (125 MHz, DMSO-d_6) data, Table 1; HR-ESI-MS *m*/*z* 561.1753 ([M + H]$^+$, calcd for $C_{31}H_{29}O_{10}$, 561.1761).

Galtamycin C (**2**): reddish-brown amorphous powder; $[\alpha]_D^{25}$ +285 (*c* 0.003, MeOH); UV (MeOH) λ_{max} (log ε) 265 (2.40), 340 (2.07) nm; IR (KBr) ν_{max} 3383, 2917, 2879, 1727, 1657, 1608, 1584, 1525, 1471, 1286, 1247, 1108, 1017, 872, 836, 716 cm^{-1}; ^1H NMR (500 MHz, DMSO-d_6) and ^{13}C NMR (125 MHz, DMSO-d_6) data, Table 1; HR-ESI-MS *m*/*z* 561.1752 ([M + H]$^+$, calcd for $C_{31}H_{29}O_{10}$, 561.1761).

Vineomycin D (**3**): yellow amorphous powder; $[\alpha]_D^{25}$ +69 (*c* 0.050, MeOH); UV (MeOH) λ_{max} (log ε) 230 (3.56), 259 (3.28), 295 (2.83) nm; IR (KBr) ν_{max} 3557, 2978, 2935, 1731, 1702, 1625, 1581, 1431, 1259, 1080, 1014, 899, 808 cm^{-1}; ^1H NMR (500 MHz, acetone-d_6) and ^{13}C NMR (125 MHz, acetone-d_6) data, Table 1; HR-ESI-MS *m*/*z* 838.3292 ([M + NH$_4$]$^+$, calcd for $C_{43}H_{52}NO_{16}$, 838.3286) and *m*/*z* 843.2838 ([M + Na]$^+$, calcd for $C_{43}H_{48}NaO_{16}$, 843.2840).

3.4. Cytotoxicity Assays, DAPI Staining Test and Flow Cytometric Analysis

The cytotoxicity evaluations of **1**–**4** against normal liver cell and hepatoma carcinoma cells were carried out using the 3-(4,5-dimethylthiazol-2-yl)-2,5-diphenyltetrazolium bromide (MTT) assay. Doxorubicin was used as positive control drug and deionized H_2O with the same DMSO concentration was used as parallel control. DAPI staining test was employed to qualitatively observe apoptosis, and the apoptotic ratio was measured by flow cytometric analysis (Becton Dickinson FACScan, San Jose, CA, USA). These tests were conducted using the methods as previously described [25,26].

4. Conclusions

Four angucycline glycosides including landomycin N (**1**), galtamycin C (**2**), vineomycin D (**3**) and saquayamycin (**4**), along with two alkaloids 1-acetyl-β-carboline (**5**) and indole-3-acetic acid (**6**), were isolated from the fermentation broth of strain *Streptomyces* sp. OC1610.4, obtained from the intertidal sediment. Galtamycin C (**2**) and vineomycin D (**3**) are rearranged angucycline derivatives respectively possessing a linear tetracyclic and a tricyclic framework of angucycline. Vineomycin D (**3**) and saquayamycin B (**4**) are isomers, comprising the same two disaccharides in the structures. Among the isolated angucycline glycosides, saquayamycin B (**4**) displayed the most potent cytotoxic activity against hepatoma carcinoma HepG-2, SMMC-7721 and plc-prf-5 cells. Although saquayamycin B was shown to induce an apoptosis in SMMC-7721 cell, its antineoplastic mechanism needs to be further investigated.

Supplementary Materials: The following are available online at http://www.mdpi.com/1660-3397/16/12/470/s1: This section includes the HR-ESI-MS, 1D and 2D NMR spectra for compounds **1**–**4**. Figures S1–S8: HR-ESI-MS, 1D and 2D NMR spectra of saquayamycin B (**4**); Figures S9–S15: HR-ESI-MS, 1D and 2D NMR spectra of landomycin N (**1**); Figures S16–S22: HR-ESI-MS, 1D and 2D NMR spectra of galtamycin C (**2**); Figures S23–S29: HR-ESI-MS, 1D and 2D NMR spectra of vineomycin D (**3**).

Author Contributions: A.P. conducted the main experiments, including the isolation and culture of strain, the isolation and structural elucidation of compounds. X.Q performed the large-scale fermentation. F.L. conducted the antitumor assay. X.L. guided the antitumor assay. E.L. guided the HPLC isolation and NMR measurement. W.X supervised the whole work and wrote the manuscript. All authors have read the manuscript and approved the final manuscript for submission.

Funding: This research was funded by the Natural Science Foundation of Shandong Province, China (ZR2014HM018) and National Natural Science Foundation of China (81872771).

Acknowledgments: We are grateful to Hong-Bo Zheng from Key Laboratory of Chemical Biology (Ministry of Education), School of Pharmaceutical Science, Shandong University, Jinan 250012, China, for recording HR-ESI-MS.

Conflicts of Interest: The authors declare no conflict of interest.

References

1. Rohr, J.; Thiericke, R. Angucycline group antibiotics. *Nat. Prod. Rep.* **1992**, *9*, 103–137. [CrossRef] [PubMed]
2. Kharel, M.K.; Pahari, P.; Shepherd, M.D.; Tibrewal, N.; Nybo, S.E.; Shaaban, K.A.; Rohr, J. Angucyclines: biosynthesis, mode-of-action, new natural products, and synthesis. *Nat. Prod. Rep.* **2012**, *29*, 264–325. [CrossRef] [PubMed]
3. Shaaban, K.A.; Ahmed, T.A.; Leggas, M.; Rohr, J. Saquayamycins G-K, cytotoxic angucyclines from *Streptomyces* sp. including two analogues bearing the aminosugar rednose. *J. Nat. Prod.* **2012**, *75*, 1383–1392. [CrossRef] [PubMed]
4. Gui, C.; Liu, Y.N.; Zhou, Z.B.; Zhang, S.W.; Hu, Y.F.; Gu, Y.C.; Huang, H.B.; Ju, J.H. Angucycline glycosides from mangrove-derived *Streptomyces diastaticus* subsp. SCSIO GJ056. *Mar. Drugs* **2018**, *16*, 185. [CrossRef] [PubMed]
5. Erb, A.; Luzhetskyy, A.; Hardter, U.; Bechthold, A. Cloning and sequencing of the biosynthetic gene cluster for saquayamycin Z and galtamycin B and the elucidation of the assembly of their saccharide chains. *ChemBioChem* **2009**, *10*, 1392–1401. [CrossRef] [PubMed]
6. Huang, H.B.; Yang, T.T.; Ren, X.M.; Liu, J.; Song, Y.X.; Sun, A.J.; Ma, J.Y.; Wang, B.; Zhang, Y.; Huang, C.G.; et al. Cytotoxic angucycline class glycosides from the deep sea actinomycete *Streptomyces lusitanus* SCSIO LR32. *J. Nat. Prod.* **2012**, *75*, 202–208. [CrossRef] [PubMed]
7. Zhu, X.C.; Duan, Y.W.; Cui, Z.M.; Wang, Z.; Li, Z.X.; Zhang, Y.; Ju, J.H.; Huang, H.B. Cytotoxic rearranged angucycline glycosides from deep sea-derived *Streptomyces lusitanus* SCSIO LR32. *J. Antibiot.* **2017**, *70*, 819–822. [CrossRef] [PubMed]
8. Helaly, S.E.; Goodfellow, M.; Zinecker, H.; Imhoff, J.F.; Sussmuth, R.D.; Fiedler, H.P. Warkmycin, a novel angucycline antibiotic produced by *Streptomyces* sp. Acta 2930. *J. Antibiot.* **2013**, *66*, 669–674. [CrossRef] [PubMed]
9. Nakagawa, K.; Hara, C.; Tokuyama, S.; Takada, K.; Imamura, N. Saprolmycins A-E, new angucycline antibiotics active against *Saprolegnia parasitica*. *J. Antibiot.* **2012**, *65*, 599–607. [CrossRef] [PubMed]
10. Panchuk, R.R.; Lehka, L.V.; Terenzi, A.; Matselyukh, B.P.; Rohr, J.; Jha, A.K.; Downey, T.; Kril, I.J.; Herbacek, I.; van Schoonhoven, S.; et al. Rapid generation of hydrogen peroxide contributes to the complex cell death induction by the angucycline antibiotic landomycin E. *Free Radical Bio. Med.* **2017**, *106*, 134–147. [CrossRef] [PubMed]
11. Korynevska, A.; Heffeter, P.; Matselyukh, B.; Elbling, L.; Micksche, M.; Stoika, R.; Berger, W. Mechanisms underlying the anticancer activities of the angucycline landomycin E. *Biochem. Pharmacol.* **2007**, *74*, 1713–1726. [CrossRef] [PubMed]
12. Fidan, O.; Yan, R.M.; Gladstone, G.; Zhou, T.; Zhu, D.; Zhan, J.X. New insights into the glycosylation steps in the biosynthesis of Sch47554 and Sch47555. *ChemBioChem* **2018**, *19*, 1424–1432. [CrossRef] [PubMed]
13. Salem, S.M.; Weidenbach, S.; Rohr, J. Two cooperative glycosyltransferases are responsible for the sugar diversity of saquayamycins isolated from *Streptomyces* sp. KY 40-1. *Acs Chem. Biol.* **2017**, *12*, 2529–2534. [CrossRef] [PubMed]
14. Huang, C.S.; Yang, C.F.; Zhang, W.J.; Zhang, L.P.; De, B.C.; Zhu, Y.G.; Jiang, X.D.; Fang, C.Y.; Zhang, Q.B.; Yuan, C.S.; Liu, H.W.; Zhang, C.S. Molecular basis of dimer formation during the biosynthesis of benzofluorene-containing atypical angucyclines. *Nat. Commun.* **2018**, *9*, 2088. [CrossRef] [PubMed]
15. Jose, P.A.; Jha, B. Intertidal marine sediment harbours Actinobacteria with promising bioactive and biosynthetic potential. *Sci. Rep.* **2017**, *7*, 10041. [CrossRef] [PubMed]

16. Zhou, T.S.; Ye, W.C.; Wang, Z.T.; Che, C.T.; Zhou, R.H.; Xu, G.J.; Xu, L.S. β-Carboline alkaloids from *Hypodematium squamuloso-pilosum*. *Phytochemistry* **1998**, *49*, 1807–1809. [CrossRef]

17. Han, X.; Hou, L.K.; Hou, J.; Zhang, Y.Y.; Li, H.Y.; Li, W.L. Heterologous expression of a VioA variant activates cryptic compounds in a marine-derived *Brevibacterium* strain. *Mar. Drugs* **2018**, *16*, 191. [CrossRef] [PubMed]

18. Uchida, T.; Imoto, M.; Watanabe, Y.; Miura, K.; Dobashi, T.; Matsuda, N.; Sawa, T.; Naganawa, H.; Hamada, M.; Takeuchi, T.; et al. Saquayamycins, new aquayamycin-group antibiotics. *J. Antibiot.* **1985**, *38*, 1171–1181. [CrossRef] [PubMed]

19. Feng, Z.M.; He, J.; Jiang, J.S.; Chen, Z.; Yang, Y.N.; Zhang, P.C. NMR solution structure study of the representative component hydroxysafflor yellow A and other quinochalcone C-glycosides from *Carthamus tinctorius*. *J. Nat. Prod.* **2013**, *76*, 270–274. [CrossRef] [PubMed]

20. Song, Y.X.; Liu, G.F.; Li, J.; Huang, H.B.; Zhang, X.; Zhang, H.; Ju, J.H. Cytotoxic and antibacterial angucycline- and prodigiosin-analogues from the deep-sea derived *Streptomyces* sp. SCSIO 11594. *Mar. Drugs* **2015**, *13*, 1304–1316. [CrossRef] [PubMed]

21. Stroch, K.; Zeeck, A.; Antal, N.; Fiedler, H.P. Retymicin, galtamycin B, saquayamycin Z and ribofuranosyllumichrome, novel secondary metabolites from *Micromonospora* sp. Tu 6368-II. Structure elucidation. *J. Antibiot.* **2005**, *58*, 103–110. [CrossRef] [PubMed]

22. Maskey, R.P.; Helmke, E.; Laatsch, H. Himalomycin A and B: Isolation and structure elucidation of new fridamycin type antibiotics from a marine *Streptomyces* isolate. *J. Antibiot.* **2003**, *56*, 942–949. [CrossRef] [PubMed]

23. Herzon, S.B. The mechanism of action of (-)-lomaiviticin A. *Accounts Chem. Res.* **2017**, *50*, 2577–2588. [CrossRef] [PubMed]

24. Zhang, X.M.; Liu, X.; Wang, Z.; Tian, Z.H.; Xie, W.D. Viridobrunnines A and B, antimicrobial phenoxazinone alkaloids from a soil associated *Streptomyces* sp. *Heterocycles* **2015**, *91*, 1809–1814.

25. Liu, S.S.; Wang, Y.F.; Ma, L.S.; Zheng, B.B.; Li, L.; Xie, W.D.; Li, X. 1-Oxoeudesm-11(13)-eno-12,8a-lactone induces G_2/M arrest and apoptosis of human glioblastoma cells in vitro. *Acta Pharmacol. Sin.* **2013**, *34*, 271–281. [CrossRef] [PubMed]

26. Zheng, B.B.; Wu, L.H.; Ma, L.S.; Liu, S.S.; Li, L.; Xie, W.D.; Li, X. Telekin induces apoptosis associated with the mitochondria-mediated pathway in human hepatocellular carcinoma cells. *Biol. Pharm. Bull.* **2013**, *36*, 1118–1125. [CrossRef] [PubMed]

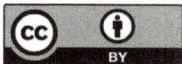

© 2018 by the authors. Licensee MDPI, Basel, Switzerland. This article is an open access article distributed under the terms and conditions of the Creative Commons Attribution (CC BY) license (http://creativecommons.org/licenses/by/4.0/).

MDPI

St. Alban-Anlage 66

4052 Basel

Switzerland

Tel. +41 61 683 77 34

Fax +41 61 302 89 18

www.mdpi.com

Marine Drugs Editorial Office

E-mail: marinedrugs@mdpi.com

www.mdpi.com/journal/marinedrugs

www.ingramcontent.com/pod-product-compliance
Lightning Source LLC
Chambersburg PA
CBHW051724210326
41597CB00032B/5598